D0068986

PHYSIOLOGY OF EXERCISE

SECOND EDITION

PHYSIOLOGY OF

EXERCISE

RESPONSES & ADAPTATIONS

David R. Lamb

Department of Physical Education,
Health, and Recreation Studies
Purdue University

MACMILLAN PUBLISHING COMPANY

New York

COLLIER MACMILLAN PUBLISHERS

London

Macmillan Publishing Company
866 Third Avenue, New York, New York 10022

Collier Macmillan Canada, Inc.

Library of Congress Cataloging in Publication Data

Lamb, David R.
  Physiology of exercise.

  Includes bibliographies and index.
  1. Exercise—Physiological aspects. I. Title.
[DNLM: 1. Exertion. 2. Physiology. WE 103 L2177p]
QP301.L27 1983   612'.044   82-9886
ISBN 0-02-367210-2   AACR2

PRINTING   91011   YEAR   89

ISBN 0-02-367210-2

To Cozette,
Michelle,
and Jason

P R E F A C E

THIS book is designed as a text for a beginning exercise physiology course. Although intended primarily as an undergraduate text, it has also proved useful to many graduate students. No previous chemistry background is assumed as a prerequisite to the use of this book, but a prior course in human or animal physiology is helpful.

As the title suggests, the main goal of the book is to describe and explain the functional responses and adaptations that accompany single and repeated bouts of physical exercise. Many examples from physical education, athletics, and medicine are included to illustrate the practical application of the concepts discussed. The mechanisms underlying the physiological responses and adaptations to exercise are emphasized throughout the text. Where appropriate, conclusive statements are made about phenomena in exercise physiology, but no attempt is made to gloss over the abundant controversies in the field. It is assumed that students at the college level should be told when problems are unresolved.

Many changes have been made in this second edition. Many of these changes have been made upon the much appreciated advice of students and colleagues. The chapters have been reorganized to focus upon cardiovascular and respiratory physiology before strength physiology and the physiology of anaerobic exercise. Given the current interest in aerobic exercise, this approach should be useful to provide early intrinsic motivation for the beginning student in exercise physiology. A new chapter on body composition and weight control has been added, and there has been a substantial expansion of many of the other chapters. The introductory chapter has been divided into two chapters to make the material conform better to the instructional time typically available in the first two class meetings. The former chapter on evaluation of muscular strength has been eliminated, and the material previously included in a chapter on muscle fiber types and fuels for exercise has been integrated into other chapters.

A feature of the second edition is a discussion of regulatory mechanisms in energy metabolism, i.e., an explanation of how the various metabolic pathways are turned on and off at appropriate times during exercise and recovery. Other advances include discussions of the lactic acid turning point ("anaerobic threshold"), the use of the Wingate anaerobic cycling test, the role of plasma volume changes in adaptation to exercise in the heat, recent information on neural control of muscular force, new findings on neuromuscular fatigue and delayed muscular soreness, and a more thorough treatment of endocrine changes with exercise and the health-related aspects of exercise.

Many recent research results have been cited in the text and included in the reference lists at the end of each chapter. These lists should prove valuable as a starting point for literature reviews used in term papers and class projects.

Professors Christine Wells, Russell Pate, Robert Kertzer and Richard Lopez provided comprehensive and helpful reviews of the manuscript, and I gratefully acknowledge their excellent contributions.

D.R.L.

C O N T E N T S

1

The Nature of Exercise Physiology
1

2

Responses and Adaptations to Exercise: General Considerations
10

3

Skeletal Muscle Structure and Function
19

4

Energy Metabolism
38

5

Nutrition and Athletic Performance
66

6

Estimation of Energy Expenditure During Exercise
99

7

Exercise, Body Composition, and Weight Control
114

8

The Physiology of Aerobic Endurance

137

9

Evaluation of Cardiovascular Function and Aerobic Endurance Performance
173

10

Training for Improved Aerobic Endurance
191

11

Temperature Regulation During Exercise
221

12

The Physiological Basis of Muscular Strength
239

13

Training for Improved Muscular Strength
272

14

Anaerobic Power and Capacity
294

15

Neuromuscular Fatigue and Delayed Muscular Soreness After Exercise

311

16

Kidney and Gastrointestinal Responses and Adaptations to Exercise

329

17

Endocrine Responses and Adaptations to Exercise
342

18

Exercise and Health
366

19

Aids and Impediments to Physical Performance: Fact and Fiction
394

APPENDIXES

A

Units of Measurement and Conversion Factors
411

B

Nutritive Values of the Edible Part of Foods
419

PHYSIOLOGY OF EXERCISE

CHAPTER 1

The Nature of Exercise Physiology

In the last 20 years there has been a dramatic worldwide acceleration, especially in the United States and Canada, in exercise and sports participation by people of all ages and of both sexes. Prior to 1960, persons seen jogging down a residential street were ridiculed as weird health freaks. In the early 1980's, on the other hand, it is estimated that more than 20 million North Americans run or jog regularly. It is now socially desirable to participate in some form of regular physical activity. However, there are some problems accompanying this generally positive development.

It is currently widely appreciated, both by physicians and laypersons, that regular exercise has many health benefits. What is not so widely appreciated is that exercise under certain conditions can be harmful and even deadly. For example, with the social appeal of participation in distance runs of 10 kilometers and even marathons, we find that many persons are totally unprepared for the stresses of such runs. As a result, they suffer severe damage to feet and legs, heat exhaustion, and heat stroke. A small number of these unprepared runners die each year. Presumably, if these persons were better educated with respect to the principles of exercise physiology, there would be far fewer serious injuries associated with our newfound enthusiasm for sports and exercise.

The participation of millions of previously inactive persons in exercise and sports has also led to problems associated with the rapid growth of the sports and exercise industry. Billions of consumer dollars are spent each year on athletic clothing, sports equipment, nutritional aids, and fitness programs. Much of this expenditure is for worthwhile purposes, but there is also tremendous advertising pressure on the consumer to purchase memberships in fitness clubs which have little to offer, to buy worthless fitness books, and to invest in useless exercise equipment at fantastic markups in price. For example, some years ago an item was marketed as an "all purpose

1

fitness improver," a claim which was patently nonsense. This device consisted of two thin metal strips about 30 centimeters (15 inches) long with small lead weights attached to one end and hand grips on the other. The instructions were to vibrate these strips back and forth, one in each hand, so that the body could "receive the strength and energy" generated by the vibration of the strips. Supposedly, all muscle groups of the body could be developed with the energy received from the vibrating strips. The manufacturer's cost for this device was about 79 cents, but the retail cost was $9.95! Obviously, these "magic strips" could develop all the muscles in the body only if the exerciser could figure out a way to vibrate them while doing pushups, situps, bench presses and other genuinely useful strength-promoting activities. A knowledge of exercise physiology can help the consumer minimize the waste of money on purchases that are physiologically unsound.

There are reasons for learning about exercise physiology other than the prevention of exercise-related injuries and the reduction of wasteful or unproductive sports-related consumer expenditures. Not the least of these reasons is the satisfaction gained from learning how one's own body responds and adapts to exercise. Before discussing some of the other reasons, though, let us first develop a common vocabulary. Specifically, let us arrive at a common understanding of what is meant by the terms "exercise physiology," "exercise science," "sports medicine," and "physical fitness." At the outset, it should be made clear that there is not universal agreement about what these terms mean. What will be described is the way the terms will be used in this book. You should consider the definitions carefully, compare them with others you have learned, see if you can develop some better ones, and decide which you prefer until some better definitions are proposed.

Exercise Physiology—What Is It?

Physiology is the study of all the functions of the body; *exercise physiology* is a subfield of physiology concerned with changes in function brought about by participation in physical exercise. In exercise physiology we study what happens to bodily functions if one exercises a *single* time, *how* these changes in function are brought about, *what changes* in function occur after *repeated* exercise sessions, *how* those changes come to pass, and, finally, what can be done to *improve* the body's response to exercise and its adaptation to repeated periods of exercise. Let there be no mystery about exercise physiology: the most complicated feature of this or any other science is the necessity to become familiar with many new terms and a few new ways of thinking. In this book that process will be simplified as much as possible.

A more concise definition of exercise physiology is as follows:

> Exercise physiology is the description and explanation of functional changes brought about by single (acute) or repeated exercise sessions (chronic exercise or training), often with the objective of improving the exercise response.

In this definition the *description of functional changes* refers to *what happens to the body,* and the *explanation* refers to understanding *how the changes occur.* For example, we now know that repeated lifting of heavy weights usually results in greater ability to lift even heavier weights. This functional change brought about by repeated bouts of exercise can be explained partly by an increased growth of muscle tissue, so that more protein threads in the muscle are available to exert contractile force, and partly by an improved ability of the nervous system to cause greater numbers of muscle fibers to contract simultaneously for the greatest possible force of contraction of the entire muscle. This understanding of how weight lifting ability develops has led to better training programs to improve the lifting response.

Note that in the concise definition of exercise physiology, the objective of improving the exercise response was qualified by the word *often*. This qualification is meant to point out that, scientifically speaking, there is no requirement that the study of exercise responses be designed to improve those responses. The basic knowledge of what happens during exercise and how it happens is important in itself, just as obtaining basic knowledge of any sort has been an important goal of human beings throughout history. It is not possible in the present to foretell what sort of knowledge will have ''practical'' benefits to mankind in the future, just as it was not understood that research in theoretical physics would lead to the development of transistors that have become part of our everyday lives in radios, television sets and computers. As it happens, a great many scientists who study the responses of the body to exercise do so with the hope of improving the capacity of heart patients to work at their jobs, helping industrial workers to work more efficiently, or establishing a new world record in the 100 meter free-style swim.

Mechanisms in Exercise Physiology

When one tries to explain *how* some change in body function comes about as a result of exercise, it can be said that one wants to know the *mechanism* underlying the response; that is, one wants to know as much as possible about the physical and chemical laws responsible for the change in function. The desire for understanding the mechanisms underlying exercise responses is governed not only by a natural curiosity, but also by the belief that knowing the details of how a response occurs will make it more likely that the response can be better predicted, better controlled, and more efficiently improved.

As an example, let us examine the relationship between regular endurance exercise (jogging, cycling, swimming, and so on) and the risk of suffering heart disease at an early age. Most studies that have compared the risk of coronary disease in groups of people who exercise regularly with the risk in groups who engage in little physical activity show that exercise seems to be protective and thus reduces the risk of suffering early heart disease. Therefore, a change in body function seems to occur as a result of regular exercise—the heart is more resistant to disease. The question in many people's minds is, ''How is this protective effect brought about?'' In other words, what is it about jogging three miles daily that enables the heart to better resist coronary artery disease? Some authorities believe that exercise has a direct effect on improving the blood-vessel supply to the heart. Others believe the exercise is beneficial because it reduces blood fat, or because it retards blood clotting in the veins, or because it causes one to lose body weight.

Hopefully, if researchers can determine the mechanism underlying the protective effect of exercise on the heart and the resultant reduction in coronary disease risk, it will be easier to prescribe exactly the right kind and amount of exercise. It may also be easier to monitor the effect of the exercise program, and it may be possible to locate the exact chemical malfunction involved, so that steps can be taken to prevent heart disease entirely by appropriate diet, medication, surgery, or radiation therapy. Although it is not always true that understanding *how* a response works makes it easier to predict, prevent, or treat, medical history books are full of examples of how such understanding has made possible far-reaching improvements in medicine. In a similar fashion, the understanding of exercise responses has made possible important gains in exercise treatment of cardiac patients, in athletic conditioning programs, and in exercise prescription for the general population.

It is also possible to ask *why* or for what *purpose* a particular physiological response to exercise occurs. For example, one may say that the heart beats faster during exercise because it must pump more blood to the working muscles, or because the skin needs more blood to help rid the body of excess heat, or because blood pressure would fall too low if the heart did not speed up, or for any number of other plausible reasons. The study of the *purposes* underlying occurrences in nature is called *teleology*. Teleological explanations of exercise responses can sometimes prove useful in helping us remember *what* and *how* things happen, but they can also impede the learning process in exercise physiology if one settles for a teleological explanation and neglects to learn *how* a response occurs. For example, a complete understanding of the heart-rate response to exercise does not stop with the declaration that the heart rate increases to provide more blood to the muscles, just as a complete understanding of an automobile's acceleration does not stop with the observation that stepping on the accelerator increases speed. One who truly understands the heart-rate response to exercise knows where the stimuli that begin the response originate and knows the nervous or hormonal steps that lie between the initial stimuli and the final speeding up of the heart. Therefore, it is more useful to think about the *how* questions rather than the *why* questions in exercise physiology.

Another problem with trying to determine why physiological responses to exercise occur is that it is usually impossible to judge objectively whether a purpose decided upon is the correct one. We don't really know, for example, whether the purpose behind a reduced amount of blood sugar after prolonged exercise is to signal the body to rest or to enable the body to use more fats for energy. It is indeed quite possible that the fall in blood sugar has no purpose but simply happens as a consequence of the depletion of sugar stores in the liver as exercise progresses.

Exercise Science

> Exercise science is the description and explanation of natural phenomena associated with physical activity and sport. Exercise science (kinesiology, movement science, and the like) includes the speciality sciences of exercise physiology, motor control, sport and exercise biomechanics, sport psychology, sport sociology and exercise biochemistry.

Human performance during exercise and sport is a composite of physiological, psychological, biomechanical, neurological, biochemical and social factors. We cannot hope to understand human performance fully until we understand all of these factors. The study of exercise and sport sciences provides the fundamental knowledge upon which we can build to improve human performance.

Sports Medicine

There are two principal understandings of the term "sports medicine" that should be discussed. The oldest understanding is that sports medicine is that branch of medical practice which deals primarily with the prevention and treatment of athletic injuries. This understanding stems largely from a tradition in many parts of the world where there are recognized specialities and training programs for physicians who wish to emphasize athletic medicine. However, in the United States no such speciality is currently recognized by the American Medical Association, the organization which certifies such specialities.

A more recent way of understanding "sports medicine" is to consider it as an umbrella term that includes everything related to exercise and sports performance, both medical and scientific aspects.

Just as most laypersons associate the general sciences of physiology, anatomy, and biochemistry with general medicine, it is not surprising that the sciences of exercise physiology, sport biomechanics, exercise biochemistry, sport psychology, etc., have gradually become associated with sports medicine. Some physicians and trainers object to this use of "sports medicine" as an umbrella term because they believe that the term should refer to the clinical aspects of the prevention and treatment of medical problems related to sport and exercise. On the other hand, some scientists object to having their work subsumed under the umbrella term "sports medicine" because they believe that this detracts from the scientific aspects of their work.

Regardless of what physicians or scientists would prefer, though, it is increasingly clear that most laypersons do think of the exercise sciences as part of "sports medicine". Also, the American College of Sports Medicine, the largest and most prestigious association of physicians, trainers, scientists, and physical educators in the world, uses "sports medicine" as an umbrella term under the belief that the best way to solve problems related to exercise is to attack them from both fronts, medical and scientific. Therefore, it appears likely that this global notion of what sports medicine is will gradually become the generally accepted understanding (Table 1.1).

Physical Fitness

There is an intimate relationship between exercise physiology and physical fitness. Just what "physical fitness" means depends upon whom one asks, but in this book the following definition seems appropriate.

> Physical fitness is the capacity to meet successfully the present and potential physical challenges of life.

TABLE 1.1
A Global View of Sports Medicine

Sports Medicine	
Scientific Aspects	Clinical Aspects
Exercise Physiology	Athletic Medicine
Sport Biomechanics	Athletic Training
Sport Psychology	Orthopedic Surgery
Exercise Biochemistry	Podiatry
Sport Sociology	Nutrition
Neuroscience	Exercise Prescription
Anatomy	Cardiology
Anthropology	Corrective Therapy
Food Science	Cardiac Rehabilitation

According to this definition, the physical fitness requirements of different individuals will vary, depending upon the nature of the physical challenges they face. For example, examine the physical fitness requirements of two persons, Peter Plowfaster, a fullback for the Baskerville Hounds professional football team, and Phillip Flaccid, librarian at the Simon Smedley School for Sick Sailors. Do these two persons have different requirements for "physical fitness"? Let us first consider the *present* physical challenges that Peter and Phillip meet in their daily lives. Peter must face the grueling challenges of professional football and must regularly work to improve and maintain his muscular strength, flexibility, anaerobic power and cardiovascular endurance. Phillip, on the other hand, leads a very sedentary existence and needs only enough strength to move an occasional box of books from one shelf to another in the library, to carry bags of groceries, and to lift the old windows in his home.

At first glance, then, it appears that Phillip needs very little in the way of regular exercise. But if we consider the *potential* physical challenges that these two characters might meet, the picture changes dramatically. The most critical potential physical challenge facing Peter, Phillip, and the rest of us is the onset of cardiovascular disease. This presents a physical challenge because those who are afflicted with heart disease or high blood pressure may be severely restricted in the physical activities they can pursue successfully, even to the extent of being unable to climb a flight of stairs without severe chest pain. There is overwhelming evidence that participation in regular exercise makes one less likely to contract early heart disease. Thus, to meet successfully the *potential* challenge of heart disease, one should participate in regular physical activity during the *present*—long before the onset of the degenerative cardiovascular disease.

Another example of a *potential* physical challenge is chronic low back pain. Millions of adults have low back pain that keeps them from vigorous recreational activities and often keeps them from their jobs. But it is clear that the risk of low back pain is much less in those who are physically active, especially those who keep their abdominal muscles strong. *Thus, even when there is no clear evidence that* present *physical challenges require regular exercise, there is ample evidence that* future *physical challenges can be met more successfully if one begins a program of regular physical activity early in life and persists in such activity throughout the years.*

Physical Fitness and Exercise Physiology

The development of physical fitness involves preparing the body for physical activity, whether that activity be surfing at the beach, shoveling snow, touching one's toes with knees locked, shooting a basketball, spiking a volleyball, or running a three-hour marathon. Therefore, because exercise physiology is the study of the body's responses to single and repeated sessions of exercise, the knowledge from exercise physiology can be used to improve physical fitness. In other words, the improvement of physical fitness is the application of the principles of exercise physiology to the improvement of one's capacity to meet successfully life's physical challenges.

For example, information gained from studies of strength-training methods can be

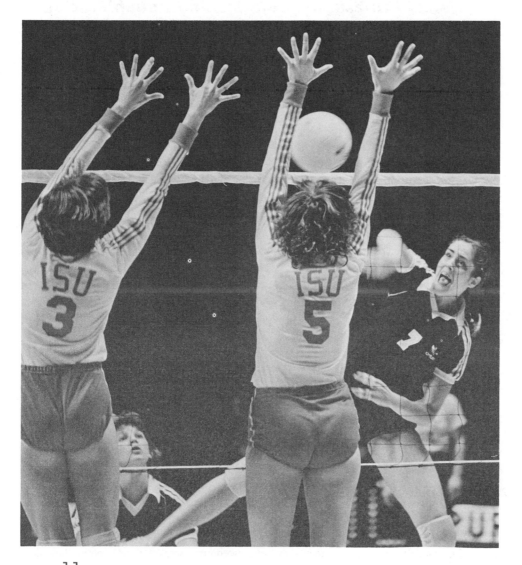

FIGURE 1.1. Physical fitness for competitive volleyball requires high levels of anaerobic power, flexibility, and strength. (Courtesy of Office of Public Information, Purdue University, West Lafayette, Indiana.)

used to design the most effective program for a person who wants to improve strength, and results of research on diet and exercise can be applied to the development of a successful weight-control program for those who are obese. It is unfortunate that many persons do not see the connection between exercise physiology and physical fitness; better physical fitness programs could be designed to meet the individual's specific fitness needs if knowledge gained from studies of exercise physiology were more frequently applied to the design of fitness programs.

Physical Fitness for Athletics and Rehabilitation

Competitive sports and athletics provide the participant with a variety of physical challenges that must be met successfully if the participant is to win a satisfactory share of the competitions. The achievement of good physical condition for athletic competition is, therefore, a special case of improving one's physical fitness. In the case of competitive volleyball, for instance, the physical challenges that must be met successfully require the development of powerful leg muscles and superior flexibility and anaerobic endurance. Successful distance running, on the other hand, primarily requires the development of aerobic (cardiorespiratory) endurance. In each competitive sport—volleyball, distance running, etc.—there are specific physical challenges that must be met by the improvement of certain aspects of physical fitness. Accordingly, the principles of exercise physiology should be applied to the improvement of physical fitness for athletes as well as for the ordinary individual.

Exercise physiology is important not only for the improvement of physical fitness for average healthy persons and for athletes, but also for those who are undergoing therapy for the treatment of problems caused by disease, accident, or birth. Thus, knowledge of the principles of exercise physiology is important for the improvement of the physical fitness of those recovering from heart attacks, suffering from diabetes, or recovering from broken bones and torn ligaments, as well as those afflicted by physical handicaps and trying to extend their capacities to meet physical challenges successfully.

The importance of the knowledge gained from exercise physiology to the improvement of physical fitness of the whole spectrum of humanity is shown in Figure 1.2. This figure is not meant to imply that only exercise physiology is important to the improvement of physical fitness; obviously psychological, biomechanical, social and other factors are also important. But exercise physiology has a dominant role to play in this field.

REVIEW QUESTIONS

1. Define the following terms as they are used in this text: exercise physiology, physical fitness, sports medicine, and exercise science.
2. List three important reasons for studying exercise physiology.
3. Explain the difference between teleological and mechanistic explanations in physiology. Give an example of each.
4. Explain how knowledge of the principles of exercise physiology is related to the improvement of physical fitness.

PHYSICAL FITNESS PROGRAMS

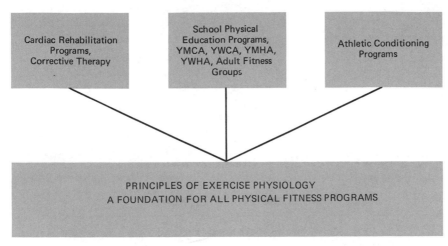

FIGURE 1.2. Relationship between exercise physiology and physical fitness.

5. If it is true that young children get all the exercise they need to meet their present physical challenges (a questionable assumption), what argument could be made for a need for additional physical activity to help them reach their optimal fitness levels?

REFERENCES

[1] Lamb, D. R. Sports medicine—what is it? *Sports Medicine Bulletin,* 1981, **16:**2–3.

[2] Hage, P. Education in sportsmedicine: coming into its own. *Physician and Sportsmedicine,* 1981, **9:**145–147.

[3] Smodlaka, V. N. Sports medicine in the world today. *Journal of the American Medical Association,* 1968, **205:**145–147.

2

Responses and Adaptations to Exercise: General Considerations

BEFORE pursuing our study of specific systems of the body and how they react to exercise stress, it should prove useful to take a more generalized approach so that we can better visualize what we hope to find in our more specific analyses. Let us begin by returning to the definition of exercise physiology presented in the previous chapter; i.e., *exercise physiology is the description and explanation of functional changes brought on by single or repeated exercise sessions, often with the objective of improving the exercise response.* In other words, we need to know what the physiological effects of exercise are and what causes those effects. We must determine what happens not only with one exercise period, but also what happens when the exercise is repeated over a period of many weeks, months, or years. At this point it is helpful to distinguish these two types of exercise effects by the introduction of two terms, "response" and "adaptation," which are used very specifically in this book.

Responses and Adaptations: The Effects of Exercise and Training

In subsequent chapters, a great deal of time is spent describing the changes in function of the body brought about by single and repeated bouts of exercise. Sometimes a single bout of exercise is called *acute* exercise, whereas repeated bouts of exercise over several days or months may be called *chronic* exercise. Also, *exercise* may be used to indicate a single episode of exercise, and *training* may be used instead of *repeated bouts* or *chronic* exercise. It is important to remember that functional changes that occur with training do not necessarily occur with a single bout of exercise. For example, a single bout of exercise does not affect one's resting heart rate, whereas regular endurance training usually reduces resting heart rate. Two other words—*response* and *adaptation*—are often used interchangeably in exercise physiology texts.

In this book the functional changes that occur when one exercises a single time are called *responses* to exercise. *Responses are the sudden, temporary changes in function caused by exercise. These functional changes disappear shortly after the exercise period is finished.* Examples of responses to exercise are the increase in heart rate, the rise in blood pressure, and the increase in breathing that accompany exercise. Each of these responses is no longer present a few minutes after the exercise is over.

An adaptation is a more or less persistent change in structure or function following training that apparently enables the body to respond more easily to subsequent exercise bouts. Ordinarily, adaptations are not seen until several weeks of training have passed, but some occur after only four or five days of training. One example of an adaptation to training is a reduction in heart rate for a submaximal exercise load that nearly always follows several weeks of training. This reduction in exercise heart rate seems to enable the heart to pump the same amount of blood to the body's tissues at a lower energy cost for the heart. Another example of an adaptation is the increased muscle size that accompanies a strenuous weight-lifting program and enables the lifter to exert greater muscular force than before training. Much of this increased strength persists for many months after the training program ends.

Homeostasis and the Negative Feedback Character of Responses and Adaptations to Exercise

Nearly all of the changes in body function brought on by exercise or training tend to reduce the stressfulness of exercise for the entire organism. For instance, contracting muscles are severely stressed as they use up oxygen, but as the heart rate and breathing rate increase, more oxygen is delivered to the working muscles to reduce that stress. As another example of this principle, consider the increase in sweat rate that accompanies repeated exercise bouts in hot environments. The heat of the environment puts a stress on all the tissues of the body, but after training in the heat, this stress is reduced because the increased sweat production helps cool the body by evaporation.

The tendency for living organisms to maintain a stable internal environment for their cells is called *homeostasis*. Thus, the human body carefully regulates the temperature, acidity, oxygen, glucose, sodium, potassium, chloride and other characteristics of its body fluids. A failure of the body to maintain homeostasis occurs, for example, when the body overheats during exercise, in spite of its best efforts to maintain a reasonable temperature by profuse sweating. The most important method used by the body to maintain homeostasis is *negative feedback regulation*. In negative feedback regulation homeostatic disturbances are sensed, integrated with other physiological input, and fed back to a physiological regulator. The regulator then causes functional changes that oppose (negate) the homeostatic disturbances.

For example, as shown in Fig. 2.1, if the homeostatic disturbance is excess carbon dioxide in the blood, negative feedback control operates as follows.

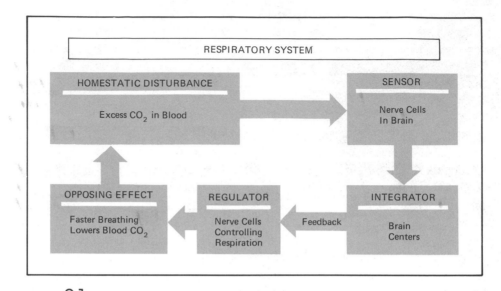

FIGURE 2.1. Example of negative feedback regulation of carbon dioxide levels in blood.

1. The carbon dioxide is sensed by specialized nerves cells in the brain.
2. The sensor in turn signals an *integrator.* The integrator in this example consists of other centers (groups of nerve cells) in the brain that process input about the optimal and current levels of carbon dioxide, oxygen, and acidity in the blood.
3. When the integrator determines that blood carbon dioxide is too high and should be reduced, an *error signal* is "fed back" to the regulator (nerve cells that regulate the muscles of breathing) to increase the rate of breathing.
4. The increased breathing causes greater exhalation of carbon dioxide so that blood levels of carbon dioxide are reduced towards normal. Thus, the initial high levels of carbon dioxide lead to functional changes (increased breathing) which oppose or negate the original homeostatic disturbance.

If the concentration of blood carbon dioxide were to go too low—because of excessive hyperventilation, for example—negative feedback regulation would oppose (negate) the disturbance in the system by reducing the breathing rate to slow the exhalation of carbon dioxide and gradually build the carbon dioxide levels back up toward homeostatically acceptable levels. Thus, through negative feedback mechanisms, factors in the chemical environment of the cells which are raised too high are soon brought down to lower, more normal levels; factors that are lowered too far are raised to higher, more normal levels. The body opposes, by negative feedback regulation, disturbances in the homeostasis of all its systems.

One should keep the principle of negative feedback regulation in mind when studying how exercise responses and adaptations to training occur. The application of this principle often helps to sort out meaningful relationships among functional changes and can be useful in predicting which responses or adaptations should occur in a given circumstance.

For example, it could be predicted that one adaptation to repeated exercise in a hot environment, if negative feedback regulation were operating, would be a better sweating response during exercise to bring the body temperature to lower, more homeostatically "correct" levels. This is precisely what occurs as one of the most important adaptations to chronic exercise in the heat.

General Patterns of Physiological Responses and Adaptations to Exercise and Training

Most physiological responses and adaptations to exercise and training are examples of negative feedback regulation apparently designed to help the body minimize changes in homeostasis during exercise. Also, most responses and adaptations fit into general patterns that often prove useful in gaining a clearer insight into those responses and adaptations. The material in this chapter is presented in the hope that it will help the reader view the various responses and adaptations to exercise within a broad physiological framework rather than as isolated facts. From the physiologist's point of view it is not enough to know that the heart rate increases with exercise; it is also necessary, for a complete understanding of this phenomenon, to know all the factors that cause the heart rate to rise. Similarly, to understand the muscular growth that accompanies weight training, it is important to know all the adaptive mechanisms involved. For the coach, physical education teacher, athletic trainer, or physician a thorough understanding of responses and adaptations to exercise can enhance the ability to explain unusual experiences that clients may report and to develop new approaches to the conditioning and care of athletes and others who wish to improve their physical fitness.

General Pattern of Exercise Responses. A simplified general pattern of physiologic responses to single exercise bouts is shown in Fig. 2.2. In this scheme exercise is the stimulus that causes a disturbance in homeostasis, that is, a change in the physical or chemical environment of the cells. Exercise may cause body temperature to rise,

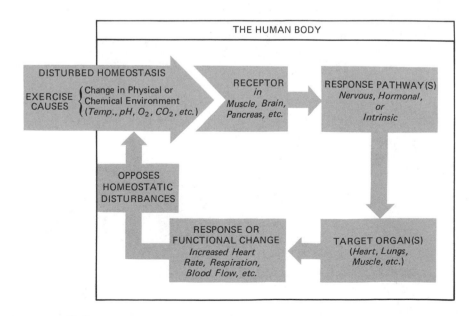

FIGURE 2.2. Simplified general scheme of physiological responses to exercise.

acidity of the blood to increase, oxygen content of the body fluids to fall, and carbon dioxide to rise, as well as many other disturbances in homeostasis to occur.

One or more of these changes in the body's internal environment are sensed by cells of the body (receptors) which then stimulate a complex response pathway. This pathway may involve changes in nerve activity (neural pathway), changes in hormones (hormonal pathway), or changes entirely within a given organ (intrinsic pathway). By means of the response pathway a "signal" is transmitted to those organs which will eventually change their functions to produce the observed response to exercise. The exercise response in turn has a negative (opposing) influence on the homeostatic disturbances caused by the exercise.

Neural Pathway. As a specific example of this general scheme, consider the body's response to the build-up of lactic acid in the blood during heavy exercise (Figure 2.3). One way to counteract this acid is to exhale more carbon dioxide from the lungs by breathing more rapidly and deeply. This works because much of this carbon dioxide comes from carbonic acid in the blood; by getting rid of carbonic acid one can reduce the effect of the increase in lactic acid. As shown in Figure 2.3, the increased acid level in the blood eventually activates the carotid bodies, clusters of specialized nerve cells in the carotid arteries high in the neck. These nerve cells signal the brain to increase the rate and depth of breathing by the lungs. As more carbon dioxide is exhaled, the acidity of the blood is reduced.

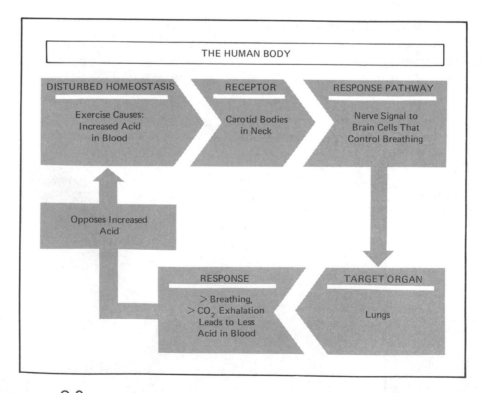

FIGURE 2.3. Example of a physiological response to exercise.

Hormonal Pathway. Some functional responses to exercise use hormonal pathways. For example, part of the explanation for an increased heart rate in response to exercise is the effect of increased secretion of epinephrine (adrenaline) and norepinephrine (noradrenaline) from the adrenal glands.

Intrinsic Pathway. An intrinsic pathway is one located within an organ, the organ serving both as receptor and target organ. A good example of an intrinsic pathway is that involved in the production of energy from carbohydrate in exercising muscles. In this case, the disturbance in homeostasis is the rapid reduction in the muscle's quick energy stores as exercise begins. However, the decreasing numbers of these energy molecules themselves activate enzymes in the muscle that cause carbohydrate to be broken down quickly to replace the quick energy stores. Note that no hormones or nerve reflexes are involved in this response; the entire process takes place in (is "intrinsic" to) the muscles themselves.

General Pattern of Training Adaptations. The general pattern of physiological or anatomical adaptations to training (Figure 2.4) is similar to that described for responses to a single exercise session, but it includes an *adaptation pathway* and arrows showing the relationships between the adaptation pathway and other elements in the scheme. The adaptation pathway is the mechanism that eventually causes a persistent change in structure or function after repeated exercise sessions. It should be noted that

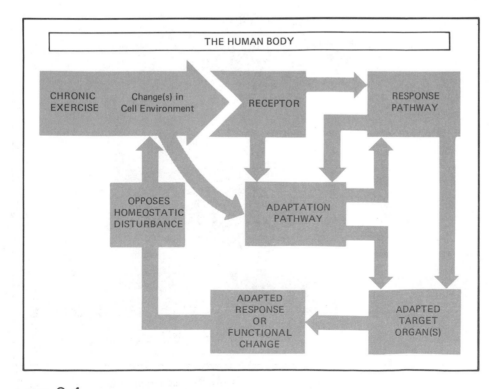

FIGURE 2.4. Simplified general scheme of physiological adaptations to training.

no one is yet certain of the entire scheme for any of the adaptations known to occur with regular physical training. Therefore, the example to follow is a bit speculative but is offered as an illustrative model.

Effect of Training on Muscle Glycogen Level. Skeletal muscle adapts to heavy running or cycling by increasing its content of glycogen, the stored form of carbohydrate energy in muscle. This is apparently an adaptation designed to oppose or compensate for the regular decrease in muscle energy stores that occurs during repeated training sessions. It appears that this adaptive increase in muscle glycogen stores is caused by an increase in the activity of one or more enzymes involved in producing glycogen [5]. The process might work in a manner similar to that illustrated in Figure 2.5.

The following explanation of glycogen adaptation refers to the numerals shown in Figure 2.5. (Numbers 1–5 refer to a typical *response* pattern.)

1. During each training session there is a reduction in the amount of chemical energy molecules in the working muscles.
2. The decrease in energy molecules during exercise is "sensed" by enzymes involved in breaking glycogen down to provide more energy.

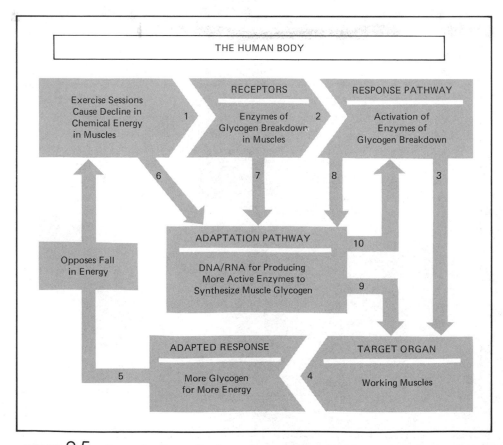

FIGURE 2.5. Example of overall scheme for a specific adaptation to exercise, i.e., increased glycogen storage in muscle.

3. The response pathway is located within the affected muscles (intrinsic pathway) and consists of an activation of the enzymes which break glycogen down for energy. This activation of enzymes increases the rate of glycogen degradation so that more energy molecules are produced.

4. The target organs are the working skeletal muscles.

5. The response is the production of new energy molecules to replace those used up during the exercise. So far we have only considered what happens during a single exercise session—*before* the training adaptation has occurred. With an adaptation to training, some chemical signal must activate the muscle's protein synthesis apparatus (DNA, RNA, etc.) so that *more enzymes are available to synthesize more muscle glycogen*. There are several ways this might work.

6. The reduced concentration of one or more chemical energy molecules may stimulate the adaptation pathway to produce more glycogen-synthesizing enzymes.

7, 8. Alternatively, chemical products of the enzymes of glycogen breakdown may stimulate the adaptation pathway.

9, 10. The adaptation pathway generally directly affects some characteristic of the target organ (in this case, by increasing the glycogen concentration in the muscles), but it may sometimes work by causing an adaptation in the response pathway to make it operate more efficiently.

Complete Explanations in Exercise Physiology

Exercise physiology has made great strides in recent years in explaining some of the responses and adaptations which accompany exercise. However, most of these responses and adaptations are still not fully understood. As one studies exercise physiology, it is important to make mental notes not only about what is known, but also about what is not known. Accordingly, it should prove useful to refer regularly to Figures 2.1, 2.2, and 2.4 to determine which pieces of the response and adaptation puzzles are present and which are missing. In this way, a more comprehensive understanding of exercise physiology will be obtained.

REVIEW QUESTIONS

1. What is a physiological "response" to exercise? Give three examples of responses to exercise.

2. Distinguish between a physiological response and an adaptation to exercise. Give three examples of adaptations to exercise.

3. What is a "homeostatic disturbance" caused by exercise? Give three examples of such disturbances.

4. What is the principal means the body uses to counteract or minimize homeostatic disturbances? Give an example of how negative feedback regulation works during exercise.

5. Persons untrained for work in high heat and humidity secrete a great deal of salt in their sweat. This loss of salt from the body fluids is potentially harmful. According to the principles of homeostasis and negative feedback regulation, what would you predict would happen to the salt concentration of sweat after a few weeks of training in the heat?

6. What are the differences between neural, hormonal and intrinsic response pathways? Make certain you can define each of these three types of pathways.

7. Explain Figures 2.1, 2.3, and 2.5 to a friend without relying on the text material.

REFERENCES

[1] Asmussen, E. Exercise: general statement of unsolved problems. *Circulation Research,* 1967, **20–21** (Supplement I): 12–15.

[2] Brooks, C. McC. The nature of adaptive reactions and their initiation. In E. Bajusz, ed. *Physiology and Pathology of Adaptation Mechanisms.* New York: Pergamon Press, 1969, pp. 439–451.

[3] Dill, D. B., ed. *Handbook of Physiology, Section 4: Adaptation to the Environment.* Washington, D.C.: American Physiological Society, 1964.

[4] Essen, B., and L. Kaijser. Regulation of glycolysis in intermittent exercise in man. *Journal of Physiology* (London), 1978, **281:**499–511.

[5] Kochan, R. G., D. R. Lamb, S. A. Lutz, C. V. Perrill, E. M. Reimann, and K. K. Schlender Glycogen synthase activation in human skeletal muscle: effects of diet and exercise. *American Journal of Physiology,* 1979, **236:**E660–E666.

C H A P T E R

3

Skeletal Muscle Structure and Function

$\mathbf{A_N}$ understanding of the structure and function of skeletal muscle is basic to an understanding of how the body responds to a single bout of exercise and adapts to physical training. That skeletal muscle is important for exercise is evident for the following reasons. First, without muscle contraction, of course, there can be no movement. Second, the period of time a movement may continue depends on the relative degree of muscular exertion and the extent of muscular fatigue. Finally, because the skeletal muscles consume most of the oxygen and require most of the body's blood during heavy exercise, the functions of other parts of the body, such as the liver, the kidneys or the stomach, are dependent upon what happens in the skeletal muscle.

The Structure of Skeletal Muscle

If one were to examine a whole skeletal muscle and gradually dissect it into its component parts, it would first be discovered that the muscle is composed of bundles of fibers. (See Fig. 3.1) *Endomysium* is the name given to the connective tissue that surrounds individual fibers and binds them together to form bundles of fibers. (See Fig. 3.2) Each bundle is called a *fasiculus* (plural: fasiculi) and is bound to neighboring fasiculi by white fibrous connective tissue, the *perimysium*. The external connective tissue that binds all the fiber bundles or fasiculi together into a whole muscle is called *epimysium* or *fascia*.

Each fiber is composed of a covering or membrane called the *sarcolemma* and a gelatin-like substance called *sarcoplasm* in which are embedded hundreds of contractile *myofibrils* and other important structures such as *mitochondria* and the *sarcoplas-*

19

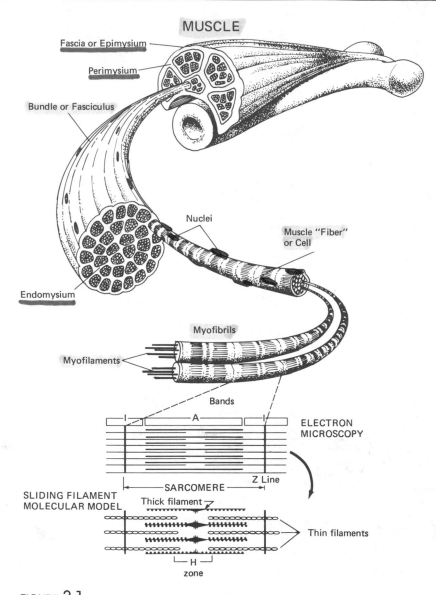

FIGURE 3.1. Skeletal muscle structure.

mic reticulum. (Fig. 3.3). Each myofibril in turn contains many fine protein threads (myofilaments). These include thin *filaments* and thick *filaments* (Fig. 3.4). When slices of muscle tissue are stained with the appropriate chemicals and observed under a microscope, they take on a banded or *striated* appearance because of the regular arrangement of the myofilaments into dark or *A bands* and light or *I bands* (Fig. 3.1, 3.4). The I bands appear light because they contain mostly the thin filaments, whereas the A bands are dark because they contain both the thin and thick filaments (Fig. 3.4). When a muscle is relaxed, the central portion of each A band appears somewhat lighter than the outer portions because the thin filaments do not meet in the center of the A band. This central, lighter area of the A band, the *H-zone*, disappears.

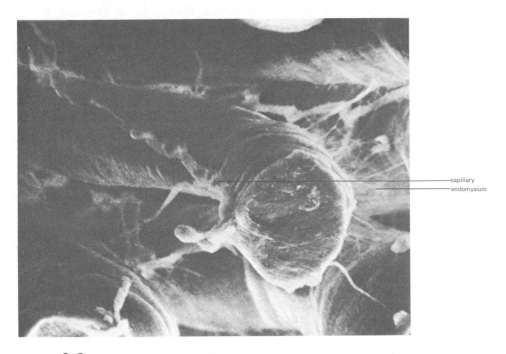

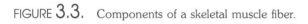

FIGURE 3.2. Stereo electron micrograph of several muscle fibers that have been teased apart to show web-like connective tissue (endomysium) between fibers. A single capillary is shown along left lower border of the central muscle fiber. (Courtesy of R. E. Carrow, W. W. Heusner and W. D. Van Huss, Michigan State University, E. Lansing, Michigan.)

FIGURE 3.3. Components of a skeletal muscle fiber.

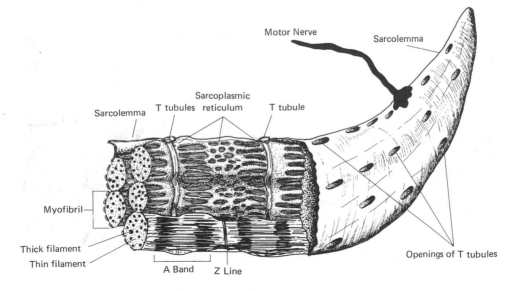

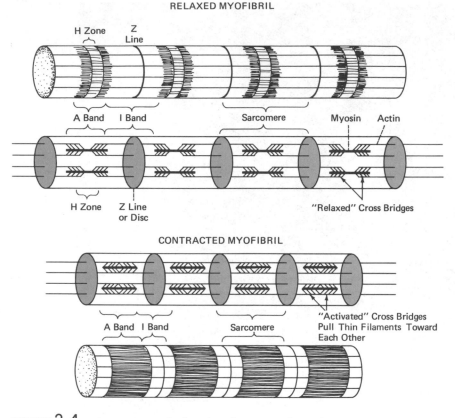

FIGURE 3.4. Appearance of relaxed and contracted muscle.

when the muscle contracts. Each I band is bisected by a *Z line* or disc which seems to anchor the thin filaments. The distance between two Z lines is known as a *sarcomere*. When a muscle fiber contracts, the Z lines move closer together and, thus, the sarcomeres shorten.

Part of the explanation of how muscle contracts involves several of the protein molecules that make up the thin filaments. The most important of these is *actin* (long strands of which are the major constituent of the thin filaments). Actin actually becomes attached to the myosin proteins of the thick filaments during the contraction cycle. However, actin and myosin cannot become attached without the cooperation of two other proteins within the thin filaments. One of these proteins is *tropomyosin*, which can block the attachment sites (binding sites) on actin where myosin attaches during contraction (Figs. 3.5, 3.6). The other protein is *troponin*, which can pull tropomyosin away from the attachment sites so that contraction may proceed (Figs. 3.5, 3.6). The function of these molecules which regulate muscle contraction is further described in the next section.

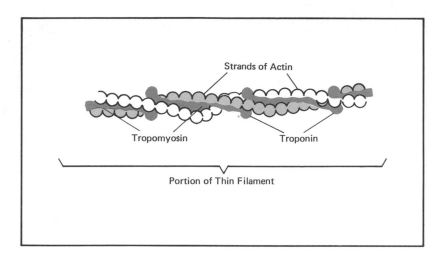

FIGURE 3.5. Sketch to show orientation of actin, tropomyosin, and troponin in a portion of a thin filament. Two strands of actin are wound together in a helix pattern. The rod-shaped tropomyosin molecules lie in the
groove between the actin strands. The troponin molecules are bound to the
actin strands at regular intervals.

Muscle Contraction

With the electron microscope, one can compare the detailed structures of relaxed
muscle fibers with those of the contracted fibers. The most common observations are
that after contraction the lengths of the A bands have not changed, whereas the I
bands are shorter and the H zones of the A bands have disappeared. These observations have led scientists to conclude that muscles contract by the sliding of thin filaments toward each other in the central parts of the A bands. As these filaments move
toward each other, the Z lines are pulled closer together so that the I bands shorten.
Also, the movement of thin filaments toward each other across the myosin filaments
causes the H zone of the A band to disappear as it becomes occupied by actin. This
notion that the thin filaments slide toward each other during contraction is called the
"sliding filament" theory of muscle contraction [23, 24, 25].

The Contractile Process

When a motor nerve fiber delivers a stimulus or *action potential* to a skeletal muscle
fiber at the motor endplate (Fig. 3.3), an action potential subsequently spreads rapidly
over the entire sarcolemma. At nearly the same instant, the action potential is transmitted down the *T-tubules* toward the interior of the fiber (Fig. 3.3). These T-tubules lie
adjacent to parts of the *sarcoplasmic reticulum,* a system of tubular channels that
spreads out over the surfaces of the myofibrils (Fig. 3.3). The transmission of the action potential down the T-tubules causes calcium to be released from the sarcoplasmic
reticulum. These calcium ions are then bound to troponin molecules. In the absence of

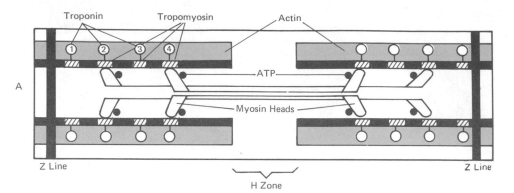

A

Troponin   Tropomyosin   Actin

ATP

Myosin Heads

Z Line   Z Line

H Zone

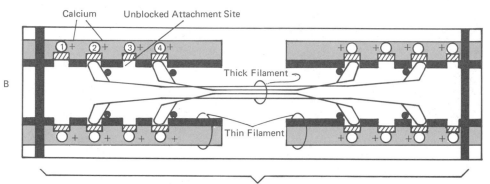

B

Calcium   Unblocked Attachment Site

Thick Filament

Thin Filament

Relaxed Sarcomere Length

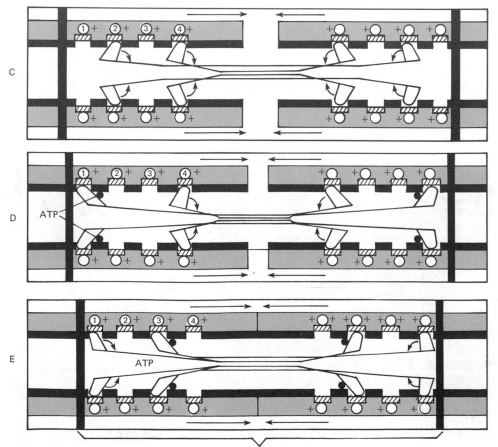

C

D

ATP

E

ATP

Contracted Sarcomere Length

calcium, tropomyosin blocks the attachment sites for myosin (Fig. 3.6A). In the presence of calcium ions, troponin changes its shape and pulls tropomyosin away from the myosin attachment sites on actin [11, 22, 32, 35] (Fig. 3.6B).

Once the myosin attachment sites on actin are unblocked, myosin molecules can form "cross bridges" with actin. The myosin molecules consist of globular "heads" and long, thin backbones. The myosin heads are movable and are somehow activated in the presence of adenosine triphosphate (ATP) so they can attach themselves to the unblocked sites on actin (Fig. 3.6B). Once the myosin–ATP complex is attached to actin, myosin can serve as an enzyme to split ATP into ADP plus phosphate (P) with the simultaneous release of chemical energy to make the myosin heads swivel toward the center of the A-band and move the thin filaments in that direction (Fig. 3.6C). This enzyme action of myosin to split ATP is called "myosin ATPase activity" or "actomyosin ATPase activity."

$$ATP \xrightarrow[\substack{\text{Myosin ATPase} \\ \text{activity}}]{} ADP + P + \text{energy for contraction}$$

As we shall see later, the amount of myosin ATPase activity in a muscle seems to determine its speed of contraction.

As hundreds of thin filaments are drawn to the center of the A-bands in a myofibril, the Z lines (to which the thin filaments are anchored) move closer together; that is, the sarcomere lengths are shortened (compare Fig. 3.6B, 3.6E). If all or most of the sarcomere lengths are shortened, the tendinous attachments of the muscle to the bone(s) will be pulled closer together to cause movement. If movement is impossible because a load is too great, the connective tissue in the muscle and the tendons will be placed under tension caused by the shortening of some of the sarcomeres.

Cross Bridge Cycling

Each time a myosin head (cross bridge) moves the thin filament toward the center of the A-band, hundreds of other myosin heads throughout the myofibril are making other attachments with thin filaments to assist in the movement. Simultaneously hundreds more are released from their attachment sites and are preparing to reattach to actin at other sites to further pull the thin filaments toward the centers of the A-bands throughout the myofibril (Fig. 3.6D,E). This repetitive attachment, release, and reattachment of myosin heads to thin filaments is called "cross bridge cycling."

FIGURE 3.6. (*Opposite*) Mechanism of muscle contraction. **A.** Myofibril at rest. Note ATP bound to myosin heads, and numbered attachment sites blocked by tropomyosin in the absence of calcium. **B.** In presence of calcium, troponin pulls tropomyosin from attachment sites so myosin/ATP can attach to actin. **C.** ATP is split to provide energy for myosin heads to swivel toward center of sarcomere and carry thin filaments with them. **D.** Myosin head that had been attached to site 2 is released from that site after combining with a fresh ATP molecule and reattaches at site 1. **E.** ATP is split at site 1 to move the thin filament to the center of the sarcomere; the head which was originally at site 4 has been released and reattached at site 3.

After a myosin head has been activated by ATP, it attaches itself to an unblocked binding site on actin and serves as an enzyme to release energy from ATP. To then disengage itself from actin, a fresh ATP molecule must be present. The myosin–ATP complex, once released from its old binding site, is free to reattach to actin at a new site closer to the Z line (Fig. 3.6CDE) to begin a fresh "cross bridge cycle." It should be emphasized that while some myosin heads are disengaging from actin, others are becoming attached to keep the contraction active. In other words, a muscle does not have to relax for cross bridge cycling to occur; this phenomenon happens during even the most intense contraction.

As an aside, it might be noted that the failure of muscle to relax in rigor mortis is caused by the lack of availability of ATP for disengagement of myosin cross bridges from the thin filaments [11].

Muscle Relaxation

When the nerve supplying a muscle fiber stops firing, the nerve stimulus no longer spreads along the sarcolemma and down the T-tubules to trigger the release of cal-

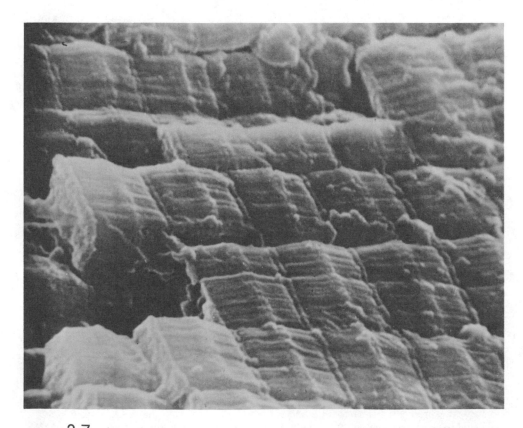

FIGURE 3.7. Stereo electron micrograph of myofibrils showing striations, z-lines. (Courtesy of R. E. Carrow, W. W. Heusner and W. D. Van Huss, Michigan State University, E. Lansing, Michigan.)

cium from the sarcoplasmic reticulum. In the absence of nerve activity, the sarcoplasmic reticulum once again binds the calcium ions that had been attached to troponin. Without calcium, troponin molecules assume their "resting" shape and allow tropomyosin to block the binding sites for myosin. This stops the attachment of myosin to actin and causes the muscle to relax until the next volley of nerve impulses.

The entire scheme of muscle contraction and relaxation is summarized in Fig. 3.8.

A knowledge of the mechanisms of muscle contraction and relaxation can aid one's appreciation and understanding of possible explanations for various physiological phenomena associated with exercise. For example, it is apparent that calcium and the sarcoplasmic reticulum system are intimately involved in the initiation of both contraction and relaxation; if there are problems with either calcium levels or sarcoplasmic reticulum function during exercise, it is easy to imagine how weakness, fatigue or cramps might result. Similarly, closely regulated levels of sodium and potassium are needed for the nerve stimulation and muscle activation, and adequate supplies of ATP must be supplied if muscle contraction is to continue normally. Also, with the knowledge that the force produced with contraction is the result of thousands of myosin heads interacting with the thin filaments, it would seem that stretching the muscle so that fewer myosin heads make contact with thin filaments would result in less force generated. Thus, there must be some optimal length of the muscle for the greatest force production. These and other phenomena will be discussed in later chapters.

SUMMARY OF MUSCLE CONTRACTION AND RELAXATION

Conditions in Relaxed Muscle:

1. Few or no nerve impulses reach muscle.
2. Calcium ions are bound to the sarcoplasmic reticulum.
3. Tropomyosin-troponin complex blocks attachment sites for myosin on actin.
4. ATP is bound to myosin heads.

Muscle Contraction:

1. Nerve impulse arrives at neuromuscular junction and causes stimulus (depolarization) to spread across sarcolemma and down transverse tubules (T tubules).
2. Depolarization of T tubules triggers the release of calcium from the sarcoplasmic reticulum. Calcium spreads to myofibrils, especially at the region of the A bands.
3. Calcium is bound by troponin. Troponin then changes shape and "pulls" tropomyosin away from attachment sites for myosin heads on actin.
4. Myosin-ATP attaches to actin at unblocked sites to form actomyosin-ATP.
5. Actomyosin-ATP is broken down to actomyosin plus ADP plus P plus energy to make myosin heads and thin filaments move toward center of A band.

Continuation of Contraction (cross bridge cycling):

6. New ATP molecules bind to myosin heads. This causes release of myosin heads from attachments to actin. In the meantime, other myosin heads have been bound to other attachment sites to maintain the contraction.
7. If other nearby attachment sites on actin are unblocked, the previously released myosin heads may be reattached; ATP is split and myosin heads plus thin filaments move further toward center of A band.
8. New ATP molecules bind to myosin heads to cause their release from actin. Cross bridge cycling continues as long as nerve impulses continue and ATP is available.

Relaxation:

1. Nerve impulse stops; this means there is no longer a depolarization stimulus across sarcolemma and down T tubules to trigger release of calcium from sarcoplasmic reticulum.
2. In the absence of a nerve stimulus, the sarcoplasmic reticulum withdraws calcium from troponin and stores it for future contractile activity.
3. In the absence of calcium, troponin changes shape and allows tropomyosin to block binding sites for myosin.
4. The muscle relaxes.

FIGURE 3.8.

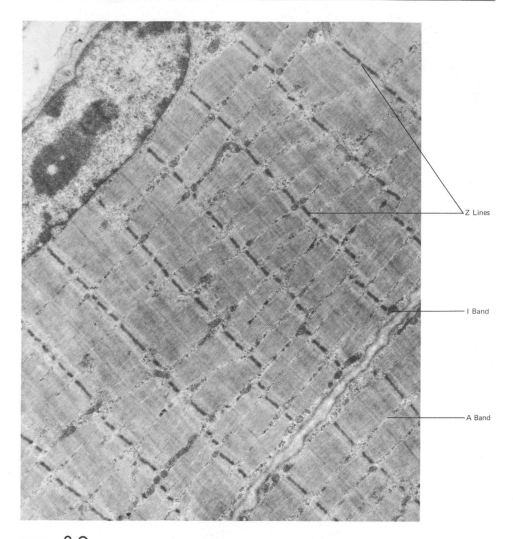

FIGURE 3.9. Electron micrograph of skeletal muscle (magnification ×7,500). (Courtesy of G. Colin Budd, Physiology Department, Medical College of Ohio, Toledo, Ohio)

Muscle Fiber Types

Skeletal muscle fibers are adapted by heredity and activity for the work they must perform. Those leg muscle fibers which are involved in prolonged contractions to maintain a human being in an upright posture have different properties than fibers used only occasionally to jump over a fence or sprint 100 meters. The major classification scheme for muscle fibers is based on how fast they produce a twitch contraction in response to an electrical stimulus. Accordingly, there are *slow twitch* (*Type I*) and *fast twitch* (*Type II*) fibers with twitch contraction times of about 110 milliseconds for slow twitch fibers and 50 milliseconds for fast twitch fibers [37]. It should be noted that, although slow twitch fibers are slower than fast ones, they still contract rapidly enough for essentially all sport activities. Slow twitch fibers tend to be smaller and produce less overall force than fast twitch fibers. But the slow fibers are more energy-efficient; they can produce more force for the same energy input [37] and are thus well adapted for prolonged exercise, when energy supply might be a limiting factor. Thus, when compared to slow twitch fibers, fast twitch fibers are easily fatigable.

Table 3.1 illustrates how different muscles in humans have different fiber-type compositions. Observe that the soleus muscle, a postural muscle of the calf, is composed almost entirely of slow twitch fibers, whereas the orbicularis oculi, an eye muscle involved in blinking, has mostly fast twitch fibers. As will be pointed out later, there is a large variability in the proportion of slow to fast twitch fibers in a given muscle among different groups of subjects. Thus, the figures shown in Table 3.1 should be considered only approximate estimates for the general population.

Myosin ATPase and Contractile Speed

It appears that the difference in speed of contraction for the two major fiber types is based largely on the fact that they have different degrees of myosin ATPase activity [37]. Since myosin ATPase is intimately involved in the muscle contraction process, it should perhaps not be surprising that fibers which have more of this enzyme activity can contract more rapidly. The difference in myosin ATPase activity in the fiber types is apparently caused by differences in the type of myosin molecule present [21, 37]; that in slow muscle is called "slow myosin", whereas that in fast muscle is called "fast myosin."

Another characteristic difference in the two major fiber types that may be related to contractile speed is that slow fibers have a very poorly developed sarcoplasmic reticulum when compared to fast muscle [37]. Since the sarcoplasmic reticulum is important for the quick release of calcium to trigger contraction, the poorly developed sarcoplasmic reticulum in slow fibers may help explain their slow response to stimulation. This

TABLE 3.1
Approximate Percentages of Slow Twitch (Type I) Fibers in Muscles from Sedentary Human Males, 20–35 Years of Age (31)

Muscle	% Slow Twitch
Soleus	87
Adductor pollicis	81
Tibialis anterior	73
Biceps femoris	67
Peroneus longus	62
First interosseus dorsales	58
Deltoid	52
Gastrocnemius mediale	50
Gastrocnemius laterale	44
Biceps brachii	43
Vastus lateralis	38
Sternocleidomastoideus	35
Triceps brachii	32
Rectus femoris lateralis	29
Orbicularis oculi	15

hypothesis is further supported by the fact that the troponin of slow muscles has a low affinity for calcium when compared to fast muscles [37]. Apparently, even when calcium is released by the sarcoplasmic reticulum, troponin in slow muscle fibers is slow to bind the calcium to initiate contraction.

Metabolic Characteristics of Different Fiber Types

Muscle fibers can be distinguished by different metabolic properties in addition to contraction times. Slow twitch fibers, for example, have a greater capacity to produce energy for long periods because they have more mitochondria with the enzymes necessary to break down fats and carbohydrates completely to carbon dioxide and water. Since this breakdown requires oxygen, it is also fortunate that slow fibers have more capillaries supplying blood to them than do fast twitch fibers [37]. Slow twitch fibers are handicapped, however, when it comes to producing energy rapidly for very intense contractions because they have little stored carbohydrate (glycogen) and little capacity to break the carbohydrate down to lactic acid for energy.

Fast twitch fibers can be subdivided into two categories based on their ability to produce energy. One subdivision, *Type IIA,* can produce energy both by complete

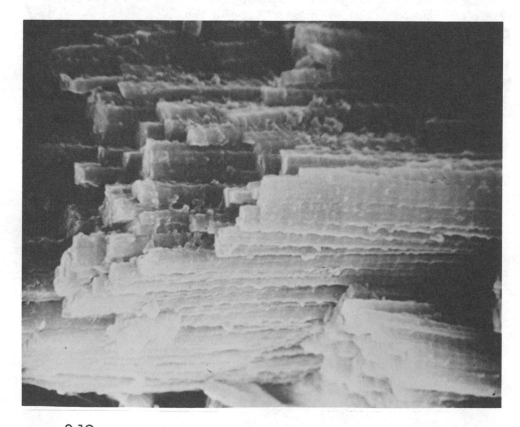

FIGURE 3.10. Stereo electron micrograph of myofibrils from a single muscle fiber. Note striations for each myofibril. (Courtesy of R. E. Carrow, W. W. Heusner and W. D. Van Huss, State University, E. Lansing, Michigan.)

oxidation, as in the slow twitch fibers, and also by breaking carbohydrate down to lactic acid. *Type IIB* fibers, on the other hand, are best adapted for short bursts of activity because they have few mitochondria and a large capacity to break down carbohydrate in the absence of oxygen. Both Type IIA and IIB fibers have large stores of glycogen for quick energy.

Neural Factors and Fiber Types

A group of muscle fibers is activated by a single motor nerve. One nerve may innervate 15–2,000 muscle fibers simultaneously. A motor nerve and all the muscle fibers it innervates are collectively called a *motor unit*. Since it has been shown that all muscle fibers within a motor unit have the same fiber type and that the fiber type is determined in large measure by the motor nerve [37], it is useful to speak of fast and slow motor units, rather than muscle fibers. Slow units are innervated by motor neurons that tend to be much smaller, both in the diameter of their axons and in the size of their cell bodies in the spinal cord, than is the case for fast motor units. Also, the nerve conduction velocity is much slower in the nerves of slow motor units [37]. The net effect of these differences in innervation is that the small neurons of the slow motor units have a lower threshold for activation than those of fast units so that the slow units

FIGURE 3.11. Fast twitch motor units are heavily recruited during jumping activities. (Courtesy of Office of Public Information, Purdue University, West Lafayette, Indiana.)

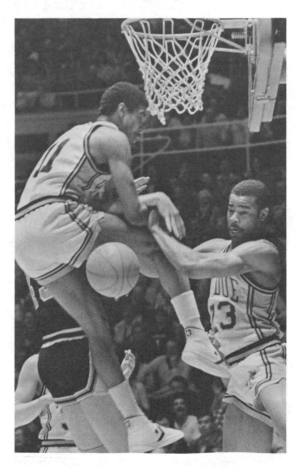

TABLE 3.2
Characteristics of Muscle Fiber Types

Characteristic	Slow (I)	Fast (IIA)	Fast (IIB)
Contractile Speed	slow	fast	fast
Size	small	large	large
Myosin ATPase Activity	low	high	high
Myosin Type	slow	fast	fast
Development of Sarcoplasmic Reticulum	poor	great	great
Troponin Affinity for Calcium	poor	great	great
Force Produced	low	high	high
Efficiency of Force Production	great	poor	poor
Fatigability	slight	great	great
Mitochondria	many	many	few
Mitochondrial Enzyme Activity	great	great	slight
Glycogen Stores	slight	great	great
Glycolytic Capacity	slight	great	great
Capillaries	many	moderate	few
Motor Neuron Size	small	large	large
Nerve Threshold for Recruitment	low	high	high
Nerve Conduction Velocity	slow	fast	fast
% in Typical Leg Muscles	45	38	16
% in Leg Muscles of Distance Runner	80	14	5
% in Leg Muscles of Sprinter	23	48	28

are recruited first for nearly all activities [37]. It is only when the intensity of activation is very great or when the slow twitch units are fatigued that the larger, more powerful fast motor units are brought into play [6, 7, 14, 15, 17, 37]. This would occur in sprinting, jumping, throwing, and other power events and toward the end of prolonged, exhaustive exercise, such as distance running or swimming.

It bears emphasizing that the smaller, more easily recruited slow motor units are activated before fast units in most activities. Even in an activity such as a high jump or shot put, slow units will usually be recruited before the fast units. Thus, it is apparently impossible to train only fast motor units; the slow ones have to be trained, too [16]. Of course, it is possible to choose training activities which will recruit the fast units more heavily than other activities [1, 12, 16, 26, 37]. For example, interval training with more intensive contractions will produce a greater involvement of fast units than long, slow, continuous training [19].

In Table 3.2 are presented some characteristics of the different fiber types and estimates of the proportions of the different types that might be found in various population groups. There is a significant variation in fiber types within groups such as distance runners, sprinters, and even untrained persons; therefore, the estimates in Table 3.2 should be considered as approximations only.

Fiber Types and Athletic Performance

After the discovery that slow twitch fibers were apparently better adapted to endurance exercise and fast twitch fibers better suited to power-related activities, many studies were done to determine whether or not athletic performance was strongly affected by the proportions of slow and fast motor units in an athlete's muscles [2, 3, 4, 10, 13, 18, 33]. It was found, for example, that elite distance runners have about 80 per cent slow twitch fibers in their leg muscles, compared to 45 per cent for nonathletes. Sprinters, on the other hand, have about 75 per cent fast twitch fibers, whereas middle-distance runners, jumpers, and throwers usually have variable proportions of the two fiber types and cannot usually be distinguished as groups from nonathletes. Females seem to have about the same proportionality of fiber types as males in athletic and nonathletic groups [4, 18, 33].

Although on average there were some marked differences in fiber types among certain athletic populations, it should be pointed out that there were many exceptions to these results [16]. Some excellent sprinters had only a modest number of fast motor units, and some elite distance runners had a normal percentage of slow units. This variability was also shown in studies in which percentages of fast and slow fibers in athletes were correlated with their individual performances. In distance runners, for example, it has been concluded that there is only a modest correlation between per cent slow twitch fibers in leg muscles and running performance [10].

There are conflicting results with respect to the relationship between fiber type and strength measures [3]. In one report, for example, no correlation was found except for leg strength during high speed contractions, when there was a significant correlation between strength and the percentage of fast twitch fibers in thigh muscles [36]. In another study on weight lifters and distance runners, for the weight lifters only, strength of a thigh muscle was related to the percentage of slow twitch fibers, whereas calf muscle strength was related to the percentage of fast twitch fibers; for the endurance runners no significant correlations were found [3]. There is also conflicting evidence on the relationship between the percentage of fast twitch fibers and strength improvements brought about with strength training [6, 30].

In summary, it appears that one is more likely to be successful in certain athletic events, especially distance running and sprinting, if the athlete is blessed with a certain muscle fiber composition. However, "ideal" fiber types do not guarantee championships; in some cases it is still possible to be successful with less than optimal fiber composition. Some portion of athletic success is determined by muscle fiber composition, but there are many other factors that are at least as important, if not more so.

Heredity and Training Effects on Fiber Types

Considering the fact that most elite endurance athletes have high percentages of slow twitch fibers, whereas most sprinters have high percentages of fast twitch fibers, one might ask whether these athletes have their peculiar fiber type distributions because of the nature of the training they pursue or because they were born with those distributions. Phrased another way, to the extent to which fiber types are important, are persons born or trained to be champions? From the results of experiments done with human subjects, the answer to this question seems to be that training does alter the metabolic characteristics of the fiber types but does not usually alter the basic contractile speed of the fibers.

In these studies, subjects undergo muscle biopsies before and after a period of training lasting from a few weeks to several months. Biopsies are usually obtained with a large needle which is similar in diameter to a drinking straw. The muscle sample, 15–45 milligrams in weight, is frozen, thinly sliced, and stained with chemicals which show myosin–ATPase activity, a reflection of fiber type, when the tissue slices are observed under a microscope. In addition to staining for ATPase activity, stains are also available to detect the metabolic characteristics of the fibers, especially the activities of mitochondrial enzymes which break down fats and carbohydrates to carbon dioxide and water. The typical result of these biopsy studies before and after endurance training is that the training enhances the mitochondrial enzyme activities of both fiber types but does not alter the myosin ATPase activity (fast or slow fiber type) [1, 12, 16, 26, 37]. More of the fast twitch fibers are classified as Type IIA after endurance training and fewer as Type IIB. These results mean that endurance training makes both fast and slow fibers better able to provide energy during prolonged work but leaves contraction times unchanged.

Contraction times (fiber types) in humans are also unchanged by strength or power training, but fast twitch fibers tend to increase in size more than slow twitch fibers [6, 30, 36]. Accordingly, fast twitch fibers are recruited heavily in strength and power activities, and the ratio of the cross-sectional area of fast fibers to the area of slow fibers increases with strength training. A similar finding occurs after heavy swim training [29].

In one study done on runners who switched from long distance training to more intensive interval training, it was observed that some slow fibers contained small amounts of "fast" myosin and fast fibers contained some "slow" myosin [21]. This suggested to the authors that these might be fibers in transition from one type to another as a result of the altered training.

It is possible that changes in fiber types occur only after years of training, but such longitudinal studies are difficult to conduct and to interpret. One problem with interpretation is that the subjects grow older during the course of the study; changes that might be caused by exercise might also be caused (or obscured) by the aging process. For the time being, therefore, the best evidence we have supports the contention that one cannot alter muscle fiber types by training and that to a certain extent many world class athletes are born and not made. Always keep in mind, though, that there are exceptions to every rule, especially when dealing with matters as complex as athletic performance.

Value of Fiber Typing for Athletes

If used indiscriminately, muscle biopsies for determining fiber types can do more harm than good. There is usually little discomfort associated with a needle biopsy, but occasionally it can cause a great deal of acute pain. More importantly, much emotional trauma can accompany the procedure if the biopsy results are interpreted as spelling the end of an athlete's career because the athlete isn't "born" to be successful in a particular event or sport. Therefore, it should be understood that there is a great deal of variability in the measurements made with the biopsy procedure—mistakes can occur quite easily if the results of a single biopsy are assumed to be infallible [16].

Although it would be unwise to base major decisions about an athlete's career on the basis of a single biopsy, the biopsy procedure has proven to be a valuable tool in research to determine energy sources for various types of exercise, limiting factors for exercise, potential mechanisms underlying fatigue and soreness, and the effects of various diets on energy stores. If used wisely, the biopsy can also prove to be a good motivator in some cases where athletes need evidence that they have the physiological capacity to be good performers. A fiber typing procedure may sometimes prove valuable if it provides some idea of whether an athlete should attempt to train for endurance rather than nonendurance events/sports if the athlete has little preference. However, fiber typing results should not be used to predict performance levels; fiber types are only poorly correlated to performance [10, 16]. A much simpler and more accurate method of predicting performance in an athletic event (at least in events that do not require the learning of major complex skills) is to have the athlete perform the event. The fastest sprinters and distance runners on a high school track team before the season begins are also likely to be the fastest sprinters and distance runners, respectively, at the end of the season.

REVIEW QUESTIONS

1. Explain how nerve stimulation to a muscle leads to contraction. What is the role of calcium in this process?
2. Sketch a segment of a myofilament showing two sarcomeres, A bands, Z lines, thin filaments, thick filaments, and H zones. Explain the difference in appearance between relaxed and contracted myofibrils on the basis of the sliding filament theory of contraction.
3. Describe the difference between a muscle fiber, a myofibril, and a myofilament.
4. Explain how the sarcoplasmic reticulum is involved in both contraction and relaxation.
5. Explain the role of tropomyosin and troponin in muscle contraction and relaxation.
6. How does cross bridge cycling account for a progressive shortening of muscle during contraction?
7. What is the function of the T-tubules in contraction?
8. How is ATP involved in both contraction and relaxation of skeletal muscle?
9. What is the relationship between myosin ATPase activity and contractile speed of a muscle fiber?
10. What are the two main fiber types in human skeletal muscle, and how do they differ?
11. Describe the recruitment pattern of fast and slow fibers in distance running, sprinting, and jumping. Is one fiber type always recruited first?
12. What anatomical and biochemical characteristics make slow twitch fibers well-adapted to endurance activties?
13. Describe some of the different characteristics for the two subdivisions of fast twitch fibers.
14. What influence does the motor nerve have on fiber recruitment for different activities?
15. What is an approximate percentage of slow fibers in the vastus lateralis of the thigh in untrained subjects, elite sprinters, and elite distance runners?
16. What is the relationship between fiber type distribution and performance in athletics? Can one accurately predict performance on the basis of fiber type?
17. What arguments could you raise against the use of muscle biopsies to determine fiber types in junior high schol athletes?
18. On the basis of the evidence presented in the text, how would you answer a question raised by a youngster who wanted to know if she could change her muscle fiber type distribution by training vigorously?

REFERENCES

[1] Andersen, P., and J. Henriksson. Training induced changes in the subgroups of human type II skeletal muscle fibres. *Acta Physiologica Scandinavica*, 1977, **99**:123–125.

[2] Bergh, U., A. Thorstensson, B. Sjodin, B. Hulten, K. Piehl, and J. Karlsson. Maximal oxygen uptake and muscle fiber types in trained and untrained humans. *Medicine and Science in Sports,* 1978, **10:**151–154.

[3] Clarkson, P. M., W. Kroll, and T. C. McBride. Maximal isometric strength and fiber type composition in power and endurance athletes. *European Journal of Applied Physiology,* 1980, **44:**35–42.

[4] Costill, D. L., J. Daniels, W. Evans, W. Fink, G. Krahenbuhl, and B. Saltin. Skeletal muscle enzymes and fiber composition in male and female track athletes. *Journal of Applied Physiology,* 1976, **40:**149–154.

[5] Curtin, N. A., and R. C. Woledge. Energy changes and muscular contraction. *Physiological Reviews,* 1978, **58:**690–761.

[6] Dons, B., Bollerup, F. Bonde-Petersen, and S. Hancke. The effect of weight-lifting exercise related to muscle fiber composition and muscle cross-sectional area in humans. *European Journal of Applied Physiology,* 1979, **40:**95–106.

[7] Edgerton, V. R., B. Essen, B. Saltin, and D. R. Simpson. Glycogen depletion in specific types of human skeletal muscle fibers in intermittent and continuous exercise. In H. Howald and J. R. Poortmans, eds., *Metabolic Adaptation to Prolonged Physical Exercise,* Basel: Birkhauser Verlag, 1975, pp. 402–415.

[8] Edman, K. A. P., G. Elzinga, and M. I. M. Noble. The effect of stretch of contracting skeletal muscle fibers. In H. Sugi and G. H. Pollack, eds., *Cross-Bridge Mechanism in Muscle Contraction.* Baltimore: University Park Press, 1979, pp. 297–309.

[9] Fitts, R. H., F. J. Nagle, and R. G. Cassens, Characteristics of skeletal muscle fiber types in the miniature pig and the effect of training. *Canadian Journal of Physiology and Pharmacology,* 1973, **51:**825–831.

[10] Foster, C., D. L. Costill, J. T. Daniels, and W. J. Fink. Skeletal muscle enzyme activity, fiber composition and $\dot{V}O_2$ max in relation to distance running performance. *European Journal of Applied Physiology,* 1978, **39:**73–80.

[11] Giese, A. *Cell Physiology,* 5th ed. Philadelphia: W. B. Saunders, 1979.

[12] Gollnick, P. D., R. B. Armstrong, B. Saltin, C. W. Saubert IV, W. L. Sembrowich, and R. E. Shepherd. Effect of training on enzyme activity and fiber composition of human skeletal muscle. *Journal of Applied Physiology,* 1973, **34:**107–111.

[13] Gollnick, P. D., R. B. Armstrong, C. W. Saubert IV, K. Piehl, and B. Saltin. Enzyme activity and fiber composition in skeletal muscle of untrained and trained men. *Journal of Applied Physiology,* 1972, **33:**312–319.

[14] Gollnick, P., R. B. Armstrong, C. W. Saubert IV, W. L. Sembrowich, and R. E. Shepherd. Glycogen depletion patterns in human skeletal muscle fibers during prolonged work. *Pflügers Archiv,* 1973, **344:**1–12.

[15] Gollnick, P., R. B. Armstrong, W. L. Sembrowich, R. E. Shepherd and B. Saltin. Glycogen depletion pattern in human skeletal muscle fibers after heavy exercise. *Journal of Applied Physiology,* 1973, **34:**615–618.

[16] Gollnick, P. D., L. Hermansen, and B. Saltin. The muscle biopsy: still a research tool. *The Physician and Sportsmedicine,* 1980, **8:**50–55.

[17] Gollnick, P. D., K. Piehl, J. Karlsson, and B. Saltin. Glycogen depletion patterns in human skeletal muscle fibers after varying types and intensities of exercise. In H. Howald and J. R. Poortmans, eds., *Metabolic Adaptation to Prolonged Physical Exercise.* Basel: Birkhauser Verlag, 1975, pp. 416–421.

[18] Gregor, R. J., V. R. Edgerton, J. J. Perrine, D. S. Campion, and C. DeBus. Torque-velocity relationships and muscle fiber composition in elite female athletes. *Journal of Applied Physiology,* 1979, **47:**388–392..

[19] Henriksson, J., and J. S. Reitman. Quantitative measures of enzyme activities in type I and type II muscle fibres of man after training. *Acta Physiologica Scandinavica,* 1976, **97:**392–397.

[20] Howald, H. Ultrastructure and biochemical function of skeletal muscle in twins. *Annals of Human Biology,* 1976, **3:**455–462.

[21] Howald, H., R. Billeter, and E. Jenny. Transitional fibres in middle distance runners. *Experientia,* 1980, **36:**747.

[22] Hoyle, G. How is muscle turned on and off? *Scientific American,* 1970, **222:**84–93.

[23] Huxley, A. F. Review lecture: Muscular contraction. *Journal of Physiology, (London),* 1974, **243:**1–43.

[24] Huxley, H. E. The structural basis of muscular contraction. *Proceedings of the Royal Society of Medicine,* 1971, **178:**131–149.

[25] Huxley, H. E., and J. Hanson. Changes in the cross-striations of muscle during contraction and stretch, and their structural interpretation. *Nature,* 1954, **173:**973–976.

[26] Jansson, E., and L. Kaijser. Muscle adaptation to extreme endurance training in man. *Acta Physiologica Scandinavica,* 1977, **100:**315–324.

[27] Jaweed, M. M., G. J. Herbison, and J. F. Ditunno, Jr. Contractile properties of rat soleus after different types of weight lifting. *International Journal of Sports Medicine,* 1980, **1:** 181–184.

[28] Komi, P. V., and J. Karlsson. Physical performance, skeletal muscle enzyme activities, and fibre types in monozygous and dizygous twins of both sexes. *Acta Physiologica Scandinavica,* 1979, (Supplementum 462).

[29] Lavoie, J.-M., A. W. Taylor, and R. R. Montpetit. Skeletal muscle fibre size adaptation to an eight-week swimming programme. *European Journal of Applied Physiology,* 1980, **44:**161–165.

[30] MacDougall, J. D., G. C. B. Elder, D. G. Sale, J. R. Moroz, and J. R. Sutton. Effects of strength training and immobilization on human muscle fibres. *European Journal of Applied Physiology,* 1980, **43:**25–34.

[31] Monster, A. W., H. C. Chan, and D. O'Connor. Activity patterns of human skeletal muscles: relation to muscle fiber type composition. *Science,* 1978, **200:**314–317.

[32] Murray, J. M., and A. Weber. The cooperative action of muscle proteins. *Scientific American,* 1974, **230:**58–71.

[33] Prince, F. P., R. S. Hikida, and F. C. Hagerman. Muscle fiber types in women athletes and non-athletes. *Pflügers Archiv,* 1977, **371:**161–165.

[34] Ridgway, E. B., and A. M. Gordon. Muscle activation: effects of small length changes on calcium release in single fibers. *Science,* 1975, **189:**881–884.

[35] Sugi, H., and G. H. Pollack. *Cross-bridge Mechanism in Muscle Contraction.* Baltimore: University Park Press, 1979.

[36] Thorstensson, A. Muscle strength, fibre types and enzyme activities in man. *Acta Physiologica Scandinavica,* 1976, (Supplementum 443).

[37] Vrbova, G. Influence of activity on some characteristic properties of slow and fast mammalian muscles. *Exercise and Sport Sciences Reviews,* 1979, **7:**181–213.

CHAPTER

4

Energy Metabolism

ENERGY is defined as the capacity to do work. Biological work includes the movement of molecules across cell membranes, the establishment of membrane potentials in nerve and muscles, the synthesis (anabolism) and degradation (catabolism) of molecules such as proteins and carbohydrates, and, most importantly for exercise physiology, the movement of thin filaments past thick filaments in muscle contraction. The energy to perform biological work comes from the energy stored within the chemical bonds of a variety of molecules. When chemical reactions cause these bonds to break, some of the energy of the bonds is released as heat and serves only to increase or maintain the body temperature; another portion of the released energy, the so called "free energy," can be used to perform biological work.

Breaking of Chemical Bonds → Heat + Free Energy

Some molecules release a great deal of free energy when their bonds are broken. These "high energy" molecules are especially useful for performing biological work. The most commonly used "high energy" molecule is adenosine triphosphate (ATP), which can release tremendous amounts of free energy when it is split into adenosine diphosphate (ADP) plus a phosphate group (P) as follows:

ATP → ADP + P + Free Energy For Biological Work

As described in the previous chapter, ATP is required to provide the energy for muscle contraction and for the recycling of the cross bridges during the contractile process; without ATP, thin filaments do not slide over the thick filaments. But there is only

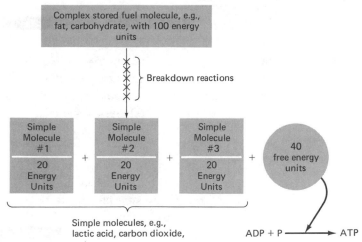

FIGURE 4.1. Release of energy from stored fuels to produce ATP.

a small store of ATP in the muscles, enough to provide for maximal contraction for about one second. Fortunately, the body has the ability to replenish ATP almost as quickly as it is broken down. This replenishment of ATP is accomplished when reserve fuel molecules, such as carbohydrates and fats, are broken down to provide free energy which can be used to join adenosine diphosphate (ADP) and phosphate (P) together to form ATP:

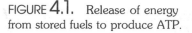

It is important to remember that stored fuels such as carbohydrate and fat *are not changed into ATP molecules*. Rather, a portion of the energy stored in the chemical bonds of the stored fuel molecules is released from those molecules, and that liberated energy then causes adenosine diphosphate (ADP) to combine with phosphate (P) to form adenosine triphosphate (ATP). In general, fuel molecules with larger amounts of energy stored in their chemical bonds are broken down into molecules with lesser amounts of energy in their bonds, and the excess energy is used to produce ATP from ADP + P. (See Fig. 4.1.) The first fuel reserve to be called upon when ATP is being used up is a molecule called *creatine phosphate* (or phosphocreatine), which is stored in the muscle fibers.

The Primary Fuel Reserve— Creatine Phosphate

Almost instantaneously as ATP is broken down to ADP + P during muscle contraction, the ATP is resynthesized at the expense of creatine phosphate. In this process creatine phosphate donates its phosphate to ADP as follows:

$$\text{Creatine phosphate} + \text{ADP} \rightarrow \text{Creatine} + \text{ATP.}$$

In this reaction, energy stored in the chemical bonds of creatine phosphate is used to cause the coupling of its phosphate to ADP to form ATP; therefore, the creatine molecule that remains contains less energy than the creatine phosphate molecule. This re-synthesis or rebuilding of ATP at the expense of creatine phosphate is especially important when extremely heavy exercise, such as sprinting, pushing an automobile, or pedaling a bicycle ergometer rapidly against heavy resistance, is sustained for less than 30 seconds. At lesser, more prolonged workloads, creatine phosphate is not depleted as rapidly as with short bursts of severe work.

The breakdown of creatine phosphate does not require the presence of oxygen delivered by the blood; therefore, it is said to be an *anaerobic* process as opposed to an *aerobic* (oxygen-requiring) process. The use of creatine phosphate for ATP re-synthesis is one of only two common anaerobic means of releasing energy for ATP production; the other is the breakdown of glucose to lactic acid. The series of chemical reactions that causes glucose to be catabolized or broken down to lactic acid is called *anaerobic glycolysis*.

Anaerobic Glycolysis

Glucose can be made available in the muscle cells for breakdown to lactic acid principally by two means: 1) the glucose molecules may pass from the blood through the sarcolemma into the cell interior or 2) the glucose can be split from glycogen stores in the muscle cell itself in a process called *glycogenolysis* (glycogen breakdown).

Glycogen molecules are nothing more than clusters of glucose molecules that are attached to each other in complex chains. (Each glucose molecule has a backbone of six carbon atoms.) The process of breaking the complex glycogen molecules down involves the removal of glucose molecules one at a time from the chain links or bonds in the glycogen molecule.

Anaerobic glycolysis consists of breaking down the six-carbon glucose molecules, which have a great deal of energy stored in their chemical bonds, into two lactic acid molecules, each having three carbons and a combined total of chemical energy less than that found in the more complex glucose molecule. Some of this difference in free energy is used to cause ADP and P to form ATP as follows:

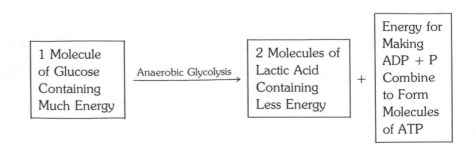

How much ATP can be produced with the energy liberated by the anaerobic break-down of glycogen or glucose? Examine Fig. 4.2, and you will note that ATP is produced in reactions F and G, and ATP is used up in reactions B and C. For the break-down of every molecule of glucose-6-phosphate that originated from blood glucose there are 4 ATP molecules produced (2 each in reactions F and G) and 2 ATP molecules used up (1 each in reactions B and C) for a *net* of 2 ATP molecules produced. Although it may not be evident from Fig. 4.2 that reaction B is involved in the derivation of glucose-6-phosphate from glycogen, the glycogen was first made from glucose that had come from the blood and undergone reaction B of Fig. 4.2. Therefore, in future calculations we will assume that the anaerobic breakdown of a glucose-6-phosphate molecule derived from either blood glucose or muscle glycogen results in a *net* production of 2 ATP molecules. (To be accurate it should be pointed out that there is another high energy molecule, *uridine triphosphate,* consumed in the production of glycogen from blood glucose. Therefore, although there is a net of two ATPs, there may actually be a net of only *one high energy molecule* produced by anaerobic glycolysis if glucose-6-phosphate is derived from glycogen. On the other hand, sometimes glycogen is not synthesized from blood glucose but from pyruvic acid or other compounds by a "reversal" of glycolysis in the muscle itself. In this case the use of an ATP in reaction B would not be required, and there would be a net synthesis of *three* ATPs or *two high energy molecules.*)

It should be noted at this point that lactic acid and pyruvic acid still have a substantial amount of energy stored in their chemical bonds. Much of this energy is available for ATP production and is released in the breakdown of lactic or pyruvic acid to carbon dioxide and water in *aerobic glycolysis,* as will be discussed later. Thus, anaerobic glycolysis is not a very efficient way to produce ATP because there is so much more potential ATP-producing energy left in the chemical bonds of lactic acid. As will be shown, the *aerobic* breakdown of the pyruvic acid left at the end of the anaerobic glycolysis of one glucose molecule can result in enough energy to produce an additional 36 molecules of ATP.

Other Considerations in Glycolysis

There are several other important aspects of glycolysis illustrated in Fig. 4.2 that need to be considered. First, note that the chemical reactions of glycolysis occur entirely in the sarcoplasm of the cell and not in the mitochondria. The reason for this is that all the enzymes that catalyze the reactions of glycolysis are located in the sarcoplasm. The enzymes for *aerobic* ATP production, on the other hand, are all located in the mitochondria.

Observe that reaction D in Fig. 4.2 is the reaction in which a molecule with six carbon atoms is first broken down into *two* molecules with three carbon atoms each.

Coenzymes and the Transfer of Electrons in Oxidation-Reduction Reactions. In reactions E and H of Fig. 4.2, molecules of NAD are involved. The letters NAD stand for the coenzyme *nicotinamide adenine dinucleotide,* an important molecule whose structure includes the B complex vitamin, nicotinic acid (niacin). A *coenzyme* is a nonprotein molecule necessary for the activity of an enzyme. NAD is impor-

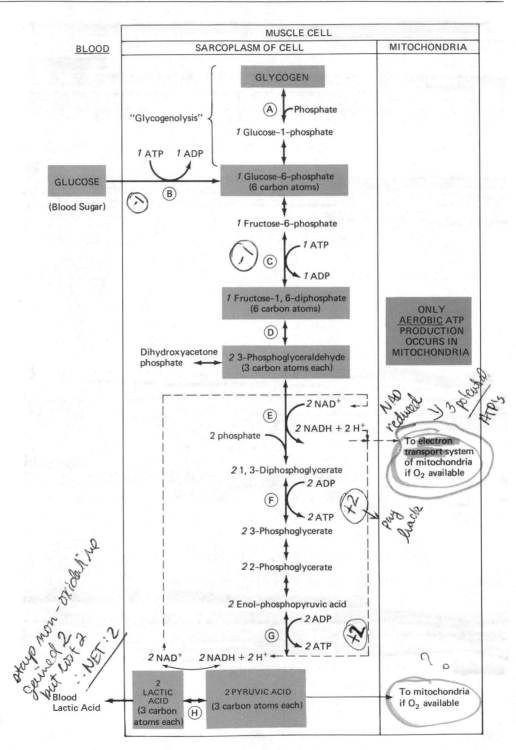

FIGURE 4.2. Anaerobic glycolysis—the breakdown of glycogen or glucose to lactic acid when oxygen supply is deficient.

in an ox. RXN, NAD gains electrons
in a red. RXN, NAD donates electrons ☆

Anaerobic Glycolysis 43

tant because it acts as an *electron acceptor* in many *oxidation* reactions of energy metabolism and an *electron donor* in *reduction* reactions. An oxidation reaction need not directly involve oxygen if an electron acceptor such as NAD is available to substitute for oxygen. (Oxygen is eventually required by animals because it is the *final electron acceptor* of metabolism, as will be discussed later.) An oxidation reaction is one in which a compound loses electrons. In biological oxidation reactions, these electrons removed by oxidation are often accompanied by hydrogen ions (H^+). In the form NAD^+, nicotinamide adenine dinucleotide can accept two negatively charged electrons ($^-$) and one hydrogen ion (H^+) as follows:

$$NAD^+ + 2(^-) + 2(H^+) \rightarrow NADH + H^+.$$

ox.
som. else is ox.
OX
for NAD

Conversely, in a *reduction* reaction (in which a compound gains electrons) NADH can donate two electrons as follows:

$$NADH \rightarrow NAD^+ + 2(^-) + H^+.$$

red. RED
for
NAD

something else is ox.

The Value of Lactic Acid for NAD Recycling. Referring again to Fig. 4.2, observe that in reaction E NAD^+ is changed to NADH. This means that NAD is accepting electrons in reaction E and, therefore, 3-phosphoglyceraldehyde is being oxidized (losing electrons). On the other hand, in reaction H of Fig. 4.2, as pyruvic acid is changed to lactic acid, NADH *loses* electrons to become NAD^+. Therefore, in H pyruvic acid is *reduced* (gains electrons) to form lactic acid, and the electrons required are donated by NADH.

Without the oxidation reaction E of Fig. 4.2, the reactions that produce ATP (F and G) could not occur. Thus, it is important to have an adequate supply of NAD^+ for reaction E to occur. As NAD^+ is used up in E, it becomes NADH. It is shown by the dotted lines that the NADH produced in E can be transformed to NAD^+ in reaction H, the production of lactic acid from pyruvic acid. This regenerated NAD^+ from reaction H can then be recycled through reaction E. Thus, the production of lactic acid is probably a *beneficial* step in anaerobic metabolism that regenerates the NAD^+ required for ATP production. It seems likely that a person deficient in the capacity to change pyruvic acid to lactic acid would have a lower than normal capacity to produce ATP by anaerobic glycolysis.

Regulatory Enzymes in Glycolysis. Another consideration in Fig. 4.2 is that the enzymes that catalyze reactions A and C, *phosphorylase* and *phosphofructokinase*, respectively, seem to be the principal enzymes that determine the maximal rate of glycogen breakdown. This means that any factors that alter the activities of these two enzymes can have profound effects on the rate of glycolysis. Some of these factors will be discussed later in this chapter.

A final point to consider about Fig. 4.2 is that nearly all of the reactions presented are reversible either directly or indirectly; that is, lactic acid or pyruvic acid under the appropriate conditions can be changed back to glycogen. In particular, reaction H is reversible so that when oxygen supply is adequate, lactic acid can be changed to pyruvic acid, which can then be further broken down to carbon dioxide and water by aerobic metabolism as will be described shortly.

Use of Lactic Acid for Energy (3)

What happens to the lactic acid produced by the muscles during exercise? A large proportion of it is changed back to pyruvic acid and broken down to carbon dioxide and water in the mitochondria. This often occurs in the muscles that produced the lactic acid. However, the lactic acid can also diffuse out of the muscles into the blood and be taken up and degraded for energy by other muscles [1,6,21]. Another way for lactic acid to be used for energy is for it to be delivered by the blood to the liver where the lactic acid can be changed into liver glycogen, essentially by a reversal of glycolysis (Fig. 4.3). The liver glycogen can then be broken down to glucose that enters the blood and is transported back to the muscles for use in glycolysis or glycogen storage. This cyclical pathway from muscle to liver and back to muscle is called the Cori cycle and is illustrated in Fig. 4.3. The Cori cycle is especially useful during prolonged exercise and for recovery because it helps to remove lactic acid, a substance which may hasten fatigue. It replenishes blood glucose for continued energy supply to the muscles.

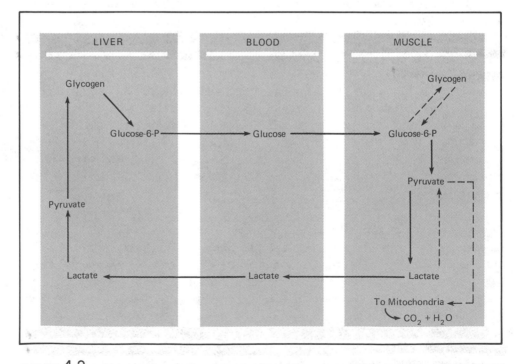

FIGURE 4.3. Major pathways for lactic acid (lactate) removal. The Cori cycle is diagrammed with solid lines.

Aerobic Carbohydrate Breakdown

Anaerobic glycolysis can produce a large amount of ATP rapidly to help meet ATP requirements during severe exercise; however, high rates of ATP production by anaerobic glycolysis cannot be sustained very long, and the severity of the exercise must be reduced if the exercise is to be continued. We are not certain why anaerobic glycolysis cannot keep the muscles working longer, but there is substantial evidence that excess acid accumulation in the muscles inactivates phosphorylase and phosphofructokinase so that glycolysis is depressed if the workload remains intense [16]. We do know that when exercise is continued for more than about 40–60 seconds, oxygen must be supplied by the blood to the working muscles for *aerobic ATP* production in the mitochondria of those muscles. In the presence of adequate supplies of oxygen the mitochondria of the cells can produce energy from carbohydrate, fat, or protein sources. Let us first consider how ATP can be produced at the expense of aerobic carbohydrate breakdown.

When oxygen supply is plentiful and the muscles are not working strenuously, the breakdown of glycogen or glucose starts in the same way as shown in Fig. 4.2 for anaerobic glycolysis. However, under aerobic conditions the pyruvic acid molecules are not converted to lactic acid, but pass instead from the sarcoplasm into the mitochondria, where a series of reactions breaks down each three-carbon pyruvic acid molecule into three molecules of carbon dioxide (CO_2) and three water (H_2O) molecules. (See Fig. 4.4.) As a result of breaking the more complex pyruvic acid molecules into simpler CO_2 and H_2O molecules, which have less energy stored in their bonds, energy is released to form 30 ATP molecules in addition to those found in the anaerobic glycolysis reactions of Fig. 4.2. Also, six extra ATP molecules are formed after electrons associated with NADH from reaction *E* in Fig. 4.2 are transported to the mitochondria as will be discussed shortly. This overall aerobic process is summarized in Fig. 4.4.

The breakdown of pyruvic acid to carbon dioxide and water in the mitochondria is a fairly complex matter, but a general knowledge of what occurs in the mitochondria should help to clarify many points in exercise physiology that will occur later in the text. Therefore, a brief explanation of aerobic carbohydrate catabolism in the mitochondria will be presented now.

First, when oxygen supply is adequate, the pyruvic acid molecules produced in the first phase of glycolysis (Fig. 4.2) diffuse from the sarcoplasm across the mitochondrial membrane to the interior of the mitochondria, where each pyruvic acid molecule loses one carbon atom and two oxygen atoms as CO_2. (See *A*, Fig. 4.5.) At the same time, each pyruvic acid molecule is oxidized in the presence of NAD^+; that is, each pyruvic acid molecule loses two electrons and two hydrogen ions. (Fig. 4.5.) These electrons are very important to ATP production as will be described later in this section.

The two-carbon molecule that is left after each pyruvic acid molecule loses its CO_2, electrons, and hydrogen ions is called an *acetyl* group. This acetyl group next combines with a molecule called *coenzyme A* (*CoA*) to form *acetyl CoA* (reaction *A*, Fig. 4.5). Each acetyl CoA molecule then enters a cyclical series of reactions called the *Krebs cycle* (citric acid cycle), shown in Fig. 4.5.

At the top of the Krebs cycle diagram, it can be seen that acetyl CoA combines with

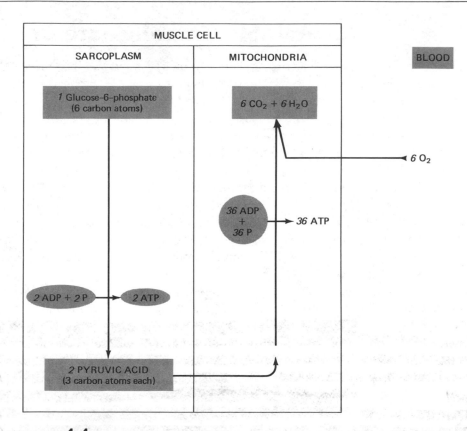

FIGURE **4.4.** Aerobic glycolysis—the complete breakdown of glucose to carbon dioxide and water in the presence of oxygen.

oxaloacetic acid and loses the coenzyme A molecule, with a molecule of citric acid resulting from this reaction. Citric acid is converted to cis-aconitic acid, which in turn is changed to isocitric acid. In reaction B, isocitric acid is oxidized (with the aid of the electron carrier, NAD^+) to oxalosuccinic acid. In reaction C, oxalosuccinic acid loses a carbon dioxide (CO_2) molecule and becomes alpha-ketoglutaric acid. The loss of a CO_2 molecule in reaction C means that we can now consider that only one of the original three carbon atoms of the pyruvic acid molecule remains. (Remember that the first carbon was lost as CO_2 in A of Fig. 4.5.) This last carbon is lost as CO_2 in the complex reaction D in which alpha-ketoglutaric acid undergoes oxidation (with NAD^+) and loss of CO_2 while producing one molecule of ATP. This is the only molecule of ATP actually produced in the Krebs cycle for *each* acetyl-CoA molecule that travels through the cycle.

After reaction D we can consider that there are no longer any of the original carbons left from pyruvic acid, and it remains only to remove four additional electrons and hydrogen ions in reactions E and F. In reaction E the electron carrier is not the usual NAD^+ molecule but, rather, a molecule called *flavin adenine dinucleotide* (FAD). In reaction F oxaloacetic acid is regenerated so that the cycle can begin anew. To produce larger amounts of ATP from the aerobic breakdown of pyruvic acid, the

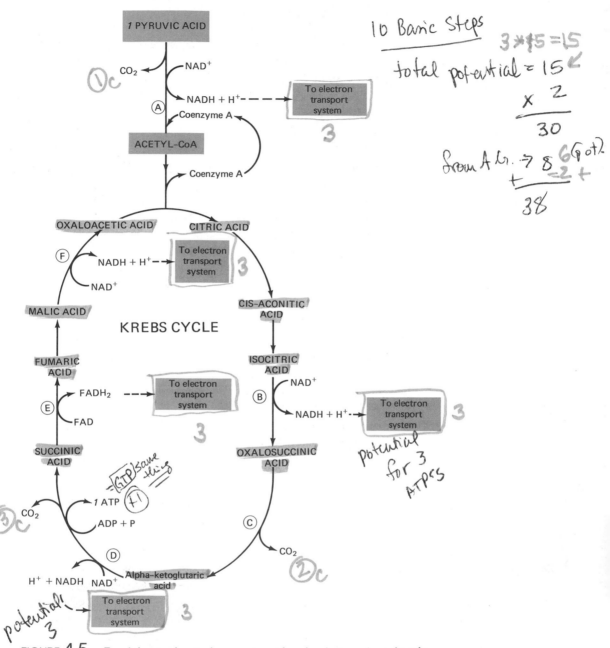

Handwritten notes:

10 Basic Steps

3 * *5 = 15

total potential = 15

$\times$ 2

30

from A.G. → 8 6(pot)
+ -2 +

38

potential
for 3
ATPSS

potential!
3

FIGURE 4.5. Breakdown of a single pyruvic acid molecule to carbon dioxide (CO_2), electrons, and hydrogen ions (H^+) in the Krebs Cycle. (Remember that *2* pyruvic acid molecules are produced by breaking down *1* glucose-6-phosphate molecule.)

electrons and hydrogen ions released to the electron carriers NAD and FAD must be transported to oxygen by way of the *electron transport system,* which is discussed in the following paragraphs.

The Electron Transport System

In the electron transport system (Fig. 4.6), as electrons and hydrogen ions are transferred from one compound to the next, chemical energy is given up at three steps (A, D, G) to provide energy for the formation of ATP from ADP and phosphate groups. That is, the loss of electrons (oxidation) that the various compounds undergo is responsible for the binding of phosphate (phosphorylation) to ADP to form ATP. Thus, the production of ATP in the mitochondria that is associated with the oxidation of successive molecules in the electron transport system is known as *oxidative phosphorylation.* It is this process that provides the greatest source of ATP for muscle contraction. Notice that the first molecule to be oxidized (reaction A) is nicotinamide adenine dinucleotide (NADH). In reaction B the flavoprotein H_2 that was reduced in A now undergoes oxidation. From this point on to step H, only electrons are transferred between compounds, whereas the two hydrogen ions (H^+) that had been bound to flavoprotein H_2 now pass into solution and can be used again in step H, the final oxidation-reduction reaction, where oxygen from the blood accepts two electrons from compound 6 (cytochrome oxidase) and combines with two dissolved hydrogen ions (H^+) to form water (H_2O).

In this scheme of electron transport it can be seen that for every two electrons (or hydrogen atoms) that pass all the way from NADH + H^+ to H_2O, three molecules of ATP are produced (at reactions A, D, G). Thus, in the aerobic breakdown of glucose or glycogen to carbon dioxide and water, every molecule of NADH that enters the electron transport system potentially can result in the production of three molecules of ATP. On the other hand, a molecule of $FADH_2$ produced by the Krebs cycle (reaction E, Fig. 4.5) enters the electron transport system at step B of Fig. 4.6 and bypasses the first ATP-producing reaction (A in Fig. 4.6). Thus, every pair of electrons delivered by $FADH_2$ results in the production of only two ATP molecules.

Total ATP Production During Aerobic Carbohydrate Breakdown

We are now in a position to determine how many molecules of ATP can be obtained from the aerobic breakdown of a molecule of glucose and where in the cell these ATP molecules are produced. If we know this, we can more easily understand the possible nature of muscle fatigue, the ways in which the body can adapt to physical training by developing its ATP-producing machinery, and many other aspects of exercise physiology.

First, refer to Fig. 4.2, the scheme of anaerobic glycolysis. As in the anaerobic breakdown of glucose, aerobic glucose breakdown still results in the production of two ATP molecules in each of two reactions (F and G of Fig. 4.2), and the expenditure of one or two ATP molecules in reactions C and B of Fig. 4.2, depending on whether glucose-6-phosphate comes from stored muscle glycogen or blood glucose, respectively. However, if oxygen is available, the two NADH molecules produced in reaction E of Fig. 4.2 are now able to transfer their electrons and hydrogen ions to the electron transport system of the mitochondria. Since three ATP molecules can be produced for every NADH molecule, a total of six ATP molecules can result from the breakdown of

ELECTRON TRANSPORT SYSTEM (CYTOCHROMES)

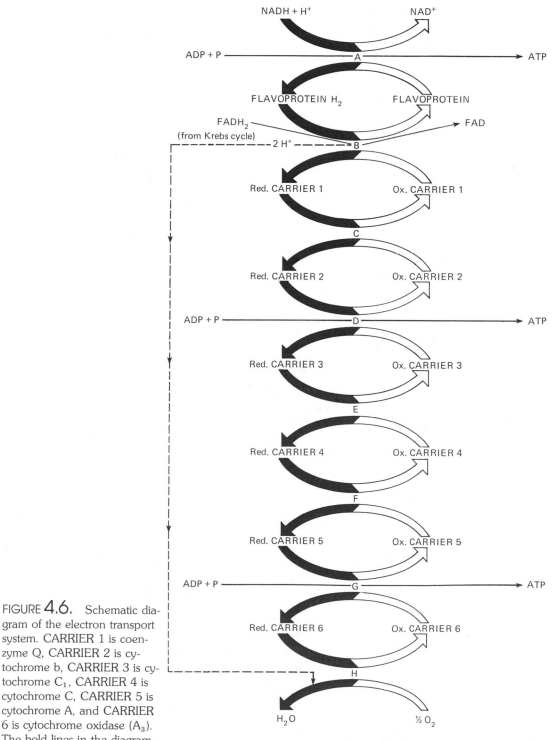

FIGURE 4.6. Schematic diagram of the electron transport system. CARRIER 1 is coenzyme Q, CARRIER 2 is cytochrome b, CARRIER 3 is cytochrome C_1, CARRIER 4 is cytochrome C, CARRIER 5 is cytochrome A, and CARRIER 6 is cytochrome oxidase (A_3). The bold lines in the diagram show the path of electrons.

SUMMARY: $\frac{1}{2} O_2 + 2 e^- + 3 ADP + 3 P \rightarrow H_2O + 3 ATP$

one glucose molecule in reaction E of Fig. 4.2. Thus, rather than the two or three ATP molecules of anaerobic glycolysis, we have shown how six more ATP molecules (a total so far of eight or nine) could result from partial aerobic glycolysis.

But this is only the beginning. Next consult Fig. 4.5, reaction A. For each of the two pyruvic acid molecules that can be derived from one glucose molecule, one NADH and, therefore, three ATP molecules can be produced for a total of six additional ATP molecules. In a similar fashion two NADH and thus six ATP molecules are produced in reactions B, D, and F of Fig. 4.5 for another 18 ATP molecules. In reaction E of Fig. 4.5, two molecules of $FADH_2$ can be sent to the electron transport system for an additional four molecules of ATP. (Remember that $FADH_2$ bypasses the first ATP production site in the electron transport system.) Finally, for each pyruvic acid molecule entering the Krebs cycle, one ATP is produced directly at reaction D of Fig. 4.5 for a total of two more ATP molecules from one glucose molecule. A grand total of 38 ATP molecules is produced aerobically. All of this is summarized as follows:

THE PRODUCTION OF ATP DUE TO ENERGY RELEASED BY THE AEROBIC
BREAKDOWN OF ONE MOLECULE OF GLUCOSE-6-PHOSPHATE

Sarcoplasm { Glycolysis (Fig. 4.2, reactions B, C, F, G: $-1-1+2+2=2$)............. 2 ATP

Mitochondria {
Krebs Cycle (Fig. 4.5, reaction D: $2 \times 1 = 2$).. 2 ATP

Electron Transport System (Oxidative Phosphorylation)

  Oxidation of $FADH_2$ (Fig. 4.5, reaction E: $2 \times 2 = 4$)...................... 4 ATP

  Oxidation of NADH (Fig. 4.2, reaction E; Fig. 4.5,
       reactions A, B, D, F: 3 ATP per
       NADH or [$10 \times 3 = 30$])............................... 30 ATP

Total Energy/Glucose-6-phosphate = 38 ATP

It should now be obvious that the production of energy (ATP) for exercise is much more efficient (from the standpoint of glucose utilization) when glucose is catabolized aerobically rather than anaerobically. As a matter of fact, the aerobic breakdown of glucose results in 19 times more ATP production per glucose molecule than does anaerobic glycolysis (38 ATP vs. 2 ATP). With adequate oxygen but a limited food supply, an organism would obviously be more apt to survive if provided with a biochemical control system that limited its ability to catabolize glucose anaerobically and increased its potential for using the more efficient aerobic process. Such a control system does exist in most higher forms of life, and without oxygen these organisms can survive at rest for no more than a few minutes and can endure heavy exercise for even less time (40–60 seconds for man). Although this natural emphasis on aerobic metabolism has undoubtedly helped early man survive prolonged periods of food deprivation and does favor his capacity for prolonged labor or athletic performance at moderate rates of energy expenditure without the need to stop for more food, it does not favor man's capacity to perform extremely heavy muscular labor for prolonged periods or his capacity to perform strenuous athletic feats such as all-out sprinting for more than a few seconds. Thus, in conditioning an athlete or laborer for *maximal* rates of work (beyond that which can be supported by aerobic metabolism alone), one must attempt to produce a physiological adaptation that will result in an ability to continue anaerobic ATP production beyond the normal limits. On the other hand, for prolonged work at lower rates of energy expenditure (for example, a marathon run or cross-country skiing), an adaptation should be produced that results in higher rates of efficient aerobic ATP production and less anaerobic glycolysis.

Adaptations of carbohydrate metabolism for various work tasks will be considered in more detail in later sections of this text. For a more thorough analysis of energy metabolism during exercise, we must now turn to the use of two other foodstuffs, fat and protein, for ATP production.

Aerobic ATP Production from Fat (Lipid)

Body fat may look ugly or beautiful depending upon the amount and where it is distributed, but no matter how it looks, it is an excellent reserve source of fuel for energy production both at rest and during exercise. In fact, one of the physiological adaptations that occurs when a person trains for long-distance running, cycling, or skiing is that fat tends to be used preferentially for ATP production during submaximal exercise while carbohydrate (glucose and glycogen) is spared. The process whereby the energy stored in the chemical bonds of fat molecules is gradually released to cause phosphate (P) and adenosine diphosphate (ADP) to combine into adenosine triphosphate (ATP) is described in the following paragraphs.

Triglyceride (Triacylglycerol)

Most of the fat (lipid) that is eaten and stored by man is in the form of triglyceride, a four-part molecule made up of one molecule of glycerol and three molecules of fatty acids as follows:

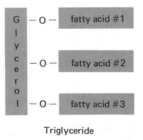

Triglyceride

The bulk of the ATP production from fat catabolism comes at the expense of fatty acid molecules that are split off from stored triglyceride molecules, transported by the blood to the muscles, and broken down by the muscles for energy. Therefore, this discussion will be restricted to ATP production from fatty acids, a process called *beta oxidation of fatty acids*. This process occurs exclusively in the mitochondria of the cells.

Oxidation of Fatty Acids

Fatty acids are long chains of carbon (C) atoms that have hydrogen (H) atoms attached to them. In humans most of these fatty acids have 16 or 18 carbon atoms.

Stearic acid has 18 carbon atoms as follows:

HOOC-CH$_2$-CH$_2$-CH$_2$-CH$_2$-CH$_2$-CH$_2$-CH$_2$-CH$_2$-CH$_2$-CH$_2$-CH$_2$-CH$_2$-CH$_2$-CH$_2$-CH$_2$-CH$_2$-CH$_3$.

There is a great deal of energy stored in all of the bonds of stearic acid, and that energy can be released only if the molecule is first activated or made more chemically reactive by a reaction with molecules of ATP and coenzyme A as indicated in reaction A of Fig. 4.7. As ATP is split into adenosine monophosphate (AMP) and two phosphate groups (PP), energy is released to bring about reaction A. In reaction B, the activated fatty acid is oxidized with flavin adenine dinucleotide (FAD) serving as the electron and hydrogen ion acceptor. In reaction C, another oxidation reaction occurs, this time with the aid of NAD$^+$.

In reaction D of Fig. 4.7 a two-carbon acetyl unit is split away from the long chain of carbons and is combined with a second coenzyme-A molecule to form a molecule of acetyl-CoA. This molecule of acetyl-CoA is indistinguishable from acetyl-CoA derived from aerobic glycolysis and thus may undergo further breakdown in the Krebs cycle (Fig. 4.5). The remaining activated fatty acid molecule now is two carbon atoms shorter than it was initially and may begin the beta oxidation cycle anew at reaction B. Reaction A is required only for the first trip through the cycle. For each cycle, two more carbon atoms are split from the fatty acid and changed to acetyl-CoA.

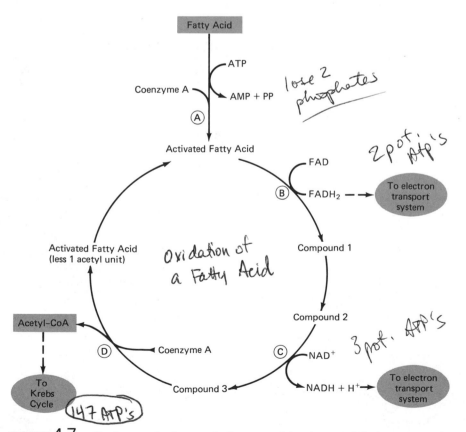

FIGURE 4.7. Oxidation of a fatty acid. Compound 1 is fatty acyl-CoA, compound 2 is β-hydroxyl acyl-CoA, compound 3 is β-keto acyl-CoA.

ATP Produced with Fatty Acid Oxidation

Let us now show how much ATP could be produced as the result of the complete breakdown of one molecule of stearic acid, which has 18 carbon atoms in its chain. In the first passage through the fatty acid oxidation cycle, one ATP is used up in activation step A in Fig. 4.7. (Since AMP is produced in step A, and it will eventually take the equivalent of 2 ATPs to provide the energy to resynthesize an ATP from AMP, some authors prefer to consider that 2 ATPs, rather than one, are used in step A.)

In reaction B one molecule of $FADH_2$ is formed which, upon passage through the electron transport system, results in the production of two ATP molecules. In reaction C of Fig. 4.7, a molecule of NADH is produced which can, via the electron transport system, cause three ATP molecules to be formed. Finally, in reaction D of Fig. 4.7, an acetyl-CoA molecule is liberated which, by way of the Krebs cycle and the electron transport system, can be used for energy to produce 12 ATP molecules. (See Figs. 4.5, 4.6 for review.) Thus, in the first cycle of the fatty acid oxidation pathway, 17 ATP molecules are produced and one is expended for a *net* of 16 ATP molecules.

Since stearic acid (18 carbons) has nine acetyl units (nine pairs of carbon atoms), it can be recycled through the oxidation cycle eight times. (On the eighth cycle, two molecules of acetyl-CoA are produced from the remaining four carbon atoms so a ninth cycle is not required.) For each cycle a two-carbon acetyl unit will be split from the fatty acid chain. Because only the first passage through fatty acid oxidation requires the loss of one ATP in reaction A, each of the next six passes through the oxidation cycle can result in the production of 17 ATP molecules. On the eighth and last passage an additional 12 ATP molecules are produced from the extra acetyl-CoA. The grand total of ATP molecules produced with the complete oxidation of stearic acid to CO_2 and H_2O thus becomes

$$16 + (6 \times 17) + 29 = 147.$$

Relative Value of Fat and Carbohydrate For Energy. To attempt a comparison between ATP production from carbohydrates and that from fat is a little like comparing a glass of milk and a bottle of beer—each is better under certain conditions. First, let us compare the energy produced per carbon atom. For the aerobic breakdown of a six-carbon glucose molecule, 38 molecules of ATP can be obtained, whereas 147 ATP molecules are produced from the breakdown of an 18-carbon fatty acid molecule. Therefore, on the basis of ATP produced per carbon atom, fat comes out ahead—8.2 to 6.3, or 30 per cent more than carbohydrate. Fat also is the winner over carbohydrate if the comparison is made between energy stored per unit of weight; a pound of fat can supply more than twice the ATP that can be produced at the expense of a pound of carbohydrate. Fat wins once again if the question concerns the supply of energy for a long duration of exercise or physical labor. The body reserves of carbohydrate are too small to sustain work for prolonged periods, but there is almost always (unfortunately for many) an overabundance of fat that can be called upon.

However, in a very important comparison—the ATP produced per unit of oxygen consumed—carbohydrate is the victor over fat. For example, 6 O_2 molecules are required to produce 38 ATP molecules during the aerobic breakdown of a molecule of glucose, whereas 26 O_2 molecules are used in the combustion of stearic acid to produce 147 ATP molecules. In this comparison carbohydrate is about 12 per cent more

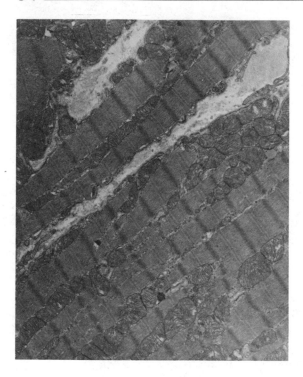

FIGURE 4.8. Electron micrograph of cardiac myofibrils showing rich supply of globular shaped mitochondria (magnification ×7,500). (Courtesy of G. Colin Budd, Physiology Department, Medical College of Ohio, Toledo, Ohio.)

efficient in terms of oxygen consumed per ATP molecule produced, and in situations where maximal performance is to a great extent limited by oxygen supply (for example, in long-distance running, cycling or skiing), it is important to oxidize carbohydrate as long as the carbohydrate supply, especially muscle glycogen, lasts.

In summary, both carbohydrates and fat are useful and important sources of reserve energy for exercise. Carbohydrate is a somewhat more efficient fuel in terms of ATP produced per molecule of oxygen consumed, but those persons engaged in long-duration physical labor or athletic events must rely also on fat in order to conserve the rather limited body reserves of carbohydrates.

Aerobic ATP Production from Protein

Proteins are complex chains of amino acids, that is, acids that have an amino ($-NH_2$) group attached to one of their carbon atoms. Some of these amino acids are, with the exception of the amino groups, almost identical to compounds that we have seen in our studies of carbohydrate metabolism. For example, the amino acids alanine, serine, and cysteine can be converted quite easily to pyruvic acid, which can then be oxidized by the Krebs cycle (Fig. 4.5) with the consequent production of ATP. Other amino acids can be converted into molecules that occur in the Krebs cycle and can, therefore, enter the Krebs cycle and be oxidized to CO_2 and H_2O.

Although many athletic coaches continue to provide their athletes with expensive pre-event meals high in protein hoping to increase their "energy supplies," it has been widely recognized by physiologists for many years that protein makes only minor contributions to ATP production during exercise unless the person who is exercising is also starving [2] or has been eating a diet low in carbohydrate [27]. This is not to say that protein cannot be used for energy (at rest, protein contributes about 5–10 per cent of the body's energy), but under normal conditions, protein is mostly used for building lean body tissue and is largely spared from energy metabolism as long as fat and carbohydrates are available. It is unusual to find any significant increase in protein use for energy during exercise when compared to rest. However, one reason for a failure to find more protein utilization during exercise may be that most investigators have not examined the protein breakdown products in sweat. Some reports suggest that a major excretion of these products occurs in sweat during prolonged exercise [27, 28].

Protein Catabolism during Exercise

Most experts agree that proteins contribute little to the total energy requirements of exercise under most circumstances. But that does not mean that proteins are not broken down during exercise. Some protein, including muscle protein, is catabolized during exercise, especially if the exercise is prolonged [3, 11, 12, 27, 28, 36]. It is not

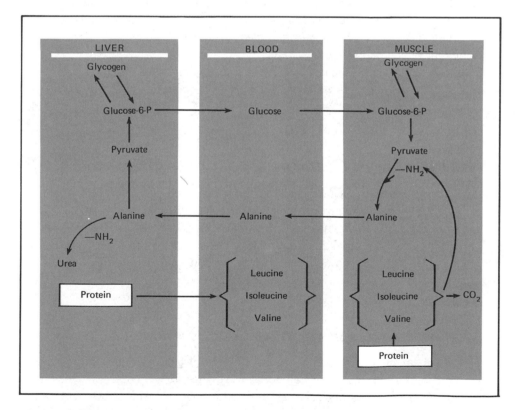

FIGURE 4.9. The glucose-alanine cycle. Glucose or glycogen is degraded to pyruvate in muscle. Amino groups ($-NH_2$) provided by amino acids from muscle or liver proteins are attached to pyruvate to make alanine. Alanine is changed to glucose after transfer to the liver.

clear, however, that the amino acids produced by this protein catabolism are used directly for fuels. Three amino acids, *leucine, isoleucine,* and *valine* are most often found to be oxidized during exercise, with leucine accounting for much of the oxidation. It appears that a principal use of the amino acids is to transfer amino groups ($-NH_2$) to pyruvic acid to produce another amino acid, *alanine* [4, 5, 11, 28]. Alanine is then delivered to the liver, where it is changed back to pyruvic acid and eventually to liver glycogen and blood glucose. This pathway is known as the "glucose-alanine cycle," and is diagrammed in Fig. 4.9. This cycle can provide an alternative to the Cori cycle (Fig. 4.3) for replenishing liver glycogen and blood glucose, especially during prolonged exercise and recovery.

Regulation of Energy Pathways

We have established that there are four main reserve energy sources that are available for replenishment of ATP used up during exercise for muscle contraction. Those sources are: 1) anaerobic breakdown of creatine phosphate, (2) anaerobic breakdown of glycogen or glucose, 3) aerobic breakdown of glycogen or glucose, and 4) aerobic breakdown of fat. How does the body know when it is time to turn on or turn off these different energy pathways? It would make sense if there were some chemical signals which could activate the appropriate pathways when they are needed and other chemicals which would inhibit the pathways when they are not needed. This is exactly what happens. *The enzymes which catalyze several key reactions in the energy pathways are sensitive to the concentrations of a number of chemicals (metabolites) which can either activate or inhibit the enzyme activity* [2, 13, 17, 18, 22, 24, 29, 31, 33, 34, 37, 38, 39, 40, 42].

Regulation of Creatine Phosphate Breakdown

Creatine kinase, the enzyme which catalyzes the breakdown of creatine phosphate, is activated by increased concentrations of ADP and inhibited by increased ATP. Therefore, as ATP is split into ADP plus P during muscle contraction, the increased levels of ADP instantly trigger the breakdown of creatine phosphate to replenish ATP. But if ample ATP is being produced by the aerobic breakdown of fats and carbohydrates, the high concentration of ATP slows down the splitting of creatine phosphate; the result is that creatine phosphate is saved for use during intense exercise.

Regulation of Glycolysis

During an activity such as sprinting, the breakdown of glycogen and glucose must occur several hundred times faster than at rest [33]. The two key enzymes involved in the regulation of glycolysis are *glycogen phosphorylase* (Fig. 4.2, reaction A) and *phosphofructokinase* (Fig. 4.2, reaction C). Phosphorylase is activated by increased amounts of adenosine monophosphate (AMP), by increased calcium, and by increased epinephrine from the adrenal glands [22, 37]. Note that this activation of phosphorylase occurs automatically for the following reasons.

1. AMP is produced faster during exercise because some of the ADP produced during contraction is directly combined to generate ATP and AMP:

$$ADP + ADP \rightarrow ATP + AMP$$

   This is called the *myokinase reaction.*
2. Calcium is released from the sarcoplasmic reticulum during contraction. This calcium can quickly affect phosphorylase.
3. Epinephrine is secreted at a faster rate as exercise becomes more strenuous.

Phosphofructokinase is activated by fructose-6-phosphate, ADP, AMP, and falling concentrations of creatine phosphate [22]. Accordingly, as more fructose-6-phosphate is produced by glycogen or glucose breakdown (Fig. 4.2, reaction C), phosphofructokinase is "turned on" to accelerate the remainder of the glycolytic process. Similarly, as muscle contraction produces more ADP, AMP, and a fall in creatine phosphate, these factors all serve to further activate the glycolytic process.

There are very limited stores of glucose and glycogen in the body compared to fat. Therefore, *exercise can be prolonged if carbohydrate breakdown is automatically decreased when fat catabolism can provide the bulk of the ATP needed to continue exercise.* Inhibition of phosphorylase and phosphofructokinase activity can have this effect of "turning off" or at least slowing down glycolysis. High concentrations of ATP relative to ADP and AMP inhibit both phosphorylase and phosphofructokinase. High ATP:ADP ratios also inhibit *pyruvate dehydrogenase,* the enzyme which breaks down pyruvic acid to acetyl CoA in the step which precedes the Krebs cycle (Fig. 4.5) [2]. If pyruvic acid is thus prevented from entering the Krebs cycle, it will accumulate and block further glycolysis. Also, as fatty acid breakdown is accelerated, citric acid accumulates in the Krebs cycle (Fig. 4.5), and *citric acid is a potent inhibitor of phosphofructokinase* [22]. Finally, fatty acids inhibit phosphofructokinase and *hexokinase,* the enzyme that changes blood glucose to glucose-6-phosphate in the muscle (Fig. 4.2, reaction B).

Regulation of Fatty Acid Breakdown for Energy

The fatty acids that are utilized for energy by contracting muscles come primarily from 1) triglyceride stored in the muscles, 2) triglyceride stored in fatty deposits throughout the body, or 3) triglyceride or fatty acids circulating in the bloodstream. The enzymes (*lipases*) responsible for splitting fatty acids from triglyceride molecules are activated by hormonal changes that accompany prolonged, vigorous exercise. Once these lipases are activated by the hormones so that large amounts of fatty acids are released into the blood and muscles, the fatty acids are rapidly burned for energy. Since more fatty acids are obtained from the blood than from intramuscular triglyceride stores during exercise, *the most important limiting factor in fat metabolism seems to be the concentration of free fatty acids in the blood, which in turn is determined by the activities of the lipases in the fat tissues, in the walls of the blood vessels, and in muscle tissue* (Figs. 4.10, 4.11) [7, 18].

The most important hormonal changes for activating the lipases and stimulating the release of fatty acids appear to be *increased* levels of *epinephrine, norepinephrine* and *glucagon* plus a *decreased* level of *insulin* [7, 25, 30, 31]. (Epinephrine and norepi-

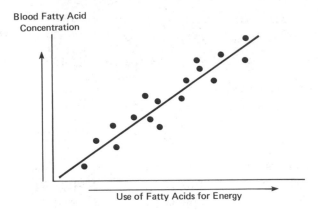

Blood Fatty Acid Concentration

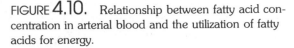

Use of Fatty Acids for Energy

FIGURE 4.10. Relationship between fatty acid concentration in arterial blood and the utilization of fatty acids for energy.

nephrine are released by the adrenal glands and by endings of the sympathetic nervous system; insulin and glucagon are released by the pancreas.) Both the depression of insulin and the increase in glucagon during exercise may be at least partly determined by the greater epinephrine and norepinephrine release; therefore, it seems that the increased activity of the sympathetic nervous system is of primary importance in stimulating the release of fatty acids from triglyceride stores in *adipose tissue* (fat tissue) and muscle. During exercise lasting an hour or more as much as a five-fold increase in fatty acid concentration in the blood has been observed [31].

There is evidence that the amount of energy derived from fatty acids during exercise can be increased by artificially elevating the concentration of fatty acids in the blood by treatment with caffeine and other drugs which result in the increased mobilization of fatty acids from fat stores [10]. This again emphasizes the importance of mobilizing fatty acids from fat tissue to promote a high concentration of fatty acids in the blood if fatty acids are to be utilized to a large degree during exercise.

Inhibition of Fatty Acid Mobilization. The mobilization or release of fatty acids into the blood from triglyceride stores is inhibited by elevated levels of lactic acid and insulin (Fig. 4.11) [17, 24, 31]. Therefore, it is not surprising that during extremely heavy exercise, when glycolysis is accelerated and lactic acid production is increased, a relatively small proportion of energy is derived from fat metabolism. This inhibition of fat metabolism during intensive exercise has some value because it is during very heavy physical activity that the ability of the body to utilize oxygen is an important limiting factor to performance. As discussed earlier, with a given amount of oxygen more energy can be produced from carbohydrate than from fat; thus, the inhibition of fat metabolism by lactate build-up is an important control mechanism during performance of activities which lead to exhaustion within 30–40 minutes.

As indicated earlier, the normal circumstance during prolonged exercise is for insulin levels to decline. Because insulin decreases lipase activity, the reduction in insulin during exercise leads to increased hormone-sensitive lipase activity and increased release of fatty acids from fat stores. However, if a high carbohydrate meal or drink is

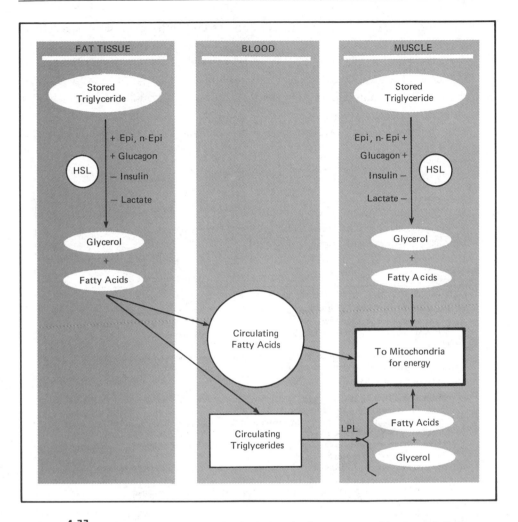

FIGURE 4.11. Regulation of fatty acid metabolism by hormones and lactic acid. Epi = epinephrine; n-Epi = nor-epinephrine; HSL = hormone-sensitive lipase; LPL = lipoprotein lipase; + = activate; − = inhibit.

consumed about an hour before exercise, blood glucose levels rise within 15–30 minutes, and more insulin is secreted from the pancreas in response to the elevated blood glucose. The increased insulin levels then cause more glucose to be used for energy by increasing the uptake of glucose from the blood into the muscles. The increased insulin also has the effect of reducing fat breakdown by inhibiting fatty acid release from triglyceride stores. Thus, glucose consumption an hour before exercise may actually decrease endurance.

Utilization of Circulating Triglycerides during Exercise. Once fatty acids have been released into the bloodstream from adipose tissue stores, 1) they may be transported to the muscles or other tissues as so-called "free fatty acids," which are only loosely bound to plasma proteins, or 2) the fatty acids may be reattached to glycerol in the blood to make circulating triglycerides, which are often bound to proteins in the blood and circulate as "lipoproteins." (Fats are known as lipids; lipid plus protein equals lipoprotein.) Before the muscles can utilize the fat from circulating triglycerides, the fatty acids must be split from the lipoprotein molecules by "lipoprotein lipase," an enzyme located in blood vessel walls in muscles and other tissues. The fatty acids can then diffuse into the mitochondria for energy production through the beta oxidation cycle. Lipoprotein lipase is also activated by epinephrine, norepinephrine, and glucagon. It is inhibited by high levels of insulin and activated during prolonged exercise [25, 30, 31].

ACTIVATION OF CREATINE PHOSPHATE BREAKDOWN

1. Decreased ratio of ATP:ADP because of splitting of ATP during muscle contraction.

INHIBITION OF CREATINE PHOSPHATE BREAKDOWN

1. Increased ratio of ATP:ADP because of increased aerobic production of ATP or decreased contraction.

ACTIVATION OF GLYCOLYSIS

1. Decreased ratio of ATP: (ADP + AMP) because of splitting of ATP during muscle contraction.
2. Decreased concentration of creatine phosphate as it is split for energy during contraction.
3. Increased calcium concentration as it is released from the sarcoplasmic reticulum during contraction.
4. Increased epinephrine and norepinephrine from the sympathetic nervous system and adrenal glands.
5. Increased fructose-6-phosphate concentration in the early steps of glycolysis.

INHIBITION OF GLYCOLYSIS

1. Increased ratio of ATP: (ADP + AMP) with greater production of ATP by aerobic mechanisms or because of decreased muscle contraction.
2. Increased citric acid concentration with greater aerobic production of ATP via the Krebs cycle, especially by fatty acid catabolism.
3. Increased concentration of creatine phosphate as it is replenished by aerobic ATP production or as exercise intensity is lessened.
4. Decreased calcium concentration as it is withdrawn to the sarcoplasmic reticulum during relaxation.
5. Decreased epinephrine and norepinephrine as the exercise intensity is lessened.
6. Reduced pH resulting from lactic acid accumulation.
7. Increased fatty acid concentration, which inhibits glucose entry into the muscle.

ACTIVATION OF FATTY ACID CATABOLISM

1. Increased concentration of fatty acids in the blood because of greater mobilization of fatty acids from adipose tissue resulting from:
   a. elevated epinephrine, norepinephrine, and glucagon as exercise is prolonged.
   b. decreased insulin as exercise continues
   c. increased caffeine and other fat-mobilizing drugs
2. Increased concentration of fatty acids in the blood because of high fat diet.

INHIBITION OF FATTY ACID CATABOLISM

1. Increased lactic acid production during heavy exercise.
2. Increased insulin concentration after carbohydrate consumption.

ACTIVATION OF OXIDATIVE PHOSPHORYLATION

1. Increased mitochondrial ADP concentration after ATP is split for muscle contraction.
2. Increased oxygen delivery to the mitochondria by the bloodstream.

INHIBITION OF OXIDATIVE PHOSPHORYLATION

1. Decreased mitochondrial ADP concentration as ADP accepts phosphate to form ATP in the electron transport system or as muscle contraction is lessened.
2. Decreased oxygen delivery to the mitochondria, especially as blood vessels are constricted during strenuous static contractions.

FIGURE 4.12. Metabolite regulation of ATP replenishment pathways during exercise.

Regulation of Oxidative Phosphorylation

Regardless of the exact mixture of fats, carbohydrates, and proteins that is to be metabolized aerobically, the electron transport system must have oxygen delivered to it by the blood to accept electrons and must have enough adenosine diphosphate (ADP) available to accept phosphate (P) and form ATP by oxidative phosphorylation. Thus, *as exercise begins, the activator of oxidative phosphorylation is the increased concentration of ADP produced by muscle contraction. As exercise reaches near maximal intensity, the availability of oxygen becomes a limiting factor in the aerobic production of ATP.*

The factors involved in the regulation of energy metabolism during exercise are summarized in Fig. 4.12.

Training-Induced Adaptations in Energy Metabolism

Physiological adaptations to training programs generally allow an exerciser to participate in subsequent exercise sessions with less severe homeostatic disturbances than in the untrained condition. Accordingly, with respect to energy metabolism, it would be logical to predict that training would result in greater energy stores and in greater activities of the enzymes involved in glycolysis, the Krebs cycle, the beta oxidation cycle, the electron transport system, and so on, so that more ATP could be replenished more quickly for a longer time. On the whole, studies have shown that these and other adaptations in energy metabolism do occur as the result of training, and exercise does become less difficult after training than before.

Adaptations Related to Creatine Phosphate

There are several published reports that suggest that training brings about modest increases in the intramuscular stores of creatine phosphate and in the activity of creatine kinase, the enzyme which splits creatine phosphate to produce ATP [2, 16, 31]. It is uncertain whether such changes, when they occur, are substantial enough to affect performance, but they are at least in the right direction to indicate that training produces a greater capacity for, and a potentially greater rate of, ATP replenishment from creatine phosphate. Also, after a training program an individual can perform the same submaximal work with less lactic acid production and a lesser fall in pH [2, 20]. To the extent that a low pH slows the resynthesis of creatine phosphate during brief recovery periods [39], this adaptation should be useful in enabling that individual to perform repeated sprints or other types of heavy, short-duration work with less fatigue.

Adaptations Related to Glycolysis

Glycogen stores are greater in trained persons [31]. This adaptation is important for endurance in activities that lead to exhaustion after 40–240 minutes [22]. Most studies have not shown increased phosphofructokinase activity after training, but there are some reports of increased glycogen phosphorylase activity [8, 16]. Thus, it appears that any training-induced changes in the rate of glycogen or glucose breakdown to lactic acid are rather small.

It is known that less carbohydrate is broken down to lactic acid during submaximal exercise after training than before, probably because the mitochondria 1) have a greater capacity to use fats for energy and 2) can replenish ATP aerobically more quickly so that less anaerobic glycolysis is required and less lactic acid is produced at the beginning of exercise [8, 20, 31]. This decrease in lactic acid production is beneficial because it results in a lesser reduction in pH and, therefore, a lesser inhibition of myosin ATPase activity and of the enzymes of glycolysis and favors fat utilization. These changes should mean delayed fatigue and increased endurance after training.

Adaptations Related to Aerobic ATP Replenishment

After endurance training the body has a greater capacity to replenish ATP aerobically and can do so at a faster rate. Part of this adaptation is caused by cardiovascular changes that allow more oxygen to be delivered to the muscles, but changes in the tissues are also important. *One of the most important overall tissue adaptations to endurance training is the doubling of the ability of the muscle mitochondria to generate ATP* [8, 31]. There are more and/or larger mitochondria in trained muscles. There is greater activity of the mitochondrial enzymes of the Krebs cycle, the electron transport system, and the beta oxidation cycle for fatty acid catabolism. Even when oxygen delivery is unchanged with training, the improved mitochondrial function can probably help the trained muscles extract and use more of the available oxygen. Thus, both fat and carbohydrate can be aerobically catabolized more effectively by trained muscles. *The effect of these changes is less reliance on inefficient ATP replenishment by anaerobic glycolysis.*

Because more work can be performed aerobically, less lactic acid is produced by trained muscles, and there is less inhibition by lactate of the lipase enzymes which mobilize fatty acids from triglyceride stores in adipose tissue and muscle. Accordingly, *endurance-trained persons have a greater ability to mobilize fat from tissues* [8, 20, 31]. Trained muscle has a greater ability to extract fatty acids from circulating triglycerides [20] and to use intramuscular triglycerides for energy [30]. The overall effect of these adaptations in fat metabolism is that trained individuals rely more on fat for energy during exercise than do the untrained [2, 8, 20, 31]. There is a tremendous storage of fat in the body compared to carbohydrate, and energy stored as fat is much lighter than an equivalent amount of carbohydrate energy. Therefore, the trained "fat-burning" person is better adapted to perform prolonged exercise than an untrained person who must rely more on limited supplies of heavy carbohydrate.

REVIEW QUESTIONS

1. We know that the air breathed in has more oxygen in it than air breathed out. What becomes of the missing oxygen?
2. In the aerobic breakdown of a molecule of glucose-6-phosphate, a net of 38 ATPs can be produced. How many of these 38 are produced in glycolysis? How many in the Krebs cycle? How many in the electron transport system?

3. Contrast the use of fat, carbohydrate and protein as exercise fuels. Consider ATP generated per volume of oxygen used up, per carbon atom, and per weight of fuel.
4. Which amino acid would be most likely to be oxidized to carbon dioxide and water during exercise?
5. Exhaled air has more carbon dioxide in it than does inhaled air. Where does that carbon dioxide come from? In what metabolic pathways is it produced? In what parts of the cell?
6. When glucose is broken down aerobically, is the glucose changed into ATP? If not, what does become of it?
7. Define the following terms: aerobic, anaerobic, glycolysis, creatine kinase, coenzyme, oxidation, reduction, Cori cycle, electron transport system, mitochondria, triglyceride, lipase.
8. If you were a coach, how would you respond to one of your athletes who insisted she must have a high protein diet to provide energy for distance running?
9. Explain the glucose-alanine cycle in Fig. 4.9.
10. Why is it important that glycolysis is automatically slowed down during prolonged exercise when fatty acids are available for metabolism?
11. Explain the apparent logic behind the fact that decreased ATP:ADP ratios accelerate energy production whereas increased ATP:ADP ratios inhibit the same processes.
12. Explain how endurance training leads to more efficient ATP production during exercise.

REFERENCES

[1] Ahlborg, G., L. Hagenfeldt, and J. Wahren. Substrate utilization by the inactive leg during one-leg or arm exercise. *Journal of Applied Physiology,* 1975, **39:**718–723.
[2] Åstrand, P.–O., and K. Rodahl. *Textbook of Work Physiology.* New York: McGraw-Hill, 1977.
[3] Bates, P. C., T. DeCoster, G. K. Grimble, J. O. Holloszy, D. J. Millward, and M. J. Rennie. Exercise and muscle protein turnover in the rat. *Journal of Physiology* (London), 1980, **303:**41P.
[4] Berg, A., and J. Keul. Serum alanine during long-lasting physical exercise. *International Journal of Sports Medicine,* 1980, **1:**199–202.
[5] Brodan, V., E. Kuhn, J. Pechar, and D. Tomkova. Changes of free amino acids in plasma of healthy subjects induced by physical exercise. *European Journal of Applied Physiology,* 1976, **35:**69–77.
[6] Brooks, G. A., and G. A. Gaesser. End points of lactate and glucose metabolism after exhausting exercise. *Journal of Applied Physiology,* 1980, **49:**1057–1069.
[7] Bukowiecki, L., J. Lupien, N. Follea, A. Paradis, D. Richard, and J. LeBlanc. Mechanism of enhanced lipolysis in adipose tissue of exercise-trained rats. *American Journal of Physiology,* 1980, **239:**E422–E429.
[8] Bylund, A.–C., T. Bjuro, G. Cederblad, J. Holm, K. Lundholm, M. Sjostrom, K. A. Angquist, and T. Schersten. Physical training in man: skeletal muscle metabolism in relation to muscle morphology and running ability. *European Journal of Applied Physiology,* 1977, **36:**151–169.
[9] Conlee, R. K., G. P. Dalsky, and K. C. Robinson. Influence of free fatty acids on glycogen supercompensation in rat heart after exercise (abstract). *Medicine and Science in Sports and Exercise,* 1981, **13:**70.
[10] Costill, D. L., G. P. Dalsky, and W. J. Fink. Effects of caffeine ingestion on metabolism and exercise performance. *Medicine and Science in Sports and Exercise,* 1978, **10:**155–158.
[11] Dohm, G. L., G. R. Beecher, R. Q. Warren, and R. T. Williams. Influence of exercise on free amino acid concentrations in rat tissues. *Journal of Applied Physiology,* 1981, **50:**41–44.
[12] Dohm, G. L., F. R. Puente, C. P. Smith, and A. Edge. Changes in tissue protein levels as a result of endurance exercise. *Life Sciences,* 1978, **23:**845–850.
[13] Essen, B., and L. Kaijser. Regulation of glycolysis in intermittent exercise in man. *Journal of Physiology,* 1978, **281:**499–511.

[14] Gaesser, G. A., and G. A. Brooks. Glycogen repletion following continuous and intermittent exercise to exhaustion. *Journal of Applied Physiology,* 1980, **49:**722–728.

[15] Gollnick, P. D., and D. W. King. Energy release in the muscle cell. *Medicine and Science in Sports and Exercise,* 1969, **1:**23–31.

[16] Gollnick, P. D., and L. Hermansen. Biochemical adaptations to exercise: anaerobic metabolism. *Exercise and Sport Sciences Reviews,* 1973, **1:**1–43.

[17] Green, H. J., M. E. Houston, J. A. Thomson, J. R. Sutton, and P. D. Gollnick. Metabolic consequences of supramaximal arm work performed during prolonged submaximal leg work. *Journal of Applied Physiology,* 1979, **46:**249–255.

[18] Hagenfeldt, L. Metabolism of free fatty acids and ketone bodies during exercise in normal and diabetic man. *Diabetes,* 1979, **28**(Supplement 1):66–70.

[19] Harris, R. C., R. H. T. Edwards, E. Hultman, L.–O. Nordesjo, B. Nylind, and K. Sahlin. The time course of phosphorylcreatine resynthesis during recovery of the quadriceps muscle in man. *Pflügers Archiv,* 1976, **367:**137–142.

[20] Henriksson, J. Training induced adaptation of skeletal muscle and metabolism during submaximal exercise. *Journal of Physiology* (London), 1977, **270:**661–675.

[21] Hermansen, L., and I. Stensvold. Production and removal of lactate during exercise in man. *Acta Physiologica Scandinavica,* 1972, **86:**191–201.

[22] Hochachka, P. W., and K. B. Storey. Metabolic consequences of diving in animals and man. *Science,* 1975, **187:**613–621.

[23] Hultman, E. Glycogen loading and endurance capacity. In G. A. Stull, ed., *Encyclopedia of Physical Education, Fitness, and Sports.* Salt Lake City, Utah: Brighton Publishing Co., 1980, 274–291.

[24] Jones, N. L., G. J. F. Heigenhauser, A. Kuksis, C. G. Matsos, J. R. Sutton, and C. J. Toews. Fat metabolism in heavy exercise. *Clinical Science,* 1980, **59:**469–478.

[25] Karlsson, J. Localized muscular fatigue: role of muscle metabolism and substrate depletion. *Exercise and Sport Sciences Reviews,* 1979, **7:**1–42.

[26] Kochan, R. G., D. R. Lamb, S. A. Lutz, C. V. Perrill, E. M. Reimann, and K. K. Schlender. Glycogen synthase activation in human skeletal muscle: effects of diet and exercise. *American Journal of Physiology,* 1979, **236:**E660–E666.

[27] Lemon, P. W. R., and J. P. Mullin. Effect of initial muscle glycogen levels on protein catabolism during exercise. *Journal of Applied Physiology,* 1980, **48:**624–629.

[28] Lemon, P. W. R., and F. J. Nagle. Effects of exercise on protein and amino acid metabolism. *Medicine and Science in Sports and Exercise,* 1981, **13:**141–149.

[29] Lithell, H., K. Hellsing, G. Lundqvist, and P. Malmberg. Lipoprotein-lipase activity of human skeletal muscle and adipose tissue after intensive physical exercise. *Acta Physiologica Scandinavica,* 1979, **105:**312–315.

[30] Lithell, H., J. Orlander, R. Schele, B. Sjodin, and J. Karlsson. Changes in lipoprotein-lipase activity and lipid stores in human skeletal muscle with prolonged heavy exercise. *Acta Physiologica Scandinavica,* 1979, **107:**257–261.

[31] McCafferty, W. B., and S. M. Horvath. Specificity of exercise and specificity of training: a subcellular review. *Research Quarterly for Exercise and Sport,* 1977, **48:**358–371.

[32] McGilvery, R. W. The use of fuels for muscular work. In H. Howald and J. R. Poortmans, eds., *Metabolic Adaptation to Prolonged Physical Exercise.* Basel: Birkhauser Verlag, 1975, pp. 12–30.

[33] Newsholme, E. A. The regulation of glycolysis in muscle during sprinting and marathon running (abstract). *International Journal of Sports Medicine,* 1980, **1:**212.

[34] Newsholme, E. A., and B. Crabtree. General principles of hormonal regulation of metabolism. In J. Poortmans and G. Niset, eds., *Biochemistry of Exercise IV.* Baltimore: University Park Press, 1981, pp. 46–58.

[35] Oscai, L. B. Effect of acute exercise on tissue free fatty acids in untrained rats. *Canadian Journal of Physiology and Pharmacology,* 1979, **57:**485–489.

[36] Refsum, H. E., L. R. Gjessing, and S. B. Stromme. Changes in plasma amino acid distribution and urine amino acids excretion during prolonged heavy exercise. *Scandinavian Journal of Clinical and Laboratory Investigation,* 1979, **39:**407–413.

[37] Richter, E. A., H. Galbo, and N. J. Christensen. Control of exercise-induced muscular glycogenolysis by adrenal medullary hormones in rats. *Journal of Applied Physiology,* 1981, **50:**21–26.

[38] Sahlin, K. Intracellular pH and energy metabolism in skeletal muscle of man. *Acta Physiologica Scandinavica,* 1978, **455**(Supplementum).

[39] Sahlin, K., R. C. Harris, and E. Hultman. Resynthesis of creatine phosphate in human muscle after exercise in relation to intramuscular pH and availability of oxygen. *Scandinavian Journal of Clinical and Laboratory Investigation,* 1979, **39:**551–558.

[40] Toews, C. J., G. R. Ward, R. Leveille, J. R. Sutton, and N. L. Jones. Regulation of glycogenolysis and pyruvate oxidation in human skeletal muscle in vivo. *Diabetes,* 1979, **28**(Supplement 1):100–102.

[41] White, T. P., and G. A. Brooks. (U-^{14}C)glucose, -alanine, and -leucine oxidation in rats at rest and two intensities of running. *American Journal of Physiology,* 1981, **240:**E155–E165.

[42] Winder, W. W., J. Boullier, and R. D. Fell. Liver glycogenolysis during exercise without a significant increase in cAMP. *American Journal of Physiology,* 1979, **237:**R147–R152.

CHAPTER

5

Nutrition and Athletic Performance

THERE is historical evidence that as early as 532 B.C., some people recognized that optimal nutrition was important for athletic performance. For example, legend has it that Milo of Croton, who won wrestling events at seven straight Olympic Games, consumed each day 20 pounds of bread, 20 pounds of meat and 18 pints of wine. It is also said that he once carried a four-year-old bull on his shoulders around the stadium at Olympia, killed it with a single blow of his fist, and then ate the whole animal in a single day.

Thus, for many centuries athletes, coaches, trainers, and physicians have passed down many radical ideas on nutrition for optimal athletic performance. Some of the more absurd ideas that held sway for many years include the practice of letting blood with leeches to remove "toxic substances" from the blood and totally restricting water intake to provide "training discipline." Most of the "wonder" diets for athletes that have been proposed over the years have no sound basis and only serve to make the athlete's life more grueling than it need be.

In one study of 171 college athletes, 98 per cent stated that performance is improved after consumption of a high protein diet [36]. In a survey 75 coaches and trainers expressed beliefs that "vitamin E is needed for building muscle," that "vitamin C is required for energy," and that "no harm can come from ingesting too many vitamins" [7]. It is unfortunate that so many coaches and athletes are poorly informed on the nutrition of athletes, because they are susceptible to misleading advertising claims and overblown testimonials from equally uninformed coaches and athletes about the value of some special dietary manipulation. Also, poor understanding of nutritional principles can lead to less than optimal performance and, more importantly, can cause illness and even death. It is the purpose of this section of the text, therefore, to provide background regarding athletic nutrition so that the reader will be better equipped to evaluate new ideas in this field and perhaps save needless expense on useless dietary supplements.

Part 1: Energy Requirements and Fuels for Exercise

Unfortunately, relatively few well-designed studies of the nutritional requirements of athletes in a variety of events have been published. Most of our knowledge of athletic nutrition, therefore, is extrapolated from the known requirements for nonathletic persons. Also, there is a difference between knowing the "minimal" requirements for athletics and knowing the "optimal" requirements. It is extremely difficult to discover optimal requirements because there are many individual differences in responses to dietary changes. Thus, what appears to be a beneficial diet for one person may not be of any aid to another.

Total Energy Requirements

The most popular common expression of energy units for human energy intake and expenditure is the large calorie (kilocalorie or Calorie), which is the energy required to raise the temperature of one kilogram of water by one degree Celsius under certain environmental conditions. In scientific work, however, there is a movement to use another unit of energy, the joule (J). One kilocalorie (kcal) is equivalent to 4,186 J, so the kilojoule (kJ), which is equivalent to 1,000 J, and the megajoule (MJ), which is equivalent to a million joules, are units which appear commonly in the literature. In this text the kilocalorie will be emphasized to facilitate understanding. An approximate conversion of kilocalories to kilojoules can be obtained by multiplying kilocalories by 4.2.

The recommended daily intake of calories, vitamins, and minerals for average persons in North America is shown in Table 5.1. As can be observed, the energy intake ranges from less than 1,300 kcal (5.4 MJ) for very small children to 2,900 kcal (12.2 MJ) for young adult males. On a body weight basis these figures translate into more than 100 kcal (419 kJ) per kilogram for infants to about 35 kcal (147 kJ) per kilogram for persons beyond age 50. For 19–22 year olds these figures are 2,900 kcal (41 kcal/kg) for males and 2,100 kcal (36 kcal/kg) for females. It is important to remember that one's daily physical activity can have an important bearing on whether these average figures lead to excessive weight gain or weight loss. In other words, a college-aged male who is extremely sedentary will probably gain weight quickly on 2,900 kcal/day, whereas a female distance runner will need substantially more than 2,100 kcal to avoid excessive weight loss.

Table 5.2 illustrates the energy expenditure for a variety of daily activities, including a number of athletic events. Note that the greatest total daily energy expenditures will occur in activities such as running and cross-country skiing, for which the body weight must be supported by vigorous muscular work for a prolonged duration. Depending upon the type and duration of athletic practice and competition engaged in, an athlete may need 400–2,000 kcal in addition to the average energy needs shown in Table

TABLE 5.]
Recommended Daily Dietary Allowances (RDA)[1]
(Designed for the maintenance of good nutrition of practically all healthy persons in the United States.)

Sex-age Category	Age (Years)		Weight		Height		Food Energy	Protein	Minerals			Vita-min A	Thia-min	Ribo-flavin	Nia-cin	Ascorbic Acid
	From	To	Kilo-grams	Pounds	Centi-meters	Inches	Calories	Grams	Cal-cium (Milli-grams)	Phos-phorus (Milli-grams)	Iron (Milli-grams)	Inter-national units	Milli-grams	Milli-grams	Milli-grams	Milli-grams
Infants	0	0.5	6	13	60	24	kg × 115 / lb × 52.3	kg × 2.2 / lb × 1.0	360	240	10	1,400	0.3	0.4	6	35
	0.5	1	9	20	71	28	kg × 105 / lb × 47.7	kg × 2.0 / lb × 0.9	540	360	15	2,000	.5	.6	8	35
Children	1	3	13	29	90	35	1,300	23	800	800	15	2,000	.7	.8	9	45
	4	6	20	44	112	44	1,700	30	800	800	10	2,500	.9	1.0	11	45
	7	10	28	62	132	52	2,400	34	800	800	10	3,300	1.2	1.4	16	45
Males	11	14	45	99	157	62	2,700	45	1,200	1,200	18	5,000	1.4	1.6	18	50
	15	18	66	145	176	69	2,800	56	1,200	1,200	18	5,000	1.4	1.7	18	60
	19	22	70	154	177	70	2,900	56	800	800	10	5,000	1.5	1.7	19	60
	23	50	70	154	178	70	2,700	56	800	800	10	5,000	1.4	1.6	18	60
	51+		70	154	178	70	2,400	56	800	800	10	5,000	1.2	1.4	16	60
Females	11	14	46	101	157	62	2,200	46	1,200	1,200	18	4,000	1.1	1.3	15	50
	15	18	55	120	163	64	2,100	46	1,200	1,200	18	4,000	1.1	1.3	14	60
	19	22	55	120	163	64	2,100	44	800	800	18	4,000	1.1	1.3	14	60
	23	50	55	120	163	64	2,000	44	800	800	18	4,000	1.0	1.2	13	60
	51+		55	120	163	64	1,800	44	800	800	10	4,000	1.0	1.2	13	60
Pregnant							+300	+30	+400	+400	18+	+1,000	+.4	+.3	+2	+20
Lactating							+500	+20	+400	+400	18	+2,000	+.5	+.5	+5	+40

[1] From *Recommended Dietary Allowances*, 9th ed., 1980, Washington, D.C.: National Academy of Sciences—National Research Council.

TABLE 5.2
Approximate Energy Costs of Various Activities[1]

Activity	kcal/hr/kg Body Weight	kcal/hr/lb Body Weight
Lying in bed	1.03	0.47
Sitting, reading	1.06	0.48
Standing	1.23	0.56
House painting	3.08	1.40
Hoeing, raking	4.09	1.86
Chopping wood	6.60	3.00
Sport Activities		
Archery	3.90	1.77
Badminton	4.0–9.0+	1.8–4.1+
Basketball, game	7.0–12.0+	3.2–5.5+
Basketball, practice	3.0–9.0	1.4–4.1
Billiards, horseshoes	2.50	1.14
Bowling	3.00	1.36
Boxing, in ring	13.3	6.04
Canoeing, rowing, kayaking	3.0–8.0	1.4–3.6
Cycling for pleasure	4.36	1.98
Cycling at 10 mph	7.0	3.18
Dancing (aerobic)	6.0–9.0	2.7–4.1
Dancing (social, square, tap)	3.7–7.4	1.7–3.4
Field hockey	8.00	3.60
Fishing from bank	3.70	1.68
Fishing while wading	5.50	2.50
Football, touch	6.0–10.0	2.7–4.5
Golf, with power cart	2.0–3.0	0.9–1.4
Golf, walking	5.10	2.32
Handball, squash	8.0–12.0+	3.6–5.5+
Racquetball, paddleball	8.0–12.0+	3.6–5.5+
Rope jumping, 60–80/min	9.0	4.09
Rope jumping, 120–140/min	11.5	5.23
Running, 12 min per mile	8.70	3.95
Running, 11 min per mile	9.40	4.27
Running, 10 min per mile	10.20	4.64
Running, 9 min per mile	11.20	5.09
Running, 8 min per mile	12.50	5.68
Running, 7 min per mile	14.10	6.41
Running, 6 min per mile	16.30	7.41
Skating, ice and roller	5.0–8.0	2.3–3.6
Skiing, snow, downhill	5.0–8.0	2.3–3.6
Skiing, cross-country	6.0–12.0+	2.7–5.5+
Skiing, water	5.0–7.0	2.3–3.2
Soccer	5.0–12.0+	2.3–5.5+
Swim breaststroke, 18 m/min	4.22	1.92
Swim breaststroke, 37 m/min	8.44	3.84
Swim freestyle, 41 m/min	7.66	3.48
Table tennis	3.0–5.0	1.4–2.3
Tennis	4.0–9.0+	1.8–4.1+
Volleyball	3.0–6.0	1.4–2.7
Walk on level, 2.3 mph (26.0 min per mile)	3.08	1.40
Walk on level, 4.5 mph (13.5 min per mile)	5.81	2.64

[1] Modified from P. B. Johnson et al., *Sport, Exercise, and You* (New York: Holt, Rinehart and Winston, 1975), and from American College of Sports Medicine, *Guidelines for Graded Exercise Testing and Exercise Prescription,* 2nd ed. (Philadelphia: Lea & Febiger, 1980).

5.1. For instance, a 70 kg (154 lb) runner who runs 10 miles (16 kilometers) daily at a pace of 7 minutes per mile requires about 1,152 kcal (4.8 MJ) of daily energy in addition to the 2,900 kcal shown in the table (14.1 kcal/hr/kg) $\times$ 70 kg $\times$ 7/6 hr = 1,152). To estimate one's daily energy needs it is possible to 1) determine the duration of various physical activities pursued during the day, 2) calculate the energy cost of those activities, and 3) add this cost to the normal caloric requirements shown in Table 5.1. In many cases, however, it is simpler to monitor body weight and adjust caloric intake accordingly. Thus, if one appears to be gaining unnecessary body weight on a particular diet, simply reduce the caloric intake. If, on the other hand, one persists in losing weight, an upward adjustment in caloric intake is indicated.

Fuels for Exercise

There are, of course, a number of foods that can be eaten to obtain a given caloric intake. The choice of foods in a diet for an athlete should essentially follow the principles of good nutrition that apply to everyone. We should consume: 1) at least 60 per cent of our daily calories as carbohydrate (80 per cent or more of these carbohydrate calories should come from starches and other complex carbohydrates and less than 20 per cent from refined sugar), 2) no more than 30 per cent of our daily calories as fat (divided equally between saturated and polyunsaturated fats), and 3) about 10 per cent of our calories as protein. Our foods should be well distributed among cereals and breads, fruits and vegetables, dairy and meat products to insure adequate intake of the essential vitamins and minerals.

However, there are some modifications in the normal diet that can be made for a given athlete for special circumstances. Some of these modifications are based upon the fuel used for a particular type of performance. With the frequent use of the muscle biopsy technique since 1966 we have come to a fairly good understanding of which fuels are used for various physical activities. The fuels used depend in large measure on the maximal rate of energy production from those fuels and the amount of the fuel stored in the tissues. Estimates of these factors are shown in Table 5.3. It should be understood that the figures presented in Table 5.3 are averages and are based on assumptions of body weight and muscle mass that may not be accurate for a given individual. However, as approximations the figures can help explain why certain fuels are required for certain activities.

Several principles can be learned from Table 5.3. First, ATP and creatine phosphate are necessary fuels for physical activities that require energy expenditures in excess of the 23 kcal/hr/kg body weight provided by anaerobic glycolysis. Maximal sprinting in track or swimming, hurling a discus, jumping, and other short-duration, intense activities demand a rate of energy release far greater than can be met by anaerobic glycolysis or by the aerobic breakdown of either carbohydrates or fats. However, it is also clear that there is so little of these fuels stored in the muscles that these intense activities cannot be maintained for more than a few seconds before the fuels are depleted.

Fatty acids, on the other hand, can provide energy at only a relatively slow rate, but because there is so much fat available, this slow rate of energy production can be

TABLE 5.3

Approximate Maximal Rates of Energy Production From Different Fuels During Exercise[1]

Fuel	Max. Rate of High Energy Phosphate Production (mmoles/sec/kg muscle)	Quantity of Fuel Available in Muscle (mmoles/kg)	Max. Rate[2] of Energy Production (kcal/hr/kg body wt)	Time for Depletion at Max. Rate[3]
ATP	6.0	6	92.6	1 sec
Creatine Phosphate	6.0	18	92.6	3 sec
Anaerobic Glycolysis	1.5	76.5	23.1	1.3 min
Aerobic				
Glycogen & Glucose	0.5	3000	7.7	100 min
Fatty Acid	0.24	Unlimited	3.7	Unlimited

[1] Modified from data in reference 43.
[2] Assuming 30 kg muscle in 70 kg person and 10 kcal/mole ATP.
[3] Assuming that no other fuels are utilized.

maintained for many hours. Compare the rates of energy production from various fuels in Table 5.3 with the energy costs of different activities in Table 5.2. Note, for example, that any of the activities requiring less than 3.7 kcal/hr/kg body weight can theoretically be supported entirely by fat breakdown alone. But carbohydrate must participate in the energy production for any activity which needs more than 3.7 kcal/hr/kg; even though there is plenty of fat available, its rate of energy release is simply too slow to meet the total demands of activities such as aerobic dancing, football, running and skiing. This explains why the depletion of glycogen in muscles results in exhaustion at high workloads; as soon as the glycogen runs out, the muscle is left with an inadequate rate of energy release when it must rely only on fat.

There is a common misconception that often accompanies the study of exercise fuels. Sometimes one is left with the impression that only one fuel is used at a time and that, for example, carbohydrate must be used up before fat is metabolized. There is probably no situation in which at least a small amount of ATP is not being replenished by the breakdown of each of the fuels we have discussed. When we say that muscle glycogen is the fuel for a given event, we mean that it is the principal fuel; but there is also at least a minor contribution to the energy supply for that event by creatine phosphate, blood glucose, and fatty acids. With this in mind, let us examine the fuels used for different types of exercise. The following discussion has been organized according to the duration of an activity leading to exhaustion; that is, when we speak of "heavy exercise for less than 40 minutes," we mean exercise leading to exhaustion in less than 40 minutes.

Maximal, Short Bursts of Exercise. When subjects pedal a bicycle ergometer at heavy loads that can be maintained for no more than one or two minutes, nearly 40 per cent of muscle creatine phosphate stores are depleted after only 10 seconds, 50 per cent after 20 seconds, and 70 per cent after 60 seconds [62]. Only very small changes in glycogen occur with such heavy work, and no significant change would be expected in blood glucose or fat stores. Nearly all the glycogen that is used is broken down anaerobically to lactic acid. A similar pattern of results would occur with any competitive athletic event lasting less than one or two minutes. The major fuels for such activities are stored ATP, creatine phosphate, and muscle glycogen [62]. Thus, throwing, jumping, and vaulting in track and field; sprints up to 800 meters; swims to 200 meters; cycling sprints; many individual gymnastics routines including apparatus routines; and weightlifting competitions would be examples of maximal, short bursts of activity that are performed chiefly at the expense of ATP, creatine phosphate, and glycogen stores. Examples from physical labor in industry would include heavy lifting activities and activities where a vigorous contraction is sustained with little movement of the joints, such as holding a heavy portable drill for brief periods (static contraction).

If maximal bursts of activity are repeated many times with brief intervening rest pauses, there will be some replenishment of ATP and creatine phosphate during the rest periods, and there will eventually be a fall in muscle glycogen levels [26, 30, 62]. There may also be some use of fatty acids from the blood. It seems that ATP and creatine phosphate are replenished during the rest pauses at the expense of glycogen, and to some extent of blood glucose and fatty acids also. Only creatine phosphate, however, is likely to be severely depleted during such repeated work-rest intervals [33, 62]. Examples of work-rest intervals that would be accompanied by progressive decreases in ATP, creatine phosphate and muscle glycogen would include football competition, repeated sprints, fast-break basketball play and repeated swim sprints.

With 15-second periods of heavy cycling exercise followed by 15-second recovery periods, the creatine phosphate stores can be replenished to about 80 per cent of the starting value within the 15-second recovery periods, but if a similar intensity of exercise is done continuously for 4–6 minutes, it takes about 3 minutes to replenish 50 per cent of the creatine phosphate stores, presumably because more lactic acid is produced during the longer exercise session [26]. This lactic acid inhibits glycolysis and fatty acid metabolism so less ATP can be produced to regenerate creatine phosphate.

If forearm muscles are forced to exercise maximally for 60 seconds, creatine phosphate is totally depleted; it takes 4 minutes before half of the creatine phosphate is replenished and 7 minutes before 95 per cent is replenished [24]. Repeated maximal contractions of the thigh muscles for 1–6 minutes leads to almost total depletion of creatine phosphate; replenishment is 50 per cent complete in about 30 seconds and 95 per cent complete in about 7 minutes [40]. This suggests that recovery intervals designed to lead to nearly total replenishment of creatine phosphate should be about 7 minutes long.

There is a rather straightforward relationship between the rate of creatine phosphate utilization and the degree of severity of the exercise. The heavier and more vigorous the activity in relation to one's capacity, the more creatine phosphate will be called upon to provide the energy necessary to replenish ATP supplies in the muscle. Creatine phosphate is always used to some degree at the beginning of any exercise, whether the work load is heavy or light for an individual; but as the loads become lighter and blood supply to the slow twitch fibers increases, less creatine phosphate and more glycogen, blood glucose, and fatty acids are utilized for energy as the slow twitch fibers take over more of the work load [62]. Thus, *the relative intensity of the exercise, which, in turn, determines how long one can persist at an activity, is an extremely important factor in the allocation of fuel.*

Heavy Exercise for Less Than 40 Minutes.   When a person exercises as hard as possible for more than two minutes but less than approximately 40 minutes, both creatine phosphate and a substantial amount of muscle glycogen are broken down for energy. The glycogen is catabolized both anaerobically and aerobically. There is still no danger of running out of glycogen in this type of activity, for example, in a 1,500–10,000 meter run or 400–2,000 meter swim, and fat would contribute probably less than 10-20 per cent of the energy cost of the exercise [62].

One rather conclusive bit of evidence that glycogen is an important fuel in this type of heavy exercise for a brief to moderate period is that subjects who have a genetic absence of glycogen phosphorylase, one of the enzymes necessary for glycogen breakdown, are unable to perform this type of exercise.

Heavy Exercise for 40–150 Minutes.   Although the anaerobic breakdown of glycogen and creatine phosphate is important at the beginning of longer heavy exercise periods, a much greater total energy contribution is made by the aerobic breakdown of glycogen, glucose, and fatty acids under these conditions. About one fourth of the energy supply for exercise that results in exhaustion within 150 minutes may be derived from the oxidation of fatty acids, whereas most of the remaining energy is supplied by the aerobic breakdown of muscle glycogen and blood glucose [62]. In long periods of heavy exercise, for example in soccer competition, distance running, skiing, swimming, and cycling, muscle glycogen may be almost totally used up and is thought to be the major limiting factor in these activities [60, 62]. Exercise physiologists have found a high correlation between the amount of glycogen stored in muscles prior to heavy exercise and one's ability to sustain the exercise for long periods. If muscle glycogen levels are increased by eating a diet high in carbohydrates, endurance also increases; with a fat diet, which lowers glycogen levels, endurance decreases [8, 62].

Muscle glycogen stores are not replenished within 24 hours following heavy endurance exercise [17]. Consequently, during successive days of heavy training, glycogen stores prior to each training session can become progressively lower (Fig. 5.1). This is a situation in which a high carbohydrate diet can help to maintain the glycogen stores to a greater degree than a normal mixed diet [19].

Another fuel for prolonged endurance exercise is lactic acid [3]. Both exercising and resting muscles and other tissues can utilize some of the lactic acid produced by the working muscles by oxidizing the lactic acid to pyruvic acid and further catabolizing the pyruvic acid to carbon dioxide and water in the mitochondria. The exact contribution of lactic acid to energy metabolism is not well established but is apparently quite substantial.

The principal reason that more fat is not used for heavy exercise is that the lactic acid produced from anaerobic glycolysis inhibits fatty acid release from triglyceride stores in fat tissue [37]. This results in a concentration of fatty acids in the blood that is inadequate to stimulate high rates of fatty acid breakdown in the muscle.

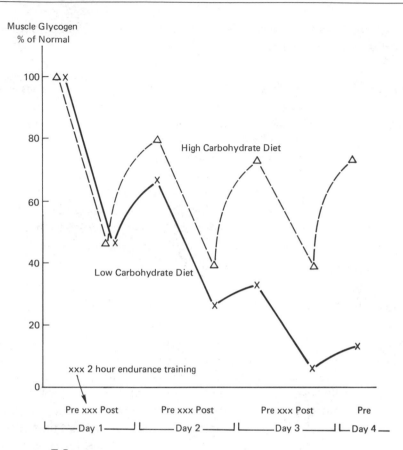

FIGURE 5.1. Progressive depletion of muscle glycogen stores over 3 days of heavy endurance training with either 40% or 70% carbohydrate diet [19].

Heavy Exercise for More Than 150 Minutes. As hard work is prolonged, for example in an endurance cycling race, an increasingly large contribution of the fuel for exercise comes from fat stored in the muscle cells and from fatty acids in the blood [1, 5, 32, 38, 39, 47, 54, 62]. This increased use of fat is a gradual process but may account for 20 per cent of the energy demands after one hour of exhaustive work and more than 50 per cent after four hours. Blood glucose is also increasingly used as exercise progresses beyond 120 minutes and is thought by many physiologists to be a possible limiting factor in such prolonged, heavy work. The answer to whether blood glucose or muscle glycogen is a more likely limiting factor in prolonged exercise may depend on the capacity of a given athlete to work for a long time at a high intensity. Accordingly, a well-trained athlete who can continue near maximum work for two or three hours probably depletes his muscle glycogen stores; this then limits his ability to continue working at the same high rate. However, a poorly trained subject may have to work at a lesser intensity in order to sustain the work for a long time, and he may suffer from a reduction in blood glucose, not muscle glycogen.

Light Exercise. With light exercise there is a much greater activation of slow twitch fibers relative to fast twitch fibers, so that nearly all the energy for ATP replenishment is released by the *aerobic* breakdown of fat, glycogen and glucose. As the duration of light exercise increases, so too does the role played by the combustion of free fatty acids for energy. For example, one who walks continuously or works at a machine in industry for eight hours may supply up to 90 per cent of his energy needs by the aerobic breakdown of fatty acids at the end of the eight hours, but only 25–50 per cent during the first four hours of the work [1, 39, 62]. This suggests an increasing recruitment of slow twitch fibers and an increasing activation of the enzymes involved in fatty acid breakdown as exercise is prolonged.

There is usually no severe depletion of fat, carbohydrate, or protein with prolonged light exercise, but occasionally blood glucose values begin to decline (Table 5.4) [47, 62]. That muscle glycogen breakdown is not essential to prolonged light exercise is demonstrated by the normal endurance to such exercise of subjects who are unable to break down glycogen.

Adaptations in Fuels Used For Exercise. It has repeatedly been shown that after serious endurance training the exerciser uses more fat and less anaerobic glycolysis for the same submaximal task when compared to the pretraining state [4, 13, 42, 62]. This increased use of aerobic metabolism to produce energy is probably related to the increased capacity of the mitochondria of the trained muscle to break down both carbohydrates and fats to carbon dioxide and water [4, 13, 62]. As more ATP is produced aerobically, there is less need for anaerobic glycolysis; this means that there will be less lactic acid produced to inhibit free fatty acid release from fat stores. Consequently, more fatty acids will be delivered to the muscles to be utilized for energy. There is also evidence that the hormone-sensitive lipase enzymes of the fat cells become more sensitive to epinephrine and norepinephrine after training [12]. Thus, a smaller increase in the hormone levels during exercise is required to stimulate fatty acid release.

The increased fatty acid use during exercise is not important for short-duration activities where the rate of energy use is so great that a large fraction of the energy must be supplied by anaerobic glycolysis. The lactic acid produced in these brief periods (less than 20 minutes) effectively limits fatty acid use by inhibiting fatty acid mobilization from fat stores.

TABLE 5.4

Degree of Depletion of Fuel Reserves with Various Types of Exercise

Fuel	Maximal, Short Bursts, Static Contractions	Heavy Inter- mittent	Heavy, Less Than 40 Min	Heavy, 40–150 Min	Heavy, Over 150 Min	Light
Creatine Phosphate	Great	Very Great	Moderate	Moderate	Moderate	Negligible
Muscle Glycogen	Slight	Moderate	Moderate	Very Great	Very Great	Negligible
Blood Glucose & Liver Glycogen	Negligible	Slight	Slight	Moderate to Great	Great to Very Great	Slight
Fatty Acids From Blood & Intracellular Triglyceride Stores	Negligible	Slight	Negligible	Negligible	Slight	Slight

In prolonged exercise in the trained state, it would be expected that less glycogen would be used in the muscles and liver and that less of a reduction in blood glucose would occur. These effects are produced because of the increased use of fat for energy.

Part 2: Dietary Manipulations of Protein, Fat, and Carbohydrate

Protein and Exercise

One of the most discussed topics among athletes and coaches is the value of high protein diets in athletic nutrition. Many years ago it was thought by some authorities that muscle protein was broken down to provide the fuel for muscle contraction during exercise. But measurements of protein breakdown products in the urine later showed no increase in excreted urinary nitrogen and presumably established that there was no significant contribution of protein to energy release during exercise [15]. However, recent determinations have shown a markedly increased excretion of protein breakdown products in the sweat [52, 53, 55]. Also, studies have provided evidence of a breakdown of actin and myosin in exercised muscle [20], of increased excretion of protein breakdown products in the urine [67], of significant alterations in amino acid distribution in the blood [9, 67], and of amino acid oxidation to carbon dioxide and water [76]. The greatest changes in protein metabolism apparently occur with prolonged exercise, especially when the subjects are calorie deprived or carbohydrate deprived [52, 53]. Calculations of the possible contribution of protein to energy production during exercise in carbohydrate-depleted subjects indicate that about 10 per cent of the energy could have been supplied by protein breakdown [52].

Although it appears likely that protein makes a small contribution to energy release during prolonged exercise if subjects are starved or fed a low carbohydrate diet, it should also be remembered that evidence of protein breakdown does not necessarily prove that the protein is used directly for energy. Much of the protein breakdown which occurs probably serves to provide amino groups for changing pyruvic acid to the amino acid alanine in the glucose-alanine cycle described in Chapter 4. In summary, it appears that protein does not supply more than 1–2 per cent of the energy needs during exercise *unless* the exerciser is calorie starved or carbohydrate depleted [64]. Protein contribution to energy during short-duration exercise can be ignored. If a coach provides pregame steaks for athletes because he hopes to improve their fuel reserves, that coach is wasting money. The provision of such meals for psychological benefits, however, may be another matter. If an athlete believes that eating meat makes him more "virile," the pregame steak may be worth the money.

Dietary Protein and Muscular Development. Another reason why supplemental protein is often considered important for athletes is that the extra protein is supposed to be valuable for building up growing muscles and bones. It is true, of course, that a daily intake of proteins is necessary for building enzymes and tissue cells, including muscle and bone. Proteins are constantly undergoing a dynamic process of being built up and broken down. When proteins are degraded, some of the nitrogen constituents of the protein are lost in the urine. These nitrogenous products can be replaced only by the dietary intake of more protein—the body cannot manufacture nitrogen. Consequently, in order to maintain body protein stores, protein must be included in the diet. The important questions are how much protein is needed daily, and to what extent can additional protein be used by the body for building extra muscle tissue?

As can be seen in Table 5.5, protein nitrogen is lost by a number of different routes from the body, and the chief increase in nitrogen loss during prolonged vigorous exercise occurs in the sweat. Most studies show no significant increase in protein nitrogen loss in the urine as a result of exercise. About 24.5 grams of total protein is lost in a day for a 70 kg (154 lb) person who does not exercise to any significant extent; this value is increased by only 7.4 grams if the person exercises heavily. If an athlete is attempting to gain muscle mass with weight training, another 7 grams of protein per day might be necessary in the diet [22]; this gives a total of about 39 grams of protein that should be ingested each day. If we add 30 per cent of this amount to account for variability among subjects, we arrive at a figure of 51 grams of protein daily for a person weighing 70 kilograms. This figure of about 0.8 grams of protein for each kilogram of body weight should meet any conceivable protein requirement during body building. Fifty-one grams of protein is equivalent to about 204 kcal of energy. If an athlete consumes 3,000 kcal daily, only 6.8 per cent of the diet would need to be protein. It is quite difficult in North America to consume less than this amount of protein; in fact, most athletes maintain diets containing more than 10 per cent protein [22].

The standard rule of thumb for protein intake is that every day a person should consume about one gram of protein for every kilogram of body weight. According to this rule, since a kilogram is about 2.2 pounds, a person who weighs 154 pounds or 70 kilograms should need about 70 grams of protein intake each day to meet the demands of tissue maintenance and growth. Although experts disagree on precisely how much protein is needed daily, very few would maintain that more than one gram of protein per kilogram of body weight is needed every day. As a matter of fact, the one gram per kilogram rule has a built-in safety factor, and most authorities believe that

TABLE 5.5

Daily Nitrogen and Protein Losses at Rest and with 2 Hours of Heavy Exercise (22)

	N₂ Lost/kg Body Weight (mg)		Protein Breakdown (g/kg)		Total Protein Breakdown (70 kg person)	
	Rest	**Exercise**	**Rest**	**Exercise**	**Rest**	**Exercise**
Urine	37	37	.231	.231	16.17	16.17
Feces	12	12	.075	.075	5.25	5.25
Skin Tissue	5	5	.031	.031	2.17	2.17
Sweat	0.1	17	.001	.107	0.07	7.49
Miscellaneous	2	2	.012	.012	0.84	0.84
TOTALS	56	73	.350	.456	24.50	31.92

about half that amount would satisfy the needs of most adults [22]. There is little evidence to support the view that a greater protein intake can increase the production of muscle in weightlifters, field events specialists, and wrestlers; most of the extra protein is simply broken down, its nitrogen is lost in the urine and sweat, and the remainder of the protein molecule is converted to fat [22, 57]. On the other hand, as long as other nutrients are not slighted, there is no known risk (other than financial) in consuming extra protein. If one is determined to have protein supplements, he should simply eat more ordinary fish, meats, and vegetables and avoid paying premium prices for such concoctions as "proteins from the sea," "high protein candy bars," "dessicated liver protein flakes," and the like. A list of protein food sources is shown in Table 5.6.

One further concept about dietary protein that should be discussed is the need for "high quality" proteins in the diet. The diet must supply all of the amino acids that are components of a protein that is to be synthesized; if one or more of these "essential" amino acids are missing from the diet, none of the protein can be synthesized. In general, protein from animal sources tends to be "high quality" protein and contains all the essential amino acids, whereas protein derived from vegetables and other foods may be deficient in one or more of these amino acids. The effects on growth of feeding various protein sources to laboratory animals are shown in Fig. 5.2. From the graph it

TABLE 5.6
Protein Food Sources

Food Serving (weight in grams)	Water (%)	kcal	Fat (%)	Carbo-hydrate (%)	Protein (%)	Approximate Amount Needed to Supply 70 Grams Protein
Chicken, fried drumstick without bone (38 grams)	55	90	10.5	Trace	31.5	6 drumsticks
Lamb chop, broiled without bone (112 grams)	47	400	29.5	0	22.3	3 chops
Ham (85 grams)	54	245	22.4	0	21.2	4 servings
Pork chop, without bone (66 grams)	42	260	31.8	0	24.2	4½ chops
Bologna, 4 slices (114 grams)	56	345	27.3	1	11.8	20 slices
Frankfurter, one (51 grams)	58	155	27.5	2	12.0	11½ franks
Tuna fish, canned (85 grams)	61	170	8.2	0	28.2	3 servings (1½ cans)
Hamburger (85 grams)	54	245	20.0	Trace	24.7	3½ servings
Steak, broiled (85 grams)	44	330	31.8	0	23.5	3½ servings
Navy beans, 1 cup (261 grams)	68	310	0.4	23	6.1	4 cups
Green beans, 1 cup (239 grams)	94	45	Trace	3.0	0.8	36½ cups
Green peas, 1 cup (160 grams)	82	115	0.6	11.9	5.6	8 cups
Peanut butter, 1 tbsp. (16 grams)	2	95	50.0	18.8	25.0	½ lb.
White bread, slice (23 grams)	36	60	4.4	50.0	8.7	35 slices
Cheese pizza, 14 inch (600 grams)	45	1480	8.0	36.0	9.3	1¼ pizzas
Skim milk, 1 cup (246 grams)	90	90	Trace	5.3	3.7	7½ cups
Yogurt, 1 cup (246 grams)	89	120	1.6	5.3	3.3	9 cups
Egg, boiled (50 grams)	74	80	12.0	2.0	13.0	11 eggs
Potato chips, 10 (20 grams)	2	115	40.0	50.0	5.0	700 chips
Watermelon, 2 lbs. (925 grams)	93	115	0.1	2.9	0.2	66 pounds
Beer, 12-oz. can (360 grams)	92	150	0.0	3.8	0.4	49 cans
Cola drink, 8 oz. (240 grams)	90	95	0.0	10.0	0.0	9,684 bottles

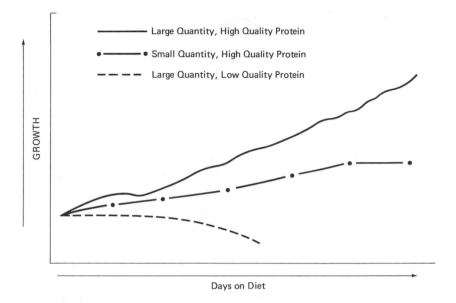

FIGURE 5.2. Effects of three different protein diets on growth of laboratory animals.

is apparent that feeding a great deal of low quality protein can retard growth much more severely than the feeding of insufficient amounts of high quality protein. It should be noted here that a diet lacking in animal protein does not necessarily have inadequate proteins; mixtures of proteins from different vegetables and grains can supply all the essential amino acids [50]. That is why vegetarians do not always show signs of protein malnutrition.

Dietary Fat and Exercise

Some fat in foods makes food more palatable to most persons, so that a total lack of fat in the diet can lead to inadequate intake of other nutrients because of poor appetite. A total lack of fat would also make adequate calorie intake very difficult for an endurance athlete because of the extremely large quantities of carbohydrates and protein that would be required to supply up to four or five thousand kcal per day. Otherwise, the principal requirement for fat arises from the need for a fatty acid called linoleic acid, which, if absent from the diet, results in symptoms such as weight loss and dry, scaly skin. Only a prolonged nonfat diet would be apt to result in linoleic acid deficiency because there is such a large store of linoleic acid in the fat depots of the body. In summary, as long as an athlete maintains his optimal weight and does not live on a fat free diet, there is little danger of his experiencing fat deficiency. On the contrary, a common problem is an excessive intake of fat that leads to obesity and may eventually lead to an increased risk of developing cardiovascular disease.

Triglyceride Feeding. Since increased fatty acid levels in the blood usually spare muscle glycogen and are associated with increased endurance time in prolonged exercise, attempts have been made to increase fatty acids by feeding triglycerides before exercise [45]. The triglyceride feedings did not increase fatty acid levels in the blood and resulted in less contribution of fat metabolism to the energy requirements of the exercise than in the control condition. Unfortunately, the triglycerides were mixed with carbohydrate cereal to make them palatable; this makes interpretation of the data difficult.

Caffeine Ingestion.   One method of increasing fatty acids in the blood is to ingest caffeine [18, 27]. Caffeine, usually about 350 milligrams, is ingested about one hour before exercise which lasts 40 minutes or longer. This amount of caffeine is equivalent to that in 2½ to 3 cups of percolator or dripolator coffee, 5 cups of freeze-dried coffee, 11 cups of tea or 5–10 12-ounce cans of caffeinated soft drinks. Subjects usually perform longer with the caffeine supplement. Also, muscle glycogen is spared, and more fats are used for energy. The exact mechanism for the usual beneficial effect of caffeine is not clear [27]. The effect can be attributed not only to elevated fatty acids, but also to a psychological lift from the caffeine and to a direct influence on the muscle to inhibit glycolysis and increase fat metabolism [27]. It should be pointed out that some persons are very sensitive to caffeine and can become disoriented and nauseated. Also, caffeine supplements do not enhance performance for everyone. Therefore, it is wise to experiment with lower doses of caffeine to determine if one is hypersensitive to its various effects.

Carbohydrates and Exercise

For optimal growth there exists only a small requirement for carbohydrates since many of the body's carbohydrates can be synthesized from protein sources. It would be very difficult for a sedentary person to devise a carbohydrate deficient diet because there is a small amount of carbohydrate in nearly all but pure fat foods (for example, corn oil or soybean oil). However, it takes time for the body to adapt to a low carbohydrate diet, and in that time period the dieter might experience unpleasant symptoms, including lack of energy. Also, anyone who performs heavy work or prolonged light work needs more than the minimal amounts of carbohydrate for optimal performance. This need for extra carbohydrates is shown in studies of the effects of diet on endurance; a high carbohydrate diet nearly always increases one's endurance to prolonged heavy exercise [62]. As a matter of fact, the consumption of a high carbohydrate diet, especially in the days just prior to competition in heavy exercise that lasts for about 40 minutes or longer, is one of the few dietary manipulations for athletes that has solid laboratory and field research evidence to support its effectiveness.

Liver Glycogen.   In studies of men subjected to liver biopsies after 24 hours on high fat and protein diets, liver glycogen was nearly 90 per cent depleted, but after two days on a carbohydrate rich diet, liver glycogen stores were about 100 per cent greater than normal, resting values (Fig. 5.3) [59, 62]. Since prolonged, heavy exercise such as a marathon race can result in a severe depletion of liver glycogen and blood glucose stores, a sound practice would be to eat a fat and protein diet for several days, and then to consume a diet rich in carbohydrates for three or four days prior to competition.

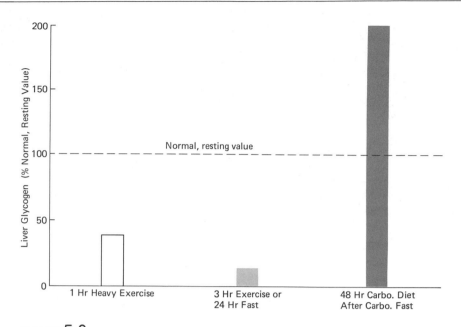

FIGURE 5.3. Effects of alterations in diet and exercise on liver glycogen. Data from reference 62.

Filling of Muscle Glycogen Stores — Diet and Exercise. One's ability to persevere at heavy exercise for about 40 to 150 minutes seems to be limited chiefly by the amount of glycogen stored in the working muscles prior to exercise [8, 19, 43, 44, 46, 62]. Therefore, for this type of work, it is important to know how best to increase muscle glycogen stores during the training period. Two factors seem to be important in this regard: diet and exercise. Research based on biopsy samples of human thigh muscles suggests that maximal filling of muscle glycogen stores occurs only after the muscles have been previously depleted of their glycogen by means of exercise coupled with a low carbohydrate diet [43, 44, 62]. With a low carbohydrate diet alone for two days, it is possible to reduce glycogen levels of resting muscle by about 30 per cent, and if this reduction is followed by three or four days of a high carbohydrate diet, the resting glycogen levels will be increased 10–50 per cent over normal values. However, when a low carbohydrate diet is accompanied by exhaustive exercise for approximately 90 minutes, glycogen is almost totally depleted from the muscles. With a subsequent high carbohydrate diet for three or four days, the glycogen then overshoots normal resting levels by up to 200 per cent (Fig. 5.5) [43, 44, 62].

Thus, to maximally fill muscle glycogen stores, it is sometimes suggested that an athlete consume a low carbohydrate diet (just enough carbohydrate to make the food palatable) for 2–3 days about 6–7 days prior to competition. Then, about 3–4 days before competition, the athlete should work to exhaustion to totally deplete glycogen stores. This should be followed by 3–4 days of light workouts and a diet rich in carbohydrates [8]. This procedure for filling the muscle glycogen stores is often called "glycogen loading," "glycogen packing," or "glycogen supercompensation."

Glycogen loading seems to be useful for many endurance athletes, but some individuals do not appear to benefit by the procedure [16, 43]. Storage of glycogen is accompanied by water retention as the water is bound to the glycogen molecules.

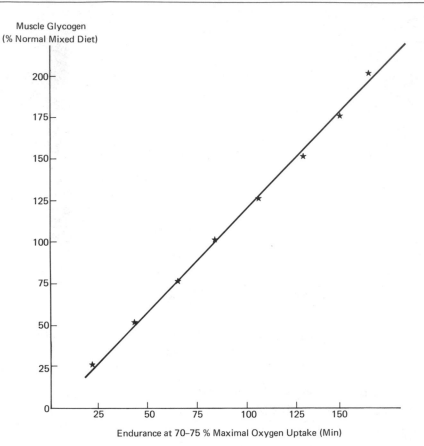

FIGURE 5.4. Relationship between endurance for heavy exercise and glycogen stores in muscle prior to exercise.

Typically, this results in a weight gain of 1–2 kilograms, with some persons gaining more and some less. If a great deal of water is retained in the muscles, a feeling of stiffness can sometimes result. On the other hand, the water released when the glycogen is broken down during prolonged exercise can be used to help maintain blood volume when body fluids are lost by sweating.

One of the practical difficulties in glycogen loading is eating the huge quantities of pasta, fruit, bread and rice required to get 70–90 per cent of one's calories from carbohydrate. Athletes can quickly decide that any diet that makes them so uncomfortable cannot possibly be good for their performances. One way to overcome this difficulty is to consume high carbohydrate liquids throughout the day. Initial studies in the author's laboratory suggest that carbohydrates in liquid form may be more effective for glycogen loading than solid diets. Presumably, the greater effectiveness of a liquid diet is caused by its more complete digestion and uptake into the bloodstream to trigger insulin secretion from the pancreas. The insulin in turn stimulates the conversion of blood glucose into muscle glycogen.

There should be few health problems associated with a high carbohydrate diet as long as a few principles are followed. 1) Most of the carbohydrate consumed should

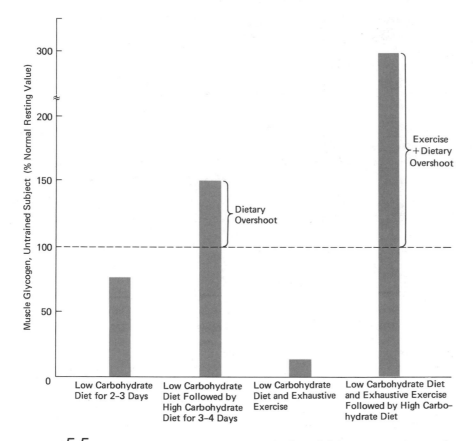

FIGURE 5.5. Glycogen overshoot in untrained subject following manipulation of diet and exercise.

consist of starch and other complex molecules rather than refined sugars. This will minimize excess tooth decay. 2) The diet should include at least 10 per cent high quality protein. 3) The diet should insure intake of the recommended daily allowances of vitamins and minerals. This latter principle can be achieved, if necessary, by ingestion of vitamin supplements.

The major problem in designing a palatable carbohydrate loading diet is to find tasty foods that include little or no fat. Experience has shown that an acceptable carbohydrate loading breakfast for most persons includes dry cereals such as corn flakes with skimmed milk and grape juice. Fruits and vegetables are essentially fat free, but must be eaten without butter, mayonnaise, and other fatty foods. Unfortunately, one must be quite creative to make pasta and rice tasty without using fat-rich tomato and cheese sauces. There are some low fat broths that can ameliorate this problem. Finally, it is good to remember that canned tuna and shellfish packed in water include little fat and provide a great deal of protein in a relatively few calories. One can design a personal carbohydrate loading diet by calculating fat, protein, and carbohydrate calories in acceptable foods from a list such as that shown in Appendix B or from the labels on foodstuffs in the supermarket. Remember that one should try to obtain 70–90 per cent of all calories from carbohydrate and 10–15 per cent from protein. Each gram of carbohydrate or protein is equivalent to 4 kilocalories, and each gram of fat is worth 9 kilocalories. By trial and error one can develop a satisfactory meal plan for carbohydrate loading.

Mechanism Underlying Glycogen Supercompensation. A number of investigations have been completed in attempts to explain how muscle glycogen is substantially increased by consumption of a high carbohydrate diet after first depleting glycogen stores with exercise and a low carbohydrate diet. It now appears that at least part of the explanation lies in changes in sensitivity of glycogen synthase, the enzyme chiefly responsible for converting glucose to glycogen [49]. After glycogen depletion the characteristics of the enzyme are altered so that synthesis of glycogen occurs more readily; however, the exact nature of the chemical changes that stimulate this enzyme adaptation is still not clear. At one time it was thought that lactic acid was the chief source of enhanced glycogen stores in muscles that had recovered from prior exercise. This now appears to be an inaccurate assumption because lactic acid disappears from the muscle (much of it being oxidized to carbon dioxide and water) within a few minutes after exercise; glycogen supercompensation in human skeletal muscle, on the other hand, is not achieved for 24–48 hours [31].

Carbohydrate Feedings Before and During Exercise. We have already established that glycogen stores are ordinarily adequate to provide energy for strenuous activities that last 40 minutes or so. Similarly, blood glucose levels typically remain quite stable for about two hours at work rates equivalent to heart rates of 100–150 beats per minute (about 30–65 per cent of maximal oxygen uptake) [2, 43]. Therefore, carbohydrate feedings should not be expected to be of any benefit for exercise that is completed within 40 minutes. (An exception of this rule is in the case of repeated daily bouts of heavy exercise. In this case, carbohydrate stores may not be fully replenished after depletion on the previous day [17, 19] Accordingly, the only logical reasons for consuming carbohydrate just before or during exercise are to spare muscle glycogen by metabolizing glucose absorbed from the intestine or to maintain stable blood glucose levels during prolonged activity.

Carbohydrate Feedings before Exercise. Because most persons prefer to exercise without much food or fluid in their stomachs, carbohydrate feedings before or during exercise are usually in the form of quickly absorbed glucose, sucrose (table sugar), or glucose polymers (chains of glucose molecules) dissolved in water. Much of the carbohydrate reaches the bloodstream as glucose within 15–45 minutes. As the blood glucose levels rise, the pancreas secretes more insulin, which is responsible for helping to transport the glucose into muscle, fat and other tissues. The insulin quickly lowers the glucose levels so that within an hour or two glucose has returned to normal or below normal values (Fig. 5.6) [19, 66]. If glycogen stores are filled by a prior high carbohydrate diet, most of the glucose will be converted to fat. Thus, there seems to be little merit in consuming carbohydrate drinks an hour or two before exercise unless it is suspected that liver or muscle glycogen stores are low. However, if glycogen stores are low because of prior competition (e.g., swim meets, track meets, twice daily football practice) or because of inadequate prior carbohydrate intake in the diet, the glu-

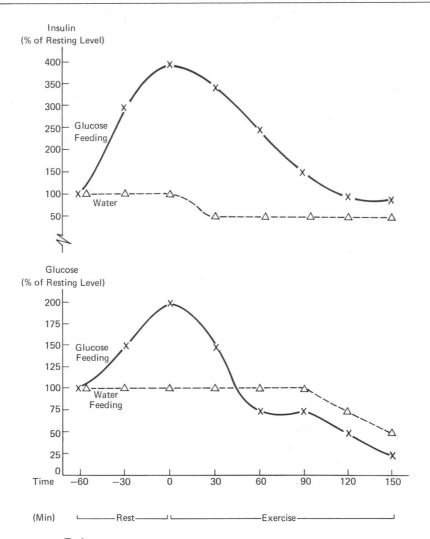

FIGURE 5.6. Effect of glucose feeding 1 hour before exercise on blood glucose and insulin levels.

cose absorbed from carbohydrate feedings before exercise may be stored as glycogen in muscle or liver and be useful for providing energy during activity.

There is another potential drawback to ingestion of carbohydrates an hour or two before exercise—the inhibiting effect of high insulin levels on fatty acid mobilization from fat stores [19, 66]. Recall that the greater the mobilization of fatty acids, the greater will be the contribution of fat to the energy demands of exercise; as more fat is used, glycogen stores can be conserved and exercise prolonged. Therefore, any major rise in insulin levels during exercise should be avoided. This means that consumption of large doses of carbohydrates before exercise should occur at least 2½–3 hours prior to activity to give insulin levels a chance to return to normal before exercise begins.

There may be one method of consuming carbohydrates before exercise that can avoid the problems related to insulin secretion. That method is to consume the carbohydrate just a few minutes before exercise. The reason that this procedure might be effective is that strenuous exercise generally produces a fall in insulin levels in the blood; thus, glucose entering the bloodstream after the start of exercise may have a minimal effect on insulin so that fatty acid mobilization is not significantly inhibited and blood glucose remains elevated. An experiment in the author's laboratory was recently conducted to test this procedure. Nine subjects exercised to voluntary exhaustion on bicycle ergometers at 65 per cent of their maximal oxygen uptakes (heart rates about 150 beats per minute) on three occasions separated by at least seven days. Five minutes before each of the three exercise sessions the subjects drank 750 milliliters (about 3 large glasses) of either a water placebo, a 4 per cent solution of glucose, or a commercially available 20 per cent solution of glucose polymers (breakdown products of corn starch). The taste, appearance, and viscosity of the drinks were indistinguishable to the subjects, and those who administered the tests did not know which drinks were being consumed on any day until the experiment was completed. Eight of the nine subjects rode longer after consuming carbohydrate drinks than after the water placebo. On average they rode for three hours after drinking the glucose polymer solution—about 29 per cent longer than after drinking water. The riders endured about 14 per cent longer after drinking the glucose solution than after drinking water. Therefore, it appears that consumption of carbohydrate drinks *immediately* before prolonged endurance exercise may be beneficial to performance.

If carbohydrate feedings are to be used, their composition should be adjusted to the environmental conditions present during exercise. In hot conditions it is more important to deliver fluid to the circulation than to deliver carbohydrate [19, 61]. Dilute solutions of carbohydrate usually empty faster from the stomach and are absorbed more rapidly into the blood than highly concentrated solutions [29]. In the heat, therefore, concentrations of sugar should be 5.0 per cent (5.0 grams per 100 milliliters) or less, and glucose polymer solutions should be 5 per cent or less to facilitate fluid replacement [19, 29]. The carbohydrate concentration in most commercial athletic drinks is 5 per cent or less [61]. In cool environments it may be more important to get glucose into the system rather than fluid. Since more carbohydrate is delivered to the blood with highly concentrated solutions, solutions as concentrated as 20 per cent can be tolerated [29]. Higher concentrations of carbohydrate in drinks tend to be syrupy and unpalatable.

The following statements summarize the state of our knowledge regarding carbohydrate feedings before exercise.

1. There is no adequate rationale to justify carbohydrate feedings before single exercise bouts lasting less than 40 minutes.
2. Carbohydrate feedings may benefit endurance exercise performance if consumed immediately before exercise.
3. Carbohydrate feedings consumed 30–120 minutes before exercise are ordinarily without benefit and may be detrimental to endurance performance.
4. If carbohydrates are to be consumed in an attempt to fill glycogen stores, they should be ingested more than 2½ hours prior to exercise to insure adequate time for digestion, for glycogen synthesis, and for the return of blood insulin to normal levels.
5. Liquids consumed before exercise in a hot environment should be isotonic or

hypotonic to body fluids. In cool environments, more concentrated carbohydrate solutions may be beneficial for endurance performance.

Carbohydrate Feedings during Prolonged Exercise. Blood glucose levels often begin to fall after about 2 hours of exercise at moderate intensities, that is, at heart rates of approximately 100–150 beats per minute [2, 43] (Fig. 5.7). The brain relies heavily upon blood glucose for its energy, and a fall in glucose to near hypoglycemic levels may account for some of the symptoms of disorientation that accompany prolonged exercise to exhaustion [10]. Blood glucose levels can be stabilized by ingestion of carbohydrate drinks at intervals during prolonged exercise [2] (Fig. 5.7). The extent to which the body utilizes the increased glucose supply provided by such carbohydrate feedings is controversial [73], but it appears that about 25 per cent of the energy expenditure during prolonged exercise may be attributed to oxidation of glucose derived from the carbohydrate ingested during exercise [64, 66].

Because of the insulin depressing effect of exercise, carbohydrate ingestion during

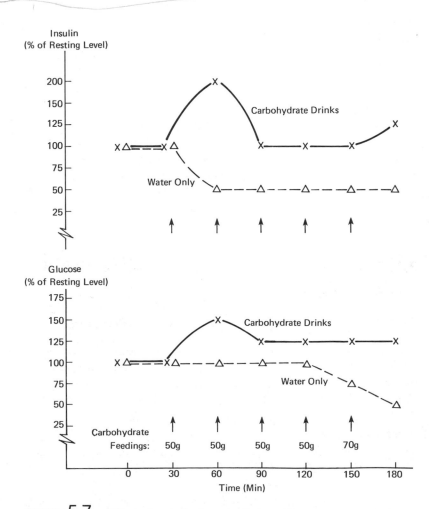

FIGURE 5.7. Effect of carbohydrate feedings at 30 minute intervals during prolonged exercise at heart rates of 150–160 beats per minute.

exercise causes a much smaller elevation of insulin than occurs at rest (Fig. 5.7), but this may still lead to a reduction of fatty acids in the blood and a diminished contribution of fat to the energy demands of activity (2). However, if the use of the increased blood glucose for energy can spare muscle glycogen somewhat [44], one might conclude that it is better to risk a reduction in fatty acid levels than a reduction in blood glucose, which is critical to the brain.

To summarize, for exercise which lasts at least 2 hours, it may be helpful to consume carbohydrate drinks, 8–12 ounces (236–235 ml) at a time, at 20–30 minute intervals during the activity. The first drink should probably be consumed about 30 minutes after exercise begins; the insulin level in the blood should have been reduced by this time so that fatty acids are mobilized for energy. The drink should be isotonic or hypotonic to body fluids to enhance the speed with which it passes from the stomach to the intestine, and it should include about 20 per cent carbohydrates (20g/100ml or 71g/12oz). Glucose polymers are probably better than simple sugars for this purpose because more carbohydrate can be included in an isotonic drink made with polymers (20 per cent vs. 6 per cent). If the environment is hot, one should probably concentrate on replacing fluid rather than adding carbohydrate. In this case, water or dilute sugar solutions (less than 5 per cent) should be used at intervals.

Glycerol Feeding.   Another approach to maintaining blood glucose levels and conserving muscle and liver glycogen during prolonged exercise is to consume glycerol [71]. Glycerol is converted to carbohydrate in the liver and is released as glucose more slowly than is the case with glucose feedings. In a study with rats, a glycerol feeding one hour before treadmill exercise helped to maintain levels of muscle glycogen, liver glycogen, and blood glucose; glycerol-fed animals ran 32 per cent longer than the control rats [71]. No studies of glycerol feedings in humans have been reported.

Part 3: Manipulation of Vitamins, Minerals, and Pre-event Meals

Vitamin Requirements for Athletes

One of the biggest gold mines for unscrupulous promoters is the sale of millions of dollars worth of unnecessary and sometimes harmful vitamin supplements. This is not to say that no one needs vitamin supplements, only that most people probably do not. The actions of many of the vitamins are required for ATP production, so many athletes and coaches are willing to try out massive doses of vitamins in the hope that more vitamins will help produce more energy.

How are vitamins used in energy metabolism? Recall in our discussions of fuel reserves how often we referred to NAD (nicotinamide adenine dinucleotide), FAD (flavin adenine dinucleotide) and coenzyme A. The basic ingredients of these compounds are the vitamins niacin (nicotinic acid), riboflavin (B_2), and pantothenic acid, respectively. Without these and other vitamins, ATP production would come to a halt. These vitamins and others serve as coenzymes that are required for the proper function of enzymes.

A list of suggested vitamin intakes is shown in Table 5.1. However, it should be noted that there are some difficulties in establishing daily vitamin and mineral allowances that are optimal for everyone. First, there is usually some variability in requirements depending on body weight, age, and metabolic peculiarities, and almost nothing is known about the effects of *severe* athletic training on vitamin levels in the body. Second, daily allowances are sometimes developed on the basis of whether or not some clinical symptom (hair loss, skin discoloration, and so on) appears with less than the recommended daily allowance; however, it may be that subclinical signs, such as changes in enzyme activities or hormone levels, occur in the absence of clinical evidence of vitamin deficiency. Consequently, recommended daily allowances may not be optimal allowances. Since the most important functions of many vitamins are not clearly understood, it is very difficult to determine optimal levels of intake for the entire population.

In spite of the difficulties present in accurately determining optimal vitamin doses, most nationally recognized figures in nutrition research maintain that nearly all Americans who consume a reasonably well-balanced diet obtain adequate vitamin intake in their foods and that athletes, too, get adequate vitamins because they eat more food and thus get more vitamins than the ordinary person. Let us take a slightly different approach and simply state that there is no unequivocal evidence that any vitamin supplement will enhance athletic performance, but some contradictory evidence concerning at least three vitamins—B_1, C, and E—does exist. Let us consider these three first.

Thiamine (B_1). From a biochemical standpoint, thiamine is involved in the reaction by which carbon dioxide is removed from pyruvic acid before pyruvic acid enters the Krebs cycle; therefore, thiamine is especially important for the breakdown of carbohydrates and fats for energy. Although the most thorough studies in the 1940's showed no effect of thiamine supplementation on work performance, the research literature contains a few others that suggest a beneficial effect of thiamine supplementation on endurance [78]. Consequently, there remains a possibility that B_1 supplements might aid performance under certain conditions, but since thiamine is rapidly excreted in the urine as soon as its concentration surpasses a threshold level in the body fluids, it seems unlikely that anyone on a well-balanced diet will benefit from thiamine supplements. There certainly is no clinical evidence, such as painful nerves, heart failure, or constipation, that physical training produces thiamine deficiency. There is also no evidence that thiamine supplements are harmful, since the excess simply enriches the urine.

Ascorbic Acid (C). Clinical signs of vitamin C deficiency do not occur until after about seven weeks on diets that contain no vitamin C. These signs include hemorrhage beneath the skin after inflation of a blood pressure cuff around the upper arm, slow healing of wounds, and bleeding of the gums. Some believe, though, that these clinical signs only show the late stages of deficiency, and that up to 5 or 10 grams of ascorbic acid per day is required for optimal functioning of the body.

Most authorities suggest that 30–60 milligrams of ascorbic acid per day are adequate. Unfortunately, the exact function of ascorbic acid is unknown, so that the argument about how much is needed each day is difficult to resolve.

Because it is suspected that ascorbic acid is involved in the production from the adrenal glands of hormones that are important for exercise, the use of ascorbic acid supplementation as an agent for improving work performance has been studied quite often. As with thiamine, however, the results of this research are contradictory with the majority of studies showing no evidence of a beneficial effect of ascorbic acid supplementation on performance [74]. One consistent result of vitamin C studies is that subjects who have been made deficient in vitamin C by ingestion of diets free of the vitamin for 30 days or more exhibit poorer performance accompanied by earlier fatigue [74]. But the diets for nearly all persons in developed countries contain 50 milligrams or more of vitamin C per day, far more than is required to prevent symptoms of deficiency. If an athlete regularly engages in prolonged strenuous activity, daily consumption of 2–4 milligrams of a vitamin C supplement per kilogram body weight (140–280 mg daily for a 70 kg person) should easily compensate for any conceivable extra requirement; massive doses of 10,000 milligrams and more per day are totally unsubstantiated by research. Although there is no proven harmful effect of consuming large quantities of vitamin C regularly, many individuals do experience nausea and diarrhea-like symptoms when this is done. There is also some evidence that the body acquires a tolerance for large doses of vitamin C, so that continued maintenance of high doses is needed to maintain body stores of the vitamin.

Alpha-tocopherol (E). Because a severe deficiency of vitamin E causes muscular weakness and a reduction of creatine in the muscles, some persons believe that vitamin E supplements should increase strength and creatine concentrations in the muscles, thereby benefiting muscular performance. Once again, however, most of the literature on the effects of vitamin E supplementation on exercise capacity does not point in this direction [25, 69]. The more authoritative studies have not provided any evidence that extra quantities of vitamin E can benefit strength or endurance. Therefore, an athlete should not be led to believe that vitamin E supplements supplied in wheat germ, for example, will improve performance.

Usually, but not always, any meaningful effect of a food supplement will be shown in nearly all the studies in which the effect has been tested. It is most likely that any beneficial effect of supplementary vitamins B_1, C, or E on athletic performance is a small effect that can easily be obscured by more important performance factors, such as training intensity and motivation.

Other Vitamins and Performance. There is no general support for the view that the supplementary intake of any vitamins can benefit athletic performance [77, 78]. Some vitamins, for example A and D, are stored to such a great extent that deficiency symptoms would not occur for months or years with a diet totally lacking in those vitamins. In fact, excessive supplements of A and D have been known to cause toxic side effects including nausea, headaches, diarrhea and even death.

Vitamin B_3 (niacin or nicotinic acid) is the major component of nicotinamide adenine dinucleotide (NAD), an important coenzyme for energy metabolism. The recommended daily allowance of this vitamin is 6.6 milligrams per 1,000 kilocalories of food intake; most of us ordinarily consume two or three times this much in normal diets. Studies have shown that ingestion of large amounts of nicotinic acid decreases the mobilization of fatty acids from fat stores so that muscle glycogen is depleted faster in prolonged exercise [78]. This can result in earlier fatigue. Accordingly, vitamin B_3 supplements are contraindicated for prolonged exercise.

Testimony from athletes indicates that many of them commonly inject huge doses of vitamin B_{12} (cyanocobalamin) in hopes of improving performance. One power lifter, when asked why he used the vitamin, said he did so "because everyone else did." When pressed for a physiological rationale for the injections, he said, "I don't know how it's supposed to work, but it sure makes my skin tingle." This case points out the blind faith that many athletes have in procedures that are recommended to them by friends and acquaintances. Actually, the principal symptom of deficiency of this vitamin is pernicious anemia. But less than 3 milligrams per day are required to prevent this rather rare type of anemia, and the typical diet includes two to five times this much [78]. There is no evidence that supplements of this vitamin increase endurance, and there is no reason to expect that B_{12} supplements would enhance strength or weight lifting performance.

The daily requirements of other vitamins (for example, folic acid, inositol, pantothenic acid, and biotin) appear to be so small that the occurrence of deficiencies during exercise or training is highly improbable. If a coach suspects that an athlete has a vitamin poor diet and has no success in improving that diet, a prudent approach would be to supply the athlete with multiple vitamin capsules on a one-per-day basis. This approach should minimize not only the expense but also the possible toxic side effects of large-dose, "fad" vitamin therapy that is unwarranted according to our present state of knowledge and is perhaps dangerous.

Mineral Requirements for Athletes

Another aspect of athletic nutrition that is sometimes exploited by commercial interests and may be relied upon by individual athletes and coaches to give a "performance edge" is the use of mineral supplements in the diet. The underlying reason why some people believe that extra minerals might benefit athletic performance is that many minerals such as magnesium, manganese, and calcium are undeniably important cofactors for the proper activity of the enzymes that are involved in energy metabolism, that is, in the production of ATP. Suggested daily mineral allowances are listed in Table 5.1.

Although there are no proven benefits of mineral supplementation for athletic performance, it is conceivable that individual athletes may have slight deficiencies in one or more minerals, depending on their training routines and diets. For individuals on diets that restrict the intake of dairy foods, for example, calcium intake may be inadequate since about 75 percent of dietary calcium usually comes from dairy products. Also, iron supplements may be beneficial for some young adult females whose dietary intake of iron is inadequate to replace the iron lost in the menstrual blood flow.

Iron Supplements. Iron intake is required to replace the daily iron loss in the feces, urine, and sweat. Iron is most important because it is used in the formation of hemoglobin in the red blood cells, myoglobin in the muscles, and some of the electron transport system components (cytochromes) in the mitochondria. The red blood cells transport oxygen to the tissues, myoglobin stores oxygen and facilitates the transfer of oxygen from the blood to the muscles, and the electron transport system, of course, is vital to the production of ATP in the mitochondria. Bone marrow and the liver store any excess iron that is absorbed from the intestine during digestion of iron-containing foods.

Prior to the beginning of a regular menstrual cycle, females have probably stored enough iron to last for about 8 years or until college age [41]. After that time, for many women the average daily intake of iron (10–12 mg) is inadequate to maintain normal body stores of iron. Although less than 2–4 per cent of college-age women are anemic (having inadequate hemoglobin formation for red blood cells), 20–33 per cent exhibit low levels of iron in the blood plasma, a condition that could eventually lead to iron-deficiency anemia and might cause reductions in myoglobin and cytochrome formation in the muscles [41]. Anemia is associated with reduced endurance performance, but diminished performance is not always seen when subjects are merely deficient in plasma iron. Iron supplementation in anemic subjects is likely to improve performance in endurance events, but most studies show no substantial effect of iron supplementation in those who have normal hemoglobin levels. If a blood testing program for anemia detection is not feasible, it appears that the rational approach is to suggest iron supplements (ferrous sulfate is quite readily absorbed) of about 15–20 mg per day for women athletes aged 19 and over who are training heavily, unless they are not menstruating regularly [41]. Women who are not menstruating regularly and males probably consume adequate iron in their normal diets to avoid substantial iron deficiencies. Excess iron, cobalt, or molybdenum supplementation can cause toxic side effects; a little may be required, but too much can be disastrous.

Deficiencies in other minerals are extremely rare in persons who consume normal diets, so it is highly improbable that mineral supplements will improve athletic performance. Extra salt and fluid intake can be important during prolonged work in the heat and will be discussed in the chapter on temperature regulation during exercise.

Pre-event Meals

Most athletes learn what they know about pre-event nutrition from their coaches, who learned it from their own coaches when they were in training. Sometimes the knowledge handed down from coach to athlete is either completely erroneous or unsubstantiated by any physiological facts. It is not uncommon, for example, to hear coaches condemn the eating of perfectly good, high carbohydrate foods such as spaghetti, macaroni and pastries, when eating high carbohydrate meals is nearly the only dietary manipulation that has been shown to be potentially effective in improving performance in high intensity, long duration events. The truth is that the main benefit of the pre-event meal is mostly a psychological one—if the athlete believes that a particular meal will benefit performance, there is a good chance it might. On the other hand, if the athlete thinks a pre-event meal will be harmful to performance, it makes little difference whether a well-balanced meal was eaten; athletic performance may be subpar.

Nearly every study of the effects of the composition of pre-event meals, the absence of a meal, or the timing of a meal before competition has failed to provide evidence of any significant beneficial or adverse effect on athletic performance. Therefore, in the absence of a proven effective routine, it is recommended that the athletic coach make the following suggestions to athletes regarding pre-event nutrition:

1. To avoid a feeling of fullness in the stomach, eat about 4 hours prior to competition. (Most food has left the stomach after 4½ hours and the small intestine after 9 hours. Total gastrointestinal transit time ranges from about 18–48 hours.)
2. Competitors in events lasting longer than about 30 minutes should eat a meal that has 80–90 per cent of its calories in the form of carbohydrates.
3. It is highly unlikely that competitors in events lasting less than 30 minutes will derive any physiological benefit from any particular composition of the pre-event meal. Thus, they should eat whatever they like as long as their experience with that food has produced no discomfort. Although most individuals would prefer not to have baked beans, cabbage and tamales before competition, if one's long experience with such foods has never produced discomfort, it is unlikely that performance will be adversely affected by such a meal.
4. Avoid eating such great quantities of food that discomfort results.
5. Sometimes, the unexpected emotional impact of forthcoming competition makes digestion uncomfortable. An athlete who feels a high level of anticipation is advised to eat only small portions of food in which he has great confidence.
6. Do not worry about the "digestibility" of foods, because little or none of the pre-event meal will be used for the immediate competition and because a substantial portion of any meal (with the possible exception of liquid diets) will still be in the gut at the time of competition, regardless of its digestibility.
7. Protein is not a significant energy source during exercise and is not recommended as a superior energy food.
8. Remember that superior performance depends on superior ability and superior training. A last minute meal or pill cannot counteract the effects of inadequate training.

REVIEW QUESTIONS

1. Describe the protein requirements of different types of athletes.
2. Explain why not all proteins are equally good from the standpoint of nutrition.
3. Review the role of carbohydrate diets in athletic performance.
4. Compare the vitamin and mineral requirements of athletes and nonathletes.
5. What pre-event nutrition plan would you recommend to various types of athletes?
6. Contrast the extra caloric requirement for distance runners with that for a sprinter.

7. What is the simplest way to determine if an athlete is obtaining the necessary caloric intake in the diet?
8. Compare the types of fuels used for the following activities: shotput, marathon run, softball game, soccer, pushups, 100 m. sprint in track or swimming.
9. Explain the fallacy underlying the notion that fuels are totally depleted in an exact sequence during exercise, e.g., creatine phosphate followed by glycogen followed by glucose followed by fatty acids.
10. What happens to lactic acid produced during exercise?
11. Why is a high carbohydrate diet especially important when an athlete works to near exhaustion for several days in a row?
12. Under what conditions does protein make a substantial contribution to energy metabolism during exercise?
13. What is the main training-induced adaptation in fuel utilization during exercise?
14. Some believe that three or four times the recommended daily allowance of protein should be consumed if one is training with weights. What evidence is there to support this proposition?
15. Why are supplements of vitamins A and D not recommended for athletes' diets?
16. What evidence is there that dietary iron supplements might be advisable for female athletes? For males?
17. What is the relationship between muscle glycogen stores and endurance in heavy, prolonged exercise?
18. Describe the protocol for "glycogen loading."
19. Using the table of nutritive values of foods (Appendix B), develop a carbohydrate loading diet for one day that you think you would find palatable. Make sure that 90 per cent of the calories are obtained from carbohydrate.
20. Summarize the evidence concerning the potential value of carbohydrate feedings prior to exercise.
21. It appears that carbohydrate feedings during exercise are more valuable than feedings before exercise. Explain why this is so.
22. What effect does caffeine have on endurance? How might this effect be brought about?
23. What principles should be followed concerning a pre-event meal for athletes?

REFERENCES

[1] Ahlborg, G., P. Felig, L. Hagenfeldt, R. Hendler, and J. Wahren. Substrate turnover during prolonged exercise in man. Splanchnic and leg metabolism of glucose, free fatty acids, and amino acids. *Journal of Clinical Investigation,* 1974, **53**:1080–1090.
[2] Ahlborg, G., and P. Felig. Influence of glucose ingestion on fuel-hormone response during prolonged exercise. *Journal of Applied Physiology,* 1976, **41**:683–688.
[3] Ahlborg, G., L. Hagenfeldt, and J. Wahren. Substrate utilization by the inactive leg during one-leg or arm exercise. *Journal of Applied Physiology,* 1975, **39**:718–723.
[4] Baldwin, K. M., G. H. Klinkerfuss, R. L. Terjung, P. A. Molé, and J. O. Holloszy. Respiratory capacity of white, red, and intermediate muscle: adaptative response to exercise. *American Journal of Physiology,* 1972, **222**:373–378.
[5] Baldwin, K. M., J. S. Reitman, R. L. Terjung, W. W. Winder, and J. O. Holloszy. Substrate depletion in different types of muscle and liver during prolonged running. *American Journal of Physiology,* 1973, **225**:1045–1050.
[6] Barac-Nieto, M., G. B. Spurr, H. W. Dahners, and M. G. Maksud. Aerobic work capacity and endurance during nutritional repletion of severely undernourished men. *American Journal of Clinical Nutrition,* 1980, **33**:2268–2275.
[7] Bentivegna, A., E. J. Kelley, and A. Kalenak. Diet, fitness, and athletic performance. *Physician and Sportsmedicine,* 1979, **7**:99–105.
[8] Bergstrom, J., and E. Hultman. Nutrition for maximal sports performance. *Journal of the American Medical Association,* 1972, **221**:999–1006.

[9] Brodan, V., E. Kuhn, J. Pechar, and D. Tomkova. Changes of free amino acids in plasma of healthy subjects induced by physical exercise. *European Journal of Applied Physiology*, 1976, **35**:69–77.

[10] Brooke, J. D. Carbohydrate nutrition and human performance. In J. Parizkova and V. A. Rogozkin, eds., *Nutrition, Physical Fitness, and Health*. Baltimore: University Park Press, 1978, pp. 42–52.

[11] Brooke, J. D., F. J. Davies, and L. F. Green. Nutrition during prolonged exercise in trained cyclists. *Proceedings of the Nutrition Society*, 1972, **31**:93A.

[12] Bukowiecki, L., J. Lupien, N. Follea, A. Paradis, D. Richard, and J. LeBlanc. Mechanism of enhanced lipolysis in adipose tissue of exercise-trained rats. *American Journal of Physiology*, 1980, **239**: E422–E429.

[13] Bylund, A.-C., T. Bjuro, G. Cederbald, J. Holm, K. Lundholm, M. Sjostrom, K. A. Angquist, and T. Schersten. Physical training in man: skeletal muscle metabolism in relation to muscle morphology and running ability. *European Journal of Applied Physiology*, 1977, **36**:151–169.

[14] Chiasson, J.-L., M. R. Dietz, H. Shikama, M. Wootten, and J. H. Exton. Insulin regulation of skeletal muscle glycogen metabolism. *American Journal of Physiology*, 1980, **239**: E69–E74.

[15] Consolazio, C. F., H. L. Johnson, R. A. Nelson, J. G. Dramise, and J. H. Skala. Protein metabolism during intensive physical training in the young adult. *American Journal of Clinical Nutrition*, 1975, **28**:29–35.

[16] Costill, D. L., P. Blom, and L. Hermansen. Influence of acute exercise and endurance training on muscle glycogen storage (abstract). *Medicine and Science in Exercise and Sports*, 1981, **13**:90.

[17] Costill, D. L., R. Bowers, G. Branam, and K. Sparks. Muscle glycogen utilization during prolonged exercise on successive days. *Journal of Applied Physiology*, 1971, **31**:834–838.

[18] Costill, D. L., G. P. Dalsky, and W. J. Fink. Effects of caffeine ingestion on metabolism and exercise performance. *Medicine and Science in Sports and Exercise*, 1978, **10**:155–158.

[19] Costill, D. L., and J. M. Miller. Nutrition for endurance sport: carbohydrate and fluid balance. *International Journal of Sports Medicine*, 1980, **1**:2–14.

[20] Dohm, G. L., F. R. Puente, C. P. Smith, and A. Edge. Changes in tissue protein levels as a result of endurance exercise. *Life Sciences*, 1978, **23**:845–850.

[21] Dressendorfer, R. H., and R. Sockolov. Hypozincemia in runners. *Physician and Sportsmedicine*, 1980, **8**: 97–100.

[22] Durnin, J. V. G. A. Protein requirements and physical activity. In J. Parizkova and V. A. Rogozkin, eds., *Nutrition, Physical Fitness, and Health*. Baltimore: University Park Press, 1978, pp. 53–60.

[23] Edgerton, V. R., B. Essen, B. Saltin, and D. R. Simpson. Glycogen depletion in specific types of human skeletal muscle fibers in intermittent and continuous exercise. In H. Howald and J. R. Poortmans, eds., *Metabolic Adaptation to Prolonged Physical Exercise*. Basel: Birkhauser Verlag, 1975, pp. 402–415.

[24] Eleff, S., D. Sokolow, A. Sapega, J. Torg, J. Leigh, and B. Chance. Non-invasive assessment of high energy phosphate metabolism in exercising muscle using nuclear magnetic resonance spectroscopy (abstract) *Medicine and Science in Sports and Exercise*, 1981, **13**:88.

[25] Entenman, C., J. A. Coughlin, and P. D. Ackerman. Substrate utilization and maximum swimming ability in rats and guinea pigs fed wheat germ oil. *Proceedings of the Society for Experimental Biology and Medicine*, 1972, **141**:43–46.

[26] Essen, B., and L. Kaijser. Regulation of glycolysis in intermittent exercise in man. *Journal of Physiology* (London), 1978, **281**:499–511.

[27] Essig, D., D. L. Costill, and P. J. Van Handel. Effects of caffeine ingestion on utilization of muscle glycogen and lipid during leg ergometer cycling. *International Journal of Sports Medicine*, 1980, **1**: 86–90.

[28] Felig, P., and J. Wahren. Fuel homeostasis in exercise. *New England Journal of Medicine,* 1975, **293**:1078–1084.

[29] Foster, C., D. L. Costill, and W. J. Fink. Gastric emptying characteristics of glucose and glucose polymer solutions. *Research Quarterly for Exercise and Sport,* 1980, **51**:299–305.

[30] Fox, E. L., S. Robinson, and D. L. Wiegman. Metabolic energy sources during continuous and interval running. *Journal of Applied Physiology,* 1969, **27**:174–178.

[31] Gaesser, G. A., and G. A. Brooks. Glycogen repletion following continuous and intermittent exercise to exhaustion. *Journal of Applied Physiology,* 1980, **49**:722–728.

[32] Gollnick, P. D., R. B. Armstrong, C. W. Saubert IV, W. L. Sembrowich, and R. E. Shepherd. Glycogen depletion patterns in human skeletal muscle fibers during prolonged work. *Pflügers Archiv,* 1973, **344**:1–12.

[33] Gollnick, P. D., R. B. Armstrong, W. L. Sembrowich, R. E. Shepherd, and B. Saltin. Glycogen depletion pattern in human skeletal muscle fibers after heavy exercise. *Journal of Applied Physiology,* 1973, **34**:615–618.

[34] Gollnick, P. D., K. Piehl, J. Karlsson, and B. Saltin. Glycogen depletion patterns in human skeletal muscle fibers after varying types and intensities of exercise. In H. Howald and J. R. Poortmans, eds., *Metabolic Adaptation to Prolonged Physical Exercise.* Basel: Birkhauser Verlag, 1975, pp. 416–421.

[35] Gollnick, P. D., K. Piehl, C. W. Saubert IV, R. B. Armstrong, and B. Saltin. Diet, exercise and glycogen changes in human muscle fibers. *Journal of Applied Physiology,* 1972, **33**:421–425.

[36] Grandjean, A. C., L. M. Hursh, W. C. Majure, and D. F. Hanley. Nutrition knowledge and practices of college athletes (abstract). *Medicine and Science in Sports and Exercise,* 1981, **13**:82.

[37] Green, H. J., M. E. Houston, J. A. Thomson, J. R. Sutton, and P. D. Gollnick. Metabolic consequences of supramaximal arm work performed during prolonged submaximal leg work. *Journal of Applied Physiology,* 1979, **46**:249–255.

[38] Hagenfeldt, L. Metabolism of free fatty acids and ketone bodies during exercise in normal and diabetic man. *Diabetes,* 1979, **28**(Supplement 1):66–70.

[39] Hagenfeldt, L., and J. Wahren. Human forearm metabolism during exercise. VII: FFA uptake and oxidation at different work intensities. *Scandinavian Journal of Clinical and Laboratory Investigation,* 1972, **30**:429–436.

[40] Harris, R. C., R. H. T. Edwards, E. Hultman, L.-O. Nordesjo, B. Nylind, and K. Sahlin. The time course of phosphorylcreatine resynthesis during recovery of the quadriceps muscle in man. *Pflügers Archiv,* 1976, **367**:137–142.

[41] Haymes, E. M. Iron supplementation. In G. A. Stull, ed., *Encyclopedia of Physical Education, Fitness, and Sports,* Vol. 2. Salt Lake City: Brighton Publishing Company, 1980, pp. 335–343.

[42] Henriksson, J. Training induced adaptation of skeletal muscle and metabolism during submaximal exercise. *Journal of Physiology* (London), 1977, **270**:661–675.

[43] Hultman, E. Glycogen loading and endurance capacity. In G. A. Stull, ed., *Encyclopedia of Physical Education, Fitness, and Sports,* Vol. 2. Salt Lake City: Brighton Publishing Company, 1980, pp. 274–291.

[44] Hultman, E. Studies on muscle metabolism of glycogen and active phosphate in man with special reference to exercise and diet. *Scandinavian Journal of Clinical and Laboratory Investigation,* 1967, **19**:Supplementum 94.

[45] Ivy, J. L., D. L. Costill, W. J. Fink, and E. Maglischo. Contribution of medium and long chain triglyceride intake to energy metabolism during prolonged exercise. *International Journal of Sports Medicine,* 1980, **1**:15–20.

[46] Johannessen, A., C. Hagen, and H. Galbo. Prolactin, growth hormone, thyrotropin, 3-, 5-, 3′-triiodothyronine, and thyroxine responses to exercise after fat- and carbohydrate-enriched diet. *Journal of Clinical Endocrinology and Metabolism,* 1981, **52**:56–61.

[47] Keul, J., G. Haralambie, T. Arnold, and W. Schumann. Heart rate and energy-yielding

substrates in blood during long-lasting running. *European Journal of Applied Physiology,* 1974, **32**:279–289.

[48] Keul, J., G. Haralambie, and G. Frittin. Intermittent exercise: arterial lipid substrates and arteriovenous differences. *Journal of Applied Physiology,* 1974, **36**:159–162.

[49] Kochan, R. G., D. R. Lamb, S. A. Lutz, C. V. Perrill, E. M. Reimann, and K. K. Schlender. Glycogen synthase activation in human skeletal muscle: effects of diet and exercise. *American Journal of Physiology,* 1979, **236**:E660–E666.

[50] Kofranyi, E., F. Jekat, and H. Muller-Wecker. The minimum protein requirements of humans, tested with mixtures of whole egg plus potato and maize plus beans. *Hoppe-Seyler's Zeitschrift fur Physiologische Chemie,* 1970, **351**:1485–1493.

[51] Langenfeld, M. E., Glucose polymer ingestion during ultraendurance bicycling (abstract). *Medicine and Science in Sports and Exercise,* 1981, **13**:84.

[52] Lemon, P. W. R., and J. P. Mullin. Effect of initial muscle glycogen levels on protein catabolism during exercise. *Journal of Applied Physiology,* 1980, **48**: 624–629.

[53] Lemon, P. W. R., and F. J. Nagle. Effects of exercise on protein and amino acid metabolism. *Medicine and Science in Sports and Exercise,* 1981, **13**:141–149.

[54] Lithell, H., J. Orlander, R. Schele, B. Sjodin, and J. Karlsson. Changes in lipoprotein-lipase activity and lipid stores in human skeletal muscle with prolonged heavy exercise. *Acta Physiologica Scandinavica,* 1979, **107**:257–261.

[55] Liappis, N., S.-D. Kelderbacher, K. Kesseler, and P. Bantzer. Quantitative study of free amino acids in human eccrine sweat excreted from the forearms of healthy trained and untrained men during exercise. *European Journal of Applied Physiology,* 1979, **42**:227–234.

[56] MacDougall, J. D., G. R. Ward, D. G. Sale, and J. R. Sutton. Muscle glycogen repletion after high-intensity intermittent exercise. *Journal of Applied Physiology,* 1977, **42**:129–132.

[57] N. L. Marable, J. F. Hickson, Jr., M. K. Korslund, W. G. Herbert, R. F. Desjardins, and F. W. Thye. Urinary nitrogen excretion as influenced by a muscle-building program and protein intake variation. *Nutrition Reports International,* 1979, **19**:795–805.

[58] Martin, B., S. Robinson, and D. Robertshaw. Influence of diet on leg uptake of glucose during heavy exercise. *American Journal of Clinical Nutrition,* 1978, **31**:62–67.

[59] Nilsson, L., and E. Hultman. Liver glycogen in man—the effect of total starvation or a carbohydrate-poor diet followed by carbohydrate refeeding. *Scandinavian Journal of Clinical and Laboratory Investigation,* 1973, **32**:325–330.

[60] Nygaard, E., P. Andersen, P. Nilsson, E. Eriksson, T. Kjessel, and B. Saltin. Glycogen Depletion pattern and lactate accumulation in leg muscles during recreational downhill skiing. *European Journal of Applied Physiology,* 1978, **38**:261–269.

[61] Patton, R. Electrolyte solutions. In G. A. Stull, ed., *Encyclopedia of Physical Education, Fitness, and Sports,* Vol. 2. Salt Lake City: Brighton Publishing Company, 1980, pp. 328–334.

[62] Pernow, B., and B. Saltin, eds. *Muscle Metabolism During Exercise.* New York: Plenum Publishing Corporation, 1971.

[63] Phinney, S. D., B. R. Bistrian, W. J. Evans, R. W. Wolfe, and G. L. Blackburn. Reduced carbohydrate oxidation during submaximal exercise by trained cyclists after adaptation to an Eskimo diet (abstract). *Medicine and Science in Sports and Exercise,* 1981, **13**: 111.

[64] Pirnay, F., M. Lacroix, F. Mosora, A. Luyckx, and P. Lefebvre. Effect of glucose ingestion on energy substrate utilization during prolonged muscular exercise. *European Journal of Applied Physiology,* 1977, **36**:247–254.

[65] Rahkila, P., J. Soimajarvi, E. Karvinen, and V. Vihko. Lipid metabolism during exercise. II. Respiratory exchange ratio and muscle glycogen content during 4 h bicycle ergometry in two groups of healthy men. *European Journal of Applied Physiology,* 1980, **44**:245–254.

[66] Ravussin, E., P. Pahud, A. Dorner, M. J. Arnaud, and E. Jequier. Substrate utilization dur-

ing prolonged exercise preceded by ingestion of 13 C glucose in glycogen depleted and control subjects. *Pflügers Archiv,* 1979, **382**:197–202.

[67] Refsum, H. E., L. R. Gjessing, and S. B. Stromme. Changes in plasma amino acid distribution and urine amino acids excretion during prolonged heavy exercise. *Scandinavian Journal of Clinical and Laboratory Investigation,* 1979, **39**:407–413.

[68] Reitman, J., K. M. Baldwin, and J. O. Holloszy. Intramuscular triglyceride utilization by red, white, and intermediate skeletal muscle and heart during exhausting exercise. *Proceedings of the Society for Experimental Biology and Medicine,* 1973, **142**:628–631.

[69] Shephard, R. J. Vitamin E and physical performance. In G. A. Stull, ed., *Encyclopedia of Physical Education, Fitness, and Sports,* Vol. 2. Salt Lake City: Brighton Publishing Company, 1980, pp. 299–310.

[70] Sherman, W. M., D. L. Costill, W. J. Fink, and J. M. Miller. Carbohydrate loading: a practical approach (abstract). *Medicine and Science in Sports and Exercise,* 1981, **13**:90.

[71] Terblanche, S. E., R. D. Fell, A. C. Juhlin-Dannfelt, B. W. Craig, and J. O. Holloszy. Effects of glycerol feeding before and after exhausting exercise in rats. *Journal of Applied Physiology,* 1981, **50**:94–101.

[72] Therriault, D. G., G. A. Beller, J. A. Smoake, and L. H. Hartley. Intramuscular energy sources in dogs during physical work. *Journal of Lipid Research,* 1973, **14**:54–60.

[73] Van Handel, P. J., W. J. Fink, G. Branam, and D. L. Costill. Fate of 14 C glucose ingested during prolonged exercise. *International Journal of Sports Medicine,* 1980, **1**:127–131.

[74] Van Huss, W. D. Vitamin C. In G. A. Stull, ed., *Encyclopedia of Physical Education, Fitness, and Sports.* Salt Lake City: Brighton Publishing Company, 1980, pp. 321–327.

[75] Wahren, J., P. Felig, G. Ahlborg, and L. Jorfeldt. Glucose metabolism during leg exercise in man. *Journal of Clinical Investigation,* 1971, **50**:2715–2725.

[76] White, T. P., and G. A. Brooks. (U-14 C)glucose, -alanine, and -leucine oxidation in rats at rest and two intensities of running. *American Journal of Physiology,* 1981, **240**:E155–E165.

[77] Williams, M. H. Vitamins A and D. In G. A. Stull, ed., *Encyclopedia of Physical Education, Fitness, and Sports,* Vol. 2. Salt Lake City: Brighton Publishing Company, 1980, pp. 296–298.

[78] Williams, M. H. The B vitamins. In G. A. Stull, ed. *Encyclopedia of Physical Education, Fitness, and Sports,* Vol. 2. Salt Lake City: Brighton Publishing Company, 1980, pp. 311–320.

C H A P T E R

6

Estimation of Energy Expenditure During Exercise

$\mathbf{K}$**NOWLEDGE** of the energy expended in various physical activities is very important for precise prescription of exercise in weight control, for the prescription of exercise used in the rehabilitation of heart disease patients, for the provision of reasonable systematic training regimens for normal subjects, and for planning sensible conditioning programs for athletes. As will be described in this chapter, the usual method of determining energy expenditure also provides information about the relative contributions of anaerobic and aerobic energy production for the exercise activity and about the type of fuel metabolized during exercise.

It is possible, but very difficult and costly, to directly measure the energy expended by a subject who exercises inside a closed chamber which has walls specifically designed to absorb and measure the heat produced. However, it is much simpler to estimate that energy indirectly by measuring the amount of oxygen consumed by the subject. Oxygen consumption (oxygen uptake) is the difference between the volume of oxygen inspired and that expired, and represents the oxygen used in the electron transport system of the mitochondria.

Each atom of oxygen utilized by the electron transport system is associated with the production of two or three molecules of ATP—two ATP molecules if electron pairs are delivered to the electron transport system by $FADH_2$ and three if delivered by NADH. Therefore, by determining the amount of oxygen consumed during exercise and recovery, we have a measurement that is directly related to ATP replenishment (energy expenditure) during exercise and recovery.

Accurate measurements of the kilocalories of heat produced as the result of oxygen utilization show that normal subjects on a mixed diet of fat, carbohydrate, and protein expend about 5 kcal of energy for each liter of oxygen they consume. Therefore, if it were known that the gallant Slavic knight, Sir Lykziz Bierlotz, consumed 15 liters of oxygen while fighting a dragon to save a beautiful princess, one could calculate that the brave fellow expended $15 \times 5 = 75$ kcal of energy.

Calculation of Oxygen Uptake and Carbon Dioxide Production

Oxygen Uptake

To calculate oxygen uptake (V_{O_2}) during a period of exercise or rest, one must subtract the volume of oxygen expired during that time period from the volume of oxygen inspired during the same time. Calculation of these two volumes requires knowledge of a) the volumes of air inspired and expired during the test period and b) the concentration of oxygen in inspired and expired air. Thus,

V_{O_2} = Volume $O_{2_{inspired}}$ − Volume $O_{2_{expired}}$, where
Volume $O_{2_{inspired}}$ = Volume $Air_{inspired}$ × Concentration $O_{2_{inspired}}$, and
Volume $O_{2_{expired}}$ = Volume $Air_{expired}$ × Concentration $O_{2_{expired}}$

By substitution of terms, we can restate the first equation as follows:

$$V_{O_2} = (\text{Vol Air}_{insp} \times \text{Conc } O_{2_{insp}}) - (\text{Vol Air}_{exp} \times \text{Conc } O_{2_{exp}}).$$

For example, if the volume of air inspired in one minute is 100 liters and the concentration of oxygen in that air is 20 per cent, then the volume of oxygen inspired

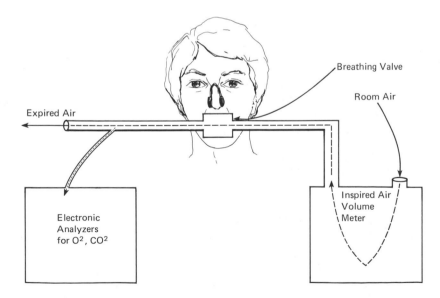

Expired Air

Breathing Valve

Room Air

Electronic
Analyzers
for O^2, CO^2

Inspired Air
Volume
Meter

FIGURE 6.1. Diagram of typical laboratory setup for measurement of energy expenditure.

in one minute is $100 \times .20 = 20$ liters of oxygen. If the volume of air expired is 100 liters and the concentration of oxygen in the expired air is 15 per cent, then the oxygen expired is $100 \times .15 = 15$ liters of oxygen. In this example, $V_{O_2} = 20 - 15 = 5$ liters of oxygen.

The concentration of O_2 in *inspired* air at sea level is a very constant 20.93% or .2093 liter O_2 per liter of air. The concentration of O_2 in a sample of the *expired* air must be measured in the laboratory with an oxygen analyzer (Fig. 6.1).

Measurement of Inspired or Expired Air Volume

Either the inspired or the expired air volume can be determined if the other is measured and if the concentration of nitrogen (N_2) in the expired air is analyzed. This calculation of one volume from knowledge of the other volume is made possible because the volume of nitrogen inspired is unchanged in the body and is, therefore, equal to the volume of nitrogen expired; that is,

$$\text{Vol } N_{2_{insp}} = \text{Vol } N_{2_{exp}}.$$

But,

$$\text{Vol } N_{2_{insp}} = \text{Vol Air}_{insp} \times \text{Conc } N_{2_{insp}},$$

and

$$\text{Vol } N_{2_{exp}} = \text{Vol Air}_{exp} \times \text{Conc } N_{2_{exp}}.$$

By substitution of terms,

$$\text{Vol Air}_{insp} \times \text{Conc } N_{2_{insp}} = \text{Vol Air}_{exp} \times \text{Conc } N_{2_{exp}}.$$

Therefore, we need to know only the nitrogen concentrations in both inspired and expired air and *either* the volume of air inspired *or* the volume of air expired to determine the other volume of air.

As an example, assume that the volume of air inspired is measured to be 100 liters, the concentration of $N_{2_{inspired}}$ is 80 per cent, and the concentration of $N_{2_{expired}}$ is 75 per cent. We can solve for the volume of air expired as follows:

$$
\begin{aligned}
100 \text{ liters} \times .80 &= \text{Vol Air}_{exp} \times .75 \\
80 \text{ liters} &= \text{Vol Air}_{exp} \times .75 \\
80 \text{ liters}/.75 &= \text{Vol Air}_{exp} \\
106.67 \text{ liters} &= \text{Vol Air}_{exp}.
\end{aligned}
$$

In normal room air at sea level the concentration of nitrogen is a constant 79.04 per cent. Therefore,

$$\text{Vol Air}_{insp} = \frac{\text{Vol Air}_{exp} \times \text{Conc N}_{2_{exp}}}{.7904}, \text{ and Vol Air}_{exp} = \frac{\text{Vol Air}_{insp} \times .7904}{\text{Conc N}_{2_{exp}}}.$$

Therefore, if the volume of *inspired* air is measured,

$$V_{O_2} = (\text{Vol Air}_{insp} \times .2093) - \left[\left(\frac{\text{Vol Air}_{insp} \times .7904}{\text{Conc N}_{2_{exp}}}\right) \times \text{Conc O}_{2_{exp}}\right].$$

However, if the volume of *expired* air is measured,

$$V_{O_2} = \left[\left(\frac{\text{Vol Air}_{exp} \times \text{Conc N}_{2_{exp}}}{.7904}\right) \times .2093\right] - (\text{Vol Air}_{exp} \times \text{Conc O}_{2_{exp}}).$$

For example, if the volume of air *inspired* during 5 minutes of exercise were 200 liters, and the concentrations of O_2 and N_2 in a sample of the *expired* air were .1700 (17%) and .7800 (78%), respectively,

$$V_{O_2} = (200 \times .2093) - \left[\left(\frac{200 \times .7904}{.7800}\right) \times .1700\right] = 7.41 \text{ liters}$$

in 5 minutes or 1.48 liters per minute. If, on the other hand, the volume of air *expired* during 1 minute of exercise was determined to be 100 liters and the concentrations of O_2 and N_2 in a sample of the expired air were .1600 (16%) and .7850 (78.5%), respectively,

$$V_{O_2} = \left[\left(\frac{100 \times .7850}{.7904}\right) \times .2093\right] - (100 \times .1600) = 4.79 \text{ liters per minute.}$$

The concentration of N_2 in expired air is usually found by subtracting the sum of the analyzed $O_{2_{exp}}$ and $CO_{2_{exp}}$ from 1.00 since there are only tiny amounts of gasses other than N_2, O_2 and CO_2 in ordinary air. Accordingly, if $O_{2_{exp}}$ and $CO_{2_{exp}}$ were analyzed as .1800 (18.00%) and .0300 (3.00%), respectively, $N_{2_{exp}}$ would be $1.00 - (.18 + .03) = .79$ (79%).

Carbon Dioxide Production

The production of carbon dioxide (V_{CO_2}) is calculated in much the same way as V_{O_2}, that is,

$$V_{CO_2} = (\text{Vol Air}_{exp} \times \text{Conc CO}_{2_{exp}}) - (\text{Vol Air}_{insp} \times \text{Conc CO}_{2_{insp}}).$$

Because the concentration of CO_2 in inspired air is only .0003 (0.03%) and is usually ignored, the equation for carbon dioxide production then becomes $V_{CO_2} = \text{Vol Air}_{exp} \times \text{Conc CO}_{2_{exp}}$ and is easily computed if the volume of expired air is measured. If the volume of *inspired* air rather than expired air is measured,

$$V_{CO_2} = \left(\frac{\text{Vol Air}_{insp} \times .7904}{\text{Conc N}_{2_{exp}}}\right) \times \text{Conc CO}_{2_{exp}}.$$

It should be mentioned at this point that the gas volumes described in this section must be converted to standard conditions of barometric pressure, temperature, and humidity so that the calculated values of oxygen uptake and carbon dioxide production can be compared to the results obtained in different environmental circumstances. Gasses expand in the heat and under low barometric pressure, but they contract in the cold and under high barometric pressure. Also, water vapor contributes to gas volumes. Therefore, it would be difficult to interpret oxygen uptakes if the volumes were not converted to universally accepted standard conditions. Those conditions are known as "STPD" conditions. The letters stand for: Standard Temperature (0°C), Pressure (760 mm Hg), and Dry. There is a table of STPD correction factors presented in Appendix E, which may be consulted for further instructions in conversion of gas volumes to STPD conditions.

Oxygen Deficit and Oxygen Debt

As stated in the preceding discussion, ATP replenishment is ultimately the result of oxygen consumption in the electron transport system of the mitochondria of the body's cells. But during the first few seconds of light exercise and for all of short-duration heavy exercise, ATP is produced primarily as a result of *anaerobic* (without oxygen) mechanisms, that is, mostly by the breakdown of creatine phosphate and muscle glycogen or glucose. Extra oxygen is then used *after the activity has been concluded* to make up for the initial anaerobic production of ATP.

There are three reasons why aerobic energy generation makes only a small contribution during heavy work and during the first part of submaximal work. First, it takes a few seconds for the circulation to deliver the required extra oxygen to the working muscles. Second, aerobic metabolism is sparked by the presence of excess ADP in the mitochondria that acts as an acceptor of phosphate to produce ATP (that is, ADP + P = ATP). Until such ADP accumulates as the result of ATP breakdown, rapid oxygen consumption and ATP production by the mitochondria do not begin [6]. Accordingly, ATP must be generated by anaerobic means until the aerobic production of ATP in the mitochondria can catch up. Finally, in heavy work the rate of demand for ATP is simply too great to be met solely by aerobic energy production during exercise; the breakdown of creatine phosphate and glycogen must occur to meet the high rate of energy use by the muscle.

The inadequacy of aerobic energy production to meet the total energy needs of the body, especially at the beginning of an exercise period, is known as the *oxygen deficit*. An additional oxygen deficit accumulates whenever energy expenditure is abruptly increased, e.g., during the sprint at the end of a race. The tendency of the body to repay this aerobic energy deficit by consuming more than usual amounts of oxygen during the period of recovery after the exercise is part of what is known as the oxygen debt (Fig. 6.2).

Operationally, the oxygen deficit is defined as the difference between the total energy cost of the work (expressed as units of oxygen) and the measured portion of the total energy cost that was met during the exercise period by aerobic energy production, that is, by oxygen consumption during the exercise period. Oxygen debt, on the other hand, is the oxygen consumed during recovery that is in excess of the amounts that normally would have been consumed at rest during an equivalent time period. To better understand these concepts, inspect Fig. 6.2 carefully. Observe the area "O_2 Consumed at Rest" at the base of the graph. This rectangle represents the resting rate of oxygen uptake, in this case 0.25 l/min., that would have occurred even if the exercise had *not* taken place. Next, observe the unshaded area under the curve between the start and finish of exercise. The area represents the *net* or excess oxygen consumption during exercise, that is, the portion of the total aerobic energy cost (above that which would have occurred during a similar period of rest) that was met during the exercise period itself. The area shaded with gray at the left of the diagram represents that portion of the total energy cost that could not be met by oxygen delivered from the lungs during exercise. In other words, *this oxygen deficit portion of the energy cost of exercise was primarily met by replenishing ATP supplies anaerobically, chiefly by the breakdown of creatine phosphate and muscle glycogen.* A portion of the oxygen deficit is also met *aerobically.* There is oxygen dissolved in blood and tissue fluids that can support some aerobic replenishment of ATP, and this oxygen utilization is not reflected in overall measurements of oxygen uptake taken at the mouth. Similarly, a small amount of oxygen is bound to *myoglobin,* a hemoglobin-like protein found in muscle; this oxygen can be released for aerobic ATP replenishment in some cases. The oxygen dissolved in body fluids and bound to myoglobin can maintain muscle contraction for perhaps 20 seconds if the work rate is not too great. Higher rates of en-

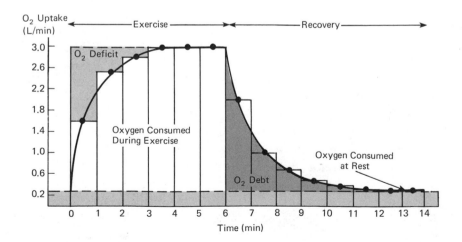

FIGURE 6.2. Energy expenditure (oxygen uptake) during exercise and recovery.

ergy expenditure require the breakdown of creatine phosphate and muscle glycogen to provide adequate rates of ATP replenishment.

The horizontal line drawn in Fig. 6.2 at 3.0 liters of oxygen uptake per minute represents the rate of total energy expenditure (in terms of oxygen) that was needed to perform this particular exercise. Notice that only during the last 3 minutes of exercise was the exerciser able to meet the total energy costs aerobically (by the uptake of oxygen). Accordingly, the oxygen deficit in this case occurred only during the first 3 minutes of exercise. For any given minute one can simply subtract the amount of oxygen consumed from the total energy expenditure to obtain the oxygen deficit for that minute. For example, for the first minute of exercise shown in Fig. 6.2, oxygen consumption was on the average about 1.6 liters (ranging from 0.25–2.20 l.), whereas the total energy use was 3.0 liters; therefore, the oxygen deficit for the first minute of work was $3.0 - 1.6 = 1.4$ liters of oxygen. For the sixth minute of exercise, on the other hand, the oxygen uptake and the energy cost were the same, 3.0 liters, so there was no additional oxygen deficit contracted during that minute.

In Fig. 6.2, the darkly shaded area shown in the recovery period illustrates the oxygen uptake after exercise that is above the normal resting level of oxygen uptake. This excess oxygen uptake during recovery is called the *oxygen debt.* Oxygen debt can be measured if one knows the total oxygen consumed during recovery and the rate of oxygen consumption that normally occurs during rest.

Causes of the Oxygen Debt

A review of Fig. 6.2 shows that the early portion of the oxygen debt (excess oxygen uptake during recovery from exercise) falls very quickly within the first minute or two, whereas the later portion falls at a more gradual rate over a prolonged time. Most authorities agree that the early portion of the excess oxygen consumed during recovery is used to regenerate depleted stores of ATP and creatine phosphate, to resupply oxygen to myoglobin in muscle, and to resupply dissolved oxygen in tissue fluids and blood [2]. Recall that these factors were depleted during the oxygen deficit period of exercise. This portion of the oxygen debt is sometimes referred to as the "alactic acid" component of oxygen debt. Alactic means "without lactic acid", and the term is used to distinguish it from the slow component of the oxygen debt which was once known as the "lactic acid" component of the debt. The lactic acid component of oxygen debt was thought to be caused by the oxidation of about 20 per cent of the lactic acid produced during exercise to provide ATP for changing the remaining 80 per cent of the lactic acid back to glycogen in the liver and/or muscles. Since the early rapid portion of the oxygen debt is not related to lactic acid metabolism, it is known as the "alactic acid" component.

It is now clear that the slow component of the oxygen debt is due to many factors in addition to lactic acid metabolism. In fact, it appears that most of the lactic acid produced is oxidized to carbon dioxide and water and that a rather small portion is used for the resynthesis of glycogen [1, 7]. This is the reverse of what early workers thought. Because of these recent findings, it is likely that the terms "alactic acid component" and "lactic acid component" will soon be replaced by "fast component" and "slow component" or "early phase" and "late phase" to describe the two portions of the oxygen debt curve.

Other Factors That Contribute to Oxygen Debt. What are some of the other factors which contribute to the excess oxygen uptake during recovery from exercise? First, the increased body temperature during exercise stimulates the mitochondria to consume more oxygen. Second, during recovery from exercise the respiratory muscles continue to work hard for some time, and the heart continues to beat above its resting rate for several minutes; both of these functions require extra oxygen. Third, epinephrine, norepinephrine, thyroxine and perhaps other hormones released during exercise stimulate the mitochondria to consume excess oxygen until the hormones are removed from the circulation. These are the most frequently mentioned factors contributing to oxygen debt, but there are undoubtedly others.

In summary, the excess oxygen uptake during recovery is not solely a function of anaerobic metabolism during exercise. There are many homeostatic disturbances caused by exercise, and some of these disturbances can cause the consumption of excess oxygen during recovery. It is not difficult to understand why the oxygen debt after severe exercise is often found to be twice as great as the oxygen deficit. The greater the homeostatic disturbance caused by exercise, the greater the oxygen debt that can be expected to result.

Estimation of Oxygen Cost, Caloric Cost, Oxygen Deficit, and Oxygen Debt

For *steady-state* work (work that can be maintained for a long period with aerobic energy production and only a brief period of anaerobic energy production at the start of the exercise bout) only oxygen uptake need be measured during rest, exercise, and recovery to enable one to estimate total energy cost, oxygen deficit, and oxygen debt in terms of oxygen units. For example, assume that a person worked as in Fig. 6.2 for 6 minutes and recovered for 8 minutes, and that the measured oxygen uptake values were as follows:

Rest: 0.25 l/min
Exercise: 1st min = 1.6 *l*, 2nd min = 2.5 *l*, 3rd min = 2.8 *l*, 4th, 5th, & 6th
            min = 3.0 *l*.
Recovery: 1st min = 2.0 *l*, 2nd min = 1.0 *l*, 3rd min = 0.7 *l*, 4th min = 0.5 *l*,
            5th min = 0.4 *l*, 6th min = 0.3 *l*, 7th min = 0.27 *l*, 8th min = 0.26 *l*.

This example will be used to show how the following equations can be used to help determine the various portions of energy expenditure as a result of exercise.

Net O_2 Cost of Exercise is the total oxygen consumed during both exercise and recovery less the oxygen that would have been consumed during the same period had the subject been at rest.

NET O_2 COST OF EXERCISE = Exercise V_{O_2} + Recovery V_{O_2}
$$- (\text{Rest } \dot{V}_{O_2} \times \text{Total Exercise \& Recovery Time})$$

It should be noted that the symbol V refers to a volume, whereas $\dot{V}$ represents a volume per unit of time, usually per minute. In the example, Exercise V_{O_2} = 1.6 + 2.5 + 2.8 + 3.0 + 3.0 + 3.0 = 15.9 l, Recovery V_{O_2} = 2.0 + 1.0 + 0.7 + 0.5 + 0.4 + 0.3 + 0.27 + 0.26 = 5.43 l, Rest $\dot{V}_{O_2}$ = 0.25 l/min, and Total Exercise & Recovery Time = 14 min. Therefore,

NET O_2 COST OF EXERCISE = 15.9 + 5.43 − (0.25 × 14)
$$= 21.33 - 3.5 = 17.83\ l\ O_2$$

Oxygen Deficit in Steady-State Exercise is the difference between the theoretical oxygen cost of the exercise (had steady-state oxygen uptake been reached instantaneously at the start of exercise) and the actual oxygen uptake observed during the exercise period. In the example shown in Fig. 6.2, the steady-state level of oxygen uptake was not reached until the third minute at 3.0 l/min. Accordingly, during the first 3 minutes the subject was replenishing ATP anaerobically and contracting an oxygen deficit.

OXYGEN DEFICIT IN STEADY-STATE EXERCISE
$$= (\text{Steady-State Exercise } \dot{V}_{O_2} \times \text{Exercise Time}) - \text{Exercise } V_{O_2}$$

In the example of Fig. 6.2, Steady-State Exercise $\dot{V}_{O_2}$ = 3.0 l/min, Exercise Time = 6 min, and the exercise V_{O_2} = 15.9 l. Accordingly,

OXYGEN DEFICIT = (3.0 × 6) − 15.9 = 18.0 − 15.9 = 2.1 liters.

Oxygen Deficit in Nonsteady-state Exercise is technically more difficult to measure accurately because the oxygen uptake during exercise never reaches a steady plateau, so that an estimated "steady-state" level of oxygen uptake must be computed. In severe exercise that can be maintained for only a few minutes, oxygen debt is much greater than oxygen deficit [4] and thus cannot be used to accurately assess oxygen deficit.

Oxygen Debt is the difference between the oxygen consumed during recovery after exercise and the oxygen that would have been consumed during the same time interval had the subject remained at rest. In Fig. 6.2, the total oxygen consumed during 8 minutes of recovery was 5.43 l, and the resting rate of oxygen uptake was 0.25 l/min. Therefore, assuming the subject would have consumed 0.25 × 8 = 2.0 l of oxygen during 8 minutes had he remained at rest, the oxygen debt shown in Fig. 6.2 was 5.43 − 2.0 = 3.43 l.

OXYGEN DEBT = Recovery V_{O_2} − (Resting $\dot{V}_{O_2}$ × Min. of Recovery)

Determination of the Caloric Equivalent of Oxygen Consumed and the Net Caloric Cost of Exercise

Caloric Equivalent of Oxygen Consumed

In exercise of short duration where a relatively small volume of oxygen is consumed, it is usually satisfactory to assume that each liter of oxygen consumed is equivalent to about 5.0 kcal. But when exercise is prolonged for an hour or more, this value could be up to 6 per cent in error. Such an error is negligible in most situations, but if greater accuracy is needed, such as to determine energy balance over a 24-hour period, a more exact caloric equivalent must be determined. This determination involves measuring the urinary nitrogen excreted, the oxygen consumed, and the carbon dioxide produced during rest, steady-state exercise, and recovery, so that a *nonprotein respiratory-exchange ratio* (R) or *respiratory quotient* (RQ) may be computed.

Respiratory Exchange Ratio

As oxygen is consumed in the mitochondria in the process of catabolizing a particular foodstuff—for example, fat, carbohydrate, or protein—the oxygen consumption is associated with a certain amount of carbon dioxide production, especially in reactions of the Krebs cycle. Each type of food broken down gives a particular ratio of the volume of CO_2 produced to the volume of O_2 consumed. This ratio, V_{CO_2}/V_{O_2}, is known as the respiratory-exchange ratio (R) or the respiratory quotient (RQ). For example, when glucose is completely oxidized ($C_6H_{12}O_6 + 6O_2 \rightarrow 6CO_2 + 6H_2O$), each volume of oxygen consumed is associated with the same volume of carbon dioxide production, so the R or RQ for glucose is $6CO_2/6O_2 = 1.0$. It takes relatively more oxygen, though, to combust a typical fat molecule ($2C_{51}H_{98}O_6 + 145O_2 \rightarrow 102CO_2 + 98H_2O$), and the R for pure fat is about $102CO_2/145O_2 = 0.70$. The R value for protein is about 0.83.

As described in Chapter 4, less oxygen must be consumed to produce a given amount of ATP from carbohydrate breakdown than from fat breakdown. This means that a liter of oxygen is associated with the production of more energy if the oxygen is used for catabolizing carbohydrate rather than fat. Therefore, for a respiratory exchange ratio of 1.0, which reflects carbohydrate metabolism, each liter of oxygen consumed should represent more kcal of energy than would be true for a respiratory exchange ratio of less than 1.0, which would reflect progressively more fat metabolism. Observe that the second column from the left in Table 6.1 contains the caloric equivalents of a liter of oxygen for different respiratory exchange ratios and that these caloric equivalents fall from 5.047 kcal/*l* for an R of 1.00 to 4.686 kcal/*l* for an R of 0.70.

Notice that the R values of Table 6.1 are labeled *nonprotein R*. This means that the volume of oxygen consumed and the volume of carbon dioxide produced as the result of the metabolism of protein during exercise must be subtracted from the

TABLE 6.1
Caloric Equivalents for Oxygen and Foodstuff Contributions to Energy for Various Nonprotein Respiratory Exchange Ratios

Nonprotein Respiratory Exchange Ratio (R or RQ)	Caloric Equivalent (kcal/liter O_2)	Approximate Contributions to Energy	
		Fat (%)	Carbohydrate (%)
1.00	5.047	0	100
0.98	5.022	6	94
0.96	4.997	12	88
0.94	4.973	19	81
0.92	4.948	26	74
0.90	4.928	32	68
0.88	4.900	38	62
0.86	4.875	47	53
0.84	4.850	53	47
0.82	4.825	62	38
0.80	4.801	68	32
0.78	4.776	74	26
0.76	4.752	81	19
0.74	4.727	88	12
0.72	4.702	94	6
0.70	4.686	100	0

total oxygen consumption and carbon dioxide production. To find the rather small contribution of protein to these gas volumes, one must measure the urinary nitrogen excreted during the exercise period and compute the amount of protein broken down plus the oxygen consumed and the carbon dioxide produced because of the protein breakdown. With short duration exercise the contribution of protein metabolism is so small that it can safely be neglected. If R values are to be used at all to determine the exact caloric equivalent of a liter of oxygen consumed, it is best to measure the protein contribution to exercise metabolism. For most practical purposes, however, the use of 5.0 as an assumed caloric equivalent for a liter of oxygen can be justified, so that neither carbon dioxide production nor urinary nitrogen needs to be measured. In many laboratories the possibility of error in using an assumed caloric equivalent of 5.0 is much less than the likelihood of error in measuring nitrogen and carbon dioxide.

Precautions Necessary in Interpreting R. Any factor which influences the production of carbon dioxide or the consumption of oxygen, but which is not directly related to the combustion of foodstuffs, can obviously result in a respiratory exchange ratio that is misleading. In heavy exercise, for example, it is not unusual to observe R values greater than 1.0 during exercise and values less than 0.7 during recovery. Such values for R are not very helpful when one is attempting to determine an accurate caloric equivalent for oxygen consumed, because even burning pure glucose or pure fat does not result in R values greater than 1.0 or less than 0.7, respectively.

Two factors are most often linked to erroneous R values. First, unnecessarily heavy breathing (hyperventilation) by an anxious subject may cause the exhalation of excess carbon dioxide that has nothing to do with energy metabolism in the mitochondria. The excess carbon dioxide artificially increases the numerator of the respiratory exchange ratio. Second, during heavy exercise a large amount of lactic acid is produced which raises the R value. This occurs for two reasons: 1) The decreased pH stimulates the brain to increase ventilation; this leads to excessive exhalation of carbon dioxide. 2) The decreased pH stimulates the breakdown of carbonic acid (H_2CO_3) in the blood to carbon dioxide and water; the carbon dioxide is exhaled by the lungs to increase R. (The breakdown of carbonic acid to water and carbon dioxide helps to minimize (buffer) the effect of lactic acid on pH.) Following heavy exercise, carbon dioxide tends to be retained by the body to replenish the stores of bicarbonate that were used to buffer the lactic acid during exercise; this retention of carbon dioxide may lower R in the recovery period to less than 0.70 for many minutes or even an hour or more.

Because unusual R values are most apt to be observed during heavy, nonsteady-state exercise, the determination of R is usually restricted to exercise of a submaximal steady-state nature. For heavy exercise a caloric equivalent of 5.0 kilocalories per liter of oxygen can be assumed so that reliance on R values is unnecessary.

Net Caloric Cost of Exercise

Net caloric cost of exercise is the total caloric cost of both exercise and recovery less the calories that would have been expended during the same period had the subject been at rest. This caloric cost is determined indirectly on the basis of measured oxygen consumption and the *caloric equivalent* of a liter of oxygen.

> NET CALORIC COST OF EXERCISE = Net O_2 Cost of Exercise (*l*)
> $\times$ Caloric Equivalent of a Liter of O_2

Assume, for example, that net oxygen cost was 17.83 liters, and the caloric equivalent was 5.0 kcal per liter. Therefore,

$$\text{NET CALORIC COST OF EXERCISE} = 17.83 \times 5.0 = 89.15 \text{ kcal.}$$

Determination of the Contribution of Various Foodstuffs to Energy Expenditure

Physical educators, doctors, coaches, dieters, and athletes are often curious about how much fat, carbohydrate, or protein is used up in various types of exercise. As was discussed in Chapter 5, a general answer is that protein breakdown is insignificant during exercise for a well-fed person, that carbohydrate is utilized most in heavy exercise, and that fat is a major source of fuel for low intensity, long duration exercise. However, a fairly precise estimate of the contributions of fat, carbohydrate, and protein to energy expenditure can be obtained from a knowledge of the volume of oxygen consumed, the volume of carbon dioxide produced, and the urinary nitrogen excreted during steady-state exercise. Table 6.2 presents equations that can be used to determine the contribution of fat, carbohydrate, and protein to energy expenditure [3].

As an illustration of how these equations could be used, suppose that Susie Sweat-socks wanted to know whether riding her bicycle to school 4 miles each way would have any impact on her massive hulk (100 kg or 220 lbs) if she rode 5 days per week for 40 weeks. Susie asked Dr. Nosemuch, the local, friendly exercise physiologist, if he would perform the appropriate tests. With the good doctor's help the following data were obtained from a one-way bicycle trip:

$$\text{Urinary nitrogen} = 0.01 \text{ g}, V_{CO_2} = 60\,l, V_{O_2} = 68\,l.$$

Thus, on a 4-mile bicycle ride Susie used $6.25 \times 0.01 = .0625$ g protein, $(4.12 \times 60) - (2.91 \times 68) - (2.56 \times 0.01) = 49.29$ g carbohydrate and $(1.69 \times 68) - (1.69 \times 60) - (1.94 \times 0.01) = 13.50$ g fat, and she expended $(3.78 \times 68) + (1.16 \times 60) - (2.98 \times 0.01) = 327$ kcal of energy. The energy expenditure associated with protein breakdown was $4.1 \times .0625 = 0.26$ kcal, with carbohydrate breakdown $4.1 \times 49.29 = 202.09$ kcal, and with fat breakdown $9.3 \times 13.50 = 125.55$ kcal.

Of the 327 kcal of energy expended on her trip to school, less than 1 per cent was because of protein breakdown, about 62 per cent because of carbohydrate break-down, and 38 per cent because of fat breakdown. In 400 trips on her bicycle, Susie would expend $400 \times 125.55 = 50,220$ kcal from fat breakdown alone and a total of $400 \times 327 = 130,800$ kcal from all sources. Although a caloric expenditure of 9,300 kcal is required to catabolize a kilogram of pure fat, only about 7,700 kcal must be spent to break down a kilogram of fat *tissue,* which contains water and connective tissue in addition to pure fat. (This translates into an expenditure of 3,500 kcal per pound of fat tissue.) Accordingly, Susie would lose $50,220/7,700 = 6.5$ kilograms (14.3 lbs.) of fat tissue from the use of fat alone in a year of cycling back and forth to school, assuming she did not alter her caloric intake. But since the other degraded foodstuffs, such as glycogen and protein, are preferentially replenished after exercise at the expense of energy derived from further fat breakdown, the actual fat loss would approach 17 kg (37.4 lbs.) (130,800/7,700). Such a weight loss would be very admi-rable and would not require any reduction in food intake. Of course, if Susie were able to reduce her caloric intake as she increased her caloric expenditure by cycling, she could lose weight even more rapidly.

TABLE 6.2
Calculation of Foodstuff Contribution to Energy Expenditure

1. Protein used during activity (g) $= 6.25 \times$ grams of urinary nitrogen excreted during activity
2. Carbohydrate used during activity (g) $= 4.12\ V_{CO_2}\ (l) - 2.91\ V_{O_2}\ (l) - 2.56$ urinary nitrogen (g)
3. Fat used during activity (g) $= 1.69\ V_{O_2}\ (l) - 1.69\ V_{CO_2}\ (l) - 1.94$ urinary nitrogen (g)
4. Energy expended (kcal) $= 3.78\ V_{O_2}\ (l) + 1.16\ V_{CO_2}\ (l) - 2.98$ urinary nitrogen (g)
5. Energy due to protein (kcal) $= 4.1 \times$ protein used (g)
6. Energy due to carbohydrate (kcal) $= 4.1 \times$ carbohydrate used (g)
7. Energy due to fat (kcal) $= 9.3 \times$ fat used (g)

In Table 6.1 are listed the approximate percentage contributions of fat and carbohydrate for various respiratory exchange ratios. If, for example, an exerciser consumed 20 liters of oxygen in an activity at an average R of 0.90, Table 6.1 shows that each of those liters of oxygen was equivalent to about 4.93 kcal, and that 32 per cent of the total caloric expenditure was the result of fat breakdown, whereas 68 per cent was due to carbohydrate. The total energy expenditure, therefore, was 20 × 4.93 = 98.6 kcal, and of this total 32 per cent or 31.6 kcal resulted from fat combustion and 68 per cent or 67.0 kcal from carbohydrate.

REVIEW QUESTIONS

1. What is the physiological basis for the estimation of energy expenditure in units of oxygen consumption?
2. Define the following terms both operationally and in terms of how they are related to aerobic and/or anaerobic energy expenditure: oxygen deficit, net oxygen cost of exercise, oxygen debt.
3. How is the respiratory exchange ratio used to determine roughly the relative contributions of fat and carbohydrate as fuels for exercise? What is the physiological basis for this technique?
4. If, as a result of an exercise bout, a subject excreted 0.005 grams of urinary nitrogen, consumed 50 liters of oxygen, and produced 45 liters of carbon dioxide, calculate the following: total energy expenditure and energy contributed by protein, fat, and carbohydrate breakdown.
5. Explain why the old concept of a "lactic acid" component of the oxygen debt is no longer valid.
6. What is the function of the fast component of the oxygen debt?
7. Explain why it is inaccurate to describe the oxygen debt solely in terms of the repayment of the oxygen deficit.
8. Haskell Schwartzkopf ran on a treadmill for 5 minutes and recovered for 10 minutes. The following data were recorded:
Subject weight: 60 kg
Caloric equivalent of oxygen: 5.0 kcal/l
Oxygen uptake at rest: 0.3 liters
Oxygen uptake during exercise:
   Minute 1:   1.2 liters
   Minute 2:   2.2 liters
   Minute 3:   2.8 liters
   Minute 4:   2.8 liters
   Minute 5:   2.8 liters
Oxygen uptake during recovery:
   Minute 1:   1.6 liters
   Minute 2:   1.0 liters
   Minute 3:   0.8 liters
   Minute 4:   0.7 liters
   Minute 5:   0.6 liters
   Minute 6:   0.5 liters
   Minute 7:   0.45 liters
   Minute 8:   0.40 liters
   Minute 9:   0.35 liters
   Minute 10: 0.30 liters
Using Haskell's data, draw a graph similar to Fig. 6.2 and calculate the following values:
a. Oxygen deficit
b. Oxygen debt

c. Net oxygen cost of the exercise
d. Net caloric cost of the exercise

REFERENCES

[1] Brooks, G. A., and G. A. Gaesser. End points of lactate and glucose metabolism after exhausting exercise. *Journal of Applied Physiology,* 1980, **49:**1057–1069.

[2] Cerretelli, P., D. Shindell, D. P. Pendergast, P. E. di Prampero, and D. W. Rennie. Oxygen uptake transients at the onset and offset of arm and leg work. *Respiration Physiology,* 1977, **30:**81–97.

[3] Consolazio, C. F., R. E. Johnson, and L. J. Pecora. *Physiological Measurements of Metabolic Functions in Man.* New York: McGraw-Hill Book Company, 1963, p. 316.

[4] Hermansen, L. Anaerobic energy release. *Medicine and Science in Sports,* 1969, **1:**32–38.

[5] Herreid II, C. F., D. A. Prawel, and R. J. Full. Energetics of running cockroaches. *Science,* 1981, **212:**331–333.

[6] Holloszy, J. O. Long-term metabolic adaptations in muscle to endurance exercise. In J. P. Naughton and H. K. Hellerstein, eds., *Exercise Testing and Exercise Training in Coronary Heart Disease.* New York: Academic Press Inc., 1973, pp. 212–222.

[7] Segal, S. S., and G. A. Brooks. Effects of glycogen depletion and work load on postexercise O_2 consumption and blood lactate. *Journal of Applied Physiology,* 1979, **47:**514–521.

CHAPTER
7

Exercise, Body Composition, and Weight Control

It is readily apparent that some persons have bodies that are more physically attractive or better adapted to certain types of athletic competition than the bodies of others. Differences in height, weight, body shape, bone lengths and weight distribution are obvious characteristics that may influence a person's appearance and athletic performance. In this chapter, however, we will consider the composition of the body, that is, the fat and nonfat components of the body, and how body composition is affected by exercise and diet.

Fat and Nonfat Components of "Typical" Man and Woman

In Table 7.1 are shown the major constituents of the autopsied bodies of typical men and women aged 20–24 years [10]. There are, of course, a number of differences in body composition between men and women, including a smaller mass of muscle and bone for women and smaller "essential" fat stores in men. Essential fat is that without which bodily function presumably begins to deteriorate. It includes fat in the myelin sheaths of nerves, in brain tissue, in bone marrow, in liver, and in all the other glands and tissues of the body. In women, the essential fat includes some of the fat in breast tissues and the uterus, as well as other sex-related fat deposits. Men and women with less than 3 per cent or 12 per cent body fat, respectively, often exhibit health problems, but there may be exceptions to this rule. There are reports, for example, of male defensive backs in football with body fat values of less than 1 per cent [10] and of female distance runners with 6 per cent body fat [22]. However, such low values may reflect errors in the indirect estimation of body fat.

TABLE 7.1
**Body Composition of Typical Young
Adult Men and Women**

Characteristic	Males	Females
Height	68.5 in	64.5 in
Weight	70.0 kg	56.8 kg
Muscle	31.4 kg	20.5 kg
	44.8 %	36.0 %
Bone	10.5 kg	6.8 kg
	14.9 %	12.0 %
Essential Fat	2.1 kg	6.8 kg
	3.0 %	12.0 %
Storage Fat	8.4 kg	8.5 kg
	12.0 %	15.0 %
Total Fat	10.5 kg	15.4 kg
	15.0 %	27.0 %
Remainder	17.7 kg	14.2 kg
	25.3 %	25.0 %

Storage fat is the fat deposited in adipose (fat) tissue throughout the body. Major fat deposits are located beneath the skin (subcutaneous fat) and around major organs such as the heart and kidneys. Storage fat serves as an energy reservoir, as insulation against the cold, and as protection from physical trauma to the body. It is the storage fat that is most subject to change with diet and exercise. Note that men and women have similar amounts of storage fat.

Determination of Body Composition

There are several methods that have been used to estimate the fat and lean constituents of the living body, but only two will be mentioned—the method of hydrostatic (underwater) weighing and the skin fold technique. The hydrostatic weighing method is used most commonly for research purposes, whereas the measurement of skin folds is a practical method for rapid screening of body composition in large numbers of subjects.

Hydrostatic Weighing

It is well known that fat tissue is lighter than muscle, bone, and other lean tissues. Fat persons float easily in water, whereas extremely lean people must exert themselves to stay afloat. Fat floats in water because its density (weight per unit volume) is less than the density of water. Therefore, if the density of a human body can be determined, it can give us some idea about the fat content of that body—the lower the density, the greater the percentage of fat. In fact, human cadavers have been tested for density and chemically analyzed for fat content so that formulas are available to convert density values to per cent fat values. Thus, if one measures a person's density, a formula can be applied to determine the per cent of fat in that person's body.

Since density is weight per unit volume, e.g., kilograms per liter, grams per cubic centimeter, or pounds per gallon, a determination of body density requires the measurement of body volume. This is done by weighing the subject on an accurate scale in air and then weighing the subject while the subject is totally submerged in water (Fig. 7.1). Since it is known that a body submerged in water is buoyed up by a force equal to the volume of water it displaces (Archimedes' principle), one need only subtract the weight of the subject under water from the weight in air to find the weight of water displaced by the subject. Then by dividing the weight of water displaced by the density of water, the volume of water displaced (body volume) is determined.

For example, if a subject weighed 70 kilograms in air and 2 kilograms under water, the weight of the water displaced by the subject was 70 minus 2 equals 68 kilograms or 68,000 grams. If the density of the water was 0.99336 grams per cubic centimeter, the volume of water displaced was 68,000/0.99336 equals 68,455 cubic centimeters, which was also the volume of the subject's body. This total body volume must be corrected for the residual volume of air in the lungs that cannot be expelled prior to underwater weighing and for the air trapped in the gastrointestinal tract (usually ignored or assumed to be 100 cc.). Let us assume that the residual lung volume was 1,500 cubic centimeters and that the gastrointestinal air was 100 cubic centimeters. This total (1,600 cubic centimeters) must be subtracted from the 68,455 cubic centimeters determined previously to give 66,855 cubic centimeters as a corrected body volume. Therefore, the subject's body density was 70,000 grams/66,855 cubic centimeters or 1.047 grams per cubic centimeter.

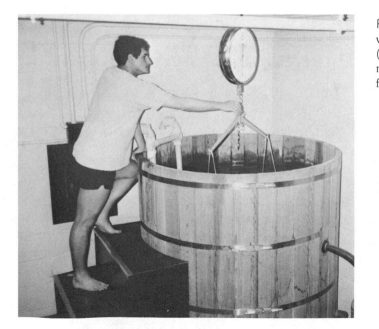

FIGURE 7.1. Estimation of body volume by underwater weighing. (Courtesy of Office of Public Information, Purdue University, West Lafayette, Indiana.)

The most popular equation for converting body density to per cent body fat is the Siri equation:

$$\% \; Fat = (495/body \; density) - 450$$

In the example just explained, % Fat = (495/1.047) − 450 = 472.78 − 450 = 22.78%.

Total body fat can be calculated by multiplying total body weight by per cent fat expressed as a decimal, e.g., Total Fat = 70 kilograms × .2278 = 15.95 kilograms.

Lean body mass can then be calculated by subtracting total body fat from total body weight, e.g., Lean Body Mass = 70 kilograms − 15.95 kilograms = 54.05 kilograms.

Equations for the body composition variables are summarized as follows.

$$Body \; Density = \frac{Weight \; in \; Air(g)}{\left[\dfrac{Wt. \; in \; Air(g) \; - \; Wt. \; in \; Water(g)}{Density \; of \; Water \; (g/cc)}\right] - (Res. \; Vol.(cc) + 100)}$$

(100 in the above equation is the assumed volume (cc) of air trapped in the gastrointestinal tract.)

$$\% \; Body \; Fat = (495/Body \; Density) - 450$$
$$Total \; Body \; Fat = (\% \; Body \; Fat/100) \times Body \; Wt. \; in \; Air$$
$$Lean \; Body \; Mass = Body \; Wt. \; in \; Air \; - \; Total \; Body \; Fat$$

Residual volume in the lungs can be accurately determined by several methods, including a fairly simple oxygen rebreathing method [23]. For general screening purposes, assumed values for residual volume can be taken from Table 7.2, but such values could lead to substantial errors in determination of body composition.

The Skin Fold Technique

Approximately 50 per cent of the store of body fat in human beings is located just beneath the skin, i.e., in the subcutaneous fat depots. Thus, if the subcutaneous fat can be estimated validly and reliably, such estimations should provide a useful indicator of total body fat. Many attempts have been made to estimate body fat by measuring the thickness of folds of skin at various sites on the body. The usual approach has been to measure body density on many subjects by underwater weighing and then to measure the thicknesses of several skin folds with special skin fold calipers. Next, on the basis of the data from underwater weighing and from skin fold thicknesses, a computer is used to develop equations which are used to predict body density (and fat) from the skin fold thicknesses. The idea is, of course, that a person who has thicker skin folds would be predicted to have a lesser body density (and more fat) than a person who has less thick skin folds.

Unfortunately, no perfect equation has been developed to predict body density or body fat on the basis of skin fold thickness, in spite of the fact that many such equations have been published [2, 3, 4, 5, 10, 18, 21]. Most of the equations have been developed for very specific populations (e.g., young sedentary males, female gymnasts) and have been based upon rather small samples of subjects. Also, it takes a

TABLE 7.2
Estimated Residual Volume of Lungs [21]

Age (years)	Residual Volume (cubic centimeters)
Females	
6–10	600
11–15	800
16–20	1000
21–25	1200
26–30	1400
Males	
6–10	900
11–15	1100
16–20	1300
21–25	1500
26–30	1700

great deal of practice to learn to measure skin folds accurately, and even among experienced technicians, differences of as great as 3 per cent can be expected with the skin fold technique [18]. Another problem with prediction equations based on skin folds and other anthropometrical measures (such as circumferences and diameters of limbs, abdomen, neck, etc.) is that they often are not sensitive enough to show differences in body fat brought on by periods of training or inactivity [18]. Accordingly, it is widely agreed that underwater weighing is a better research tool than measurement of skin fold thicknesses for estimating body fat changes over a period of time. Nevertheless, skin fold techniques are useful for screening subjects who may be grossly overfat or underfat and can serve as an effective motivating tool in physical education, athletics, and fitness programs.

Generalized Prediction Equations for Body Composition. As suggested earlier, most equations designed to predict body density on the basis of skin fold thickness and other measurements should only be used for very specific populations of subjects, i.e., subjects similar to those used for the development of the prediction equations. Some of these equations are described in the reference list at the end of this chapter. However, equations have been derived that can apparently be applied quite generally [3, 4]. Two of these equations are presented here to show how they are used.

Prediction of Body Density in Women Aged 18–55 Years [4]. The thickness of skin folds was measured in millimeters vertically at the back of the arm (triceps) and at the front of the thigh, and obliquely at the side just above the iliac crest (supra-ilium). The equation that was developed to predict body density (BD) used the sum of these three skin folds (A), the square of this sum (B) and the subject's age in years (C):

$$BD = 1.0994921 - 0.0009929\,A + 0.0000023\,B - 0.0001392\,C$$

For example, assume that a female athlete is 20 years old, weighs 50 kilograms, and has skin fold thicknesses of 8 millimeters at the triceps, 10 millimeters at the thigh, and 20 millimeters at the suprailium site. The sum of the three skin folds would be 38 millimeters, the square of that sum would be 1,444 millimeters, and her body density would be calculated as follows:

$$BD = 1.0994921 - (0.0009929 \times 38) + (0.0000023 \times 1444)$$
$$- (0.0001392 \times 20)$$
$$BD = 1.0622991$$

This athlete's body density value could then be used in the Siri equation (see previous section on hydrostatic weighing) for determining her per cent body fat as follows:

$$\% \text{ Body Fat} = (495/1.0622991) - 450$$
$$\% \text{ Body Fat} = 15.97 \%$$

Next, the per cent body fat just computed can be used to determine total body fat:

$$\text{Total Body Fat (kg)} = (\% \text{ Body Fat}/100) \times \text{Body Weight (kg)}$$
$$\text{Total Body Fat (kg)} = (15.97/100) \times 50$$
$$\text{Total Body Fat} = 7.985 \text{ kilograms}$$

Finally, the athlete's lean body mass can be calculated:

$$\text{Lean Body Mass (kg)} = \text{Body Weight (kg)} - \text{Total Body Fat (kg)}$$
$$\text{Lean Body Mass} = 50 - 7.985 = 42.015 \text{ kilograms}$$

This generalized equation for prediction of body fat in women is closely related to body fat estimated by hydrostatic weighing (correlation coefficient of about 0.84) and usually will come within 4 per cent of the per cent body fat value calculated from hydrostatic weighing [4]. However, the equation may be somewhat less accurate for women over 40 years of age than for younger women [4]. The equation should prove quite useful for screening purposes and for following changes in skin fold thickness (but not necessarily changes in body fat) with training and diet restriction.

that's good?

Prediction of Body Density in Men Aged 18–61 Years [3]. In the development of equations to predict body density in men, the thickness (mm) of skin folds was determined vertically at the front of the thigh, horizontally at the abdomen adjacent to the umbilicus, and vertically along the midaxillary line on the side at the level of the fifth rib [3]. The body density equation derived from the sum of these three skin folds (A), the square of this sum (B), and the age of the subject in years (C) is as follows:

$$BD = 1.1093800 - 0.0008267 \text{ A} + 0.0000016 \text{ B} - 0.0002574 \text{ C}$$

The equation for men is utilized in the same way as that previously illustrated for women. The prediction of body density with the equation for men has a correlation coefficient of 0.90 with estimation of body density by hydrostatic weighing [3].

Imperfections of Indirect Estimates of Body Composition

Both underwater weighing and skin fold techniques provide indirect estimates of body fat. Underwater weighing provides more accurate values for body density than does the skin fold technique. However, these body density values are then used in equa-

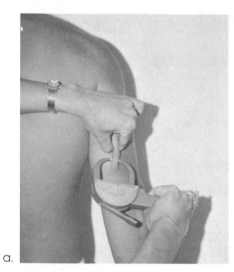

a.

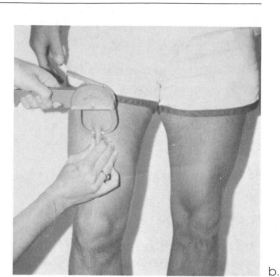

b.

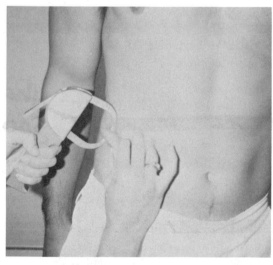

c.

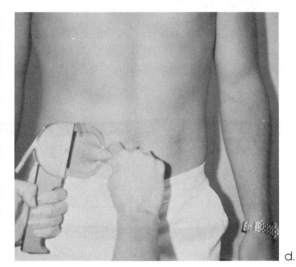

d.

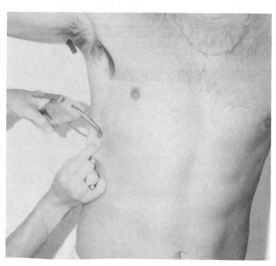

e.

FIGURE 7.2. Skinfold sites: a. triceps, b. thigh, c. suprailiac, d. abdominal, e. midaxillary line.

tions to estimate indirectly the per cent of body fat. The equations for converting body density to per cent body fat were derived from direct measures of body density and body composition on human cadavers. Unfortunately, the most popular equations were derived from analyses performed only on cadavers of white males. The equations may, therefore, lead to substantial errors when used to predict body fat from body density in females and nonwhites, regardless of the accuracy of the determination of body density by underwater weighing or skin fold testing [12].

Development of Body Fat During Growth and Aging

Body fat (adipose tissue) consists of many cells filled to a greater or lesser degree with triglyceride fat molecules. In young persons the total mass of fat tissue can be enlarged by increasing the amount of fat stored in each cell (hypertrophy) or by increasing the number of cells in adipose tissue (hyperplasia). In general, the number of fat cells seems to increase up to about 16 years of age, after which increased fat ordinarily accumulates because of increases in the size of cells already present [10, 14]. Fat cell number does not decrease with weight loss, but the size of the cells can be dramatically reduced by diet and exercise [10]. The per cent body fat for women aged 16–25 averages about 25, whereas that for men is about 13–15 per cent [10]. In women aged 30–68 body fat is increased to 29–34 per cent, and in men aged 27–59 body fat is 22–27 per cent [10].

However, just because a typical 40-year-old woman has 30 per cent body fat and most 40-year-old men have more than 20 per cent body fat does not mean that these are ideal values. Rather, it makes sense that the percentage of body fat in young adults, i.e., 15 per cent for men and 25 per cent for women, should be maintained or decreased in middle and later adulthood. Body fat greater than about 30 per cent for 40-year-old women or 20 per cent for 40-year-old men should be viewed as an indication of the onset of obesity.

It should be noted that a more consistent pattern of physical activity distinguishes those who are lean from those who develop moderate obesity. In other words, many persons become obese not because they eat more than their lean counterparts but because they expend less energy to burn up the food consumed [10]. Therefore, the fostering of regular physical activity habits early in childhood can play an important role in the maintenance of a healthful body composition throughout life.

Obesity and Weight Control

Obesity is a condition characterized by excessive fat storage. The degree of overfatness that is labeled "obesity" is arbitrary, but an excellent case has been made for establishment of an obesity criterion of 20 per cent body fat for males and 30 per cent for females [10, 14]. These criteria for obesity represent one standard deviation (5 per cent) above the mean average fatness for active young adult males (15 per cent fat) and females (25 per cent fat), respectively. It is true that average older persons have more fat than these percentages would indicate, but it seems likely that these higher values for fatness with aging are not beneficial to health; therefore, the values for younger adults are more logically used as baselines for determination of obesity.

Obesity of Childhood Onset and Adult Onset

There are two general types of obesity—childhood onset and adult onset. Obesity of childhood onset is the most severe and is characterized by adipose tissue which contains 4–5 times the number of fat cells as in normal persons, with little increase in cell size compared to normals [14]. Approximately 80 per cent of obese children remain obese as adults. Adult onset obesity, on the other hand, is characterized by an increased size of fat cells, but not an increase in cell number. Although treatment of obesity by diet and exercise often gives discouraging long-term results, the results are much more likely to be positive with adult onset obesity than with obesity that begins in childhood.

Obesity as a Risk Factor in Disease

Obesity is associated with an increased risk of high blood pressure, heart disease, diabetes, kidney disease, gall bladder disease, and joint disease [10, 14, 15]. Consequently, because more than 110 million people in the United States are too fat [10], any effect that exercise and diet can have on obesity will make a significant impact on the health status of the population.

Causes of Obesity—The Caloric Balance Equation

There are different specific causes of obesity in different individuals, and the physiological mechanisms involved are extremely complex. However, in all cases the energy consumed in the diet must exceed the energy expended in daily activities for excess fat to be deposited. Conversely, if the energy expenditure is greater than the energy consumption, fat will eventually be metabolized and weight will be lost. This idea that body weight changes are caused by imbalances between caloric intake and caloric expenditure (Fig. 7.3) has been an extremely useful concept in nutrition and weight control, but in practice it is sometimes difficult to demonstrate that the concept is valid. For example, rather dramatic short-term changes in body weight can be caused by very small changes in caloric balance accompanied by large changes in body water. Also, calculations of the number of dietary calories required to decrease or increase body weight are often foiled by unsuspected changes in the body's resting rate of metabolism—resting metabolic rate may decrease with caloric restriction and increase with caloric excess [20].

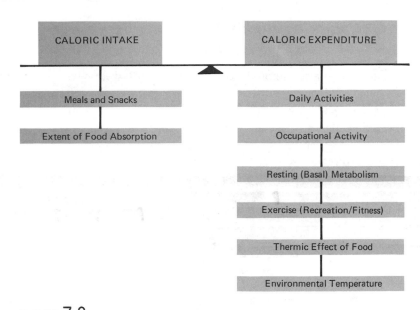

FIGURE 7.3. Some factors involved in caloric balance equation.

Caloric Deficit or Excess Required to Alter Body Weight

The standard rule of thumb for weight control is that if a person is currently maintaining a fairly stable weight, to lose 0.45 kilograms (1 pound) of fat tissue one must either increase energy expenditure or decrease energy intake (or some combination of the two) by 3,500 kilocalories. (A pound of pure triglyceride has an energy equivalent of 4,227 kilocalories, but a pound of fat tissue contains water and connective tissue in addition to triglyceride.) Similarly, a person with a stable body weight must decrease energy expenditure and/or increase energy intake by a total of 3,500 kilocalories to increase body fat by one pound. However, this figure of 3,500 kilocalories per pound of fat should only be used as a rough guideline for a one-pound loss or gain in body weight. One reason for this is that changes in body weight are not necessarily changes in fat tissue. During the early phases of dieting, for example, most of the weight loss is water; in this case, a caloric deficit of only 2,000 kilocalories or less may be required to produce a weight loss of one pound [20]. A pound of weight lost through exercise is likely to represent a greater loss of fat than will the same weight loss produced by dieting [10, 15]. In addition to disturbances in water balance, some factors that may contribute to discrepancies in *actual* compared to *predicted* weight changes include alterations in the basal metabolic rate, the energy expended in daily activities, the energy expended due to the thermic effect of food, and the energy expended for body temperature regulation. These factors are shown in Fig. 7.3.

Changes in Basal Metabolic Rate and Daily Physical Activity

Some individuals fail to lose the predicted amount of body weight when subjected to severe diets because their bodies adapt by reducing resting energy expenditure as much as 30 per cent and daily physical activity as much as 50 per cent [11, 20]. Thus, certain individuals adapt to low calorie diets by reducing their daily energy expenditure. Such persons may find it extremely difficult to lose weight even on a very strict diet, and some may even *gain* weight [11].

In contrast to calorie restriction, moderate exercise training is not likely to cause a decreased resting metabolic rate. In fact, exhaustive exercise may elevate metabolic rate for up to 12 or even 24 hours after exertion [21]. This is one of the apparent advantages of weight loss through exercise; the effect of increased caloric expenditure may last long after the exercise is completed. However, there may be some individuals who do experience a decreased resting metabolic rate and/or who minimize their daily physical activity when undertaking an exercise training program. This could perhaps account for the minimal effects of exercise on weight reduction in some persons. Research adequate to answer this question has not been completed.

Changes in the Thermic Effect of Food and in Environmental Temperature

If oxygen uptake at rest is measured after a 12-hour fast and then an hour or two after a meal, the oxygen uptake (resting metabolic rate) is 10–35 per cent greater after the meal [10, 24]. This phenomenon is called the "thermic effect" of food. The increased oxygen uptake is used for digestion and assimilation of the food and for the synthesis of proteins and other molecules following uptake of the food by the body's cells. Proteins have a greater thermic effect than fat or carbohydrate. Therefore, if a person begins a diet containing less protein than was previously consumed, it might be expected that the new diet would be associated with a lower thermic effect; this decreased energy expenditure may slightly offset the decreased caloric intake and result in less weight loss than predicted. Also, it is known that energy expenditure during exercise after a meal is greater by 10 per cent or more than energy expenditure during similar exercise while fasting [11, 24].

A minor but potentially significant factor which affects energy balance is the effect of environmental temperature on resting metabolism. Body heat production, which requires energy expenditure, tends to increase markedly in a cold environment and slightly in a hot, humid environment. Consequently, if a diet and/or exercise progiam is begun in an environment different from that in which the baseline measurements of energy balance (stable body weight) were made, the effect of the program might be somewhat greater or lesser than predicted because of the change in environmental temperature. As an extreme example, if a stable body weight for a subject were maintained on a daily caloric intake of 3,000 kilocalories during an Alaskan winter, perhaps only 2,500 kilocalories would be required to maintain the same weight if the subject moved to Tennessee. Thus, this subject could undergo a 500-kilocalorie dietary restriction upon moving to Tennessee and find that no body weight was lost.

In summary, there are many factors which can complicate the question of how many calories should be removed from the diet or added to an exercise program to accomplish a given goal of body weight and fat reduction. For most obese persons, a figure of 3,300–3,500 kilocalories per pound of body weight and fat will be reasonably correct. But in those cases where the calculated weight or fat loss is more or less than that predicted, changes in factors such as resting metabolic rate, daily activity, thermic effects of food and environmental temperature may help to explain the discrepancy.

The Role of Exercise in Weight Reduction Programs

Most obese persons find it extremely difficult to sustain a weight reduction program for a prolonged period. It is not unusual for eight out of ten persons who attempt to lose weight by dietary restriction to discontinue the program within one year. The few who manage to lose the desired amount of weight often fail to maintain the desired body weight for more than a year or two [1, 10, 15]. There are no comprehensive studies which answer the question of whether weight loss through a combination of diet and exercise is more likely to have a long-lasting effect than weight loss through diet alone. However, there are some positive aspects of exercise which suggest that this might be the case.

Exercise and Appetite. It is commonly believed that appetite is increased after exercise so that food intake is always greater in those who exercise than in those who are sedentary. This conception is accurate only to a limited degree. It is true that those who regularly perform exhaustive physical training or occupational labor do eat more than sedentary persons [15]. However, this extra food intake does not result in greater body weight or body fat, i.e., its energy content either matches or is less than the energy expended through exercise. Distance runners, for example, certainly eat more than most sedentary persons of the same age; a failure to compensate for most of the extreme amounts of energy expended through running would soon result in illness. But distance runners are extremely lean compared to their sedentary counterparts [10, 22]. Therefore, even though they may consume more calories on an absolute basis, such athletes eat less relative to their energy expenditure than the typical sedentary person. The same must be true for most high-level athletic groups, since all but ice hockey players and weight throwers (shot, discus, hammer, javelin) usually have less relative fat than the sedentary population (Tables 7.3, 7.4). Thus, at the very least, heavy occupational labor maintains the ratio of energy intake to energy expenditure, and intensive exercise training results in a relative suppression of appetite.

There is some evidence that certain types of exercise are associated with an absolute reduction in appetite when exercisers are compared to sedentary controls [13, 15, 17]. Male (but not female) rats who exercise regularly for intensive, brief workouts eat less than sedentary controls, and factory workers in jobs requiring moderate physical labor were shown to consume fewer calories than workers in sedentary jobs [15]. Therefore, there is no reason to believe that the increased caloric expenditure caused by regular physical exercise will be completely offset by increased food intake; in fact, exercise may actually cause a slight reduction in food intake.

TABLE 7.3
Per Cent Body Fat in Champion Male Athletes[1]

Athletes	Range of Per Cent Body Fat
Elite Marathon Runners	2.7–4.3
Elite Middle/Long-Distance Runners	1.4–5.0
Olympic Jumpers	6.8–8.2
Olympic Gymnasts	7.0–9.9
Olympic Track Sprinters/Hurdlers	8.2–10.1
Olympic Wrestlers (bantam & featherweight)	1.2–12.7
Olympic Basketball Players	8.4–13.2
Olympic Swimmers	9.0–12.0
Olympic Rowers	14.1–15.4
Olympic Decathloners	13.4–18.0
Olympic Throwers (shot, discus, hammer)	29.4–30.9
Professional Football Players	
Offensive Backs and Receivers	9.4
Defensive Backs	9.6
Linebackers	14.0
Offensive Linemen and Tight Ends	15.6
Defensive Linemen	18.2
Baseball Players	11.8–14.2
Jockeys	14.1
Ice Hockey Players	15.1
Body Builders	6.6–9.3
Power Lifters and Olympic Lifters	9.7–13.9

[1] From data compiled from various sources in references 6, 10, 22.

Effects of Exercise and/or Diet on Body Composition. For most persons either regular exercise or calorie-restricted diets can be successfully used to reduce body fat. One advantage of exercise in weight reduction programs is that weight loss accomplished through exercise is almost entirely due to fat loss with a maintenance or gain in lean tissue. On the other hand, weight loss through diet restriction often includes a large loss of water and some lean tissue, especially early in the weight reduction program [1, 10, 15]. With severe caloric restriction, weight loss for the first few days of the diet may be as great as 0.8 kilograms (1.8 pounds) per day, but this weight loss con-

TABLE 7.4
Per Cent Body Fat in Champion Female Athletes[1]

Athletes	Range of Per Cent Body Fat
Olympic Track Sprinters/Hurdlers	12.4–13.7
Olympic Jumpers	8.4–14.1
Olympic Divers	11.5–13.9
Olympic Gymnasts	11.0–14.7
Olympic Swimmers	14.5–16.6
Distance Runners	15.2–16.8
Volleyball Players	25.3
Shot, Discus and Javelin Throwers	27.0–33.8

[1] From data compiled from various sources in references 10, 22.

sists of about 70 per cent water, 25 per cent fat, and 5 per cent protein [20]. One reason why so much water is lost in the early stages of a severe diet is that glycogen from the liver and muscles is depleted for energy; each gram of glycogen binds about three grams of water which is released as the glycogen is utilized for fuel. This can account for about two kilograms (5 pounds) of water. An illustration of the effects of diet alone or diet plus exercise on the composition of body weight loss is shown in Figs. 7.4 and 7.5.

However, in some circumstances diet alone may be more effective than exercise alone in bringing about weight and fat loss. In those obese persons who have large numbers of fat cells (hyperplastic obesity), exercise without diet control may be totally

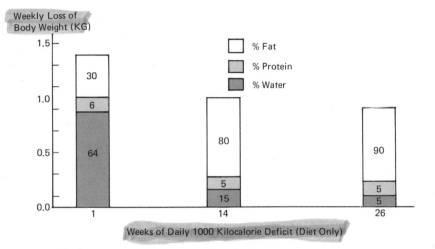

FIGURE 7.4. Schematic representation of composition of weight loss produced by caloric restriction of 1000 kcal daily.

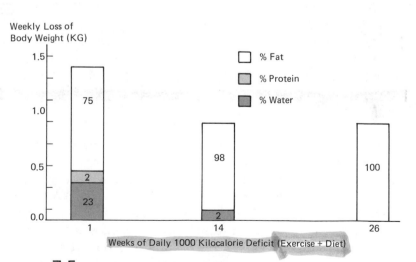

FIGURE 7.5. Schematic representation of composition of weight loss produced by 500 kcal caloric restriction plus 500 kcal increased energy expenditure through exercise.

ineffective in reducing body weight or body fat [8]. Presumably, these obese persons increase their food intake to counteract the caloric expenditure of exercise.

It should also be noted that exercise alone may produce much slower fat loss than diet alone [8] because a greater daily caloric deficit can ordinarily be achieved through diet restriction than through exercise, especially in obese persons, who often experience joint and muscle pain upon exercise. For example, an obese person may tolerate a 2,000 kilocalorie reduction in daily food intake but may not tolerate more than 500 kilocalories of exercise daily. However, the severe dietary restriction will probably result in greater loss of lean tissue than will the more moderate caloric deficit produced by exercise.

Importance of the Severity and Duration of Exercise and Diet. The amount of body fat lost through diet or exercise depends on many factors, the most important of which is the *degree* of caloric restriction by diet or excess caloric expenditure through exercise. Obviously, one would expect a greater loss of fat with severe dieting or exercise than with a minimal diet or exercise program. An exercise regimen in which a person works with greater intensity, for a longer duration per session, and for more sessions per week will produce a greater fat loss than a lesser exercise program [10].

The total *duration* of the exercise program or diet regimen is also important for predicting fat loss. With exercise programs lasting only a few weeks a significant change in body composition may not occur; in general, the longer the training program, the greater the loss of fat that can be expected. This principle holds true, of course, only so long as the caloric expenditure resulting from exercise and daily activities exceeds the caloric intake in the diet; once the energy intake and energy expenditure are in balance, body weight and body fat will stabilize. Modest exercise regimens may lead to a loss in weight of only one or two kilograms and a reduction in relative body fat of only 1 per cent. More rigorous exercise programs often lead to weight losses of three kilograms or more with changes of relative fat of 5 per cent or more, especially in individuals who have substantial amounts of excess fat at the beginning of the exercise program [2, 10]. With weight loss programs which rely only on caloric restriction, the duration of the diet is especially important in determining the amount of fat lost. This is so because in the early phase of dieting, much of the weight loss experienced is water, not fat. As the duration of the diet is lengthened, the loss of water decreases and that of fat increases [1, 10].

Exercise and Lean Body Mass. It is common for persons who have not exercised vigorously for many months or years to increase their lean tissue weight as they participate in a new exercise program. Sometimes the increase in lean body mass will offset the loss of fat tissue so that body weight remains stable, a phenomenon which can be discouraging to those who mark the success of an exercise program solely by the weight loss it produces. Such an increase in lean body mass may occur even with jogging and running programs [1, 10], which ordinarily do not stimulate muscle growth in more fit persons. In relatively fit individuals lean tissue can be increased by weight training, gymnastics, wrestling, and other types of heavy resistance exercise. Those who participate in weight training often exhibit body weights 20–30 per cent greater than the typical values listed in life insurance tables for persons of the same height [6]. Nearly all of this "excess" weight consists of extra muscle mass. Thus, exercise programs can alter body composition not only by reducing body fat, but also by increasing lean body mass [15].

Body Fat in Athletes. Numerous studies have been completed to characterize the body composition of various groups of athletes. The relative fat (% body fat) of champion athletes can serve as a rough guideline for the amount of fat athletes should be expected to carry for the greatest likelihood of success in a given event. For example, good distance runners almost invariably have a low percentage of body fat; to carry more fat than necessary will deter performance in distance running and in many other sports where moving the body mass requires a significant expenditure of energy. Values found for different groups of male and female athletes are shown in Tables 7.3 and 7.4.

Several points should be noted after inspection of Tables 7.3 and 7.4. First, the values reported are average values from one or more groups of athletes; there is a wide range of individual variation within these groups. For example, some of the best female distance runners have only 6 per cent body fat, a value less than that for many male distance runners [22]. Thus, these average values of per cent body fat are not necessarily the best values to enhance the probability of success in a specific event; some athletes excel with less or greater body fat percentages. Second, most of the groups of athletes had less relative body fat than the average of about 15 per cent for young adult males and 25 per cent for young adult females. Because few would question that such athletes are "healthier" than nonathletes, it may be that even the 15 per cent and 25 per cent values for body fat are too high for optimal health. Third, it is apparent that some very heavy athletes are not necessarily overly fat. Individual professional football players and weightlifters are usually much heavier than nonathletes relative to their heights. However, these athletes are heavier by virtue of greater lean tissue mass (muscle and bone) and not because of greater relative fat. Therefore, standard life insurance height and weight tables often unfairly penalize athletes for excess weight because those tables do not consider body composition.

Similarly, athletic trainers, coaches, and recruiters for the military, police, and firefighters may reject candidates for positions or require them to lose excessive weight if body composition is not taken into account. Body composition testing by skin fold or underwater weighing techniques is becoming increasingly common in screening candidates for such occupations. Such tests are also used for following the changes in skin folds or body composition of employees over a period of time.

Health Benefits of Exercise versus Dietary Restriction.

One important attribute of exercise in a weight reduction program is that regular exercise ordinarily produces improvements in cardiovascular function, muscular strength and endurance, ligament and bone strength, and flexibility. Such health benefits do not accrue to those who attempt to lose weight through diet alone. In addition, exercise can be recreational in nature to provide added incentive to maintain the weight reduction program. Weight loss through exercise can be enjoyable; weight loss through caloric restriction generally is not.

Guidelines for Establishing a Weight Reduction Program. There are several logical steps that should be followed if one is serious about losing weight and maintaining the new body weight. These steps are shown in Table 7.5.

Determination of the Desired Body Weight. Typically, one determines how much weight is to be lost rather arbitrarily. For example, Lilly Lumpylines may decide to lose weight until her red dress fits again, or George Grossegaster may strive to lose "5 or 10 pounds". A better procedure is to determine one's current lean body mass, decide what the ideal percent body fat would be, and calculate the desired body weight with the assumption that all weight lost will be fat. Mathematically, this procedure is expressed as follows:

$$\text{DESIRED BODY WEIGHT} = \frac{100 \times \text{CURRENT LEAN BODY WEIGHT}}{100 - \% \text{ BODY FAT DESIRED}}$$

Lean body mass is determined by either the underwater weighing technique or by the skin fold technique as described earlier in this chapter. The per cent body fat desired will ordinarily be at or below the average level for young adults, that is, 15 per cent for males and 25 per cent for females. However, if an athlete wishes to achieve optimal weight for performance in, for example, distance running, he or she may decide that 5 per cent is the desired percentage of body fat since champions in distance running typically exhibit this low level of fat. Let us assume that Lawrence Lardlegs currently weighs 90 kilograms (198 pounds), 20 per cent of which is body fat as determined by the skin fold technique. This means that Lawrence has a lean body weight of 72 kilograms (80 per cent of 90 kilograms). If Lawrence wishes to achieve a body fat percentage of 13 per cent, the calculation of his desired weight would be:

$$\text{DESIRED BODY WEIGHT} = \frac{100 \times 72}{100 - 13} = 7200/87 = 82.8 \text{ kg}$$

TABLE 7.5
Procedures for Weight Reduction Programs

Step 1: Determine what final body weight is desired and the length of time appropriate to reach that weight.

Step 2: Estimate the daily caloric intake which maintains the current body weight.

Step 3: Estimate the current daily caloric expenditure.

Step 4: Calculate the daily caloric deficit required to reach the desired body weight in the appropriate time period.

Step 5: Decide how the caloric deficit established in Step 4 will be achieved, i.e., the exercise expenditure and the dietary deficit.

Step 6: Keep careful records of body weight, food intake, and energy expenditure.

Step 7: Adjust the diet and/or exercise program as needed to achieve or maintain the weight reduction goal.

This means that Lawrence must reduce his current body weight of 90 kilograms by 7.2 kilograms (15.8 pounds) to achieve his desired body fat.

Optimal Rate of Weight Loss.   How much time is reasonable for a slimming program to achieve the desired body weight? What is the optimal rate of weight loss? Most authorities suggest that rapid crash diets are not satisfactory as more gradual programs over a prolonged duration. In other words, most people who attempt to lose weight by a starvation diet or other type of crash diet do not achieve and maintain their desired weights as often as those who lose weight more gradually. The usual guideline is that one should attempt to lose about 0.45 kilogram (1 pound) per week. Thus, Lawrence Lardlegs should plan to lose his 7.2 kilograms over at least a 16-week period (7.2/0.45 = 16).

Estimation of Daily Caloric Intake Which Maintains Current Body Weight.   Before the appropriate amount of caloric restriction for a reducing diet can be accurately determined, it is important to know how many calories are being consumed at the current body weight. In other words, it is important to know the baseline daily calorie consumption before deciding how many calories are to be eliminated from the diet. The most practical method of determining this baseline energy intake is by maintaining a dietary record. In this procedure the prospective dieter writes down the type and quantity of all food and drink consumed during meals and snacks over a period of 10–14 days. Next, the total energy value of the food and drink eaten is calculated with the aid of a table such as that found in Appendix B. Finally, the total energy consumption is divided by the number of days the dietary record was maintained; this gives an average daily caloric intake. Assuming that body weight has not changed significantly during the period of dietary recall and that the recall days were truly representative of the dieter's eating habits, this estimate of baseline caloric intake should provide a satisfactory value upon which to base an effective plan for weight reduction.

Estimation of Current Daily Caloric Expenditure.   As long as body weight has remained stable during the dietary recall period, one can be relatively certain that the daily caloric expenditure during that period was about the same as the caloric intake. Since determination of caloric intake by dietary record is usually more accurate than estimation of energy expenditure by physical activity recall, it is usually best to assume that energy expenditure will be similar to energy intake during a period of stable body weight. If, however, body weight is likely to be unstable during the dietary record period, the prospective dieter should also carefully record the nature and duration of all physical activity engaged in during the dietary record period. The caloric value of this activity can then be estimated with the use of a table of energy costs of different activities such as Table 5.2.

Another good reason to estimate the energy cost of daily physical activity prior to undertaking a weight loss program is to be able to determine whether the program has any effect on daily activity that might be reflected in a lesser or greater loss of body weight than predicted. For example, if less weight is being lost than expected, one could complete a second physical activity recall to determine if the dieter is becoming less active during the diet period.

Finally, it may be important to predict the type of exercise that will be pursued in the near future. In this way, if greater or lesser energy expenditure is projected in the near future, the weight reduction program can be adjusted accordingly. Thus, if one were planning a cross-country bicycle trip within a month of beginning a weight reduction plan, this extra caloric expenditure should be estimated and included as part of the plan.

If one wishes to have the option of finding out whether resting metabolic rate has changed as a function of the weight reduction program, it is also important to estimate resting energy expenditure before beginning the program. This is done in a laboratory or hospital setting where oxygen uptake can be measured for 10 minutes or so in the supine resting state after a 12-hour fast and a 30-minute period of undisturbed rest. The oxygen uptake can then be converted into kilocalories of energy expended per hour of rest per square meter of body surface area, the usual method of expressing basal or resting metabolic rate. It is rare that such direct measurements will be available, however. Unfortunately, attempts to estimate basal or resting metabolic rate indirectly are subject to a substantial amount of error. This makes it unlikely that any procedure other than direct measurement of daily resting metabolism will be useful.

Calculation of the Daily Caloric Deficit Required to Achieve the Desired Body Weight. Once the desired body weight has been determined, the appropriate rate of weight loss has been decided, and the current level of caloric intake and energy expenditure have been estimated, it is a simple matter to calculate the daily caloric deficit needed to bring about the desired change in weight. The steps required are outlined below.

1. Determine kilograms or pounds of body weight to be lost:

Total Weight Loss = Current Weight − Desired Weight

2. Determine the rate at which weight is to be lost. Usually this will be 0.45 kilograms (1 pound) per week. Otherwise, compute the rate as follows:

Weekly Rate of Weight Loss = Total Weight Loss/Weeks Available

3. Determine the daily caloric deficit required.

Daily Caloric Deficit = Weekly Rate of Weight Loss (kg) × 1,100

or

Weekly Rate of Weight Loss (lb) × 500

(The assumption is that a deficit of 7,700 kilocalories is required to lose a kilogram of fat tissue and 3,500 kilocalories to lose a pound of fat tissue. One seventh of these values is used to correct weekly rates to daily rates. It is usually better to think in terms of the daily deficit rather than a weekly or monthly deficit because working on a daily plan helps to establish a more regular pattern of monitoring food intake and energy expenditure.)

For example, if a woman currently weighs 70 kilograms (154 pounds) and wishes to achieve a weight of 60 kilograms (132 pounds), she would need to lose 10 kilograms (22 pounds). If she decided to attempt to lose 0.45 kilograms (1 pound) per week, she would have to establish a caloric deficit of 0.45 times 1,100 equals 495 kilocalories daily. If, on the other hand, she wished to lose 10 kilograms in a 10-week period, she would have to establish a caloric deficit of (10/10) times 1,100 equals 1,100 kilocalories per day.

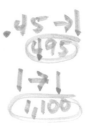

Establishing the Desired Caloric Deficit—Exercise. Most authorities believe that a combination of diet and exercise is the optimal approach to weight and fat reduction, but there is no fast rule about the exact proportions of diet and exercise in such a program.

If one enjoys exercise and is willing to find the time to exercise, most of a moderate caloric deficit (300–600 kcal/day) can be achieved by exercise. For those who do not enjoy exercise or cannot discipline themselves to participate in exercise, a greater emphasis must be placed on caloric restriction. A typical recommendation is that 50 per cent of the deficit be established through exercise and the remainder through diet.

There are many types of exercise and combinations of intensities, durations and frequencies that are appropriate to weight control programs. A good starting point is to consult a table of energy costs of various activities similar to Table 5.2. If one wishes to minimize exercise time, one should select an activity which ranks high in energy cost per hour. But if there are no time constraints, a low intensity exercise such as walking can be extremely useful in weight reduction; one simply has to walk for long durations. In addition to walking, activities such as jogging, cycling, cross-country skiing, swimming, tennis, racquetball, handball, and squash have all proved to be satisfactory in weight control programs [1, 11, 15]. These activities are especially valuable because they also bring about important cardiovascular benefits.

Establishing the Desired Caloric Deficit—Diet. There are a few guidelines that should be followed when establishing a weight control diet. First, avoid starvation diets, crash diets, and fad diets. These have health risks associated with them and generally do not produce satisfactory results for most dieters [10]. Second, there should be about 0.9 grams of protein in the diet for each kilogram of body weight; ordinarily, protein calories will constitute about 10–20 per cent of the total caloric intake in a moderate diet scheme. Second, about 60 per cent of the calories in the diet should come from carbohydrates, and most of these should be complex carbohydrates such as potatoes, rice, fruit, and vegetables, with little sugar. Third, no more than 30 per cent of the calories in the diet should be derived from fat, and unsaturated fat should make up about one half of the fat calories.

One can become fairly precise in counting the calories in the diet by referring to a table of caloric values of foods such as that in Appendix B. Such tables are quite comprehensive and allow one to calculate not only caloric intake but also the distribution of protein, carbohydrate, and fat in the diet.

Record Keeping and Weight Reduction Program Adjustment. It is important to maintain daily records of body weight, food intake, and exercise patterns, especially for those who have difficulty in adhering to the prescribed weight loss program. If weight is not lost as predicted, it is valuable to have careful records of caloric intake and exercise habits to determine whether the problem with the weight loss regimen lies with a failure to control caloric intake adequately, a failure to complete the required exercise program, or some change in resting metabolic rate or normal daily physical activity. Having determined where the problem exists, one need only adjust the exercise upward and/or the food consumption downward to continue the program on a revised basis. Of course, if the weight loss is much greater than expected, one can eat a little more or exercise a little less to decrease the rate of weight loss.

For those persons who need to lose only a few kilograms, it may be unnecessary to keep careful records of caloric intake and expenditure. Such individuals simply must concentrate on eating slightly less for meals and snacks and adhering to a regular program of exercise.

Weight Gain.   In contrast to the usual problem of overweight and overfat, some persons, especially young male athletes, wish to gain weight. There are no easy answers to this problem, since most persons will want to gain lean tissue with minimal fat. In some cases a person's resting metabolic rate may increase by 50 per cent in response to a high calorie diet so that little or no weight gain occurs [11]. Note that this is the reverse of what often happens in overweight persons who attempt to lose weight by caloric restriction.

The usual advice for those who wish to gain weight is to consume a high calorie diet and to perform regular weight lifting exercises to maximize the production of lean muscle and minimize the production of excess fat. Weight gain diets should contain at least 1.0–1.5 grams of protein daily per kilogram of body weight to insure adequate protein intake for increased muscle protein synthesis. The diet should also have a somewhat greater content of calorie-rich fat than normal or weight reduction diets. However, before embarking on such a program, one should consider the implications for cardiovascular health of prolonged consumption of a diet high in fat.

"Spot" Reducing.   It is often thought that fat can be removed from specific regions of the body, such as the thighs, arms, or abdomen, by exercising muscles in those regions. Thus, people perform situps in the hope of reducing abdominal fat and leg exercises to reduce thigh fat. Unfortunately, the deposition of fat in particular regions of the body is determined primarily by heredity. The fuel for situps may be derived from fat stores in the arms or the liver and have absolutely no effect on subcutaneous fat around the abdomen. Also, if the exercise is intense, most of the fuel may be glucose and glycogen with very little degradation of fat unless carbohydrate calories are restricted. Most studies have shown no change in fat cell size as a result of localized exercise [1, 7, 21]. Situps can reduce abdominal circumference, but this effect is due to increased muscle tone, not to decreased fat. The best way to rid the body of subcutaneous fat is by a combination of diet and exercise of many large muscle groups in activities such as running, walking, cycling or swimming.

REVIEW QUESTIONS

1. Explain why some body fat is essential to health.
2. What argument can you propose against the definition of obesity as excess body weight for height?

3. What health burdens does obesity impose?
4. Explain the principle underlying the determination of body fat by hydrostatic weighing.
5. Contrast the percentage of body fat in most athletic groups relative to the sedentary population.
6. Describe how body composition testing can be useful in testing athletes, policemen, firemen, and other groups. Of what value is body composition evaluation in weight control?
7. With respect to body composition changes, what advantage is there to weight loss by exercise rather than diet?
8. Why is diet important in weight control programs, especially in cases where large amounts of weight must be lost?
9. What are the prospects for a person who begins a weight control program to continue on the program for more than a few weeks or months?
10. Why is the weight lost during the first few days of a diet likely to be much greater than that lost later in the program?
11. When body weight is stable, caloric intake and expenditure are in balance. List the factors which are included in the determination of caloric expenditure.
12. Why is it recommended that one should attempt to produce a weekly caloric deficit of only about 3,500 kcal in a weight control program?
13. How can changes in resting metabolism confound efforts to lose or gain weight?
14. Explain the relationship between exercise and appetite. Does appetite necessarily increase when one exercises more?
15. What are some health benefits of losing body weight by exercise rather than by diet only?
16. Assume that your body weight currently contains 30 per cent fat. Using your current body weight, design a weight control program which would allow you to attain a value of 20 per cent body fat over a period of 100 days.
17. Explain why spot reducing usually is ineffective.

REFERENCES

[1] Franklin, B. A., and M. Rubenfire. Losing weight through exercise. *Journal of the American Medical Association,* 1980, **244:**377–379.
[2] Holland, G. J. A review of in vivo quantitative analysis of body composition. In R. H. Cox and J. K. Nelson, eds., *AAHPERD Research Consortium Symposium Papers.* Washington, D.C.: American Alliance for Health, Physical Education, Recreation and Dance, 1980, pp. 46–75.
[3] Jackson, A. S., and M. L. Pollock. Generalized equations for predicting body density of men. *British Journal of Nutrition,* 1978, **40:**497–504.
[4] Jackson, A. S., M. L. Pollock, and A. Ward. Generalized equations for predicting body density of women. *Medicine and Science in Sports and Exercise,* 1980, **12:**175–182.
[5] Katch, F. I., and V. L. Katch. Measurement and prediction errors in body composition assessment and the search for the perfect prediction equation. *Research Quarterly for Exercise and Sport,* 1980, **51:**249–260.
[6] Katch, V. L., F. I. Katch, R. Moffatt, and M. Gittleson. Muscular development and lean body weight in body builders and weight lifters. *Medicine and Science in Sports and Exercise,* 1980, **12:**340–344.
[7] Krotkiewski, M., A. Aniansson, G. Grimby, P. Bjorntorp, and L. Sjostrom. The effect of unilateral isokinetic strength training on local adipose and muscle tissue morphology, thickness, and enzymes. *European Journal of Applied Physiology,* 1979, **42:**271–281.
[8] Krotkiewski, M., K. Mandroukas, L. Sjöstrom, L. Sulivan, J. Wetterqvist, and P. Bjorntorp. Effects of long-term physical training on body fat, metabolism, and blood pressure in obesity. *Metabolism,* 1979, **28:**650–658.
[9] Liepa, G. U., E. J. Masoro, H. A. Bertrand, and B. P. Yu. Food restriction as a modulator of age-related changes in serum lipids. *American Journal of Physiology,* 1980, **238:**E253–E257.

[10] McArdle, W. D., F. I. Katch, and V. L. Katch. *Exercise Physiology: Energy, Nutrition, and Human Performance.* Philadelphia: Lea & Febiger, 1981.

[11] Miller, D. S. Food intake and energy utilization. In J. Parizkova and V. A. Rogozkin, eds., *Nutrition, Physical Fitness, and Health.* Baltimore: University Park Press, 1978, pp. 3–8.

[12] Moore, M. Percent body fat testing: 'A two-edged sword.' *Physician and Sportsmedicine,* 1980, **8:**79–81.

[13] Nikoletseas, M. M. Food intake in the exercising rat: a brief review. *Neuroscience & Biobehavioral Reviews,* 1980, **4:**265–267.

[14] Oscai, L. B. Obesity. In G. A. Stull, ed., *Encyclopedia of Physical Education, Fitness, and Sports: Training, Environment, Nutrition, and Fitness.* Salt Lake City, Utah: Brighton Publishing Co., 1980, pp. 356–361.

[15] Oscai, L. B. The role of exercise in weight control. *Exercise and Sport Sciences Reviews,* 1973, **1:**103–123.

[16] Phinney, S. D., E. S. Horton, E. A. H. Sims, J. S. Hanson, E. Danforth, Jr., and B. M. LaGrange. Capacity for moderate exercise in obese subjects after adaptation to a hypocaloric, ketogenic diet. *Journal of Clinical Investigation,* 1980, **66:**1152–1161.

[17] Rolls, B. J., and E. A. Rowe. Exercise and the development and persistence of dietary obesity in male and female rats. *Physiology & Behavior,* 1979, **23:**241–247.

[18] Sinning, W. E. Use and misuse of anthropometric estimates of body composition. *Journal of Physical Education, Health and Recreation,* 1980, **51:**43–45.

[19] Staff. Weight reduction in wrestling. *Physician and Sportsmedicine,* 1981, **9:**79–96.

[20] Van Itallie, T. B., and M.-U. Yang. Diet and weight loss. *New England Journal of Medicine,* 1977, **297:**1158–1161.

[21] Wilmore, J. H. *Athletic training and physical fitness.* Boston: Allyn and Bacon, 1977.

[22] Wilmore, J. H., C. H. Brown, and J. A. Davis. Body physique and composition of the female distance runner. *Annals of the New York Academy of Sciences,* 1977, **301:**764–776.

[23] Wilmore, J. H., P. A. Vodak, R. B. Parr, R. N. Girandola, and J. E. Billing. Further simplification of a method for determination of residual lung volume. *Medicine and Science in Sports and Exercise,* 1980, **12:**216–218.

[24] Zahorska-Markiewicz, B. Thermic effect of food and exercise in obesity. *European Journal of Applied Physiology,* 1980, **44:**231–235.

[25] Zambraski, E. J. Weight loss for sports competition. In G. A. Stull, ed., *Encyclopedia of Physical Education, Fitness, and Sports: Training, Environment, Nutrition, and Fitness.* Salt Lake City, Utah: Brighton Publishing Co., 1980, pp. 369–376.

CHAPTER

8

The Physiology of Aerobic Endurance

ENDURANCE or staying power in some physical activities such as basketball, soccer, distance running, swimming, and cycling is limited by the capacity of the circulatory system (heart, blood vessels, and blood) and the respiratory system (lungs) to deliver oxygen to the working muscles and to carry chemical waste products away from them. Such activities are classified as "cardiovascular," "cardiorespiratory," or, as in this text, "aerobic" endurance activities.

The degree to which circulation and respiration limit one's performance depends on many factors, chief of which are the intensity of the exercise, the duration of the activity, and the amount of static muscle contraction involved. In general, the lesser the intensity, the longer the duration, the lesser the amount of static contraction involved, the more that performance in the activity will be limited by the functioning of the heart, blood vessels, blood and lungs. Distance running, for example, is a relatively low-intensity, long-duration activity consisting mostly of rhythmic, nonstatic muscle contractions and is limited mainly by aerobic capacity. Weight lifting performance, on the other hand, is limited mostly by the strength and endurance of a few muscles that are contracting statically to a large extent. These static contractions tend to close off blood vessels and restrict blood flow to the working muscles, so that the muscles must work in the presence of very little oxygen. Therefore, weight lifting would be categorized as an activity requiring relatively little aerobic endurance.

Some events, such as running from 400 to 800 meters or swimming for 200 meters, fall in between weight lifting and distance running. Middle-distance running and swimming events are not limited so much by endurance of a few muscle groups or by oxygen transport to working muscles as by a combination of oxygen transport capacity and capacity for anaerobic energy (ATP) production in *many* large muscle groups. Thus, all "endurance" activities have both aerobic and anaerobic compo-

137

nents, the shorter events having a larger anaerobic component and the longer events being more aerobic in nature. Table 8.1 shows one way of classifying some activities based on the degree to which the energy for these activities is derived from anaerobic sources within the working muscles or from aerobic sources requiring the transport of oxygen to the muscles. Note that the classification of staying power for an activity as "anaerobic" or "aerobic" is somewhat arbitrary and depends only on the extent to which muscular endurance is limited by anaerobic or aerobic energy production.

Part 1: Cardiac Function

It is known that a period of aerobic endurance training is followed by an increased ability to tolerate long-distance running or swimming; that is, the trained person can run or swim farther and faster. Many physiologists believe that this increased endurance can be explained almost entirely by the improved functioning of the trained heart and that other functional changes in the circulatory, respiratory, and muscular systems are of little significance. Because the heart maintains circulation, and therefore all organic function, it is certainly understandable that many have used cardiac function as the single criterion for determining endurance capacity and training effectiveness. However, as described later in this and subsequent chapters, factors other than heart

TABLE 8.1
Aerobic and Anaerobic Energy Production in Various Activities[1]

Activity	% Anaerobic Energy	% Aerobic Energy	Activity Classification
25 m. Swim 50 m. Sprint	95	5	Speed, Strength
50 m. Swim 100 m. Sprint	85	15	Speed, Strength
100 m. Swim 200 m. Sprint	80	20	Speed, Strength, Anaerobic Endurance
200 m. Swim 400 m. Sprint	70	30	Anaerobic Endurance, Speed, Strength
400 m. Swim 800 m. Run	60	40	Anaerobic Endurance, Aerobic Endurance, Speed
800 m. Swim 1500 m. Run	40	60	Aerobic Endurance, Anaerobic Endurance
1600 m. Swim 3000 m. Run Basketball (Fast Break Style) Soccer Fullback	15	85	Aerobic Endurance, Anaerobic Endurance
Marathon (26 mi.)	<1	>99	Aerobic Endurance

[1] Exact percentages depend on the state of training of the individual, and upon natural endowment in such factors as muscle fiber types, speed, muscle size, and body weight.

function are also important in circulorespiratory endurance performance and must not be overlooked.

Cardiac Output at Rest and During Exercise

At rest the heart pumps four to six liters of blood into the arteries of a healthy college student each minute. This rate of pumping is known as the *cardiac output.* It may be increased about four times to approximately 22 liters per minute in normal young men and 15 liters per minute in average young women [26, 27]. In highly trained male athletes cardiac outputs as high as 30 liters per minute have been measured [46].

A resting cardiac output of five liters per minute may be achieved if the heart rate is 65 beats per minute and if the stroke volume (amount pumped per beat) is 77 milliliters ($65 \times 77 = 5005$ milliliters $= 5.005$ liters). During vigorous exercise, the cardiac output may be increased to 30 liters per minute by a tripling of heart rate to 195 beats per minute and a doubling of stroke volume to 154 milliliters ($195 \times 154 = 30.030$ liters). Therefore, the increased cardiac output that accompanies exercise is due to increases in both heart rate and stroke volume (Fig. 8.1) [46, 47].

If one were to record heart rate at rest just prior to, during, and for several minutes after a vigorous bout of running or swimming, one would discover an anticipatory rise in heart rate just prior to exercise, a gradual leveling off during exercise (if the work is not maximal) and a slow decline back toward resting values following exercise (Fig. 8.1). Before attempting to explain how these changes in heart rate are brought about, it may be useful to review briefly some of the factors known to affect the heart rhythm.

Control of Heart Rate

The heart is normally controlled by neural, hormonal, and intrinsic factors. Of these general control classifications, the control of heart rate by the nervous system is the most important.

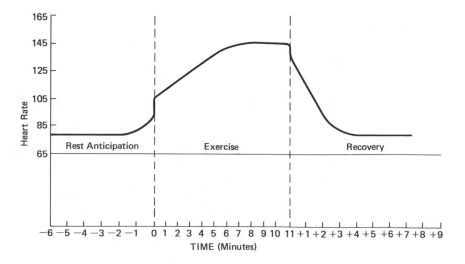

FIGURE 8.1. Heart rate response before, during, and after moderate exercise.

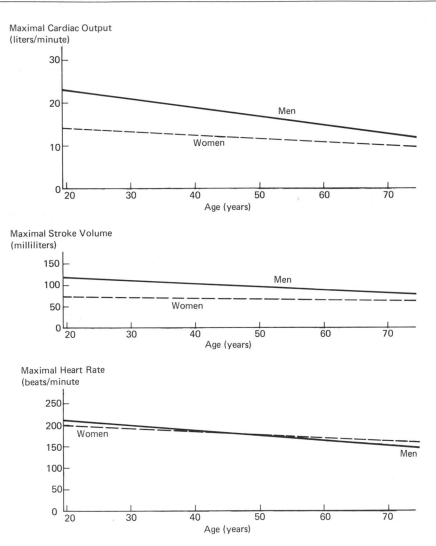

FIGURE 8.2. Maximal cardiac output, stroke volume and heart rate for adult men and women [26, 27].

Neural Factors in Heart Rate Control. The heart is supplied with nerves from both sympathetic and parasympathetic divisions of the autonomic nervous system. The sympathetic *cardiac accelerator* nerves secrete norepinephrine (noradrenaline) and some epinephrine (adrenaline) at their endings on the heart to make the heart speed up. The parasympathetic *vagus* nerve endings secrete acetylcholine, which slows the rhythm of the heart. The firing of the cardiac accelerator nerves and vagus nerves is controlled by nerve centers in the brain, primarily in the medulla. These cardiac control centers can be stimulated by emotional excitement, by nerve reflexes sensitive to changes in muscle chemistry, blood pressure, and arterial pH, and by many other factors. Some circumstances call for the cardiac accelerator nerves to be activated, whereas others call for the vagus nerves to slow the heart. However, there is always some activity of both accelerator and vagus nerves; normally, no situations exist when either the vagus or the cardiac accelerator nerves are totally silent.

The heart rate at rest is ordinarily much more powerfully influenced by the vagus nerves than by the sympathetic nerves. Thus, the heart speeds up markedly if the vagus nerves are cut, but the heart slows only modestly if the function of the accelerator nerves is interrupted. To speed the heart up, therefore, it is feasible to increase the activity of the accelerator nerves or to decrease the output of the vagus nerves or to do some of both. In fact, it is likely that *most of the increase in heart rate during exercise is caused by inhibition of the normal vagal activity;* there is increased accelerator nerve firing during exercise, but it is less significant overall than decreased vagal activity.

Hormonal Factors in Heart Rate Control. Hormones circulating in the blood can directly affect the heart rhythm. Epinephrine and norepinephrine secreted from the adrenal gland are the most powerful of these circulating hormones; they increase the heart rate. Hormones from the thyroid gland also increase the heart rate.

Intrinsic Factors in Heart Rate Control. If the heart muscle is warmed, it beats more rapidly; cold slows it down. Increased filling of the heart chambers with blood stretches the sinoatrial node, the "pacemaker" of the heart; this stimulates the node to set a faster heart rhythm. Changes in the balance of electrolytes such as potassium and sodium in the heart tissue can either increase or decrease the heart rate. Each of these factors—temperature, stretch, and electrolyte balance—operate directly on the heart without the intervention of the nervous system or hormones. Consequently, these are considered *intrinsic* factors in heart rate control.

Anticipatory Rise in Heart Rate

The pre-exercise anticipatory rise in heart rate is thought to be caused by an "emotional" stimulation of the cardiac accelerator centers at the base of the brain. The origin of the excitement or anxiety before exercise is the *limbic system* of the brain (the limbic lobe of the cortex and the hypothalamus). The limbic system activates nerve fibers leading to the cardiac control centers of the medulla; this increases the firing of the cardiac accelerator nerves and decreases firing of the vagus nerves.

This anticipatory rise in heart rate may also be caused in part by increased circulating epinephrine and norepinephrine from the adrenal glands and sympathetic nerves that have been stimulated by the limbic system. As one would expect, the anticipatory rise in heart rate is much greater during a highly competitive situation than during, for example, a noncompetitive practice session.

Exercise Heart Rate

Even in the absence of an anticipatory rise in heart rate, experts have detected that the heart beats faster almost instantaneously when exercise starts [44]. The first beat of the heart after exercise begins is faster than the preceding ones. The speed with which this response occurs makes it apparent that it is caused by a nerve reflex, probably at least partly originating from receptors in the working muscles and/or joints [44, 49]. Free nerve endings, muscle spindles, and receptors in joint capsules have been suggested as the receptors responsible for this instantaneous cardioacceleration as exercise begins. Thus, as muscles begin to contract and joints begin moving through a range of motion, impulses are generated in the muscles and joint receptors; these impulses then pass to the spinal cord and to the cardiac regulating center of the brain. There the vagus nerves are inhibited so that a rise in heart rate occurs.

"Central Command" and Exercise Heart Rate. As the motor areas of the cortex of the brain become activated during voluntary movement, those areas send impulses not only to the working muscles, but also to the cardiac regulatory centers of the medulla of the brain to excite the cardiac accelerator nerves and inhibit the vagus nerves. This effect is similar to that occurring when the limbic system is activated during the anticipatory rise in heart rate prior to exercise. The control of cardiovascular and respiratory responses to exercise by higher centers of the brain is called control by "central command" [49].

Muscle Chemoreceptors and Exercise Heart Rate. As muscles contract, potassium, lactic acid, and a number of other chemicals leave the intracellular space and accumulate in the tissue fluid. It is thought that potassium leakage from muscle cells may stimulate free endings of small nerve fibers in the blood vessels or connective tissue of the muscle tissue. These nerve fibers may then transmit signals to the cardiac control centers of the brain to increase heart rate [23, 45, 49]. During severe static (isometric) contractions which cause blood flow to be greatly restricted, a lack of oxygen (hypoxia) in the tissue may also stimulate nerve endings reflexly to increase heart rate [49].

Arterial Chemoreceptors and Exercise Heart Rate. There are nerve endings in the walls of the carotid arteries and the aorta that respond to changes in blood oxygen, carbon dioxide, and pH. The role of these chemoreceptors in heart rate control during exercise is probably minimal because arterial oxygen and carbon dioxide do not ordinarily change in a direction which would be expected to excite the chemoreceptors. A reduction in arterial pH accompanies the lactic acid increase in the blood during severe exercise. However, any small effect of this fall in pH on heart rate is probably mediated indirectly by an increased breathing rate [49]. In other words, there is no firm evidence that arterial chemoreceptors play a significant role in the increased heart rate that occurs during exercise.

Circulating Hormones and Exercise Heart Rate. As exercise exceeds moderately high intensity (at a heart rate above 150) for 20 minutes or more, epinephrine, norepinephrine, and perhaps free thyroid hormone levels rise progressively in the blood. These hormones increase the heart rate during prolonged heavy exercise.

Intrinsic Factors and Exercise Heart Rate. Finally, there seem to be factors in the heart itself that increase its rate of contraction during exercise. This is suggested by the fact that even when the nerves to the heart are blocked chemically or surgically, the heart still beats faster in response to exercise. Persons who have had their cardiac nerves blocked are not capable of working quite as hard as normal persons, but their heart rates can rise to 120 or so during treadmill running. One of the intrinsic factors is the increased rate of firing of the sinoatrial node in response to its being stretched as more blood returns to the right side of the heart during rhythmic exercise. Another intrinsic factor is the effect of temperature on the speed with which action potentials can be initiated in the heart. As the temperature of the heart rises during vigorous exercise, the heat causes a faster rate of development of the electrochemical impulses which stimulate the heart to beat. This effect can be observed also in the absence of exercise by drinking a hot drink and recording the gradual rise in one's heart rate as the heat passes through the body fluids from the warmed esophagus to the nearby heart.

Heart Rate After Exercise

The heart slows rapidly when exercise stops. With a fall in accelerating influences from the limbic system and motor cortex, from muscle and joint mechanoreceptors, and from muscle chemoreceptors, it is easy to understand why the heart rate declines, but it is not so easy to understand why it doesn't return to normal even faster than it does. The accelerator effect of increased levels of epinephrine and of increased temperature of the heart may continue to operate until the body cools and the epinephrine is metabolized. Other unknown intrinsic mechanisms may also be operating. It also seems likely that potassium and other metabolites which are produced by the working muscles affect the cardioregulator centers of the medulla to maintain a high heart rate until the levels of these chemicals in the body fluids return to resting values. A summary of the probable factors involved in heart rate changes before, during, and after exercise is shown in Table 8.2.

TABLE 8.2
Summary of Probable Factors Involved in Heart Rate Changes Before, During, and After Exercise

Factor	Anticipatory Rise	Exercise Rise	Postexercise Fall
Neural Activity Originating in the Brain			
1. Activity of the limbic system	Increase	Increase	Decrease
2. Activity of motor cortex		Increase	Decrease
Peripheral Nerve Reflexes			
1. Muscle/joint mechanoreceptor reflexes		Increase	Decrease
2. Muscle chemoreceptor reflexes		Increase	Decrease
Circulating Hormones			
Epinephrine, thyroxine, norepinephrine	Increase	Increase	Decrease
Intrinsic Factors			
1. Stretch of sinoatrial node		Increase	Decrease
2. Temperature effect		Increase	Decrease

Stroke Volume

The amount of blood pumped into the aorta with each beat of the heart is known as the stroke volume, and the stroke volume increases up to twice that at rest when one exercises strenuously in an upright posture—for example, when running or cycling [46]. This increased stroke volume is probably a result of increased stimulation of the heart muscle by epinephrine and norepinephrine from the sympathetic nervous system and the adrenal glands. These two hormones cause the heart not only to beat faster but to contract more forcefully and completely, thus ejecting more blood with each contraction. Also, the effect of increased amounts of blood returning to the heart as a result of muscle action on veins may cause the fibers of the heart to be stretched. This results in a more forceful contraction of those fibers because of a more effective overlap of actin and myosin filaments. The effect is known as the Frank-Starling phenomenon and causes a more complete emptying of the heart with each beat during exercise [54].

The increased stroke volume that occurs during exercise in an upright posture is not always seen when a person performs exercise while in a prone or supine position [47]. For example, a swimmer would experience an increased cardiac output, but mostly because of a greater heart rate; stroke volume changes very little when going from a resting prone or resting supine condition to an exercising prone or exercising supine position. The explanation for this is that in a horizontal posture, the stroke volume is near maximal even at rest. The effect of upright exercise is simply to bring the stroke volume up to the value it would have achieved had the person been at rest in a prone or supine position (Fig. 8.3).

Possible Heart Damage Because of Sudden Heavy Exercise—Value of Warmup

The value of warmup prior to strenuous physical activity has usually been attributed to the prevention of muscular or connective tissue injuries, or to a better circulation of oxygen and nutrients to the working muscles. However, a much more important value

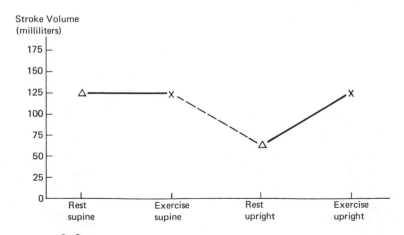

FIGURE 8.3. Effects of posture and exercise on cardiac stroke volume.

of warmup may be the prevention of heart damage during the first few seconds of strenuous exercise. This has been suggested by studies which show that subjects who undertook sudden, strenuous treadmill exercise with no prior warmup exhibited electrocardiographic abnormalities [6] or other signs of abnormal function of the left ventricle [20]. It appears that sudden strenuous exercise causes an insufficiency of blood flow to the heart muscle. These signs that the hearts of the subjects were not obtaining a large enough blood supply were nearly all abolished when the strenuous run was preceded by a 2-minute warmup run on the treadmill. The warmup precaution is advisable for everyone who engages in strenuous exercise and especially for older subjects who have a greater risk of heart damage.

Part 2: Circulation

During running, swimming, and other aerobic endurance activities, the working muscles may use oxygen at a rate ten to twenty times greater than when at rest. To supply the extra oxygen required, not only must cardiac output increase, but the circulation of blood through the working muscles must be dramatically increased. This increased cardiac output is delivered to working muscles by two changes in the vascular system — 1) dilation of blood vessels in the working muscles and 2) constriction of blood vessels to reduce blood flow and then allows dilation of those vessels to increase flow.

Blood Flow in Working Muscles

In resting leg muscles, blood flows at a rate of about 5 milliliters of blood per 100 grams of muscle per minute. Thus, in a gastrocnemius muscle weighing 500 grams (a little over a pound) blood flows through at 25 milliliters (about 5 teaspoons) per minute. During heavy rhythmical exercise such as running, the blood flow in this muscle may increase by 15 times, up to 375 milliliters per minute [2]. This enhancement of circulation is shown in Fig. 8.4, which also shows that blood flow falls sharply as the muscles contract and rises when they relax. This pattern of flow is caused by the rhythmical muscle contraction and relaxation, which alternately compresses the blood vessels to reduce blood flow and then allows dilation of those vessels to increase flow.

Control of Blood Flow in Skeletal Muscle. Blood flow to skeletal muscle is determined 1) by the arterial pressure which drives the blood into the vessels of the muscle, 2) by the degree to which the blood vessels are dilated (opened) to receive the blood, and 3) by the extent to which the blood is able to leave the muscle through the venous system so that the inflow of more blood is not blocked.

Blood Pressure and Blood Flow to Active Muscles. The major factor which elevates blood pressure during exercise is the increased cardiac output. The tendency for arterioles to constrict in tissues other than skeletal muscle helps to maintain the high arterial pressure. As will be described later in this chapter, blood vessels in the liver, the kidney, the digestive organs, and perhaps other tissues are relatively constricted during heavy exercise. This vasoconstriction in tissues other than the working muscles in-

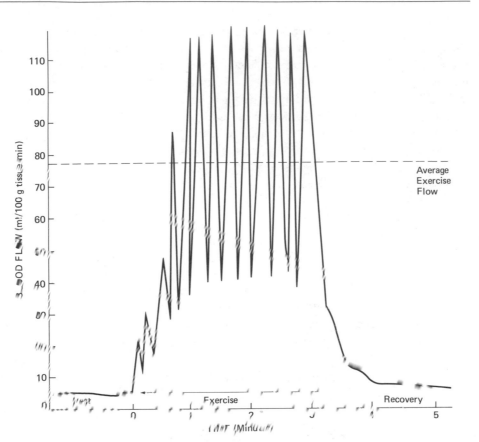

FIGURE 8.4. Blood flow in working muscles.

creases the resistance to blood flow in those tissues and diverts the blood into the vessels of the working muscles. A rise in blood pressure is especially important in exercise because the increased pressure is needed to overcome the tendency of contractions to close off arterioles in the muscle itself.

Vasodilation and Blood Flow to Active Muscles. Figure 8.5 shows the anatomy of a capillary bed in skeletal muscle. The arterioles that deliver blood to capillary networks have smooth muscle cells in their walls. If this smooth muscle is contracted, the arterioles constrict and reduce blood flow. If the smooth muscle relaxes, the arterioles dilate to let more blood pass into the muscle. There are also smooth muscle cells (precapillary sphincters) located at the entrances to individual capillaries (Fig. 8.5). These precapillary sphincters act as valves to close off capillaries when the sphincters are contracted and to allow flow when they are relaxed. It is clear that the increased blood flow to active skeletal muscle is primarily caused by a massive relaxation of the smooth muscle cells at the arterioles and at the capillary openings. However, exactly how this relaxation is controlled is not so clear.

The smooth muscle of blood vessels is controlled by three factors:

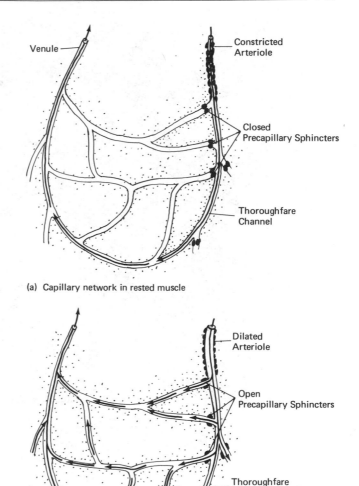

(a) Capillary network in rested muscle

FIGURE 8.5. Local blood flow through skeletal muscle.

(b) Capillary network in exercising muscle

sic nerve activity, intrinsic nerve activity, and *metabolite concentrations.* The extrinsic innervation consists of sympathetic vasoconstrictor fibers and sympathetic vasodilator fibers. The vasoconstrictor fibers secrete norepinephrine, which makes the smooth muscle cells contract. The vasodilator fibers secrete acetylcholine, which relaxes the smooth muscle. The extrinsic innervation is of minor importance in the vasodilation that occurs in working skeletal muscle because cutting of these nerves has little or no effect on the increased blood flow. However, *the sympathetic extrinsic nerves may be important in any anticipatory elevation in blood flow that may occur* [24].

Intrinsic Nerves. The intrinsic nerves in the walls of arterioles have only recently been demonstrated. These nerves have their cell bodies in the arterioles, not in the spinal cord, and appear to be responsible for almost all of the early vasodilation in

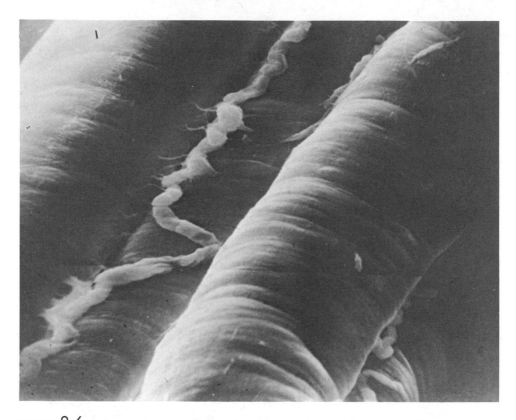

FIGURE **8.6.** Stereo electron micrograph showing surfaces of three muscle fibers. A twisted white capillary is shown on surface of central muscle fiber. (Courtesy of R. E. Carrow, W. W. Heusner and W. D. Van Huss, Michigan State University, E. Lansing, Michigan.)

working muscle [24]. As these intrinsic nerves cause the arteriolar smooth muscles to relax, blood flow begins to increase within one-half second and continues to build for another 30–45 seconds until a plateau is reached. As exercise stops, the intrinsic nerve activity stops very rapidly and is not responsible for the continued high blood flow during recovery [24]. It appears that the major factor in greater blood flow to exercising skeletal muscle is dilation of the arterioles, which occurs within five seconds of the start of contraction. Once the arterioles are dilated, the flow in the capillaries is determined passively by factors such as capillary size, red cell size, and blood viscosity [25].

Metabolites. Because cutting of the extrinsic nerves was known to have little effect on the exercise-induced vasodilation in skeletal muscle, it was widely agreed for some years that the vasodilation must be caused by local chemical factors that relax the smooth muscle cells of the arterioles. Indeed, a number of chemical changes that occur in working muscle are capable of causing vasodilation. In particular, decreased oxygen, increased potassium, increased adenosine, increased carbon dioxide, decreased pH, and increased phosphate have been suggested as the best candidates for metabolite control of circulation [15, 24, 28]. However, it is now apparent that the

TABLE 8.3
Summary of Vasodilator Influences in Contracting Skeletal Muscle

Time	Extrinsic Nerves	Intrinsic Nerves	Metabolites
Anticipation of Exercise	Yes	No	No
Initiation of Exercise	No	Yes	No
Prolongation of Exercise	No	Yes	Yes
Recovery	No	No	Yes

changes in these chemicals occur too slowly to account for the initial increase in blood flow during exercise [24, 25]. Nevertheless, it seems likely that such *chemical changes may contribute to the maintenance of increased flow during prolonged exercise and during recovery from exercise* [24]. A summary of factors involved in vasodilation during exercise is shown in Table 8.3.

Venous Drainage in Active Muscles. If blood gets "dammed up" in capillaries because it cannot leave the muscle, blood flow is diminished. If muscles contract statically, some veins may be closed by the mechanical pressure of the contracting muscles, and blood flow may be reduced. In dynamic, rhythmic activities such as running or swimming, however, the alternate contraction and relaxation of the muscles serves to massage the blood vessels and accelerate the venous drainage from the muscles back toward the heart. This helps to increase the flow of blood through the muscles.

Blood flow gradually returns to normal during recovery from exercise (Fig. 8.4) as the circulation carries away vasodilator substances and brings oxygen to the muscles. One reason for "tapering off" by slow jogging after an exercise bout is to allow the circulation to remove substances such as bradykinin that may later contribute to muscle stiffness or soreness. A more important reason is to prevent the accumulation of blood in the legs that might cause inadequate venous return and inadequate cardiac output. Inadequate blood flow to the brain could then result in fainting.

It should be noted that the patterns of blood flow described in this chapter refer only to rhythmic work of an endurance nature. With static contractions blood flow is increased with light loads but is increasingly occluded by the compression of the vessels caused by more severe muscle contraction. Thus, flow may be completely shut off above 60–70 per cent of one's maximal voluntary contraction strength [2].

Blood Flow in Nonworking Muscles

If all vessels of the circulatory system were dilated at the same time, there would be an insufficient amount of blood to fill them, venous return to the right side of the heart would fall, cardiac output would fall, and the organism would be in a state of circulatory shock and in danger of death. Thus, although there are about 6 quarts of blood in an adult, the potential circulatory capacity may be 15–20 quarts. Therefore, if blood vessels in working muscles are dilated, blood vessels in visceral organs and skin must constrict if cardiac output is to be maintained or increased.

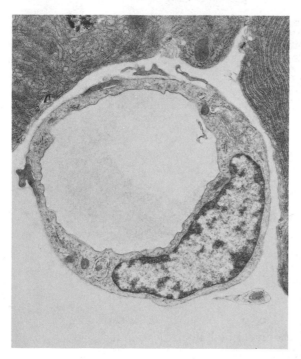

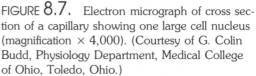

FIGURE 8.7. Electron micrograph of cross section of a capillary showing one large cell nucleus (magnification × 4,000). (Courtesy of G. Colin Budd, Physiology Department, Medical College of Ohio, Toledo, Ohio.)

In the past it was thought that blood flow to nonworking muscles was reduced by sympathetic vasoconstriction so that some of the blood in the resting muscles could be delivered to the active ones [11]. More recent reports, however, show that blood flow to resting muscles not only does not decrease, but it actually increases during heavy work by other muscles [21].

Blood Flow in the Viscera

Blood volume is shifted to working muscles from liver, spleen, stomach, intestines, and kidneys. Blood flow to these organs can be reduced by up to 80 per cent during severe exercise, probably by the action of the sympathetic nervous system on the blood vessels serving these organs [47]. One might wonder how an organ such as the liver can survive several hours of exercise with only 20 per cent of its normal blood flow. The answer is that although the liver and gut ordinarily receive about one fourth of the total cardiac output of 5 liters per minute, they remove only about 10 to 25 per cent of the available oxygen from the blood. Thus, these organs seem to be able to afford a drastic shutdown of their blood supply without any significant harmful effects; they simply extract a greater percentage of the smaller amount of available oxygen.

It should be pointed out that the degree of vessel constriction to these internal organs depends to a great extent on the *relative* severity of the exercise for a given individual [47]. For example, an athlete capable of running a marathon race (26.2 miles) in three hours might experience an 80 per cent reduction in blood flow to his internal organs if he completed the marathon in three hours, but only a 30 per cent decrease in circulation if he ran the same distance in five hours. In other words, it is not necessarily true that all distance runners or other endurance athletes have a marked fall in blood flow to their internal organs when they compete. The extent of the circulation to the internal organs depends on the athlete's capacity and on how strenuously he competes.

It is not known how the body can precisely regulate blood flow to nonworking tissues depending on the relative severity of the workload for a given person. It seems that there must be a nerve reflex pathway originating in the working muscles. Some receptor in these muscles may be stimulated by a chemical such as lactic acid that is produced in greater quantities as the work becomes more strenuous [47]. Unfortunately, such a reflex remains speculative.

Skin Blood Flow

After an initial small decline in skin blood flow as submaximal exercise begins, an endurance athlete ordinarily shifts some of the blood volume to the skin to carry away excess body heat; the extent of this shift may involve a skin blood flow during exercise of four to seven times that at rest [2] (Fig. 8.8). However, with exhaustive, prolonged exercise, the working muscles apparently have first call on the blood, and some of the increased skin blood flow may be shifted back to the muscle [47]. This phenomenon would occur in an athlete whose skin becomes more pale as he approaches an exhausted state. With heavy work lasting only a few minutes, skin vessels are constricted so that little or no increased flow to the skin occurs [47].

The shift of blood flow to the skin to remove heat is accomplished by the action of the hypothalamus. The hypothalamus is stimulated by the increasing temperature of the blood circulating through the hypothalamus during exercise and by increasing skin temperature if work is performed in a hot environment. The hypothalamus, in turn,

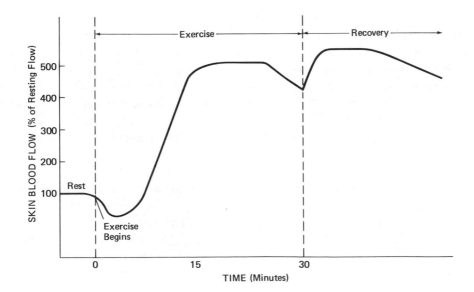

FIGURE 8.8. Skin blood flow during prolonged exhaustive work.

stimulates the nerves to the blood vessels of the skin by way of the medulla of the brain. These nerves cause relaxation of the smooth muscle around the vessels and a resultant dilation of those vessels so that more blood can flow to the skin. At the beginning of exercise and at exhaustion, some unknown reflexes cause vasoconstriction of skin vessels.

Coronary Blood Flow

As the heart muscle works increasingly harder during exercise, its demand for more oxygen is met by an increase of blood flow through the coronary arteries up to five times the resting value [2]. This increased flow is especially important for the heart because the heart normally removes 70–80 per cent of the oxygen from the blood of the coronary arteries. The coronary blood supply is enhanced by the action of epinephrine and norepinephrine, which are associated with a dilation of the coronary arteries. Even more important are the dilating effects of a reduced amount of oxygen in the heart and the greater aortic blood pressure that forces more blood into the coronary arteries. (The coronary arteries originate in the aorta as it leaves the left ventricle.) This increased coronary flow occurs mostly during diastole (relaxation) of the ventricles because ventricular contraction (systole) collapses coronary vessels. Because physical training causes the heart to beat less frequently during submaximal exercise, the heart is resting more, so that greater coronary flow can be achieved.

Blood Flow to Lungs, Adipose Tissue, and Brain

The increased output of blood from the left ventricle during exercise obviously must first pass from the right ventricle through the lungs. Therefore, if cardiac output increases fourfold, the blood flow in the pulmonary circulation must also increase fourfold.

Blood Flow to Adipose Tissue. Blood flow to adipose (fat) tissue beneath the skin and around the kidneys has been measured in human beings during prolonged exercise [9]. Perhaps surprisingly, the flow to subcutaneous adipose tissue increased by as much as 400 per cent and that to fat depots around the kidneys by 700 per cent. The mechanism underlying the increased flow is unknown, but it apparently does not require increased body temperature [9]. Presumably, the increased flow to adipose tissue is valuable in prolonged exercise to help deliver fatty acids mobilized from triglyceride stores to the working muscles.

Blood Flow to the Brain. There seems to be no change in overall blood flow to the brain, but at least in dogs there is evidence of a 30 per cent increase in flow to local areas of the brain associated with motor control [22]. Blood flow to the motor cortex, the cerebellar cortex, and the spinal cord was increased in dogs that ran on a treadmill. The increased flow to these discrete areas is apparently due to the accumulation of metabolites associated with increased brain activity in these regions.

Summary of Blood Flow Changes During Exercise. In summary, blood flow during rhythmical exercise is increased to organs that must function at a rate greater

TABLE 8.4
**Summary of Regional Blood Flow Changes During
Relatively Intense, Prolonged, Rhythmic Exercise**

Blood Flow to:	Exercise Blood Flow		
	Increased	No Change	Decreased
Working Muscles	X		
Nonworking Muscles	X or	X	
Skin	X		
Coronary Circulation	X		
Kidneys			X
Liver, Spleen			X
Gastrointestinal Tract			X
Lungs	X		
Brain		X (Local changes)	
Adipose Tissue	X		

than that occurring during rest—that is, to working skeletal muscles, heart, skin, adipose tissue, and lungs—but is decreased to kidneys, liver, stomach, and intestines. Localized changes occur in the brain (Table 8.4). These shifts in blood flow are accomplished both by mechanisms involving the hypothalamic, temperature-regulating nerve centers and the medulla of the brain and by local changes in the environment of the blood vessels, especially in the working muscle.

Blood Pressure During Exercise

Arterial blood pressure changes can be caused by alterations in cardiac output, blood vessel size, and blood volume. Increased cardiac output increases the flow of blood into arteries; this causes greater pressure within the vessels. Constriction of arterioles causes greater resistance to blood flow, so that the heart must pump more forcefully to drive blood through the narrowed arteries; this raises pressure. Vasodilation reduces arterial pressure. Greater blood volume increases arterial pressure and lesser volume decreases it, if other factors do not compensate for the volume changes.

During dynamic endurance exercise, such as running or cycling, the dilation of thousands of blood vessels in the working muscles reduces the arterial resistance to blood flow more than the vasoconstriction in nonworking tissues increases resistance. Therefore, the net effect of changes in blood vessel size during exercise is to *decrease* blood pressure. Simultaneously, however, cardiac output is increasing during exercise, and that increased cardiac output causes a greater systolic blood pressure that more than counteracts the tendency toward reduced pressure caused by vasodilation in the working muscles. Since only a slight fall in blood volume sometimes accompanies exercise, the *overwhelming effect of exercise on blood pressure is to increase systolic pressure, primarily because of the increased cardiac output.*

The effect of dynamic exercise, such as exhaustive cycling or distance running, on systolic and diastolic arterial blood pressure is shown in Fig. 8.9. As is shown, there is usually only a slight rise or no change in diastolic pressure during dynamic exercise.

In static exercise both systolic and diastolic pressure can rise sharply, even when a finger or hand is contracting isometrically [4, 5]. The marked rise in blood pressure

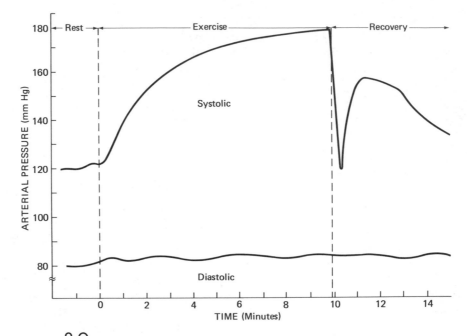

FIGURE 8.9.   Systolic and diastolic blood pressure during dynamic exercise to exhaustion.

during static contractions seems designed to help drive more blood into the strongly contracting muscles, and is apparently caused by a nerve reflex arising in the working muscles [33]. A greater than normal rise in blood pressure is also observed when one works dynamically with only small groups of muscles (for example, arms instead of legs), especially when one performs arm work with the arms above waist level [4]. Such work is experienced by carpenters, painters and other tradesmen who must often work overhead. Because of the inordinately high blood pressures produced by static or overhead dynamic arm work, this type of work is contraindicated for those with cardiovascular disease [4].

Fig. 8.9 also shows a marked fall in systolic blood pressure immediately after completion of an exhaustive bout of dynamic exercise. Such a fall in pressure is not uncommon, especially if the exerciser is in an upright posture and stops all muscular activity immediately after completing the exercise. The fall in pressure can be explained by a pooling of blood in the still dilated blood vessels of the legs because of a cessation of the pumping action of the leg muscles on the veins of the legs. Since less blood returns to the heart, cardiac output may drop precipitously, and the exerciser may faint because of a lack of blood flow to the brain. This type of collapse can be observed after exhaustive work on a bicycle ergometer or after completion of a grueling endurance-type athletic event. The drastic fall in pressure can be avoided if the exerciser continues muscular activity at a reduced level for a few minutes after completion of the athletic event or work task, so that the vascular system has a chance to gradually adjust the flow of blood from working muscles and dilated skin vessels to the central circulation. If the exerciser is too exhausted to continue at a low level of work, he should be advised to lie down to avoid fainting.

The rise in blood pressure that accompanies exercise is related to the severity of the task so that heavier workloads are associated with higher blood pressures [5]. Exercise blood pressure also tends to be higher in older subjects, who also usually have higher resting blood pressures [5].

Part 3: Blood

The characteristics of the blood are very important for aerobic endurance exercise. Since hemoglobin in the red blood cells carries oxygen, it is obvious that the number of red blood cells and the amount of hemoglobin in those cells are important in determining how much oxygen can be transported to the working muscles. This fact has been amply demonstrated by the diminished endurance observed in subjects who have had some of their blood withdrawn [14]. Blood is also vital for carrying away lactic acid, carbon dioxide, and other products of metabolism produced in the tissues during both rest and exercise.

The changes in the characteristics of the blood after a single bout of exercise or after physical training are not always easily predicted. There is a wide range of normal values for most of the constituents of blood at rest, and this range becomes even wider after exercise and training. The inconsistent effects of exercise and training on the makeup of the blood can be partly attributed to normal variation even at rest, partly to variations in exercise regimens and training programs, and partly to differences in methodology for blood analysis. At any rate, it is inaccurate to state that any tissue, and especially the blood, of all subjects responds in exactly the same manner to all types of exercise and training. When discussing "typical" responses of the blood to exercise, therefore, one must understand that there are many exceptions to those responses, usually only in terms of the magnitude of the response, but sometimes also in the direction of the response.

With the above qualifications in mind, let us examine Table 8.5, which describes some of the reported changes in the characteristics of the blood that occur with a single bout of maximal exercise and with endurance training. Except where indicated, maximal exercise refers to exercise at greater than 60 per cent of maximal oxygen uptake (heart rate about 150 beats/minute) prolonged for an hour or longer.

Exercise and Blood Volume

The effect of exercise on blood volume seems to depend on the type of exercise, the intensity of exercise, and the state of training and acclimation to work in the heat. First, it should be made clear that a single bout of exercise does not affect the number of red blood cells in the circulatory system. These cells are too large to leak out of the capillaries, and increased production of red blood cells cannot occur rapidly enough to increase their numbers in circulation in the course of a few hours or less. Accordingly, any acute change in blood volume must be caused by a shift of plasma water out of the vascular system (if blood volume is diminished) or into the vascular system (if blood volume is increased). A shift of plasma out of the blood vessels is known as

TABLE 8.5

Effects of Maximal Exercise and Physical Training on Characteristics of Blood in Young Adults[1]

Blood Characteristics	Untrained		Trained	
	Male	Female	Male	Female
Total Blood Volume (liters)				
Rest	5.7	4.3	6.2	4.6
Maximal Exercise, Cycling	5.2	4.0	6.3	4.7
Maximal Exercise, Running	5.7	4.3	6.4	4.8
Total Hemoglobin (grams/kilogram body weight)				
Rest	10.5	9.4	11.0	10.0
Maximal Exercise	No Change		No Change	
Hemoglobin Concentration (grams/100 ml blood)				
Rest	16.0	14.0	15.4	13.4
Maximal Exercise, Cycling	18.4	16.2	15.0	13.0
Maximal Exercise, Running	16.0	14.0	15.0	13.0
Red Blood Cell Count (millions of RBC/mm³)				
Rest	5.4	4.6	5.2	4.4
Maximal Exercise, Cycling	6.2	5.3	5.1	4.3
Maximal Exercise, Running	5.4	4.6	5.1	4.3
Total Red Blood Cells (trillions)				
Rest	30.8	19.8	34.6	22.1
Maximal Exercise	No Change		No Change	
Hematocrit (%)				
Rest	46.0	42.0	44.2	40.3
Maximal Exercise, Cycling	52.9	48.3	43.0	39.0
Maximal Exercise, Running	46.0	42.0	43.0	39.0
White Blood Cell Count (thousands of WBC/mm³)				
Rest	7.0	7.0	No Change	
Maximal Exercise	15.0	15.0	No Change	
Arterial Oxygen Content (ml O_2/100 ml blood)				
Rest	19.5	16.8	No Change	
Maximal Exercise	No Change		No Change	
Arterial Oxygen Partial Pressure, P_{aO_2}, (mm Hg)				
Rest	100	100	No Change	
Maximal Exercise	100	100	95–100	
Oxygen Content in Femoral Vein (ml O_2/100 ml blood)				
Rest	9.0	9.0	No Change	
Maximal Exercise with legs	3.0	3.0	1.4	1.8
Oxygen Partial Pressure in Femoral Vein, P_{vO_2}, (mm Hg)				
Rest	30.0	30.0	No Change	
Maximal Exercise with legs	13.0	14.0	10.0	11.0
Oxygen Content in Right Atrium (ml O_2/100 ml blood)				
Rest	13.0	11.0	No Change	
Maximal Exercise	5.5	5.5	4.0	4.0
Oxygen Partial Pressure in Right Atrium, $P_{\bar{v}O_2}$, (mm Hg)				
Rest	40.0	40.0	No Change	
Maximal Exercise	18.0	19.0	15.0	16.0
Difference Between Arterial O_2 Content and Mixed Venous Blood (R. Atrium) O_2 Content, (A–$\bar{V}$ O_2 Difference), (ml O_2/100 ml blood)				
Rest	6.5	5.8	No Change	
Maximal Exercise	14.0	11.3	15.5	12.8
Arterial CO_2 Partial Pressure, P_{aCO_2}, (mm Hg)				
Rest	40.0	40.0	No Change	
Maximal Exercise	38.0	38.0	No Change	

TABLE 8.5 **(continued)**

Blood Characteristics	Untrained		Trained	
	Male	**Female**	**Male**	**Female**
Femoral Vein CO_2 Partial Pressure, $P_{\bar{v}CO_2}$, (mm Hg)				
Rest	47.0	47.0	No Change	
Maximal Exercise	63.0	63.0	70.0	70.0
Right Atrium CO_2 Partial Pressure, $P_{\bar{v}CO_2}$, (mm Hg)				
Rest	45.0	45.0	No Change	
Maximal Exercise	60.0	60.0	67.0	67.0
Lactic Acid in Arteries & Veins (mg/100 ml blood)				
Rest	12.0	12.0	No Change	
Submaximal Exercise (6 mph run)	50.0	50.0	18.0	18.0
Maximal Exercise	120	120	140	140
pH of Blood in Femoral Vein				
Rest	7.37	7.37	No Change	
Maximal Exercise	7.10	7.10	6.90	6.90
pH of Blood in Arteries				
Rest	7.40	7.40	No Change	
Maximal Exercise	7.20	7.20	7.0	7.0
Blood Temperature				
Rest	37.6°C	37.6°C	No Change	
Maximal Exercise	40.0°C	40.0°C	41.2°C	41.2°C

[1] There are wide individual and group differences for many of these blood characteristics. Values given should be considered as rough approximations only. Data from many sources, principally references 2, 5, 30, 36, 42, 46, 52 and 53.

"hemoconcentration," and a shift of water from the interstitial or intracellular spaces into the blood vessels is called "hemodilution."

Bicycle Exercise and Blood Volume. Blood volume is decreased during bicycle exercise, especially in untrained persons. The heavier the load while cycling, the greater is the hemoconcentration effect [52]. The maximal reduction in plasma volume is about 15 per cent, which means that total blood volume would be decreased about 8 per cent. (Blood contains about 54 per cent plasma and 46 per cent red blood cells.) There are two phenomena which seem to explain the hemoconcentration effect during bicycle exercise. First, as the muscles contract, veins are compressed so that less blood leaves the capillaries than enters through the arteries. This raises the pressure in the capillaries and forces some plasma out of the capillaries into the tissue spaces. (The accumulation of water in the tissue spaces is responsible for the so-called "pumping up" of the muscles that accompanies repeated rapid lifting of dumbbells or barbells. Shortly after the exercise period, the excess water in the muscle tissue makes its way back into the blood. As the blood volume returns to normal, so does the size of the muscles.)

The second explanation for hemoconcentration during bicycle exercise is that osmotically active metabolites such as potassium, phosphate, and lactic acid accumulate in the tissue spaces and draw plasma water from the capillaries. This helps explain the relationship between exercise intensity and hemoconcentration; as the exercise gets more difficult, more lactic acid and other metabolites are produced to draw water from the capillaries.

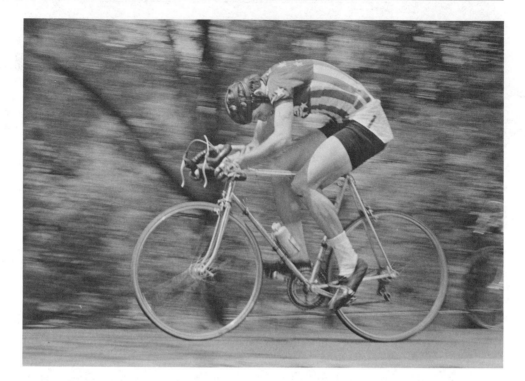

FIGURE 8.10.   Blood volume is usually decreased more during cycling than during running. (Courtesy of Office of Public Information, Purdue University, West Lafayette, Indiana.)

Treadmill Exercise and Blood Volume.   Changes in plasma and whole blood volume are quite unreliable when subjects perform running exercise; sometimes there is a hemoconcentration, sometimes a hemodilution, and often no change at all [52]. The reasons for the different effects on blood volume between running and cycling are unclear, but two are offered for consideration. First, cycling uses a smaller muscle mass to accomplish the same rate of work; therefore, it may be that veins are more compressed during muscle contraction when cycling than when running. Accordingly, this may cause greater leakage of water from the capillaries. Second, for the same energy expenditure lactic acid begins accumulating earlier in cycling than in running [52]. Thus, when a subject is cycling, osmotically active lactic acid molecules may have longer to act to draw water from the capillaries.

Effect of Training on Blood Volume.   Endurance training causes approximately an 8 per cent increase in resting blood volume. This change is caused by a 12 per cent increase in plasma volume and smaller increases in red blood cell volumes [5, 10]. The increased plasma volume seems to be caused by a retention of more plasma proteins, chiefly albumin [10, 50]. There is not a greater concentration of protein in the blood but simply more total protein to hold more water in the vascular system by osmosis [10]. The mechanism for the increase in red blood cells is unknown.

During exercise, trained persons often exhibit hemodilution, especially if the training is done in hot, humid conditions [19, 50, 51]. This expansion of plasma volume during exercise is valuable, particularly if prolonged work must be performed in hot environments. Some of the blood volume is shifted to the skin and away from working muscles in hot conditions, and heavy sweating can reduce plasma volume. Persons with expanded blood volumes are better able to meet the circulatory needs of both the working muscles and the skin than are those who are untrained.

The mechanism for plasma volume expansion during exercise in trained persons seems to hinge on an increased delivery of proteins from the lymph to the blood and a decreased loss of proteins from the plasma to the tissue fluids in trained persons [19, 50, 51]. Lymph has high concentrations of protein, and lymph flow to the vascular system is almost doubled during exercise [41]. If trained persons can retain more protein in the blood plasma, this protein can draw water from the tissue fluids into the capillaries to expand the plasma volume. Trained persons shift less of their blood volume to the skin vasculature during a standard bout of exercise because they lose heat better than the untrained by virtue of an improved sweating response. Therefore, it has been hypothesized that untrained persons are more likely to lose plasma volume (hemoconcentration) because more protein tends to be lost from the capillaries in the skin than from other tissues [19].

"Sports Anemia". Some investigators who have noted decreased hematocrit values in trained persons have suggested that sports training leads to a type of anemia. (The hematocrit is measured by centrifuging a blood sample in a tube until the red blood cells settle to the bottom. The hematocrit is the percentage of the entire blood volume that consists of red blood cells. Thus, a hematocrit of 46 means that 46 per cent of the blood consists of red cells.) If plasma volumes are not measured, a fall in hematocrit could be suggestive of a decreased red blood cell production or an increased destruction of red blood cells. Either of these circumstances could lead to a reduced oxygen transporting capacity in the blood. However, when plasma volumes are measured after exercise in trained persons or at rest in trained, heat acclimated persons, it is usually found that there is no deficiency in red blood cells; rather, the decreased hematocrit is caused by a beneficial increase in plasma water. Accordingly, the term "sports anemia" should not be used unless it is shown that reduced hematocrits and hemoglobin values are not a function of an expanded plasma volume.

Exercise and Hemoglobin

Hemoglobin is a large protein complex within the red blood cell. Hemoglobin is obviously vital to exercise because it transports oxygen from the lungs to the working muscles. Since red blood cells do not ordinarily leave the vascular space during exercise, it is not surprising that *total* hemoglobin does not change with exercise. Hemoglobin *concentration* during exercise reflects the extent of any hemoconcentration or hemodilution; hemoglobin concentration will rise with hemoconcentration and fall with hemodilution.

Endurance training is associated with a small increase in the production of red blood cells. Therefore, total hemoglobin increases slightly with such training. The concentration of hemoglobin at rest declines slightly with training because the increase in plasma volume is somewhat larger than the increase in red cells. Expansion of plasma volume in trained persons further reduces hemoglobin concentration *during* exercise.

Exercise and Red Blood Cells

The red blood cell count is a measure of the concentration of red cells in a small volume of blood. Thus, it is a measure of the concentration of red cells. If hemoconcentration occurs during exercise, the red cell count will increase. With hemodilution, the count will decrease. The total number of red cells does not change during exercise because the cells do not leave or enter the vascular compartment to a significant extent. With training, however, the total number of red cells will increase somewhat.

Exercise and Hematocrit

Since the hematocrit is a measure of the concentration of red cells in the total blood volume, the hematocrit will increase with hemoconcentration and decrease with hemodilution. There is usually little or no change in hematocrit with training in a cool environment because both plasma and red cells increase to some extent. In hot environments training may cause hemodilution and thus a fall in hematocrit.

Exercise and White Blood Cells

The increased white blood cell count that often is seen after exercise is usually explained as an effect of the greater circulation during exercise "washing out" the white blood cells from their storage places in the lungs, bone marrow, liver and spleen [30]. Such an explanation seems reasonable for the lungs and perhaps bone marrow, but blood flow in liver and spleen tends to decline with exercise. This white cell response is of no special benefit to the organism during exercise, and the white blood cell count resumes its normal value within a few hours after completing physical activity.

Exercise and Arterial Oxygen

It is important to observe the lack of an appreciable exercise effect on arterial oxygen content and partial pressure. The lungs function so effectively that even under conditions of maximal exercise, most studies show little or no change in arterial oxygen levels. Likewise, physical training has no reproducible effect on arterial oxygen, and there is no good evidence to support the conclusion that regular exercise improves the ability of the lungs to deliver oxygen to the blood.

Exercise and Venous Oxygen

The reason that oxygen levels are lower in the femoral venous blood than in the arterial blood during leg exercise is that mitochondria of the leg muscles are using oxygen to carry away electrons and hydrogen ions in the electron transport system of aerobic metabolism. As the oxygen combines with hydrogen, water is formed so that the venous blood has less oxygen to deliver back to the heart and lungs. Oxygen in the right atrium of the heart is called *mixed venous oxygen* because venous blood from working muscles is mixed with venous blood from nonworking tissues. Accordingly, oxygen levels are higher in mixed venous blood than in venous blood from working muscles because there is a greater usage of oxygen in working muscles than in nonworking organs.

Exercise and Arterio-Venous Oxygen Difference

The difference between the oxygen content of arterial blood and mixed venous blood ($A-\overline{V}$ O_2 Difference) represents the amount of oxygen extracted from the blood and used by the tissues. Consequently, when the muscles are actively consuming oxygen during exercise, the arteriovenous oxygen difference increases. Training is sometimes associated with increased arteriovenous oxygen differences after maximal exercise, probably because trained muscles have more mitochondria that can better utilize oxygen that is delivered to the muscles [47]. These mitochondrial changes also explain the training-induced decreases in oxygen levels of femoral and mixed venous blood.

Exercise and Blood Carbon Dioxide

Carbon dioxide values are greater in venous blood than in arterial blood because the mitochondria of the tissues produce carbon dioxide as a product of aerobic energy metabolism. Training increases the output of carbon dioxide during maximal exercise because training causes an increased production of mitochondria that can, in turn, generate more carbon dioxide.

Exercise and Blood Lactate

Lactic acid is a product of anaerobic glycolysis and is, therefore, found in greater amounts in the blood during exercise that is heavy enough to demand some anaerobic energy production. The trained person produces less lactic acid during submaximal work because he relies more upon aerobic metabolism as a result of increased effectiveness of skeletal muscle mitochondria. During *maximal* work, on the other hand, the trained individual can produce greater amounts of lactic acid because he has greater stores of muscle glycogen to break down to lactic acid, and/or because he can better tolerate increased levels of acid with improved motivation or some unknown physiological adaptations.

Exercise and Blood pH

The acidity or pH of the blood during exercise is a direct reflection of the increased production of lactic acid. Accordingly, the lower pH (greater acid) in the blood of athletes during maximal exercise is caused by the greater lactic acid generated in trained individuals.

Exercise and Blood Temperature

Blood temperature increases during exercise because some of the chemical energy released by the breakdown of carbohydrates and fats in the muscle is lost as heat energy and because the process of muscle contraction itself produces heat. The trained person can generate more heat because he can work longer with heavier workloads than untrained individuals, and his muscles can, therefore, create more heat.

Exercise and Oxygen Release from Hemoglobin

The increased temperature and greater acidity of the blood circulating through the working muscles cause oxygen to be released somewhat more rapidly from the hemoglobin of the red blood cells. Thus, exercise changes in the muscles serve to increase oxygen delivery to those muscles. The increased carbon dioxide content of the blood does not have much effect on the release of oxygen from hemoglobin during prolonged exercise [53].

Blood Doping

The fact that physical performance is known to be poor after blood loss or withdrawal has led to experiments designed to discover whether *more* blood can enhance performance. In these studies subjects have a pint or more of their blood withdrawn and frozen. After 5–6 weeks during which their bodies replace the lost blood, the previously withdrawn red blood cells are reinjected into the circulation. The rationale for this procedure, "blood doping," is that the extra red blood cells may be able to deliver more oxygen to the working muscles to improve their endurance.

Blood doping is illegal under international athletic rules, but testimonial evidence suggests that many endurance performers, especially in Europe, have used the procedure. Roughly two out of every three scientific experiments show that blood doping has some beneficial effect on athletic performance [61]. It appears that the critical factor is to withdraw at least 800–1,200 milliliters (2–3 pints) of blood. In one well-designed double-blind study, 5–mile run times for average road runners improved by about 50 seconds after blood doping [61]. It is not clear whether a similar effect would occur with elite athletes.

Regardless of the relative effectiveness of blood doping, it seems to be an artificial means of gaining a possible performance edge that should not become accepted practice. One can imagine the logical extension of such procedures to include surgical manipulations of the nerve supply to muscles in an attempt to form more slow twitch fibers or surgical alterations of tendon insertions to provide a more effective angle of pull. Such procedures are not in the best interests of individual athletes or of sport.

Part 4: Pulmonary Function

During aerobic endurance activities, more oxygen must be delivered from the lungs to the working muscles, and excess carbon dioxide must be removed from the muscles. These processes require an accelerated exchange of oxygen and carbon dioxide between the lungs and the blood; they are accomplished by an increased flow of blood through the lung capillaries (increased pulmonary perfusion), by an increased rate and depth of breathing (ventilation), and by an increased rate of diffusion of oxygen from the lungs into the blood and of carbon dioxide from the blood to the air in the lungs.

Pulmonary Perfusion

The right ventricle pumps more blood to the lungs during exercise at the same time that the left ventricle delivers more blood to the working muscles and to the rest of the body. Even though there may be five times more blood pumped through the lungs during maximal exercise than at rest, there is only a slight rise in blood pressure within the lung capillaries [36]. This slight rise in blood pressure means that there must be many more open capillaries in the lungs during exercise than at rest, and that the millions of tiny air sacs (alveoli) in the lungs must be much better perfused with blood. As a consequence of this increased perfusion or distribution of blood to the alveoli and of the increased rate of flow of blood through the lungs, more oxygen can diffuse into the pulmonary blood, and more carbon dioxide can diffuse out of the blood into the alveolar air.

Ventilation

At rest, the lungs are ventilated at approximately six liters per minute. This six liters is the result of breathing about 12 times per minute with the volume of each breath (*tidal volume*) being about one-half liter. During prolonged "steady state" endurance exercise, maximal ventilation is about 80–100 liters per minute in young adult males and 45–80 liters per minute in females, who have smaller lungs than males. With brief maximal exercise, such as an 800-meter run, ventilation rates in excess of 120–140 liters per minute may be observed [5]. Breathing frequency increases from about 12 times per minute at rest to 45 times per minute during heavy exercise. For a person weighing 70 kilograms, the tidal volume increases from about 0.5 liter at rest to 2.5 liters during exercise. Smaller persons have smaller tidal volumes.

Vigorously increased breathing is known as "hyperpnea." The hyperpnea of exercise operates so effectively that even during maximal exercise, the arterial oxygen content is not different from resting values, and, if anything, the arterial carbon dioxide content is slightly less than at rest.

Control Mechanisms in Exercise Hyperpnea

Exercise hyperpnea has been studied for more than 100 years, yet we still cannot fully explain how increased rates of muscle contraction lead to increased breathing. Many investigators have noted an extremely rapid onset of hyperpnea as exercise begins and a rapid reduction in breathing at the end of exercise (Fig. 8.11). It was deemed impossible that any *humoral* substances such as lactic acid or carbon dioxide could be released rapidly enough to account for these rapid components of the breathing response. (Humoral substances are those found in body fluids.) Consequently, it has been thought that there must be at least a *neurogenic* component (arising from the

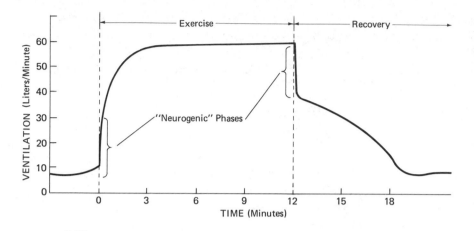

FIGURE 8.11. Ventilation response to mild exercise.

brain or from nerve reflexes not initiated by humoral factors) to exercise hyperpnea, and some have suggested that the nervous system can account for the entire exercise hyperpnea response. On the other hand, with prolonged exercise there seems to be a gradual increase in ventilation that is likely to be caused by changes in some humoral factor(s) (Fig. 8.11). As with the neurogenic theory, some researchers have found evidence that the entire hyperpnea response to exercise can be fully accounted for by humoral factors. Let us review some of the neurogenic and humoral possibilities for control of ventilation during exercise.

Neurogenic Factors in Exercise Hyperpnea. *Central Commands.* It is possible that some of the exercise hyperpnea is caused by signals initiated in the motor cortex or some other center in the brain [31]. These signals could affect the control centers for respiration, which are located in the medulla of the brainstem. This theory is difficult to test in human beings, but an interesting study on cats has been reported [16]. In this study cats who had their cerebral cortices removed walked on a treadmill. It was found that hyperpnea began shortly before the animals began to walk and was increased as the cats walked more vigorously. The hyperpnea occurred even when all feedback from muscles and joints and from receptors in the carotid arteries and aorta was eliminated. There were no changes in blood chemistry that could account for the hyperpnea. The authors concluded that exercise hyperpnea in cats can be caused by signals descending from the level of the hypothalamus [16].

Muscle and Joint Receptors. In experiments on anesthetized dogs and cats it has presumably been possible to remove all humoral influences on respiration by circulating the experimental animal's blood to another animal and replacing the experimental animal's blood with that from a third animal. When the leg muscles of the animal are then stimulated electrically, it should be possible to determine whether humoral influences are required for the ventilation response. Some studies have reported that exercise hyperpnea in these animal preparations does not require humoral stimuli but does require information feedback to the brain from muscles and joints;

when the spinal cord is cut, little or no hyperpnea occurs [12, 31]. Other experiments, however, suggest that exercise hyperpnea in these animal experiments can be fully accounted for by changes in unknown humoral factors [32] or by changes in carbon dioxide delivery to the lungs [58]. Especially damaging to the hypothesis that receptors in the limbs play a major role in exercise hyperpnea are human experiments which show that varying the pedaling rate while cycling does not substantially affect ventilation [55, 59].

It is probably premature to dismiss totally any effect of neural feedback from the muscles and joints on exercise hyperpnea. Studies on anesthetized animals or humans working on a bicycle ergometer in the laboratory certainly cannot reproduce all the physiological phenomena experienced by a volleyball player or marathon runner. However, the bulk of the available evidence does not implicate muscle and joint receptors as major factors in exercise hyperpnea.

Humoral Factors in Exercise Hyperpnea. Receptors that are sensitive to oxygen lack, carbon dioxide excess, and/or pH decrease are known to exist in the medulla of the brain, the carotid bodies of the carotid arteries, and the aortic bodies of the aortic arch. Since muscles consume oxygen and produce carbon dioxide and lactic acid, it was logical to investigate whether these chemoreceptors were important to exercise hyperpnea. It has been found that the central pH-sensitive chemoreceptors in the medulla [7] and the aortic chemoreceptors are not important to the hyperpneic response to exercise [59]. However, *the carotid bodies are vital to the fine regulation of exercise hyperpnea during mild to moderate exercise and are the only factor of importance for the rapid increase in ventilation with heavy exercise* [55, 59]. Some of the best evidence to support the importance of the carotid bodies is that obtained in patients who have had their carotid bodies removed. These patients do experience hyperpnea during moderate exercise, but the hyperpnea develops very slowly; they do not exhibit the marked increase in breathing that ordinarily occurs during heavy exercise [59].

There appears to be no major contribution of epinephrine or norepinephrine to exercise hyperpnea since chemical blockade of the receptors for these hormones does not alter the hyperpnea response [17].

Arterial Carbon Dioxide Set-point Theory. One group of investigators has performed many experiments, primarily on humans, that suggest a major role for carbon dioxide in exercise hyperpnea [42, 55, 56, 58, 59]. They have concluded that for mild to moderate exercise the body regulates arterial carbon dioxide levels around a constant set-point, much as a thermostat is used to regulate temperature at some preset level. Some of the evidence supporting this position includes the fact that only insignificant changes occur in arterial carbon dioxide pressure during exercise until the exercise intensity is great enough to cause marked increases in blood lactic acid levels. Furthermore, if the resting levels of arterial carbon dioxide are altered by chronic treatment with acid or base, the body regulates carbon dioxide around these new resting levels during exercise [42].

Wasserman and his colleagues believe that the initial rapid phase of exercise hyperpnea can be explained by a greater flow of carbon dioxide to the lungs [56]. This may at first seem improbable, because there is inadequate time for the increased carbon dioxide produced by the muscles to get to the known sensors of carbon dioxide in the aorta, carotid arteries, and brain. However, we know that cardiac output increases instantaneously with the onset of exercise [44]. Therefore, even if the *concentration* of carbon dioxide does not change instantly, the *total delivery* (concentration times blood flow) of carbon dioxide to the lungs does increase rapidly. Unfortunately, there are no known receptors for carbon dioxide flow located in the arterial circulation. The carotid bodies help to fine tune this system during moderate exercise, but there seem to be other receptors which are more important for the overall effect. One study on dogs suggests that humoral receptors other than the carotid bodies are important to exercise hyperpnea and that these receptors are not located within the brain [32].

During *heavy* exercise, the carotid bodies are quickly activated by the decreased pH associated with increased lactic acid. The carotid bodies then stimulate the respiratory centers of the medulla to markedly influence the rate of breathing [55, 59]. The relationship between heart rate and ventilation during exercise is shown in Fig. 8.12. As is shown in the figure, ventilation increases linearly with the exercise intensity (as reflected by heart rate) until it rises rapidly at a heart rate of about 150 beats per minute. At this time most subjects are working at about 60 per cent of their maximal oxygen uptakes, and lactic acid has accumulated in the blood to about 2 millimoles per liter of blood. This upward breaking point in ventilation and lactic acid production is sometimes called the "anaerobic threshold" and will be discussed in more detail in the next chapter.

The various factors thought to influence exercise hyperpnea are summarized in Fig. 8.13.

Pulmonary Diffusing Capacity

The pulmonary (lung) diffusing capacity for a gas such as oxygen represents the rate of diffusion of the gas between the air sacs (alveoli) of the lungs and the blood of the lung capillaries. This capacity varies with many factors, including the thickness of the lung

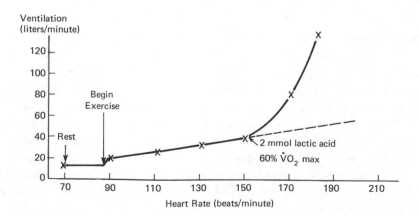

FIGURE 8.12. The relationship between heart rate (a reflection of exercise intensity) and ventilation.

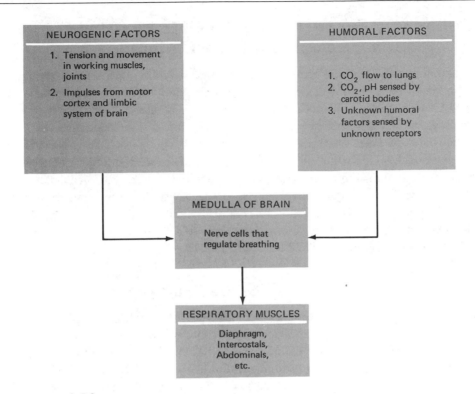

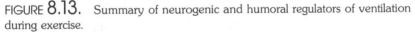

FIGURE 8.13. Summary of neurogenic and humoral regulators of ventilation during exercise.

tissue, the thickness of the red blood cell membrane, the amount of plasma between the air sac and the red blood cell, and most importantly, the surface area of contact between alveoli and blood in the pulmonary capillary.

There is up to a 300 per cent increase in pulmonary diffusing capacity for oxygen during maximal exercise [36]. This change is thought to be brought about almost entirely by the increased perfusion of blood around the air sacs of the lungs. At rest in an upright posture, many of the pulmonary capillaries are closed, especially at the top of the lungs, because gravity tends to cause blood to pool in the lower parts of the lungs. Therefore, there is little or no diffusion of oxygen from many of the alveoli surrounded by the closed capillaries. However, as an elevated cardiac output during exercise forces more blood into the pulmonary artery, most of the pulmonary capillaries that were closed at rest become filled with blood. This creates a greater surface area for diffusion of oxygen from alveolar air to the pulmonary blood and accounts for the increase in pulmonary diffusing capacity for oxygen during exercise.

Although the pulmonary diffusing capacity for carbon dioxide also increases during exercise as a result of a better perfusion of blood through the lungs, this phenomenon is of little consequence. The diffusion of carbon dioxide proceeds about 20 times faster than the diffusion of oxygen and would be rapid enough even if there was no exercise effect on the carbon dioxide diffusion capacity.

Pulmonary Function As a Possible Limiting Factor in Circulorespiratory Endurance

Most authorities believe that under normal circumstances in young persons, the lungs are perfectly capable of meeting the demands imposed by even the heaviest types of exercise stress [5, 36]. The levels of oxygen and carbon dioxide in the arterial blood delivered from the left ventricle during maximal exercise are usually unchanged from resting values, and one's maximal voluntary ventilation capacity of 120–180 liters per minute is not strained during long duration exercise where values of 60–100 liters per minute are commonly observed. Thus, the changes in lung perfusion, ventilation, and diffusing capacity for oxygen during exercise are usually sufficient to keep arterial oxygen and carbon dioxide at values essentially unchanged from those at rest. However, elderly persons have lower maximal pulmonary ventilation rates, and their maximal oxygen uptakes may thus be limited by lung function.

"Hypoxic" Swim Training

Many swim coaches ask their swimmers to hold their breath or breathe as infrequently as possible during practice swims. They reason that this will cause hypoxia in the tissues because the delivery of oxygen in the blood will be diminished. Further, it is believed that the metabolic energy systems of the tissues will be able to adapt to this hypoxia so that subsequent competitive swims can occur with greater rates of ATP production in hypoxic situations. It has been shown, however, that such breath control techniques do not result in hypoxia and do not affect oxygen uptake during the practice swims [13]. Any benefit of such procedures may result from an elevated arterial carbon dioxide content, which does occur. Perhaps swimmers learn to tolerate high carbon dioxide levels so that the drive to breathe causes less discomfort.

Summary

The physiological responses of the heart, lungs, and blood vessels are of primary importance in determining the ability of one to persist at prolonged physical activity. These responses are described in this chapter, and the mechanisms which bring about the responses are explained. A failure of any of these mechanisms to provoke the appropriate responses may lead to diminished aerobic endurance performance, whereas improved responses can produce improved performance.

Exercise causes greater cardiac output by increasing both heart rate and stroke volume. A limited blood volume is effectively diverted to the working muscles by means of a widespread constriction of blood vessels supplying nonworking organs, and a dilation of blood vessels in the working muscles. A large increase in cardiac output overwhelms a small net decrease in peripheral resistance and is responsible for an elevated arterial blood pressure that provides the force to drive blood through the tissues during exercise. Pulmonary ventilation and diffusion of oxygen and carbon dioxide both increase so effectively during exercise that normal young persons are not ordinarily limited in their aerobic endurance by an inadequacy of the lungs. Values of oxygen, carbon dioxide, lactic acid, and other chemicals in the blood during exercise reflect not only the changes in oxygen uptake and the production of carbon dioxide and lactic acid by the working muscles, but also a commonly observed hemoconcentration that occurs when high intracapillary pressures force fluid from the capillaries into the tissue spaces.

REVIEW QUESTIONS

1. What is meant by the terms *neurogenic, humoral,* and *intrinsic* in explanations of physiological changes?
2. Describe two factors that are probably involved in the immediate rise in heart rate at the start of exercise.
3. List two humoral stimuli that may cause a gradual rise in heart rate as exercise progresses.
4. Describe and explain the changes in stroke volume that accompany postural changes and exercise.
5. Explain why shifts in regional blood flow are required during exercise.
6. How is it possible for an organ such as the liver to sustain an 85 per cent decrease in blood flow during exercise and yet suffer no apparent damage?
7. Which is more important in determining arterial pressure during rhythmic exercise: changes in vascular resistance or changes in cardiac output? Explain your answer.
8. Examine Table 8.5 and explain each sex difference in blood characteristics and each exercise-induced and training-induced change in blood characteristics.
9. List two neurogenic factors and two humoral factors which may be involved in the ventilation response to exercise.
10. Explain why pulmonary function in healthy subjects is ordinarily not considered a limiting factor in aerobic endurance performance.

REFERENCES

[1] Andersen, P. Capillary density in skeletal muscle of man. *Acta Physiologica Scandinavica,* 1975, **95**:203–205.
[2] Anderson, K. L. The cardiovascular system in exercise. In H. Falls, ed., *Exercise Physiology.* New York: Academic Press, Inc., 1968, pp. 79–128.
[3] Asmussen, E. Ventilation at transition from rest to exercise. *Acta Physiologica Scandinavica,* 1973, **89**:68–78.
[4] Åstrand, I. ST depression, heart rate, and blood pressure during arm and leg work. *Scandinavian Journal of Clinical and Laboratory Investigation,* 1972, **30**:411–414.
[5] Åstrand, P.-O., and K. Rodahl. *Textbook of Work Physiology,* 2nd ed. New York: McGraw-Hill, 1977.
[6] Barnard, R. J., G. W. Gardner, W. V. Diaco, R. N. MacAlpin, and A. A. Kattus. Cardiovascular responses to sudden strenuous execise—heart rate, blood pressure, and ECG. *Journal of Applied Physiology,* 1973, **34**:833–837.
[7] Bisgard, G. E., H. V. Forster, B. Byrnes, K. Stanek, J. Klein, and M. Manohar. Cerebrospinal fluid acid-base balance during muscular exercise. *Journal of Applied Physiology,* 1978, **45**:94–101.
[8] Brodal, P., F. Ingjer, and L. Hermansen. Capillary supply of skeletal muscle fibers in untrained and endurance-trained men. *American Journal of Physiology,* 1977, **232**:H705–H712.
[9] Bulow, J., and J. Madsen. Human adipose tissue blood flow during prolonged exercise II. *Pflügers Archiv,* 1978, **376**:41–45.
[10] Convertino, V. A., P. J. Brock, L. C. Keil, E. M. Bernauer, and J. E. Greenleaf. Exercise

training-induced hypervolemia: role of plasma albumin, renin, and vasopressin. *Journal of Applied Physiology,* 1980, **48**:665–669.

[11] Costin, J. C., and N. S. Skinner, Jr. Competition between vasoconstrictor and vasodilator mechanisms in skeletal muscle. *American Journal of Physiology,* 1971, **220**:462–466.

[12] Dejours, P. Control of respiration in muscular exercise. In W. O. Fenn and H. Rahn, eds., *Handbook of Physiology, Section 3: Respiration,* Vol. 1. Washington, D.C.: American Physiological Society, 1964, pp. 631–648.

[13] Dicker, S. G., G. K. Lofthus, N. W. Thornton, and G. A. Brooks. Respiratory and heart rate responses to tethered controlled frequency breathing swimming. *Medicine and Science in Sports and Exercise,* 1980, **12**:20–23.

[14] Ekblom, B., A. N. Goldbarg, and B. Gullbring. Response to exercise after blood loss and reinfusion. *Journal of Applied Physiology,* 1972, **33**:175–180.

[15] Eklund, B. Influence of work duration on the regulation of muscle blood flow. *Acta Physiologica Scandinavica,* 1974, (Supplementum 411).

[16] Eldridge, F. L., D. E. Millhorn, and T. G. Waldrop. Exercise hyperpnea and locomotion: parallel activation from the hypothalamus. *Science,* 1981, **211**:844–846.

[17] Fagard, R., T. Reybrouck, P. Lijnen, A. Amery, E. Moerman, and A. De Schaepdryver. Alpha- and beta-adrenoceptor blockade does not affect ventilation during exercise in man. *Medicine and Science in Sports and Exercise,* 1980, **12**:375–379.

[18] Fortney, S. M., E. R. Nadel, C. B. Wenger, and J. R. Bove. Effect of acute alterations of blood volume on circulatory performance in humans. *Journal of Applied Physiology,* 1981, **50**:292–298.

[19] Fortney, S. M., and L. C. Senay. Effect of training and heat acclimatization on exercise responses of sedentary females. *Journal of Applied Physiology,* 1979, **47**:978–984.

[20] Foster, C., J. D. Anholm, C. K. Hellman, J. Carpenter, M. L. Pollock, and D. H. Schmidt. Left ventricular function during sudden strenuous exercise. *Circulation,* 1981, **63**:592–596.

[21] Greenleaf, J. E., L. D. Montgomery, P. J. Brock, and W. Van Beaumont. Limb blood flow: rest and heavy exercise in sitting and supine positions in man. *Aviation, Space, and Environmental Medicine,* 1979, **50**:702–707.

[22] Gross, P. M., M. L. Marcus, and D. D. Heistad. Regional distribution of cerebral blood flow during exercise in dogs. *Journal of Applied Physiology,* 1980, **48**:213–217.

[23] Hnik, P., N. Kriz, F. Vyskocil, V. Smiesko, J. Mejsnar, E. Ujec, and M. Holas. Work-induced potassium changes in muscle venous effluent blood measured by ion-specific electrodes. *Pflügers Archiv,* 1973, **338**:177–181.

[24] Honig, C. R. Contributions of nerves and metabolites to exercise vasodilation: a unifying hypothesis. *American Journal of Physiology,* 1979, **236**:H705–H719.

[25] Honig, C. R., C. L. Odoroff, and J. L. Frierson. Capillary recruitment in exercise: rate, extent, uniformity, and relation to blood flow. *American Journal of Physiology,* 1980, **238**:H31–H42.

[26] Hossack, K. F., R. A. Bruce, B. Green, F. Kusumi, T. A. DeRouen, and S. Trimble. Maximal cardiac output during upright exercise: approximate normal standards and variations with coronary heart disease. *American Journal of Cardiology,* 1980, **46**:204–212.

[27] Hossack, K. F., F. Kusumi, and R. A. Bruce. Approximate normal standards of maximal cardiac output during upright exercise in women. *American Journal of Cardiology,* 1981, **47**:1080–1086.

[28] Hudlicka, O. Effect of training on macro- and microcirculatory changes in exercise. *Exercise and Sport Sciences Reviews,* 1977, **5**:181–230.

[29] Ingjer, F., and P. Brodal. Capillary supply of skeletal muscle fibers in untrained and endurance trained women. *European Journal of Applied Physiology,* 1978, **38**:291–299.

[30] Karpovich, P. V., and W. E. Sinning. *Physiology of Muscular Activity,* 7th ed. Philadelphia: W. B. Saunders, 1971.

[31] Levine, S. Ventilatory response to muscular exercise. In D. G. Davies and C. D. Barnes, eds., *Regulation of Ventilation and Gas Exchange.* New York: Academic Press, Inc., 1978, pp. 31–68.

[32] Levine, S. Ventilatory response to muscular exercise: observations regarding a humoral pathway. *Journal of Applied Physiology,* 1979, **47:**126–137.

[33] Lind, A. R., G. W. McNicol, and K. W. Donald. Circulatory adjustments to sustained (static) muscular activity. In K. Evang and K. L. Anderson, eds., *Physical Activity in Health and Disease.* Baltimore: William and Wilkins, 1966, pp. 38–63.

[34] Longhurst, J. C., and J. H. Mitchell. Reflex control of the circulation by afferents from skeletal muscle. In A. C. Guyton and D. B. Young, eds., *Cardiovascular Physiology,* Vol. 3. Baltimore:University Park Press, 1979, pp. 125–148.

[35] Longhurst, J., and R. Zelis. Cardiovascular responses to local hindlimb hypoxemia: relation to the exercise reflex. *American Journal of Physiology,* 1979, **237:**H359–H365.

[36] Margaria, R., and P. Cerretelli. The respiratory system and exercise. In H. Falls, ed., *Exercise Physiology.* New York:Academic Press, Inc., 1968, pp. 43–78.

[37] Matell, G. Time-courses of changes in ventilation and arterial gas tensions in man induced by moderate exercise. *Acta Physiologica Scandinavica,* 1963, **58**(Supplementum 206).

[38] Maxwell, L. C., T. P. White, and J. A. Faulkner. Oxidative capacity, blood flow, and capillarity of skeletal muscles. *Journal of Applied Physiology,* 1980, **49:**627–633.

[39] McCloskey, D. I., P. B. C. Matthews, and J. H. Mitchell. Absence of appreciable cardiovascular and respiratory responses to muscle vibration. *Journal of Applied Physiology,* 1972, **33:**623–626.

[40] Mohrman, D. E., and H. V. Sparks. Myogenic hyperemia following brief tetanus of canine skeletal muscle. *American Journal of Physiology,* 1974, **227:**531–535.

[41] Olszewski, W., A. Engeset, P. M. Jaeger, J. Sokolowski, and L. Theodorsen. Flow and composition of leg lymph in normal men during venous stasis, muscular activity and local hyperthermia. *Acta Physiologica Scandinavica,* 1977, **99:**149–155.

[42] Oren, A., K. Wasserman, J. A. Davis, and B. J. Whipp. Effect of CO_2 set point on ventilatory response to exercise. *Journal of Applied Physiology,* 1981, **51:**185–189.

[43] Osnes, J.-B., and L. Hermansen. Acid-base balance after maximal exercise of short duration. *Journal of Applied Physiology,* 1972, **32:**59–63.

[44] Petro, J. K., A. P. Hollandee, and L. N. Bouman. Instantaneous cardiac acceleration in man induced by a voluntary contraction. *Journal of Applied Physiology,* 1970, **29:**794–798.

[45] Petrofsky, J. S., C. A. Phillips, M. N. Sawka, D. Hanpeter, A. R. Lind, and D. Stafford. Muscle fiber recruitment and blood pressure response to isometric exercise. *Journal of Applied Physiology,* 1981, **50:**32–37.

[46] Roskamm, H. Myocardial contractility during exercise. In J. Keul, ed., *Limiting Factors of Physical Performance.* Stuttgart: Georg Thieme, Publishers, 1973, pp. 225–234.

[47] Rowell, L. B. Circulation. *Medicine and Science in Sports,* 1969, **1:**15–22.

[48] Rowell, L. B. Human cardiovascular adjustments to exercise and thermal stress. *Physiological Reviews,* 1974, **51:**75–159.

[49] Rowell, L. B. What signals govern the cardiovascular responses to exercise? *Medicine and Science in Sports and Exercise,* 1980, **12:**307–315.

[50] Senay, L. C. Effects of exercise in the heat on body fluid distribution. *Medicine and Science in Sports,* 1979, **11:**42–48.

[51] Senay, L. C., and Kok, R. Effects of training and heat acclimatization on blood plasma contents of exercising men. *Journal of Applied Physiology,* 1977, **43:**591–599.

[52] Senay, L. C., G. Rogers, and P. Jooste. Changes in blood plasma during progressive treadmill and cycle exercise. *Journal of Applied Physiology,* 1980, **49:**59–65.

[53] Thomson, J. M., J. A. Dempsey, L. W. Chosy, N. T. Shahidi, and W. G. Reddan. Oxygen transport and oxyhemoglobin dissociation during prolonged muscular work. *Journal of Applied Physiology,* 1974, **37:**658–664.

[54] Upton, M. T., S. K. Rerych, J. R. Roeback, Jr., G. E. Newman, J. M. Douglas, A. G. Wallace, and R. H. Jones. Effect of brief and prolonged exercise on left ventricular function. *American Journal of Cardiology,* 1980, **45:**1154–1160.

[55] Wasserman, K., B. J. Whipp, R. Casaburi, M. Golden, and W. L. Beaver. Ventilatory con-

trol during exercise in man. *Bulletin Europeén de Physiopathologie Respiratoire*, 1979, **15:**27–47.

[56] Wasserman, K., B. J. Whipp, and J. Castagna. Cardiodynamic hyperpnea: hyperpnea secondary to cardiac output increase. *Journal of Applied Physiology*, 1974, **36:**457–464.

[57] Weil, J. V., E. Byrne-Quinn, I. E. Sodal, J. S. Kline, R. E. McCullough, and G. R. Filley. Augmentation of chemosensitivity during mild exercise in normal man. *Journal of Applied Physiology*, 1972, **33:**813–819.

[58] Weissman, M. L., B. J. Whipp, D. J. Huntsman, and K. Wasserman. Role of neural afferents from working limbs in exercise hyperpnea. *Journal of Applied Physiology*, 1980, **49:**239–248.

[59] Whipp, B. J. The hyperpnea of dynamic muscular exercise. *Exercise and Sport Sciences Reviews*, 1977, **5:**295–311.

[60] Williams, M. H., A. R. Goodwin, R. Perkins, and J. Bocrie. Effect of blood reinjection upon endurance capacity and heart rate. *Medicine and Science in Sports*, 1973, **5:**181–186.

[61] Williams, M. H., S. Wesseldine, T. Somma, and R. Schuster. The effect of induced erythrocythemia upon 5-mile treadmill run time. *Medicine and Science in Sports and Exercise*, 1981, **13:**169–175.

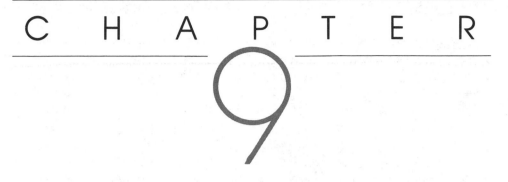

C H A P T E R
9

Evaluation of Cardiovascular Function and Aerobic Endurance Performance

THE principal limiting factor for most types of exercise that last longer than three or four minutes is the capacity of the heart, lungs, and circulation to deliver oxygen to the working muscles. Therefore, a physical educator, coach, or physician who wishes to evaluate one's circulorespiratory fitness or one's capacity for aerobic activity should try to estimate the maximal functional capacity of the heart, lungs, and circulation of the student, athlete, or patient. This maximal functional capacity of the circulorespiratory system is best evaluated with a test of the body's capacity to consume oxygen at a maximal rate, that is, with a maximal oxygen uptake test.

Maximal Oxygen Uptake

The rate of maximal oxygen uptake is abbreviated $\dot{V}_{O_2}$ max, where the V_{O_2} represents the volume of oxygen consumed, usually in liters or milliliters, and the dot over the V is a notation that tells us that this volume is to be expressed per unit of time, usually per minute. Thus, the expression $\dot{V}_{O_2}$ max $= 3$ l/min means that a person can maximally consume oxygen at a rate of 3 liters per minute. The term *maximal oxygen uptake* is synonymous with the terms *maximal oxygen consumption, maximal oxygen intake,* and *maximal aerobic power* and represents the greatest difference between the rate at which inspired oxygen enters the lungs and the rate that expired oxygen leaves the lungs (Fig. 9.1). Therefore, to measure maximal oxygen uptake one must know the amount of oxygen inspired and the amount expired; the difference between these two values is the amount of oxygen that has been taken up and used by the electron transport system of the mitochondria to produce energy for the active tissues.

It is not unusual for oxygen uptake to increase about 10 or even 20 times when one passes from a condition of rest (about 0.25 l/min) to heavy endurance exercise (about 2.5 to 5.0 l/min). For young adult women maximal oxygen uptake is about 2.3 l/min, whereas men are apt to consume about 3.4 l/min under maximal exercise conditions [27]. There is a fairly broad range of values for maximal oxygen uptake, depending on such factors as state of physical training, age, and sex. For example, the maximal oxygen uptake of typical college females may range from less than 1.7 to greater than 3.0 l/min, and for college males from less than 2.7 to greater than 4.0 l/min [27]. Outstanding men and women cross-country skiers in Scandinavia have had values reported as high as 6.0 and 4.0 l/min, respectively [4].

Because oxygen is used by all the body tissues, a larger individual has a greater oxygen uptake than a smaller one both at rest and during exercise. Accordingly, it is better for comparative purposes to record oxygen uptake values on the basis of body weight, ordinarily in terms of milliliters of oxygen per kilogram of body weight. Therefore, since a kilogram is equivalent to approximately 2.2 pounds, a man who weighs 154 pounds (70 kilograms) and has a maximal oxygen uptake of 2.8 l/min (2800 ml/min) can also be said to have a maximal oxygen uptake of 2800/70 = 40 ml/kg/min. When expressed in this fashion, typical maximal oxygen uptake values for college men and women are about 48 and 40 ml/kg/min, respectively [27]. Expressing the same data in terms of lean body mass or fat-free body weight is not usually advisable because such an expression unjustifiably penalizes those who are less fat [16].

Some Factors That Determine Maximal Oxygen Uptake

Let us review some of the physiological functions that are involved if one is to have a normal maximal oxygen uptake capacity. *First,* the heart, lungs, and blood vessels must be functioning adequately so that oxygen inhaled into the lungs is delivered to the blood. *Second,* the process of oxygen delivery to the tissues by the red blood cells must be normal; that is, there must be normal heart function, blood volume, red blood cell count, and hemoglobin concentration, and the blood vessels must be able to shift blood from nonworking tissues to the working muscles where the oxygen demand is greatest. *Third,* the tissues, especially the muscles, must have a normal capacity to use the oxygen that is delivered to them. In other words, they must have normal energy metabolism and mitochondrial function. As we have seen previously, the lungs of a healthy person do not limit the ability to consume oxygen [4]. Also, a routine blood test can determine whether the characteristics of the blood are normal. *Therefore, heart function, the ability to circulate blood to the active tissues, and the ability of the tissues to extract and utilize oxygen remain as factors to be evaluated by tests of maximal oxygen uptake in nonelderly persons who do not have pulmonary disease.*

Heart function is reflected by cardiac output (CO). Both the ability of the circulatory system to transfer blood from inactive to active regions and the ability of the tissues to extract oxygen from the blood are reflected by the difference in the content of oxygen between arterial and venous blood (arteriovenous O_2 difference, A-$\overline{V}$ O_2 Diff.). A person who can shift most of the blood to working muscles during exercise will have a

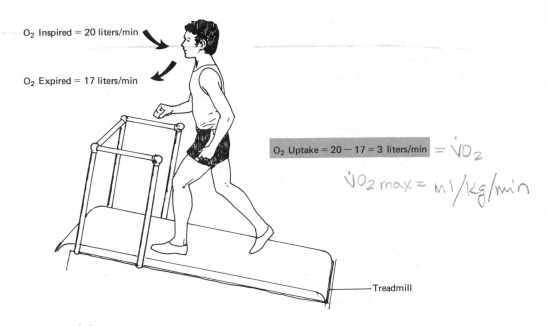

FIGURE 9.1. Schematic view of how oxygen uptake is measured.

large arteriovenous oxygen difference because the active muscles will be able to extract more oxygen from the blood than would inactive tissues of the body. Likewise, one whose muscles have highly active mitochondria will be able to extract oxygen from the blood supply quite readily. A large proportion of slow twitch fibers can be important in this regard.

Assuming that the lungs and blood characteristics are normal, maximal oxygen uptake is a function of maximal cardiac output and maximal arteriovenous oxygen difference. This fact can be expressed in a simple equation as follows: $\dot{V}_{O_2}$ max = max CO × max A-$\overline{V}$ O_2 Diff. [31]. Let us assume that a subject's maximal cardiac output is 25 liters per minute, that the oxygen content of the blood in the arteries is 20 milliliters of oxygen per 100 milliliters of blood, and that the oxygen content of the mixed venous blood sampled in the right atrium is 5 milliliters of oxygen per 100 milliliters of blood. The subject's max A-$\overline{V}$ O_2 Diff. is 20 − 5 = 15 ml/100 ml or 0.15 liters of oxygen per liter of blood. Accordingly, this subject's maximal oxygen uptake is 25 × 0.15 = 3.75 liters per minute. Remember that the cardiac output represents the amount of blood potentially available for oxygen delivery to the active tissues each minute. The arteriovenous O_2 difference represents the degree to which the oxygen contained in the blood pumped out of the heart is used by the active tissues for aerobic energy metabolism.

Maximal Oxygen Uptake and Endurance Performance

While it is true that a person's maximal oxygen uptake reflects the maximal functional capacity of the cardiovascular system, and the maximal functional capacity of the cardiovascular system is usually the most important determinant of one's performance in physical activity of an aerobic nature, it is not true that a person with a great maximal oxygen uptake is necessarily an outstanding endurance performer [4, 22, 27].

The ability to perform for long durations at a high *percentage* of maximal oxygen uptake appears to be crucial for championship caliber endurance performance. As an illustration of this principle consider two distance runners, Agatha Allout and Christina Cruzalong. Agatha has a maximal oxygen uptake of 50 ml/kg/min, and Christina has a maximal oxygen uptake of only 46 ml/kg/min. However, Christina can run a marathon at an average oxygen uptake of 36.8 ml/kg/min (80 per cent of her maximal oxygen uptake), but Agatha can run for long distances at only 35 ml/kg/min, 70 per cent of her maximal oxygen uptake. It is not surprising, therefore, that Christina can usually beat Agatha in distance races, even though Christina has a lower maximal oxygen uptake. Elite distance runners [29] and cross-country skiers [23] can perform at greater than 85 per cent of their maximal oxygen uptakes without accumulating large amounts of lactic acid, whereas untrained persons have difficulty maintaining more than 65 per cent of their maximal oxygen uptakes for long periods. Also, in groups of experienced distance runners, all of whom have high maximal oxygen uptakes, the best runners seem to be those who have the lowest oxygen uptakes for standardized submaximal runs [9]. Presumably, the greater efficiency of the better athletes is caused by a greater ability to use the minimum number of motor units to perform the run.

Many other factors such as motivation and technique play a role in endurance performance. Thus, although an outstanding endurance athlete must have a relatively high maximal rate of oxygen uptake, it does not always follow that the best performer in a group of excellent performers has the greatest maximal oxygen uptake. A track coach who knows the maximal oxygen uptakes of all the freshman track candidates will be able to select those athletes who have the *physiological* potential to become good endurance performers, but the coach will not be able to predict very accurately from a test of oxygen uptake which of these potentially good performers may finally become champions. The *emotional, psychological,* and *technical* characteristics of the athletes must also be considered.

Maximal Oxygen Uptake and Cardiovascular Health

Although a test of maximal oxygen uptake can be useful to the physical educator or coach to determine those who are most fit for cardiorespiratory endurance activities, a much more important use of this test from the health standpoint is its use in the detection of cardiovascular disease and in the assessment of one's capacity for exercise prior to the undertaking of an exercise program. The test is useful for normal fitness purposes as well as for the rehabilitation of patients who have suffered heart attacks or show clinical signs of cardiovascular disease. In recognition of the value of exercise testing, physicians, exercise physiologists, and physical educators throughout the world are establishing testing and exercise centers where trained exercise technicians administer graded exercise tests, usually to those over 35 years of age. The results of these tests are used in the diagnosis of cardiovascular disease and in the prescription of exercise training programs that are conducted by skilled exercise leaders [2, 28].

Principles of Testing Maximal Oxygen Uptake

Routine testing of maximal oxygen uptake has been accomplished chiefly with three methods of exercise: treadmill exercise, bicycle ergometer exercise, or bench stepping [6, 27]. There are certain advantages to each of these procedures. A stepping bench is inexpensive and portable. A bicycle ergometer can be used to measure the quantity of work performed very accurately. Furthermore, in cycling, the upper body is relatively motionless for easy monitoring of electrocardiogram, blood pressure, and other physiological measurements. Treadmill tests produce the highest values for maximal oxygen uptake and are subject to the least differences in skill and efficiency between subjects [27]. One of the greatest problems inherent in the use of step tests is that at higher workloads for normal, active, and well-trained subjects, the height of the step and the rate of stepping become so great that it becomes increasingly difficult to maintain one's balance and the appropriate stepping cadence [27]. Both step tests and bicycle ergometry tend to place a great deal of stress on a relatively few leg muscles, so that performers often are forced to stop working because of muscle pain before maximal oxygen uptake has been achieved [27]. Consequently, the treadmill test has achieved great popularity in the United States when precise measurements of maximal oxygen uptake are desired. That is not to say, however, that other procedures are not acceptable. The step test may be useful for testing patients with low capacities, and the bicycle ergometer is excellent as long as it is understood that it will probably underestimate maximal oxygen uptake by about 5–10 per cent, both because of the muscle pain factor and perhaps because of the smaller amount of muscle tissue involved in bicycle work than in treadmill exercise [27].

Criteria for Establishing That Maximal Oxygen Uptake Was Achieved. Probably the most important criterion for determining that one has achieved maximal oxygen uptake for a given test procedure is whether oxygen consumption reaches a plateau or perhaps declines slightly with increasing workloads (Fig. 9.2). Because it is known that oxygen uptake increases linearly with increasing workloads up to the maximal rate of oxygen uptake, a plateau of oxygen uptake with an increasing workload is a sure sign that the subject has achieved his maximum. Sometimes the plateau is very brief, and a fall in oxygen uptake may be observed with progressively greater workloads (dashed line in Fig. 9.2). This fall in oxygen uptake is caused by decreased cardiac output. This happens because the stroke volume falls in response to increased delivery of the blood to the skin as exhaustion approaches. In the absence of a plateau or a fall in oxygen uptake, one cannot be certain that the highest, or *peak,* oxygen uptake is indeed the subject's *maximal* oxygen uptake. Other evidence that may support the conclusion that a peak oxygen uptake is also the maximal uptake for a given subject might include a high level of blood lactic acid (above 70–80 mg/100 ml blood) and achievement of near maximal heart rate (Table 10.1) [4]. Both of these factors usually are observed at the time of maximal oxygen uptake.

Additional factors to be considered in determining that maximal oxygen uptake is recorded for a particular test are exercise posture, muscle mass used in the exercise, exercise intensity, exercise duration, mechanical efficiency for the task, and the motivation of the subject [27, 31]. *Posture must be upright,* either sitting or standing, be-

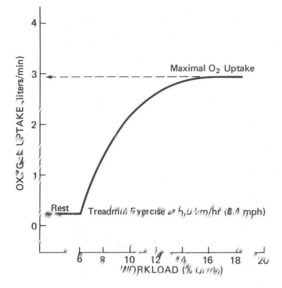

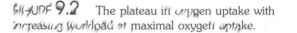

FIGURE 9.2 The plateau in oxygen uptake with increasing workload at maximal oxygen uptake.

...use the highest oxygen uptakes observed in a horizontal posture while pedalling a bicycle ergometer or during swimming are almost always 6-29 per cent less than the highest uptakes for the same subjects on the treadmill [4, 26]. World class swimmers, however, are capable of matching their bicycle maximal oxygen uptakes while swimming, but their swimming values are still 6-7 per cent lower than treadmill values, perhaps because swimming may require use of a smaller muscle mass than running [20].

Because the increased activity of skeletal muscles accounts for most of the increased oxygen uptake during exercise, it is obvious that large muscles must be used if maximal oxygen uptake is to be attained. In other words, one should not expect to ... as great an oxygen uptake from arm work as from leg work, and arm work combined with leg work should give a somewhat greater oxygen uptake than either leg work by itself [17, 33]. About 50 per cent of the total muscle mass must be exercise before maximal oxygen uptake can be achieved [31].

Both exercise intensity and duration must be great enough to elicit a near ... response of the cardiovascular system if maximal oxygen uptake is to be ... minimum of about three or four minutes of running on the treadmill is ... achieve maximal oxygen uptake, whereas treadmill walking up progress... ... may require 20 minutes or longer to elicit a maximal response [2, ... of the workload is increased progressively in tests of maximal o... ... that eventually the intensity must reach a level sufficient to bring ab... ...

Finally, a good test of maximal oxygen uptake should not depe... motivational levels of the subject [21]. It would be absurd to choose ... measure oxygen uptake, for example, because of the high levels ... ... required to perform such a task. Even in a simple task such ... ergometer, differences in efficiency among individuals can be ... Walking is a familiar task to most, and there are only negligi...

efficiency among individuals [27]. Some tasks, such as fast running on a treadmill, also suffer from the fact that many persons are either fearful of or are unwilling to persist in those activities. For both efficiency and motivational reasons treadmill walking up progressively greater inclines is a commonly used test of maximal oxygen uptake [5]. Walking tests that are more prolonged in nature, that is, in which the intensity is only gradually increased, seem to be tolerated better than briefer walking tests, even though similar values in maximal oxygen uptake are achieved by both methods [13]. For some subjects, however, shorter progressive treadmill running tests produce nearly 10 per cent greater oxygen uptakes than prolonged treadmill walking, perhaps because blood flow to the skin increases during prolonged exercise, and this may reduce blood and oxygen supply to the working muscles [15].

Selection of Exercise Loads for Evaluation of Aerobic Capacity. There is no commonly used protocol for testing maximal oxygen uptake that is satisfactory for all populations of subjects. A test used primarily in hospital settings is of little value for trained endurance athletes, and tests designed for athletes are too strenuous for cardiac patients. Regardless of the subject population, the exercise test should progress from initial exercise loads which can be accomplished without difficulty to more difficult loads which lead to maximal exercise in a reasonably short time, usually 10–20 minutes. Tables 9.1 and 9.2 show the approximate rates of energy expenditure required to perform various exercise loads on motor driven treadmills and bicycle ergometers. Note that for cycle ergometry (Table 9.2) the oxygen cost *per kilogram of body weight* is lower for heavier persons. The *total* oxygen cost at a given load is approximately the same for everyone because body weight is largely supported by the seat of the ergometer; therefore, the oxygen cost per unit of body weight is less for heavier people. It should also be understood that any treadmill test or cycle ergometer

TABLE 9.1

Approximate Energy Costs for Treadmill Walking and Running (ml O$_2$/kg/min)[1][2]

Speed (mph[2])	Treadmill Grade (%)							
	0.0	2.5	5.0	7.5	10.0	12.5	15.0	17.5
1.7	8.0	10.2	12.2	14.4	16.1	18.2	20.3	22.4
2.0	8.8	11.2	13.6	16.1	18.6	21.0	23.1	25.6
2.5	10.2	13.3	16.1	19.2	22.0	25.2	28.4	31.2
3.0	11.6	15.0	18.9	22.4	25.9	29.8	33.2	36.8
3.4	12.6	16.8	20.6	24.8	29.0	33.2	37.1	41.3
3.75	13.6	18.2	22.8	27.3	31.8	36.4	41.0	45.1
5.0	30.1	33.2	36.0	39.2	42.0	45.2	48.3	—
6.0	35.7	39.2	43.0	46.6	50.0	53.9	57.4	—
7.0	41.0	45.2	49.4	53.6	57.8	62.0	66.2	—
7.5	43.8	48.3	52.8	57.4	62.0	66.5	71.0	—
8.0	46.6	51.4	56.4	60.9	65.8	70.7	75.6	—
9.0	51.8	57.0	62.6	67.9	73.5	78.8	84.4	—
10.0	57.0	63.0	69.0	74.9	81.2	87.2	93.1	—

[1] To convert to METS (multiples of the resting metabolic rate), divide the tabled value by 3.5.
[2] To convert to meters/minute, multiply the tabled value by 26.82.

TABLE 9.2
Approximate Energy Costs for Cycle Ergometry (ml O_2/kg/min)[1][2]

Exercise Load		Body Weight (kg[2])					
(kgm/min)	(watts)	50	60	70	80	90	100
300	50	17.8	15.0	13.0	11.2	10.2	9.1
450	75	24.2	20.0	17.2	15.0	13.3	11.9
600	100	31.2	24.8	21.4	18.9	16.8	15.0
750	125	36.0	30.1	25.6	22.4	20.0	17.8
900	150	42.0	35.0	30.1	26.2	23.4	21.0
1050	175	48.0	39.9	34.3	30.1	26.6	24.2
1200	200	53.9	45.2	38.5	33.6	30.1	27.0
1350	225	59.9	50.2	42.7	37.2	33.5	30.2
1500	250	65.9	55.1	46.9	40.8	36.9	33.4
1650	275	72.0	60.2	51.2	44.5	40.4	36.7
1800	300	78.3	65.5	55.7	48.4	44.1	40.2
1950	325	84.3	70.6	60.0	53.1	47.6	43.6
2100	350	90.4	75.6	64.4	56.8	51.2	47.0

[1] To convert to METS (multiples of resting metabolic rate), divide the tabled value by 3.5.
[2] To convert to pounds, multiply by 2.2.

test should be preceded by adequate warmup and brief practice for the types of exercise to be performed. This is especially true for treadmill walking and running, which can be extremely disorienting during the first attempt at this type of exercise.

Test Protocols for Cardiac Patients. A cardiac patient should begin an exercise test at a load which demands about 8 ml O_2/kg/min. An additional 3–4 ml O_2/kg/min should be required to perform each successive stage of the test, and each stage should last for 3 minutes. A protocol for cardiac patients is shown in Table 9.3. The test should continue until a prescribed end-point (usually a specified heart rate) has been reached, until the patient's symptoms (chest pain, labored breathing, etc.)

TABLE 9.3
Treadmill Test Protocol for Cardiac Patients

Stage No.	Speed (mph)	Grade (%)	Time (min)	O_2 Cost (ml/kg/min)
1	1.7	0.0	3	8.0
2	1.7	5.0	3	12.2
3	1.7	10.0	3	16.1
4	2.5	7.5	3	19.2
5	3.0	7.5	3	22.4
6	3.0	10.0	3	25.9
7	3.0	12.5	3	29.8
8	3.4	12.5	3	33.2
9	3.4	15.0	3	37.1
10	3.75	15.0	3	41.0
11	3.75	17.5	3	45.1

cause the patient to voluntarily stop exercising, or until the test is terminated by the physician or technician conducting the test because of observed inadequacies in the patient's cardiovascular response (poor response of blood pressure, heart rate, electrocardiogram, etc.) [2, 6, 7, 8, 15, 28].

Test Protocols for Normal, Healthy Subjects. Normal, presumably healthy persons can usually begin at a workload requiring about 25 ml O_2/kg/min. Accordingly, most treadmill tests for normal persons start at a walking pace of 3.4 or 3.75 mph and a grade of 5.0 or 7.5 per cent, and cycling tests begin at 75 or 100 watts. Increments of 3–7 ml O_2/kg/min in energy requirements should occur in successive stages of the test. Average persons can ordinarily reach maximal oxygen uptake during walking tests, but the steep treadmill grades required to call forth energy demands of 30–45 ml O_2/kg/min may result in back pain and localized thigh muscle pain for those less fit. Consequently, if maximal values are not likely to be obtained at a grade of 12.5 per cent or less, it may be advisable to reduce the grade to 5 per cent or 7.5 per cent after the 12.5 per cent walking grade and to increase the speed of the treadmill to 5 mph. Most nonathletic subjects will begin jogging or running to maintain a speed of 5 mph.

It is recommended that two minutes be the duration of the early stages of the test for normal nonathletic subjects to insure a gradual increase in physiological demands. The later stages should be one minute in length to minimize the possibility of muscular fatigue before maximal oxygen uptake is achieved. A treadmill protocol for normal nonathletic persons is shown in Table 9.4.

Test Protocols for Endurance Athletes. Well-trained endurance athletes can be expected to achieve maximal oxygen uptakes of greater than 50 ml O_2/kg/min, and they should have no difficulty running at a 9 or 10 mph pace. Consequently, a test for such athletes can be started at an energy cost of 30 ml O_2/kg/min and can progress every minute by 3–7 ml O_2/kg/min. A suggested protocol for testing endurance athletes is shown in Table 9.5.

TABLE 9.4
**Treadmill Test Protocol for Normal,
Healthy Subjects**

Stage No.	Speed (mph)	Grade (%)	Time (min)	O_2 Cost (ml O_2/kg/min)
1	3.4	7.5	2	24.8
2	3.4	10.0	2	29.0
3	3.4	12.5	2	33.2
4	3.4	15.0	2	37.1
5	3.75	15.0	1	41.0
6	5.0	12.5	1	45.2
7	7.0	5.0	1	49.4
8	7.0	7.5	1	53.6
9	7.0	10.0	1	57.8
10	7.0	12.5	1	62.0

TABLE 9.5
Treadmill Test Protocol for Endurance Athletes

Stage No.	Speed (mph)	Grade (%)	Time (min)	O_2 Cost (ml/kg/min)
1	5.0	5.0	1	36.0
2	5.0	7.5	1	39.2
3	6.0	5.0	1	43.0
4	6.0	7.5	1	46.6
5	7.0	5.0	1	49.4
6	7.0	7.5	1	53.6
7	8.0	5.0	1	56.4
8	8.0	7.5	1	60.9
9	8.0	10.0	1	65.8
10	8.0	12.5	1	70.7
11	9.0	10.0	1	73.5
12	9.0	12.5	1	78.8
13	9.0	15.0	1	84.4
14	10.0	12.5	1	87.2
15	10.0	15.0	1	93.1

Prediction of Maximal Oxygen Uptake from Physiological Responses to Submaximal Tests

During exercise of submaximal intensity, heart rate and ventilation rate increase approximately in proportion to increases in oxygen uptake. Consequently, numerous attempts have been made to predict maximal oxygen uptake from heart rate, ventilation rate, and other variables during standardized submaximal exercise loads [14, 27]. In this way, an estimate of maximal cardiovascular function can be achieved without undue stress on subjects who may have unknown cardiovascular disease, without the need for the high levels of motivation required in tests that push subjects to near maximal levels, and without the need for complex, time-consuming direct determinations of oxygen uptake. Although these tests can usually provide a close approximation of maximal oxygen uptake, they are subject to a prediction error of around 10 per cent or greater [27]. Thus, these tests often underestimate or overestimate maximal oxygen uptake by about 10 per cent for a given subject. Since the reproducibility of routine direct tests of maximal oxygen uptake is in the neighborhood of 2–4 per cent, the prediction from submaximal test results is not entirely satisfactory. Some of the submaximal tests are terminated when the subject reaches a predetermined heart rate that represents a certain percentage (often 85 per cent) of predicted maximal heart rate for that subject. Unfortunately, there is a wide range of maximal heart rates for a given age group, so that prediction of maximal heart rate is often poor [6]. This accounts for some of the poor predictions of maximal oxygen uptake obtained with submaximal tests.

Even though submaximal tests to predict maximal oxygen uptake are not satisfactory for research purposes, their use to assess maximal cardiovascular capacity is justified in situations where financial, personnel, subject safety, and time considerations prohibit direct determinations of maximal oxygen uptake. One of the simplest of these submaximal tests that has been validated for untrained college males is one where the subject pedals a bicycle ergometer at a speed of 60 revolutions per minute with a workload of 150 watts (900 kilopond meters per minute) for five minutes [14]. Heart rate is measured during the fifth minute of the ride (HR_{150}), and maximal oxygen uptake is predicted from the following equation: $\dot{V}_{O_2}$ max (l/min) $= 6.3 - .01926\,HR_{150}$. Accordingly, if a subject's heart rate during the fifth minute were 160 beats per minute, his predicted maximal oxygen uptake would be $6.3 - .01926\,(160) = 3.218\ l$/min.

Other popular submaximal exercise tests include the Physical Working Capacity-170 test [37] and the Åstrand-Rhyming test [3]. These tests are more time consuming than the Fox test for predicting maximum aerobic power, but have been more widely used with various populations. Both use heart rate during submaximal exercise to predict maximal oxygen uptake.

Prediction of Maximal Oxygen Uptake from Running Performance

Because it is widely accepted that performance in distance running is dependent to a great extent upon cardiovascular function, several tests have been designed to estimate maximal oxygen uptake from running performance either on the treadmill or in the field. These performance measures include maximal running time on the treadmill [5, 7, 15]; best time for running 600 yards, 1 or 1½ miles [1], or 2 miles [30]; and maximal distance covered in 9 [1] or 12 minutes [1, 10]. Performance on distance runs was initially reported to have a very strong relationship to maximal oxygen uptake [10], but later studies with more homogeneous populations (all subjects having similar ages, body weights, and physical condition characteristics) have showed rather poor predictions of maximal oxygen uptake from 12-minute runs [16, 22, 27]. One reason for this is that in addition to maximal cardiovascular function, factors such as motivation and pain tolerance are important in determining maximal run performance. It has also been demonstrated that maximal treadmill running time can be improved without any improvement in maximal oxygen uptake [15]. Consequently, running performance does not seem to be an especially good predictor of maximal oxygen uptake and probably should not be used to estimate maximal cardiovascular function except as that function is involved in running performance. In other words, tests such as the 12 minute run can only roughly assess cardiovascular function, but they are likely to give a very good indication of one's ability to persist at distance running.

In the physical education class or on the athletic field, however, the distance run with all its drawbacks is undoubtedly the best *practical* indicator of cardiovascular function. Treadmill and bicycle work tests, whether maximal or submaximal, are simply too impractical to use with large numbers of students or athletes. Norms for performance on the 12 minute run are provided in a popular format along with *exercise programs* designed to improve cardiorespiratory fitness [11].

Prediction of Aerobic Endurance Performance

The ability to perform well in aerobic endurance activities such as distance running, cycling, and swimming is best tested by having the subject engage in the actual activity for which he has been, or will be, trained. In other words, if one wished to know which of 100 girls were the best candidates for distance running training, all the prospective trainees should compete in a distance run, perhaps 1,500 or 3,000 meters (1 or 2 miles), to find out which candidates were the fastest finishers. This type of test measures not only cardiovascular function, but also motivation, pain tolerance, running efficiency, sense of pace, and race strategy—all of which contribute to performance in distance running. Likewise, cyclists should be tested by cycling, swimmers by swimming, and other performers by participation in their chosen event.

The physical educator or coach must be aware that such a test, if used to predict future performance, is biased in favor of those with greater experience. Therefore, if a mediocre finisher is obviously handicapped by a poor sense of pace, by poor mechanical skills, or by ineffective race strategy, the physical educator or coach should consider such handicaps carefully before deciding to expend too much effort on faster finishers who may have more nearly approached their maximal performance capacities. It would be unwise to conclude that performance on running tests could be used to predict accurately endurance performance in other types of activity. There are too many differences between performances in running and swimming, for example, for an accurate prediction of one based on knowledge about the other.

Running Economy, Lactic Acid Levels, and Ventilation Breaking Point ("Anaerobic Threshold")

It is widely appreciated that a relatively high level of maximal oxygen uptake is *necessary* for high level aerobic endurance performance but is *not sufficient* to guarantee successful performance in competition with other athletes who also have relatively high maximal oxygen uptakes [9, 25, 29]. Endurance athletes must also be capable of exercising efficiently for prolonged times at *high percentages* of their maximal oxygen uptakes. For example, it has been shown that 10-kilometer running times for a group of highly trained runners with similar maximal oxygen uptakes could be predicted quite accurately from their oxygen uptakes at running speeds of 9 or 10 mph [9]. Runners who used less oxygen at these submaximal loads had faster 10-kilometer times. It appears that the best endurance athletes learn to use the smallest possible muscle mass (for the smallest oxygen demand) to accomplish their performances [29].

Lactic Acid Levels and Endurance Performance. Another characteristic of elite endurance athletes is that they can exercise at high percentages (80 per cent or more) of their maximal oxygen uptakes for long periods without accumulating large amounts of lactic acid in their blood [23, 25, 29, 32, 35]. As a matter of fact, it seems that the ability to exercise at high levels without the excessive accumulation of lactic acid is another possible predictor of success in distance running. One study reported very high correlations between maximal running speed for 5 to 12 miles (8–20 kilometers) and the running speed at which lactic acid accumulated to a level of 2.2 mmoles/l (20 mg/100 ml blood) [25]. Thus, if a coach had access to a treadmill or bicycle ergometer, the coach could obtain blood samples from the fingertip or earlobe during a progressive exercise test and have the samples analyzed for lactic acid at a local hospital. The results might prove useful for monitoring training progress.

The onset of blood lactic acid accumulation has traditionally been thought to reflect the point at which the demand for energy in the muscles was so great or the oxygen delivery so poor that anaerobic glycolysis caused lactic acid to accumulate in the blood [38]. However, we now know that the *production* of lactic acid is not the only factor that can contribute to lactic acid accumulation in the blood. It is possible to accumulate lactic acid if the *removal* of lactic acid from the blood is diminished or if there is a reduced *utilization* of lactic acid for energy. It is known, for instance, that blood flow to the liver (where some of the lactic acid is removed from the blood) is progressively reduced as exercise becomes more intense; this factor by itself could cause lactic acid accumulation in the blood without an increased rate of production of lactic acid by the muscles. Also, the accumulation of lactic acid could simply reflect the increased recruitment of fast twitch motor units that have poor capacities for aerobic energy production [35]. Some [21, 24], but not all, reports [32] show a positive correlation between the percentage of slow twitch muscle fibers in subjects and the running speed at which blood lactic acid accumulates.

The lack of association between the production of lactic acid in the muscle and the accumulation of blood lactic acid is suggested by a report of widely different levels of *muscle* lactic acid in different subjects when *blood* concentrations of 4 mmoles/*l* (36 mg/100 ml blood) were reached [36]. Thus, it is likely that several factors in addition to the rate of lactic acid production affect the rapidity with which blood lactic acid accumulates during exercise.

Ventilation Breaking Point and "Anaerobic Threshold." It has been known for many years that up to a point the rate of pulmonary ventilation increases regularly in a linear manner as exercise loads become more and more difficult. During these early stages of progressive exercise, ventilation increases in parallel with oxygen uptake. However, as the load reaches a point where a heart rate of about 150 beats per minute is achieved, ventilation begins to increase more sharply than oxygen uptake with continued increases in exercise load. This is the so-called "ventilation breaking point" (Fig. 9.3, middle and upper graphs). This point typically occurs at about 40–60 per cent of maximal oxygen uptake and is associated with an upward break in blood lactic acid accumulation to a concentration of 2 millimoles per liter (Fig. 9.3, lower graph) [35]. A second, more drastic breaking point in both ventilation and lactic acid often can be detected at a heart rate of 170–190 beats per minute. At this time one can observe an oxygen uptake equivalent to 65–90 per cent of maximum and a lactic acid concentration of 4 millimoles per liter (Fig. 9.3) [35].

Mechanism of Ventilation Breaking Point. The most likely explanation for this exercise response is that it is caused by the lactic acid which begins to accumulate in the blood at this time (Fig. 9.3, lower graph). The excess hydrogen ions associated with the acid are "neutralized" or buffered by bicarbonate in the blood. This buffering occurs because hydrogen ions (H^+) are combined with bicarbonate ions (HCO_3^-) to

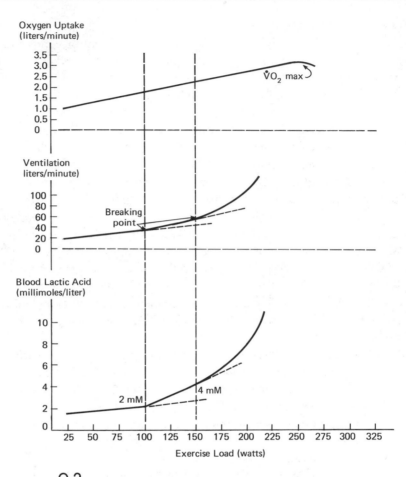

FIGURE 9.3. Oxygen uptake, ventilation, and blood lactic acid at ventilation breaking point ("anaerobic threshold").

form carbonic acid; the carbonic acid then breaks down into carbon dioxide and water as follows:

$$H^+ + HCO_3^- \rightarrow H_2CO_3 \rightarrow CO_2 + H_2O.$$

It is thought that the excess carbon dioxide stimulates the carotid body chemoreceptors or some unknown receptors to bring about a reflex increase in ventilation [38]. This extra breathing rids the body of the excess carbon dioxide. To complicate matters, though, it has been shown that the ventilation breaking point exists in patients who have a deficiency of the glycogen-degrading enzyme, phosphorylase; these patients cannot produce lactic acid because they cannot break down glycogen for energy [19]! It may be that the association between the increased lactic acid and the increased ventilation is only circumstantial and that some unknown factor operates to stimulate the extra ventilation.

"Anaerobic Threshold." Because it was thought that the increased lactic acid levels at the ventilation breaking point were caused by the onset of anaerobic conditions in the exercising muscles, the breaking point was called the "anaerobic threshold" [38]. As described earlier in this chapter, the anaerobic threshold concept is an oversimplification of the physiological facts because at least a portion of the increased lactic acid may be related to factors other than increased production of lactic acid, Accordingly, most investigators in this field now avoid reference to the term "anaerobic threshold" and instead emphasize the "ventilation breaking point" or the "onset of blood lactic acid accumulation." Incidentally, most experiments with athletes arbitrarily assign the value of 4 millimoles per liter (4mM) as the onset of blood lactate accumulation. This value seems to be more reproducible than the 2 mM value usually observed at the first upturn of the lactic acid curve (Fig. 9.3, lower graph). Also, athletes can exercise for many hours with lactic acid levels lower than 4 millimoles per liter, so the 2 millimolar concentration is of little practical importance for trained athletes [23, 32].

Practical Significance of Ventilation and Lactic Acid Breaking Points. Regardless of the physiological mechanism underlying the breaking points in ventilation and lactic acid concentration, these points may be better indicators of aerobic endurance performance and of training progress than maximal oxygen uptake. In addition, they may be useful in determining training intensities for optimal improvements in aerobic endurance [23]. It has already been pointed out that maximal oxygen uptake is a poor predictor of aerobic performance among good athletes as long as the maximal oxygen uptake is relatively high for all. Also, most of the improvements in maximal oxygen uptake are seen within the first few months of training. Continued improvement in performance is not associated with increased maximal oxygen uptake. Although it is a relatively simple matter to monitor ventilation and oxygen uptake and thus obtain the ventilation breaking point in the laboratory, it is more practical to obtain sequential blood samples for lactate analysis from earlobes or fingertips while athletes are exercising in the field at carefully monitored rates. In this way more athletes can be tested under conditions similar to those experienced in competition. Accordingly, most investigators have been reporting blood lactate results rather than ventilation breaking point results.

Use of Lactate Accumulation Data for Placement of Athletes in Endurance Events. Running speed achieved at the 2 millimolar [25] and 4 millimolar [21] lactic acid concentrations and the average mechanical power achieved at the 4 millimolar lactic acid level [24] have been shown to be highly correlated with endurance performance. Although these results do not support prediction of success in aerobic performance by lactic acid testing (it being far simpler to run time trials), they do show an association between performance level and the onset of lactate accumulation. Lactic acid tests may be useful in determining why an athlete with a high maximal oxygen uptake has difficulty in performing prolonged exercise. Such tests may help the coach place athletes in events more suited to their physiological attributes. As an illustration, a runner with a high maximal oxygen uptake but a low running speed at which lactate accumulates may be better suited to 1500–3000 meter events than longer races. On the other hand, a runner with a mediocre maximal oxygen uptake but a high running speed before lactic acid accumulates may be best suited to the marathon distance.

Lactate Accumulation as an Indicator of Training Progress. The potential value of lactic acid accumulation tests for evaluating training progress is shown by the fact that strenuous training improves the athlete's ability to perform at high levels before lactic acid accumulates to the 2 or 4 millimolar level [12, 34, 35]. These improvements are greater than those seen in maximal oxygen uptake and generally can be observed to progress throughout the duration of the training; maximal oxygen uptake levels off within the first few months of training. If the training is done at exercise loads much below those which elicit lactic acid concentrations of about 4 millimolar, improvements in either maximal oxygen uptake or lactic acid threshold are less likely to be seen [35]. It appears that lactic acid tests performed every few months during the training season might be useful to determine if the lactic acid turning points are occurring at greater exercise loads or if the training load should be increased to stimulate the lactate adaptation.

Use of Lactate Turning Points to Determine Training Intensity. Finally, it has been proposed that lactic acid turning points should be monitored regularly during training to provide information relative to training intensity [23]. It is suggested that training loads should be heavy enough to elicit lactic acid levels of about 4 millimolar to get the most benefit from training. The best way to do this is to have the athlete train at the speed, not at the heart rate, at which the 4 millimolar lactate level occurs [23]. The reason for not using the heart rate is that the heart rate increases as exercise duration increases; thus, if one begins to exercise at a heart rate of 170 beats per minute, the speed will have to be reduced as the exercise continues. This results in too much lactic acid production at the beginning of the training session and an exercise load which is too light at the end of the session [23].

REVIEW QUESTIONS

1. Describe the factors which determine maximal oxygen uptake.
2. Explain why maximal oxygen uptake can be used to evaluate maximal cardiovascular function in subjects who have no pulmonary disease. Write the equation that illustrates the relationship between maximal oxygen uptake and cardiovascular function.
3. Why is it not possible to predict aerobic endurance performance accurately from knowledge of a subject's maximal oxygen uptake?
4. List the principles of testing for maximal oxygen uptake and the criteria used to determine whether one's maximal oxygen uptake has been achieved.
5. List several performance tests that have been used to predict maximal oxygen uptake. What are some advantages and disadvantages of such tests?
6. Explain why the term "anaerobic threshold" has fallen into disfavor.
7. What evidence is there that an athlete's ability to exercise for a prolonged time at a high percentage of maximal oxygen uptake may be more highly related to aerobic endurance than maximal oxygen uptake?
8. How can tests of blood lactic acid levels be used to help determine appropriate training intensities for endurance athletes?
9. What is the currently accepted explanation for the ventilation turning point which occurs with progressively increasing exercise loads?
10. List some of the major differences in treadmill test protocols suggested for cardiac patients, normal subjects, and endurance athletes.

References 189

REFERENCES

[1] American Alliance for Health, Physical Education, Recreation, and Dance. *AAHPERD Youth Fitness Test Manual,* Rev. ed. Washington, D.C.: American Alliance for Health, Physical Education, Recreation, and Dance, 1976.

[2] American College of Sports Medicine. *Guidelines for Graded Exercise Testing and Exercise Prescription,* 2nd ed. Philadelphia: Lea & Febiger, 1980.

[3] Åstrand, I. Aerobic work capacity in men and women with special reference to age. *Acta Physiologica Scandinavica,* 1960, **49** (Supplementum 169).

[4] Åstrand, P.-O., and K. Rodahl. *Textbook of Work Physiology,* 2nd ed. New York: McGraw-Hill Book Company, 1977.

[5] Balke, B., and R. Ware. An experimental study of physical fitness of Air Force personnel. *U.S. Air Force Medical Journal,* 1959, **10**:675–688.

[6] Bruce, R. A. Methods of exercise testing. Step test, bicycle, treadmill, isometrics. *American Journal of Cardiology,* 1974, **33**:715–720.

[7] Bruce, R. A., R. Kusumi, and D. Hosmer. Maximal oxygen intake and nomographic assessment of functional aerobic impairment in cardiovascular disease. *American Heart Journal,* 1973, **85**:546–562.

[8] Cardus, D. Exercise testing: methods and uses. *Exercise and Sport Sciences Reviews,* 1978, **6**:59–103.

[9] Conley, D. L., and G. S. Krahenbuhl. Running economy and distance running performance of highly trained athletes. *Medicine and Science in Sports and Exercise,* 1980, **12**:357–360.

[10] Cooper, K. H. A means of assessing maximal oxygen intake. Correlation between field and treadmill testing. *Journal of the American Medical Association,* 1968, **203**:201–204.

[11] Cooper, K. H. *The New Aerobics.* New York: Bantam, 1970.

[12] Davis, J. A., M. H. Frank, B. J. Whipp, and K. Wasserman. Anaerobic threshold alterations caused by endurance training in middle-aged men. *Journal of Applied Physiology,* 1979, **46**:1039–1046.

[13] Falls, H. B., and L. D. Humphrey. A comparison of methods for eliciting maximum oxygen uptake from college women during treadmill walking. *Medicine and Science in Sports,* 1973, **5**:239–241.

[14] Fox, E. L. A simple, accurate technique for predicting maximal aerobic power. *Journal of Applied Physiology,* 1973, **35**:914–916.

[15] Froelicher, Jr., V. F., H. Brammell, G. Davis, I. Noguera, A. Stewart, and M. G. Lancaster. A comparison of three maximal treadmill exercise protocols. *Journal of Applied Physiology,* 1974, **36**:720–725.

[16] Gitin, E. L., J. E. Olerud, and H. W. Carroll. Maximal oxygen uptake based on lean body mass: a meaningful measure of physical fitness? *Journal of Applied Physiology,* 1974, **36**:757–760.

[17] Gleser, M. A., D. H. Horstman, and R. P. Mello. The effect on VO_2 max of adding arm work to maximal leg work. *Medicine and Science in Sports,* 1974, **6**:104–107.

[18] Graham, T. E., and G. M. Andrew. The variability of repeated measurements of oxygen debt in man following a maximal treadmill exercise. *Medicine and Science in Sports,* 1973, **5**:73–78.

[19] Hagberg, J. M., E. F. Coyle, J. M. Miller, J. E. Carroll, and W. H. Martin. Ventilatory threshold without increasing blood lactic acid levels in Mcardle's disease patients—anaerobic threshold? *Medicine and Science in Sports and Exercise* (abstract), 1981, **13**:115.

[20] Holmer, I., A. Lundin, and B. O. Eriksson. Maximum oxygen uptake during swimming and running by elite swimmers. *Journal of Applied Physiology,* 1974, **36**:711–714.

[21] Jacobs, I., B. Sjodin, and R. Schele. Muscle fiber composition and enzymes as determinants of marathon performance and onset of blood lactate accumulation (abstract). *Medicine and Science in Sports and Exercise,* 1981, **13**:114.

[22] Jessup, G. T., H. Tolson, and J. W. Terry. Prediction of maximal oxygen intake from Ås-

trand-Rhyming test, 12-minute run, and anthropometric variables using stepwise multiple regression. *American Journal of Physical Medicine,* 1974, **53:**200–207.

[23] Kindermann, W., G. Simon, and J. Keul. The significance of the aerobic-anaerobic transition for the determination of work load intensities during endurance training. *European Journal of Applied Physiology,* 1979, **42:**25–34.

[24] Komi, P. V., A. Ito, B. Sjodin, and J. Karlsson. Lactate breaking point and biomechanics of running (abstract). *Medicine and Science in Sports and Exercise,* 1981, **13:**114.

[25] LaFontaine, T. P., B. R. Londeree, and W. K. Spath. The maximal steady state versus selected running events. *Medicine and Science in Sports and Exercise,* 1981, **13:**190–192.

[26] Magel, J. R., G. F. Foglia, W. D. McArdle, B. N. Gutin, G. S. Pechar, and F. I. Katch. Specificity of swim training on maximum oxygen uptake. *Journal of Applied Physiology,* 1975, **38:**151–155.

[27] Nagle, F. J. Physiological assessment of maximal performance. *Exercise and Sport Sciences Reviews,* 1973, **1:**313–338.

[28] Naughton, J. P., and H. K. Hellerstein, eds., *Exercise Testing and Exercise Training in Coronary Heart Disease.* New York: Academic Press, Inc., 1973.

[29] Pollock, M. L. Submaximal and maximal working capacity of elite distance runners. Part I: cardiorespiratory aspects. *Annals of the New York Academy of Sciences,* 1977, **301:**310–322.

[30] Ribisl, P. M., and W. A. Kachadorian. Maximal oxygen intake prediction in young and middle-aged males. *Journal of Sports Medicine and Physical Fitness,* 1969, **9:**17–22.

[31] Rowell, L. B. Human cardiovascular adjustments to exercise and thermal stress. *Physiological Reviews,* 1974, **54:**75–159.

[32] Rusko, H., P. Rahkila, and E. Karvinen. Anaerobic threshold, skeletal muscle enzymes and fiber composition in young female cross-country skiers. *Acta Physiologica Scandinavica,* 1980, **108:**263–268.

[33] Secher, N. H., N. Ruberg-Larsen, R. A. Binkhorst, and F. Bonde-Petersen. Maximal oxygen uptake during arm cranking and combined arm plus leg exercise. *Journal of Applied Physiology,* 1974, **36:**515–518.

[34] Sjodin, B. Training effects on onset of blood lactate accumulation and muscle enzyme activities (abstract). *Medicine and Science in Sports and Exercise,* 1981, **13:**114.

[35] Skinner, J. S., and T. H. McLellan. The transition from aerobic to anaerobic metabolism. *Research Quarterly for Exercise and Sport,* 1980, **51:**234–248.

[36] Tesch, P. Muscle lactate accumulation at onset of blood lactate accumulation (abstract). *Medicine and Science in Sports and Exercise,* 1981, **13:**114.

[37] Wahlund, H. Determination of the physical working capacity. *Acta Medica Scandinavica,* 1948, (Supplementum 215).

[38] Wasserman, K., B. J. Whipp, S. N. Koyal, and W. L. Beaver. Anaerobic threshold and respiratory gas exchange during exercise. *Journal of Applied Physiology,* 1973, **35:**236–243.

CHAPTER 10

Training for Improved Aerobic Endurance

THERE are two principal reasons for wishing to improve one's ability to persist in performing physical activities that demand an efficient heart, lungs, and circulation. An endurance athlete is obviously interested in improving aerobic endurance to enhance athletic performance. But a more important consideration is the desire of many persons to improve their aerobic endurance in an effort to minimize their chances of becoming victims of heart disease early in their lives. Some of the evidence that suggests endurance exercise may offer some protection against the early onset of heart disease is presented in a later chapter. We will now describe the generally accepted principles of training for aerobic endurance improvement and explain some of the physiological adaptations that are commonly observed in trained individuals.

Part 1: Principles of Training for Aerobic Endurance

Before any strenuous training program is started, it is important to know if the trainee has any medical problems that might be aggravated by vigorous exercise or that might preclude a successful training outcome. Ideally, each trainee should undergo a complete physical examination, including an electrocardiogram taken during exercise, before engaging in the training program. Practically speaking, this ideal is rarely met because of financial considerations and the lack of medical personnel and facilities for stress testing. However, those with known symptoms of cardiovascular disease and all previously inactive individuals over the age of 35 should undergo a thorough physical examination (including exercise ECG) by their physicians to detect undisclosed cardiovascular disease [4]. Young, healthy trainees should be carefully monitored during the first stages of a training program so that any signs of inability to cope with the exercise stress can be detected before the stress becomes overwhelming. Extremely labored breathing, failure to keep up with one's peers, and any obvious symptoms of extreme physical discomfort should be taken as signs that a medical examination should be required and/or that the level of exercise for the individual should be reduced. Such signs of undue stress should, however, be rare occurrences if training programs are tailored to individual capacities as described in the next section.

Training Should Be Individualized and Should Progress Slowly

That there are great differences in aerobic endurance capacities among individuals should be recognized when undertaking or designing training programs. The program of the world champion distance runner, Farely Fleetfoot, is not appropriate for Pasquale Plumprump, whose most impressive distance performance is a train ride from Cucamonga to Kalamazoo. Training can be individualized in many ways, but two of the most commonly used procedures are to modify the exercise load according to a person's heart rate increase or to base the target times for exercise on past performances. With these two procedures, trainees with lesser aerobic capacities will train at lower intensities than those with greater endurance. Trainees who work according to their capacities are not discouraged by their inabilities to meet unrealistic training goals. They are also less apt to experience minor medical ailments or, in the case of those with cardiovascular disorders, to precipitate a heart attack.

Another way to minimize the risk of heart attacks, muscle and joint injuries, and muscular soreness is to begin the training program at a very low level and to progress very slowly for the first 2–3 weeks of training. This precaution is especially important for those over 35 who have not been in training for two years or more, and for any person with cardiovascular disease symptoms. Even young participants are more likely to continue a training program if they can avoid severe muscular soreness at the start of the program. *One simple criterion for minimizing the risk of exercising at too great an intensity is to work at levels that will allow one to carry on a normal conversation during the exercise.* If breathing becomes too labored to continue speaking comfortably, the pace should be slowed.

Aerobic Training Should Impose Unaccustomed Demands Upon One's Potential for Aerobic ATP Replenishment

The ability to persist in prolonged rhythmic exercise depends largely on the potential of the cardiovascular system to deliver oxygen to the muscles and upon the potential of those muscles to utilize the delivered oxygen for ATP replenishment by aerobic metabolism. Just as confinement to a bed for several weeks reduces demands on the cardiovascular and muscular systems and diminishes aerobic endurance, increased demands imposed by vigorous exercise will stimulate adaptations in cardiovascular and muscular function which will enhance aerobic endurance [8, 19, 54, 70]. What exercise load is sufficient to bring about greater aerobic endurance? Any *regular* program of exercise that moderately elevates one's heart rate and breathing rate above resting values for at least 5–10 minutes will lead to some aerobic endurance benefits [28, 70]. At low levels of training, these benefits may consist only of an enhanced ability to exercise without obvious physical discomfort. With more vigorous training programs, marked improvements in maximal oxygen uptake may occur. Those who are less fit may be satisfied with the endurance improvements brought on by a program of walking [28, 33], whereas endurance athletes will submit themselves to unbelievably rigorous training routines in efforts to compete successfully in aerobic endurance performances.

For those who are familiar with the strenuous training routines engaged in by endurance athletes, it is easy to be derisive about programs consisting of walking, mild calisthenics, and slow swimming or jogging. Although such moderate training routines cannot produce world-class endurance performers, they can improve the trainee's ability to exercise comfortably, and they may bring about measurable improvements in cardiovascular function and sometimes even in maximal oxygen uptake [70]. Subjects in poor physical condition should be encouraged to do some type of endurance exercise. No matter how mild the program, it will undoubtedly be better than no program at all.

Training Activities Should Be Rhythmic in Nature

Improvements in maximal oxygen uptake and cardiac function consistently occur if the exercise training utilizes rhythmic, large-muscle activities such as walking, jogging, cycling, swimming, hiking, rowing, cross-country skiing, skating, rope skipping, tennis, squash, racquetball, handball, soccer, and badminton [4, 5, 70]. Weight training and other activities which rely on many static (isometric) muscle contractions are less likely to cause significant improvements in maximal oxygen uptake. Cooper [20, 21] has produced a practical method of equating different types of exercise for their cardiovascular benefits, in which a variety of points are awarded for completion of various intensities and durations of activity.

Oxygen Uptake Can Be Stressed Maximally by Working at Less Than Maximal Intensity

To place stress on the cardiovascular and muscular mechanisms that bring maximal improvements in maximal oxygen uptake, it is not necessary to work at maximal intensity. It has been demonstrated that maximal oxygen uptake is reached at about 95 per cent of maximal heart rate or at about 80 per cent of maximal performance speed for a given training distance [8, 70]. Determining the appropriate speed for stressing maximal oxygen uptake at a given training distance becomes a simple matter if either maximal heart rate or fastest time for the distance is known. Thus, if Bjorn Blookerfeist has a maximal heart rate of 200 beats per minute and a best time of 120 seconds for the 800-meter run, he could run repeat 800's at a heart rate of $200 \times 0.95 = 190$ beats per minute. Since Bjorn's maximal speed for the 800 meters is $800/120 = 6.67$

m/sec, he could run repeat 800's at 80 per cent of that speed (.80 × 6.67 = 5.34 m/sec). At this speed, Bjorn's training time for each 800-meter run would be 800/5.34 = 150 seconds to insure that maximal oxygen uptake would be reached during most of the exercise periods (assuming short recovery intervals). A simpler method of calculating the training time is to divide the best time for the training distance by 0.8.

$$100\% \; \dot{V}O_2 \; max. \; Time \; (sec) = Best \; Time \; (sec)/0.8$$

For example, if the best time for a 100-meter swim is 60 seconds, the 100-meter training time approximately equivalent to 100 per cent $\dot{V}O_2$ max. is 60/0.8 = 75 sec. Training at speeds faster than this will tax the anaerobic systems to a great extent, and fewer repeats can be accomplished to stress the aerobic mechanisms.

As stated previously, it is not necessary to work at 95 per cent of maximal heart rate to bring about *some* improvement in maximal oxygen uptake. This type of high intensity work is needed only by those who want to get the greatest possible improvement in maximal oxygen uptake in the shortest possible time.

Aerobic Training Should Be Progressive

As with any form of fitness training, aerobic conditioning programs are most effective when the exercise routines become progressively more difficult with increasing weeks and months of training. The reason for this is that the body adapts only to unaccustomed stress; as adaptations to one level of exercise training are made, that level no longer provides an unaccustomed stress, so what was once difficult becomes relatively easy. Therefore, the cardiovascular system and other organ systems that have adapted to one intensity of exercise must be overloaded by greater intensities of exercise if greater adaptations are desired.

There are two common methods used to ensure the progressive nature of an aerobic training program. One is to predict (guess) the appropriate times to increase the exercise load, duration, and frequency on the basis of past experiences with similar trainees. This is the method used by some athletic coaches who plan a detailed training schedule for their athletes for the entire season without the slightest bit of evidence that those athletes will have adapted to each step of the training routine. While it is possible that experienced coaches may be very successful with this sort of program, it is also probable that some individual trainees in such a program would be better suited to an individualized approach, based on physiological evidence that adaptations to one level of training were achieved before subsequent levels were attempted.

A second method of ensuring the progressive nature of aerobic training is to base the training intensity upon a certain exercise heart rate, that is, 95 per cent of maximal heart rate, 50 per cent of maximal heart rate, heart rate of 130 beats per minute, 170 beats per minute, and so on. The principle underlying this training scheme is that as the body adapts to exercise, the resting heart rate and the heart rate for a given submaximal exercise load will be reduced [8]. Therefore, as the individual becomes better trained, a greater exercise load will be required to elicit a given heart rate. For an untrained person, it takes very little activity to bring about a heart rate of 150; up to a point, a much greater work load is required to elicit a heart rate of 150 after a period of training. Likewise, 80 per cent of maximal heart rate can be achieved by a smaller intensity of exercise before training than after some weeks of training. This technique of basing exercise load on heart rate obviously requires that the trainee become accustomed to measuring heart rates several times during each workout.

At that point in a training program when one has increased the maximal oxygen uptake to its hereditary limit, a plateau will be reached at which there is no longer a reduction in heart rate for a given exercise load, no matter how long one trains at that load. At this point, a training program based solely upon exercising at a given heart rate (with the possible exception of extremely high rates such as 95 per cent of maximum) will no longer insure the attainment of progressive increases in exercise load and aerobic endurance capacity. When, after a few weeks of training at a given load, the trainee finds that exercise need not be done at a faster rate or with a heavier load to attain the same exercise heart rate, the trainee must conclude that he or she has reached a heart rate plateau. The trainee must then work at a higher level that will elicit a faster heart rate if the trainee is to continue improving the capacity to persist in exercise at a high percentage of maximal oxygen uptake. (Even though one reaches a limit in $\dot{V}_{O_2}$ max improvement, one can continue to enhance the ability to work for longer times at greater percentages of that $\dot{V}_{O_2}$ max.)

Progression Based on Improvements in Maximal Oxygen Uptake and/or Threshold for Lactic Acid Accumulation. If it is feasible to test an athlete's maximal oxygen uptake and/or threshold for lactic acid accumulation regularly (see previous chapter), these markers of training improvement should be used in the determination of training progression. If heart rate, oxygen uptake, and lactic acid levels are simultaneously monitored during a progressive maximal treadmill or bicycle ergometer test, it is possible to find the heart rate corresponding to a given percentage of maximal oxygen uptake and/or the heart rate corresponding to the accumulation of lactic acid. As training causes improvements in maximal oxygen uptake and lactic acid threshold, heart rates at 100 per cent of maximal oxygen uptake and at lactate threshold will also increase; these increased heart rates may then be used as target heart rates during training. It is recommended that maximal oxygen uptake and lactate threshold be tested at intervals of 3–4 months.

Minimal Intensity, Duration, and Frequency of Exercise Required to Improve Maximal Oxygen Uptake

What is the minimal amount of exercise required to bring about measurable improvements in maximal oxygen uptake, the most commonly accepted measure of aerobic endurance fitness? Investigations of this matter have considered as little as 3 minutes of mild exercise per day to as much as an hour or more of heavy daily exercise [12, 15, 28, 33, 70, 79, 84]. Subjects for most of the studies on exercise threshold for aerobic endurance enhancement have been adult males, and the training programs have usually emphasized continuous rather than interval exercise. A general conclusion that can be drawn from this research is that for most healthy young or middle-aged adults some improvement in maximal oxygen uptake can be expected if 1) the exercise intensity is at least that required to bring the heart rate above 135 beats per minute, 2) the duration of each exercise period at this intensity is at least 10 minutes, and 3) the frequency of training is at least three times per week. This minimum of 30 minutes per week does *not* include warmup time, does *not* include training for anything other than aerobic endurance fitness, and does *not* produce increases in maximal oxygen uptake for *every* trainee. If one wished greater assurance that training would improve maximal oxygen uptake, exercise heart rate should be about 150 beats per minute, exercise duration should be at least 30 minutes per session, and training sessions should be conducted at least 3 times each week.

Suggested Ranges of Exercise Heart Rates for Aerobic Endurance Training

The practice of prescribing a single exercise heart rate, for example 135 or 150 beats per minute, for aerobic training ignores the fact that such an exercise load might be too mild for a well-conditioned individual who wishes to achieve a *maximal* training effect but too severe for a trainee with cardiovascular disease. Even among normal untrained subjects there is a wide range of resting, submaximal, and maximal exercise heart rates, depending upon age, sex, and heredity, so that exercise at a common heart rate will produce different relative intensities of work and different training effects [8, 83].

Older persons have lower exercise heart rates for comparably strenuous exercise loads than young persons; accordingly, a threshold heart rate of 130 beats per minute for young adults may be equivalent to only 110–120 beats per minute for elderly persons [5]. An exercise heart rate of 130 beats per minute could be too stressful for an untrained elderly person.

As shown in Fig. 10.1, the exercise load at any given heart rate will be relatively easier for many females compared to many males [8]. For example, a heart rate of about 128 beats per minute will be equivalent to 50 per cent of the maximal oxygen uptake for the average fit young adult male, but only 42 per cent for the average female. The reason for this difference is that the female has a smaller heart, has less hemoglobin in her blood, and transports less oxygen at a given cardiac output; thus, relative to the male, her heart must beat faster to reach any given percentage of her maximal oxygen uptake. On average, females must exercise at heart rates about 8–10 beats faster than males if exercise loads are to be of similar relative severity.

Percentage of Maximal Heart Rate for Exercise Prescription. Another technique sometimes used for prescribing exercise intensity is to have subjects train at *some percentage of predicted maximal heart rate*. For example, it may be thought that everyone should exercise at 70 per cent of maximal heart rate. However, this practice suffers from two drawbacks—maximal heart rate undergoes changes with age, and there is a fairly large variation in maximal heart rate even among subjects of the same age [8]. Therefore, unless maximal heart rate is directly measured, prediction of maximal heart rate is subject to substantial error. Accordingly, an exercise load equivalent to 70 per cent of predicted maximal heart rate will be relatively too severe for some

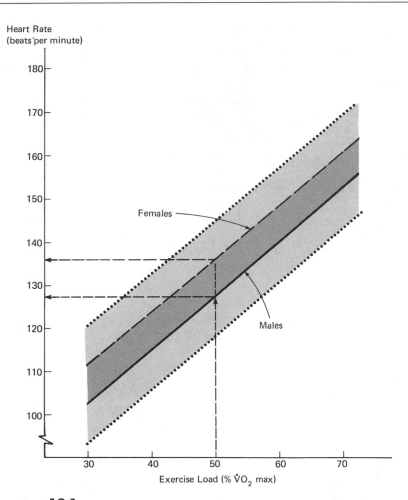

FIGURE 10.1. Approximate relationship between heart rate and exercise load (expressed as a percentage of maximal oxygen uptake) for healthy, fit young adults. Shaded areas represent standard deviations. Note the overlap between sexes as shown by the more darkly shaded area. Modified from Astrand and Rodahl [8].

and too mild for others [27]. This concept is particularly important when prescribing exercise loads for heart patients, whose maximal heart rates may be very low as a result of disease processes.

The Karvonen Formula for Prescribing Exercise Heart Rate. One way to facilitate exercise prescription is to estimate exercise intensity *in relation to one's maximal oxygen uptake.* Since at submaximal work loads, there is a linear relationship between heart rate and oxygen uptake [8], one can prescribe exercise at a heart rate that represents a given percentage of one's maximal oxygen uptake (Fig. 10.1). Heart rates representing 40–75 per cent of maximal oxygen uptake have been suggested as target heart rates for aerobic training of nonathletic groups [27, 59, 71, 76, 82, 83]. Unfortunately, it is not an easy matter to determine maximal oxygen uptakes for everyone who wishes to undertake an aerobic endurance training program. Consequently, an alternative method of prescribing target heart rates for training has been based on the difference between resting and predicted maximal heart rates and has found widespread acceptance [59].

Karvonen [59] proposed that exercise heart rate should be at least the sum of the *heart rate at rest* plus *60 per cent of the difference between maximal and resting heart rates,* that is,

$$HR_{Ex} = HR_{Rest} + 0.60\,(HR_{Max} - HR_{Rest}).$$

Accordingly, if one's resting heart rate were 65 and maximal heart rate were 205, the training heart rate should be greater than $65 + 0.60\,(205 - 65) = 149$. The basis for this technique is that the difference between resting and maximal heart rates for a given person represents the reserve of the heart for increasing cardiac output. Exercise at a heart rate representing a high percentage of this reserve should then be adequate to bring about appropriate cardiovascular adaptations. The exercise heart rate as determined by the Karvonen formula represents about 50 per cent of maximal oxygen uptake in untrained males and 45 per cent in females. In trained persons, the Karvonen heart rate represents approximately 60 per cent and 55 per cent of maximal oxygen uptake in males and females, respectively [8]. After training one relies more on stroke volume and less on heart rate to deliver oxygen.

The Karvonen technique is not without its detractors. It has been pointed out that the prediction of maximal heart rate, even when adjusted for age, is subject to error, especially when dealing with cardiac patients [50]. For those in good health, however, the Karvonen technique seems to be a good compromise solution to the problem of exercise prescription.

In Table 10.1 are illustrated suggested ranges of exercise heart rates for aerobic endurance training of persons with various ages and resting heart rates. In each case, the low end of the range was determined by 1) subtracting the resting heart rate from the predicted maximal heart rate for subjects of various ages [8, 83], 2) multiplying the difference so obtained by 0.6 (60 per cent of "cardiac reserve"), and 3) adding the value found in 2) to the resting heart rate to find the training heart rate. The high end of each range was calculated as 95 per cent of the trainee's predicted maximal heart rate. If a trainee were 15 years old with a resting heart rate of 80 beats per minute, the heart rate during exercise periods should be maintained above 155 ($205 - 80 = 125; 0.6 \times 125 = 75; 75 + 80 = 155$). The exercise heart rate so determined should represent a minimal or threshold intensity of training for the individual to insure that the training will be strenuous enough to cause some adaptations of the heart and circulation and perhaps measurable improvements in maximal oxygen uptake [28, 29, 33, 50, 61, 70]. For greater assurance of improvements in maximal oxygen uptake, one should exercise at greater than threshold levels. For the same 15-year-old trainee, the maximal training heart rate should be about 195 beats per minute ($205 \times 0.95 = 195$). By exercising at 95 per cent of predicted maximal heart rate, one should reach maximal oxygen uptake during exercise [8, 70]. This high intensity of exercise is most often used in athletic training and is usually too high for ordinary conditioning programs.

If one exercises at an intensity greater than 95 per cent of maximal heart rate, maxi-

TABLE 10.1

Suggested Ranges of Exercise Heart Rates for Aerobic Endurance Training.[1]

Age (years)	Estimated Max. H.R.	Heart Rate While Standing At Rest				
		50	60	70	80	90
5	205			151–195	155–195	159–195
10	210			154–200	158–200	162–200
15	205		147–198	151–195	155–195	159–195
20–25	200	140–190	144–190	148–190	152–190	156–190
30	195	137–185	141–185	145–185	149–185	153–185
35	190	134–180	138–180	142–180	146–180	150–180
40	185	131–176	135–176	139–176	143–176	147–176
45	180	128–171	132–171	136–171	140–171	143–171
50	175	125–166	129–166	133–166	137–166	140–166
55	170	122–162	126–162	130–162	134–162	137–162
60	165	119–157	123–157	127–157	131–157	134–157
65	160	116–152	120–152	124–152	128–152	131–152
70	155	113–147	117–147	121–147	125–147	128–147

[1] Training at low heart rates should improve endurance but may not increase maximal oxygen uptake. Training at high heart rates will maximize rate of improvement in endurance and maximal oxygen uptake; it is recommended for athletes.

mal oxygen uptake will not increase further, but anaerobic metabolism will produce high levels of lactic acid, and less work will be accomplished during the training period. However, training at greater than 95 per cent of maximal heart rate is necessary for improving the *anaerobic* capacity of distance athletes, so that sprints at the start and finish of a race may be prolonged.

Maximal heart rate at different ages can be roughly estimated by subtracting one's age in years from 225 or 220. For example, if a person is 50 years old, maximal heart rate should be 175 (225 minus 50 equals 175) or 170 beats per minute (220 minus 50 equals 170). Regardless of the method used to estimate maximal heart rate, the chances that the estimate will be in error by 5–10 beats per minute or more are great [8]. Accordingly, one should not hope to be too precise in exercise prescription by any technique that depends on estimation rather than direct determination of maximal heart rate. In most instances, precision is not important. In the case of heart patients, it is wise to be conservative in the estimate of maximal heart rate if it cannot be measured directly.

There are substantial individual differences in what constitutes the optimal exercise intensity for aerobic conditioning. The suggested ranges of exercise heart rates shown in Table 10.1 should encompass the optimal values for all trainees, with the possible exception of some patients with cardiovascular disease and some elderly persons who should perhaps exercise at lower heart rates [50]. Exercise prescription has not been developed to the point where a simple measure can be used as the sole basis of a precise prescription for all individuals. It remains for the individual trainee, the exercise leader, the physician, the physical educator, and the coach to use judgement based on knowledge of the trainee to select the appropriate exercise heart rate within the ranges shown in Table 10.1 or to modify the ranges as necessary for unique individuals and circumstances. A training program for older persons is shown in Table 10.2.

TABLE 10.2
**A Beginning Aerobic Training Program for Persons
50 Years of Age and Older [30]**

The deVries Jog-walk Program for Older Persons			
Days[1]	Jog	Walk	Number of Sets[2]
1–6	50 steps	50 steps	start at 5; build to 10
7–12	50 steps	40 steps	start at 5; build to 10
13–18	50 steps	30 steps	start at 5; build to 10
19–24	50 steps	20 steps	start at 5; build to 10
25–30	50 steps	10 steps	start at 5; build to 10
31–36	75 steps	10 steps	start at 5; build to 10
37–42	100 steps	10 steps	start at 5; build to 10
43–48	125 steps	10 steps	start at 5; build to 10
49–54	150 steps	10 steps	start at 5; build to 10
55–60	175 steps	10 steps	start at 5; build to 10
61–66	200 steps	10 steps	start at 5; build to 10

67 and later: Proceed with individualized program based on Karvonen technique

[1] Based on 3 training sessions per week
[2] Increase the number of sets by one each day at each level

Range of Expected Improvements in Maximal Oxygen Uptake

Trainees who begin a conditioning program with a relatively high maximal oxygen uptake can expect either no changes or only minor improvements with mild to moderate training, whereas those who are in poor condition may experience increases of 30 per cent or more in maximal oxygen uptake [70, 72, 73]. The usual improvement shown in maximal oxygen uptake for young and middle-aged subjects is about 15–20 per cent [70].

Interval Training

If exercise is performed without stopping during a training session, the exercise is said to be of the "continuous" type. If intervals of exercise are interspersed with rest or recovery periods, it is classified as "interval" training. An illustration of hypothetical changes in oxygen uptake and oxygen deficit during an interval training session is shown in Fig. 10.2. In this example both exercise and recovery intervals are 3 minutes long. If total energy expenditure is the same, both continuous and interval training seem to produce similar changes in aerobic endurance measures, and both can be successfully used to improve aerobic endurance and aerobic performance [8, 22, 34]. Interval training is particularly important for improving the ability to maintain sprints at the beginning and end of a race. Nearly all successful endurance athletes include both continuous and interval types of training in their programs.

The high end of the ranges for exercise heart rates shown in Table 10.1 can be used to indicate interval training heart rates for athletes and others who desire high levels of aerobic fitness. When using *interval* training for the maximal improvement of aerobic

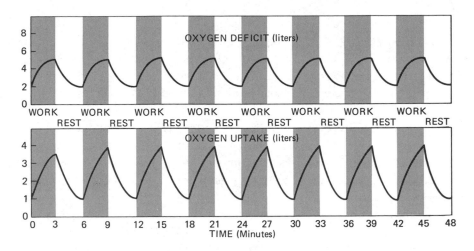

FIGURE 10.2. Hypothetical rise and fall of oxygen uptake and oxygen deficit during an interval training period designed to enhance aerobic endurance.

FIGURE 10.3. Interval training procedures can be used successfully in training for soccer. (Courtesy of Office of Public Information, Purdue University, West Lafayette, Indiana.)

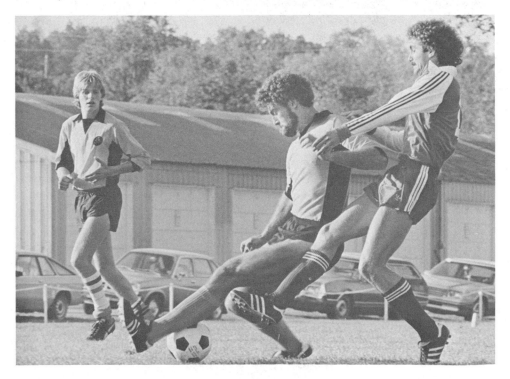

potential, it is important to achieve maximal or near maximal oxygen uptakes during each exercise period, but not to exceed the exercise intensity that will provoke maximal oxygen uptake. The reason for this is that heavier loads must be met by progressively greater contributions of anaerobic metabolism; consequently, exhaustion ensues more quickly to reduce the total work performed during the training session.

Principles for Aerobic Interval Training.   There are two important assumptions in the rationale for including interval training in an aerobic training program for general fitness or athletic training. The first is that interval training is better than continuous training for *adapting the nervous system to the movement patterns experienced in competition.* The second assumption is that interval training allows one to exercise longer at the limits of aerobic metabolism than does continuous training; this should cause more beneficial *adaptations in the aerobic metabolic systems in the muscles.* These assumptions are based on the fact that one cannot maintain the exercise intensity of competition throughout a training session that utilizes continuous exercise exclusively. A competitive pace for 3,000 meters, for example, cannot be sustained over the course of a 2-hour continuous training session. Therefore, it is reasoned, the neural patterns reinforced during *continuous* training will be those used at a *slower* pace than the one used in competition. Also, with slow continuous training the mitochondrial systems for replenishing ATP will not be stressed to the extent possible with shorter, more intensive exercise periods. In other words, with continuous training one becomes most adapted to a pace slower than the competitive pace.

With *interval* training, the *exercise* intervals are designed so that the exercise pace is similar to that used in competition; the *recovery* intervals are designed so that many of these high quality exercise intervals can be completed during the training session. This approach presumably causes maximal adaptation of both the nervous system and the metabolic system for performance at the competitive pace.

The underlying rationale for interval training appears sound. However, comparisons of the effectiveness of the interval approach and the continuous approach to *aerobic* endurance training have generally shown little difference between the two [22, 34]. For *anaerobic* endurance, it is widely accepted that interval training is the better approach. Perhaps the reason for the similarity in effectiveness between interval and continuous exercise in *aerobic* training is that at the longer competitive distances, athletes can begin to approach the competitive pace in practice sessions. Thus, good distance runners and swimmers can perform for an hour or longer at paces equivalent to 85–90 per cent of their maximal oxygen uptakes. Any advantage gained from interval training at 95–100 per cent of maximal oxygen uptake may be difficult to detect. Even if it is only equally effective to continuous training routines, interval training should be included in aerobic athletic training programs; interval training can improve performance in the early and late sprint phases of competition and can help relieve the boredom associated with the use of only one type of training.

Suggested Durations of Exercise and Recovery Intervals for Aerobic Interval Training.   The duration of exercise intervals for aerobic training should be long enough to allow the trainee to reach maximal oxygen uptake during most of the exercise intervals and short enough to minimize early fatigue. However, convincing evidence that short work intervals produce lesser improvements in aerobic potential than longer intervals is not available. Although most trainees should be able to achieve maximal oxygen uptakes more consistently with 3–5 minute work periods [8], actual comparisons of adaptations in maximal oxygen uptake induced by short and long periods have produced discordant results [40, 62]. The data of Knuttgen and his coworkers [62] suggested that 3-minute exercise periods interspersed with 3-minute recovery periods produced greater gains in maximal oxygen uptake than did a 15-second exercise and 15-second recovery regimen. On the other hand, Fox and his colleagues [40] found greater improvements in trainees who completed shorter work intervals (8–40 seconds) than in those who trained for longer durations (2½–5 minutes). Because of differences in subject populations, strict comparisons between the two studies are not possible. Therefore, it is suggested that both brief and longer periods be included in interval training programs to provide variety, to enhance anaerobic potential, and to improve aerobic potential. However, the emphasis should be placed on equal work and recovery periods of 3–5 minutes duration to enable more trainees to maintain maximal oxygen uptake during more of the workout period [8]. If shorter work intervals are used, the rest intervals should also be shortened to help maintain high oxygen uptakes throughout the training session [8].

Figure 10.2 illustrates the theoretical rise and fall of oxygen uptake and oxygen deficit during an aerobic interval training period. Note that the trainee's maximal oxygen uptake of 4.0 liters is reached during all but the first of the 3-minute exercise periods, and that oxygen deficit is not allowed to accumulate to the subject's maximal oxygen deficit capacity of 6.0 liters.

Suggested Intensity of Recovery Intervals for Aerobic Training. The intensity of recovery intervals is one of the variables that can be manipulated during interval training. For example, it would be possible to lie down, stand, walk, jog, or run during recovery from a running interval. It has been shown that exercise at approximately 30–40 per cent of maximal oxygen uptake is best for hastening the removal of accumulated lactic acid from the blood [13]. This intensity represents a heart rate of about 100–115 for young fit males and 105–120 for females [8]. Thus, a continuation of mild exercise during recovery is recommended as the main form of recovery interval for aerobic interval training.

Loss of Aerobic Fitness upon Cessation of Training

If one who has become conditioned to aerobic forms of exercise stops training, most of the benefits of training may be lost within two weeks to three months [17, 32, 42, 68, 71]. Values of maximal oxygen uptake, heart rate response to submaximal exercise, heart rate recovery after exercise, and resting heart rates usually revert to pretraining levels faster than the total capacity for submaximal work. Thus, part of the increased endurance to submaximal work tasks that is brought on by training must result from such "psychological" factors as increased tolerance to pain, greater motivation, or reduced anxiety, in addition to improvements in cardiovascular and muscular function [7, 42]. The "psychological" improvements seem to persist longer than the cardiovascular changes. The fact that aerobic fitness is transient in nature illustrates the need for *regularity* in exercise training. It is not possible to retain a moderate level of aerobic fitness by playing golf once a week or even daily during the summer months alone. It does not make sense to plan for aerobic fitness during only four or five months of the year. On the other hand, training during the summer, providing it progresses slowly, is better than no training at all, and absence from a training program because of prolonged illness does not mean that prior training was necessarily wasted. The evidence simply suggests that *regularity* in exercise programs should be the goal of all types of fitness conditioning.

Maintenance of Previously Acquired Aerobic Fitness

A general principle of fitness programs is that it takes less activity to maintain an established level of fitness than to acquire it in the first place. This principle also is applicable to aerobic fitness. Several studies have reported that after vigorous conditioning programs, aerobic fitness (usually assessed by measures of maximal oxygen uptake) can be maintained by workouts 30–60 minutes long, one to three times weekly [17, 41, 52, 71]. These studies have included training and maintenance programs conducted for relatively short periods, and it is unknown whether low-level maintenance programs can maintain fitness for a year or longer. From the data available, however, we conclude that a conservative recommendation for maintenance of aerobic fitness is a 30-minute training session three times weekly, with an exercise load similar to that used originally to acquire aerobic fitness. Although this recommendation may include more work than is absolutely essential, it seems advisable to risk such an error than to risk advising a program that may not be adequate to maintain fitness.

Part 2: Adaptations to Aerobic Endurance Training

The physiological effects of physical training with continuous, rhythmic exercise have been frequently studied for many years. Although contradictory reports have resulted from these studies, there are, nevertheless, some generally accepted accounts of "typical" or expected adaptations to regular endurance training. As these adaptations are described, the reader should keep in mind that factors such as age and fitness level can minimize or enhance the likelihood that any given adaptation will occur.

Cardiovascular Function During Maximal Exercise

It is widely recognized that aerobic endurance training can improve physical performance by causing substantial changes in cardiovascular function during maximal exercise. Because of the widespread interest in discovering means to prevent the early onset of degenerative heart disease, the role of exercise in improving cardiovascular function has come under increasing scrutiny. The most accepted measure of the effectiveness of exercise training in enhancing cardiovascular function is the nearly universal increase in maximal oxygen uptake that occurs with training.

Factors Influencing Improvement in Maximal Oxygen Uptake. As described in the previous chapter, maximal oxygen uptake depends upon the ability of the heart to deliver blood to the working muscles and the ability of the circulation to shift blood from nonworking regions of the body to working muscles. Therefore, maximal oxygen uptake can be viewed as a measure of maximal cardiovascular function, and improvements in maximal oxygen uptake after exercise training are ordinarily caused to some extent by improved maximal cardiovascular function.

Changes in maximal oxygen uptake as a result of aerobic training range from no improvement to increases as great as 43 per cent and more [70]. The extent of any training effect depends on many factors, including physical condition prior to initiation of training, age, mode of exercise during assessment of maximal oxygen uptake, heredity, and type of training program. Both males and females respond to aerobic training with similar increments in maximal oxygen uptake, so *sex of the trainee is not an important factor in predicting improvements in maximal oxygen uptake* as long as other factors, especially the type of training, are equal [70]. Whether or not training at a high altitude has a beneficial effect, compared with sea-level training, on maximal oxygen uptake is controversial. There seems to be no value in training at 2,300 meters as opposed to sea level [2], but this altitude may be below the threshold altitude (3,000 m.?), above which benefits have been observed in other studies [24, 31].

Physical Condition Prior to Training. Increases in maximal oxygen uptake in response to a training program are the least in those persons who are most fit and the greatest in those who are least fit before the training program begins [8, 70, 73]. Subjects who have been bedridden for several weeks or completely inactive for several years can expect to achieve a 30 per cent increase in maximal oxygen uptake [73], whereas fit endurance athletes may experience no further gains in maximal oxygen uptake with an additional training period [72]. The underlying basis for this phenomenon is that each individual has a certain potential for optimal cardiac development, circulatory function, and muscular development, so that inactive persons have further to go to achieve their potentials than do habitually active persons. Most studies of changes in maximal oxygen uptake caused by aerobic endurance training in untrained men have shown improvements of 15–20 per cent [70, 73].

Age. Comparisons of improvements in maximal oxygen uptake for various age groups is somewhat difficult because of the scarcity of literature describing changes in very young and very old subjects and because it is rare that very young or old subjects train at the high intensities often achieved by young and middle-aged adults. Thus, training programs are often not strictly comparable. From the evidence available, it appears that youths 10–15 years of age can achieve the same percentage increments in maximal oxygen uptake as adult subjects [35, 66], but that elderly trainees can expect somewhat lesser improvements in aerobic power [70, 73]. Elderly trainees do not experience as great a percentage of improvement in maximal oxygen uptake because they have lower maximal cardiac outputs; maximal heart rate falls from 200 in youth to about 160 at age 65 [8]. Also, maximal pulmonary ventilation during exercise of short duration is lowered from 140–160 l/min at age 25, to 80 l/min or less in those 65 years of age and older [75]. This reduction in maximal exercise ventilation is probably due to connective tissue changes in the joints of the rib cage that lead to stiffening of those joints. Gradual deterioration in lung and bronchial structure follows so that airway resistance is increased [75].

It should be emphasized once again that part of the lesser improvement in maximal oxygen uptake observed in elderly trainees is probably accounted for by the fact that exercise programs for the elderly tend to be very conservative with rather mild intensities of work prescribed. It may be that an older subject who engages in *heavy* training may experience just as great an improvement in aerobic power as a younger person.

Mode of Exercise During Assessment of Maximal Oxygen Uptake. The magnitude of any effect of aerobic endurance training on maximal oxygen uptake depends to some extent on whether the exercise task used to evaluate oxygen uptake is similar to the exercise used in training. For example, if one trains by cycling but is tested for maximal oxygen uptake on a treadmill, smaller gains in aerobic power are apt to be observed than if the trainee were tested on a bicycle ergometer [69]. Likewise, training by swimming increases maximal oxygen uptake when measured during tethered swimming, but not when measured with a treadmill test. The apparent reason for different maximal oxygen uptake adaptations when different types of exercise tests are used is that muscles specifically trained in one type of exercise (for example, arm muscles in swim training) do not have the same involvement in one form of exercise test as in another. Consequently, training-induced adaptations in the ability of muscles to extract oxygen from the blood or improvements in local circulation to the working muscles may not be evaluated properly with an exercise test that does not specifically stress those muscles.

A practical consequence of this phenomenon of exercise specificity in maximal oxygen uptake adaptations is that aerobic endurance training in one form of exercise is not necessarily of benefit when the trainee performs another type of physical activity requiring the use of untrained muscles. This is the common experience of many who, thinking themselves to be in "good shape" because they practiced basketball regularly, find that they become rapidly fatigued in a game of squash, in swimming, or in some other activity for which they have not specifically trained.

Heredity. Not all trainees of the same environmental, social, economic, and educational background improve their maximal oxygen uptakes to the same extent with the same type of training. In other words, there seem to be some inborn factors that predispose certain individuals to have greater adaptations to training than others [70]. Whether differences in populations of muscle fiber types, pain thresholds, emotions, enzyme systems, or some other differences in biological characteristics will eventually be shown to explain the variability in maximal oxygen uptake adaptations to training remains to be seen.

Type of Training. Previously in this chapter, we learned that marked differences in the degree of change in maximal oxygen uptake are associated with differences in training programs. A program consisting of 5–10 minutes of walking twice per week will almost certainly produce no change in maximal oxygen uptake, whereas large increases in oxygen uptake can be produced as adaptations to more strenuous types of training [70].

Maximal Cardiac Output, Heart Rate, and Stroke Volume. In *previously sedentary young adults* about 50 per cent of the increase in maximal oxygen uptake that occurs with endurance training is associated with an increased *maximal cardiac output,* and 50 per cent with an increased *maximal arteriovenous oxygen difference* [8, 22, 72, 73]. In *fit young males and older subjects* nearly all of the increase in maximal oxygen uptake has been attributed to a greater maximal cardiac output [8, 72, 73]. Accordingly, it can be stated that the improvement in maximal cardiac output with aerobic training is at least as important as any other change in maximal cardiovascular function and may be the *only* significant change observed in some subjects [72].

The maximal cardiac output typically rises from untrained values of 22 or 16 l/min in young adult males and females, respectively, to 24 and 18 l/min after aerobic endurance training [8, 73]. This training-induced rise in maximal cardiac output is *not* a function of a greater maximal heart rate after training because, if anything, the maximal heart rate declines slightly with training [8, 70, 73]. Consequently, the greater maximal cardiac output after training must be the result of a greater stroke volume [8, 72, 73]. Pretraining maximal stroke volumes of 110 and 80 ml for young adult males and females, respectively, typically increase to 122 and 96 ml after several months of aerobic training [8, 73].

Mechanisms for Improved Stroke Volume. The greater stroke volume in hearts of trained persons at rest and during exercise has been attributed to three mechanisms acting separately or together.

1. Greater stroke volume may be caused by greater diastolic filling of the chambers of an enlarged heart so that the heart has a greater blood volume to force out when it contracts. This mechanism has been reported to occur in both males and females [78, 87]. Often, the mass of the left ventricle is enlarged [58, 87]. Increased ventricular wall thickness appears to be most likely to occur in activities such as weight training, in which the heart is forced to work against high resistance caused by strenuous muscle contractions [58].

2. Greater stroke volume at rest and during submaximal exercise may be indirectly caused by greater diastolic filling of the ventricles in response to a reduced heart rate [86]. As heart rate is reduced with training, the chambers of the heart have longer to fill with blood. Greater filling stretches the muscle fibers, causes better overlap of thick and thin filaments, and results in a greater contractile force. This mechanism cannot explain the greater stroke volume observed in trained persons during *maximal* exercise because training typically does not reduce the maximal heart rate.

3. Greater stroke volume may be caused by improved contractility of the heart muscle [10, 11, 74, 78, 80]. Many studies have shown greater stroke volumes without increased heart volumes. Therefore, the trained heart must be able to contract more completely to eject a greater fraction of the blood within its chambers. Studies on rats suggest that training causes an adaptation in the sarcolemma of the heart muscle fibers to allow the sarcolemma to bind more calcium from the extracellular fluid [80]. This extra sarcolemmal calcium is then made available to troponin in the muscle cell to initiate more cross bridge formation and more forceful contraction.

The majority of the evidence available supports the conclusion that at least a portion of the training-induced improvement in stroke volume is caused by improved cardiac contractility. Whether greater heart size is a common or rather rare phenomenon in human beings awaits improvements in techniques used to evaluate cardiac dimensions in living subjects.

The heart requires less oxygen if it pumps the same cardiac output with a slower heart rate. Therefore, since the improved stroke volume associated with aerobic training allows the heart to beat more slowly at rest and during submaximal exercise, the heart requires a smaller blood flow through its coronary arteries and consumes less oxygen [11]. However, there is no persuasive evidence that *maximal* blood flow to the heart is increased after training [11].

Maximal Arteriovenous Oxygen Difference, Muscular Blood Flow, and Oxygen Extraction. Fifty per cent or more of the greater maximal oxygen uptake associated with aerobic training may be caused by an improved maximal arteriovenous difference in oxygen content [22, 73]. This greater arteriovenous oxygen difference could be produced by training if a greater fraction of the cardiac output were shifted to the working muscles, but this does not seem to happen [72]. Although there may be a greater maximal blood flow to trained working muscles (a point of controversy [19]), there is also more blood delivered to nonworking regions [72]. The problem of whether training increases maximal muscular blood flow remains unresolved because of technical difficulties in measuring this flow, but evidence that maximal blood flow is *not* increased by training is accumulating [53].

Accordingly, the increase in maximal arteriovenous oxygen difference caused by training must be the result of some factor(s) that increase the rate of oxygen extraction from the blood by the working muscles. The precise mechanism by which this increased oxygen extraction is accomplished is unknown. Three of the possibilities that have been suggested include: 1) an *enhanced diffusion of oxygen* from capillary to muscle *because of greater stores of myoglobin* in trained muscles, 2) a *greater number of capillaries* for each muscle fiber so that oxygen can diffuse more readily to the working fibers, and 3) a *greater ability of skeletal muscle mitochondria to make use of delivered oxygen* [72].

There is evidence that aerobic training does result in greater myoglobin concentrations in trained muscles [53]. However, the role of myoglobin in promoting diffusion of oxygen during exercise is not proved.

Several studies have shown that trained laboratory animals and human beings have slightly increased numbers of capillaries per unit of muscle cross-sectional area or per muscle fiber [3, 16, 57]. Although these results suggest that increased capillarity may account for some of the improved ability of trained muscles to extract oxygen from the blood, there is not necessarily any relation between greater capillarity and greater blood flow or oxygen uptake [67]. Therefore, *one cannot make a strong argument that increased capillarity is an important adaptation for improving maximal oxygen uptake.*

Holloszy [53] has speculated that the greater maximal arteriovenous oxygen difference observed after training may be the result of an increased number and/or size of mitochondria. He illustrates this possibility by citing a hypothetical case wherein oxygen delivery to an *untrained* muscle working maximally would be adequate to allow the mitochondria of that muscle to consume 98 per cent of the oxygen that those mitochondria could potentially consume. If during the training the number and/or size of mitochondria in the muscle cells increased 50 per cent, the oxygen level in the muscles during maximal exercise might fall to the point where the mitochondria could consume oxygen at a rate equal to only 75 per cent of their maximal potential. Assuming that the maximal oxygen-consuming capacity of the untrained mitochondria was 100, then oxygen consumption of these *untrained* mitochondria during maximal exercise was $0.98 \times 100 = 98$. *After training,* the maximal capacity of the mitochondria increased by 50 per cent to 150, so that when working at 75 per cent of capacity during maximal work, the oxygen consumption of the trained mitochondria was $0.75 \times 150 = 112.5$, an increase of 14.8 per cent in oxygen consumption over the 98 found in the untrained muscles (Table 10.3). This 14.8 per cent hypothetical increase in maximal oxygen consumption was accomplished by a 50 per cent increase in mitochondrial mass, a very reasonable estimate [53]. Thus, even though blood flow to the working muscles may ultimately limit maximal oxygen uptake [9, 26, 37], it is possible that mitochondrial adaptations can allow greater extraction of the delivered oxygen in trained muscles to increase maximal oxygen uptake.

It is clear that there are, in fact, many mitochondrial adaptations that accompany aerobic endurance training [53, 54]. The *mass of the mitochondria* in a given amount of skeletal muscle is much greater in trained laboratory animals and human beings. Also, the *activities and amounts of many of the enzymes* involved in the Krebs cycle, the fatty acid oxidation cycle, and the electron transport system are increased up to twice the untrained values. It is not clear how repeated exercise results in the greater net synthesis of mitochondrial enzyme proteins. However, many of the molecules (cytochromes) of the electron transport system require the production of a heme protein, and the activity of the enzyme needed to synthesize heme may be 3–4 times as great in trained animals as in untrained animals [55]. This critical enzyme, *delta-aminolevulinic acid synthetase,* may be a vital link in the production of mitochondrial proteins. Further work must be done to find out how exercise triggers the activity of this enzyme and other important enzymes in the mitochondria.

Blood Pressure During Maximal Exercise.   There is no evidence that blood pressure during maximal exercise is changed with training. We know that maximal cardiac output is raised and that blood volume is somewhat increased after training; therefore, if blood pressure during maximal exercise is unaffected by training, the total peripheral resistance (primarily dependent on the diameters of the arterioles) must be

TABLE 10.3

Hypothetical Changes in Mitochondrial Oxygen Uptake per Unit Mass of Skeletal Muscle (53)

	Pretraining	Posttraining
Mitochondrial Mass	100%	150%
$\dot{V}_{O_2}$ max for Mitochondria	100	150
%$\dot{V}_{O_2}$ max Achieved with Available Oxygen	98	75
Total Mitochondrial $\dot{V}_{O_2}$	98	112.5
Calculations	$(.98 \times 100 = 98)$	$(.75 \times 150 = 112.5)$

decreased. It seems likely that one of the effects of training is that during maximal exercise arterioles are opened more completely in tissues such as kidneys, liver, and skin. This vasodilation would decrease peripheral resistance. Because more maximal work can be done after training at the same pretraining blood pressure, the trained person has a lower blood pressure per unit of work accomplished.

Maximal Aerobic Endurance Performance

Improvements in performance of such aerobic activities as running, swimming, and cycling cannot be entirely accounted for by improvements in maximal oxygen uptake. As Saltin [73] has pointed out, endurance athletes of recent years have maximal oxygen uptakes quite similar to those of endurance athletes of the 1930's. But contemporary competitive endurance performance records are substantially improved over the older records. Also, the improvement in maximal oxygen uptake with training is usually restricted to about 15–20 per cent in healthy persons, but performance times often can improve by 30 per cent or more in this same training period. Both of these observations support the contention that factors other than improved maximal cardiovascular function are involved in the improved performances that accompany aerobic endurance training. It seems likely that two of those additional factors are an improved anaerobic capacity and an enhanced tolerance to the physical and psychological discomfort experienced during heavy work. For work lasting longer than about 10 minutes, another important factor may be an improved ability to work at high percentages of one's maximal oxygen uptake with a lesser contribution of anaerobic metabolism. Support for this hypothesis includes evidence that marathon running times are highly correlated with the running speed at which blood lactic acid begins to accumulate rapidly [77]; as one becomes better trained, it is possible to run faster without significant accumulation of lactic acid.

Cardiovascular Function During Submaximal Exercise

Except for athletes, a more important consideration than adaptations during *maximal* exercise are adaptations resulting from aerobic training that enable one to persist at higher levels of *submaximal* exercise with less disturbance of homeostasis. Such adaptations enable one to perform occupational labor more easily at higher rates, perform work around the home or garden with less distress, and engage in more demanding recreational pursuits for longer periods with more gratification.

Oxygen Cost of Submaximal Exercise (Mechanical Efficiency). For a simple task such as walking at 2.5 miles per hour, it is generally conceded that the trained person requires the same amount of oxygen to perform the task as he did before training [8, 53]. This means that training in a task such as walking produces no great change in *mechanical efficiency* (calories of work produced/calories of energy expended to produce the work). For fast running or for more complex tasks such as swimming, shoveling or lifting, improvements in efficiency do result from training as the trainee gradually learns to use only the necessary musculature required to accomplish the task [23]. In this way, oxygen consumption by extraneous motor units is eliminated.

It might also be expected that the reduced reliance on anaerobic energy production in trained persons would reduce total oxygen cost. The theoretical oxygen cost of removing lactic acid during recovery is twice as great as the oxygen equivalent of the energy released by the lactic acid production [51]. However, actual measurements show a 1 to 1 relationship between oxygen deficit and oxygen debt in steady-state, short duration exercise [43]. In other words, substitution of aerobic for anaerobic ATP production does not change the total energy (O_2) cost of exercise. Thus, with submaximal exercise where no skill learning is involved, oxygen uptake *during exercise* increases due to greater aerobic contributions to ATP replenishment, but oxygen uptake in *recovery* is reduced since less oxygen deficit is accumulated in the trained state [46]. The *total* oxygen uptake is unchanged by training.

Cardiac Output, Heart Rate, and Stroke Volume During Submaximal Exercise. Most experiments show that there is no significant training effect on cardiac output during submaximal exercise, but some show a small reduction of cardiac output in the trained state [8, 73]. Heart rate during the exercise is nearly always reduced and the stroke volume increased with training [8, 73]. The decrease in exercise heart rate may be caused by increased parasympathetic activity of the vagus nerves. Training does cause a reduction in plasma epinephrine and norepinephrine at submaximal exercise loads, but this decrease in hormones is not closely associated with the decrease in exercise heart rate [85]. The increased stroke volume is probably the result of a greater heart volume and/or improved cardiac contractility [10]. Accordingly, if a subject could run at 7 miles per hour with a cardiac output of 14 liters per minute, a heart rate of 165 beats per minute, and a stroke volume of 80 milliliters before training, he might be able to run at the same pace with the same cardiac output, but with a heart rate of 150 and stroke volume of 93 milliliters after several months of aerobic training.

Arteriovenous Oxygen Difference, Muscle Blood Flow, and Oxygen Extraction During Submaximal Exercise. As discussed previously, oxygen cost is usually unchanged, and cardiac output during standard submaximal exercise is unchanged or slightly reduced with training. Therefore, arteriovenous oxygen difference must increase during the exercise to account for an increased contribution of aerobic energy production as a result of training [8]. Contrary to popular opinion, blood flow to submaximally working muscles after training is somewhat reduced from the values found before training [19]. Accordingly, the greater arteriovenous oxygen differences found in trained subjects exercising at a standard load cannot be caused by a greater shift of blood volume to the working muscles; training must cause a greater extraction of oxygen by those muscles. This greater extraction of oxygen during submaximal work is simply the result of the increased diffusion gradient for oxygen from the blood to the muscle as the partial pressure of oxygen in the muscle cell and tissue fluid is reduced by mitochondrial activity. In other words, there is a reserve of blood flow to the working muscles that can be reduced by training with no adverse effects; the decreased flow is compensated for by more rapid diffusion of the decreased oxygen supply. During submaximal work, oxygen delivery is not limiting for muscular work.

Blood Pressure During Submaximal Exercise. Systemic arterial blood pressure during a standard submaximal work task has been found to be either decreased [18], unchanged [8], or slightly increased as an effect of training. A decreased blood pressure could be the result of reduced peripheral resistance as more blood flows through nonworking regions [72]. An increased pressure could be viewed as a means of providing greater force to drive blood into contracting muscles. After training, cardiac output is either unchanged or reduced with submaximal work, blood flow to nonworking regions of the body is increased [72], and the blood volume is only slightly greater [8]. Therefore, it appears that any increased blood pressure must be caused by a decreased vasodilation in the working muscles. This hypothesis is consistent with reported reductions in muscle blood flow during submaximal work [19].

Pulmonary Function During Submaximal Exercise

At very light exercise loads the endurance athlete may breathe less frequently and more deeply [8] with slightly less overall ventilation [65]. This reduced ventilation for a given light exercise load is thought to be caused by a reduced sensitivity of the arterial and brain chemoreceptors which respond to carbon dioxide levels in the blood [65]. Evidence suggests that this reduced chemosensitivity may be inherited and that training per se does not change it [65]. At heavier work loads, the ventilation rate for a standard exercise task and the ventilation rate per liter of oxygen uptake are less after training [8, 65]. This adaptation is explained by the reduced level of lactic acid in the blood of the trained person, who relies more on aerobic metabolism. Since lactic acid stimulates ventilation, trained persons have less of a ventilatory drive than do untrained people.

Endurance for Submaximal Exercise Loads

A universal adaptation associated with training is that the completion of previously difficult tasks becomes easier and progressively greater work loads can be accomplished without undue discomfort and fatigue. The mechanisms underlying this adaptation probably vary with exercise intensity. With mild exercise where there is no substantial accumulation of oxygen deficit or lactic acid, it seems likely that improvements in 1) mechanical efficiency (for complex skills only) and 2) psychological tolerance to the work are mostly responsible for an enhanced ability to persist at a given task. After training only with legs subjects indicate lower ratings of perceived exertion (a marker of psychological tolerance) with submaximal *leg* exercise, but not with *arm* exercise [64]. Similarly, subjects who train only with arms can more easily tolerate arm exercise, but not leg exercise, after training. These findings suggest that the mechanism for reduced perceived exertion ratings is located in the trained muscles [64]. Perhaps the reduced lactic acid levels in the trained muscles cause less of an adverse sensation after training.

With heavier exercise that relies to a moderate extent on anaerobic glycolysis for ATP replenishment, that is, exercise that is tolerated for 10 minutes to 1 hour or more, additional factors that contribute to increased endurance are 1) greater anaerobic capacity, 2) greater glycogen stores, 3) improved temperature regulation, and 4) greater mitochondrial capacity for aerobic ATP replenishment. Improvements in glycogen storage with training and diet were described in Chapter 5, and improvements in anaerobic capacity and temperature regulation will be described in subsequent chapters. The enhanced mitochondrial capacity for aerobic energy production deserves further comment.

Mitochondrial Adaptations and Submaximal Exercise

It has been conclusively shown in laboratory animals and humans that aerobic endurance training causes a substantial increase in the numbers and/or sizes of mitochondria in trained muscles [53, 56]. These structural changes are accompanied by greater capacities of the trained mitochondria to produce ATP as a result of greater activities of enzymes of the Krebs cycle, the electron transport system, and other metabolic systems related to ATP production [53]. These mitochondrial changes can explain how trained muscles produce less lactic acid for submaximal exercise than do untrained muscles. First, one should recall that important enzymes of glycolysis are stimulated by a buildup of ADP in the sarcoplasm of the muscle; the greater the concentration of ADP, the faster the rate of glycolysis and subsequent production of lactic acid. Therefore, any factor that leads to a *reduced* level of ADP in the sarcoplasm can reduce the rate of glycolysis and lactic acid production. Second, it is known that the consumption of oxygen by mitochondria (and the associated production of ATP) is dependent upon the presence of ADP. Thus, for a given steady-state level of oxygen consumption by a single mitochondrion, there must exist a certain mitochondrial concentration of ADP. This ADP diffuses into the mitochondria from the sarcoplasm. Accordingly, in a trained muscle with *more* mitochondria or a greater number of electron transport assemblies in *larger* mitochondria, each mitochondrion or electron transport assembly would have to consume proportionately less oxygen, at lower concentrations of ADP, to produce the same *total* oxygen consumption in the entire muscle. Because a lower concentration of ADP is thereby required, aerobic ATP replenishment can reach a steady state more rapidly with less oxygen deficit, less anaerobic glycolysis, and less lactic acid production (Fig. 10.4) [46, 53].

As an illustration, assume that before training, a small muscle had 100 mitochondria and that this muscle could perform a certain type of exercise with a total oxygen uptake of 1,000 atoms of oxygen per minute. Thus, each mitochondrion consumed 10 atoms of oxygen per minute. Assume, further, that there had to be 5,000 ADP molecules in the sarcoplasm of the muscle to provide for diffusion of enough ADP into each mitochondrion to stimulate oxygen consumption at a rate of 10 atoms per minute. After training, assume that the muscle had twice as many (200) electron transport assemblies, either because of more mitochondria, more assemblies in larger mitochondria, or both. In this trained state, each mitochondrion of the muscle had to consume oxygen at only 5 atoms per minute to achieve that same total oxygen uptake of 1,000 atoms per minute for the submaximal work load. But since a lower concentration of ADP is required to stimulate an oxygen uptake of 5 atoms per minute by each electron transport assembly, perhaps only 2,500 ADP molecules were needed in the sarcoplasm of the muscle to provide adequate delivery of ADP to the mitochondria. There-

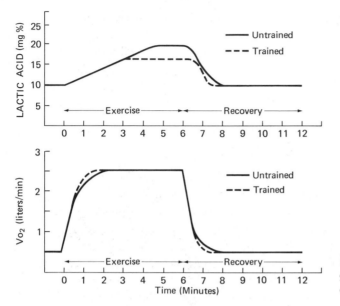

FIGURE 10.4. Effect of training on oxygen uptake and lactic acid accumulation during submaximal exercise.

fore, a steady state of oxygen uptake to balance ATP breakdown could be achieved faster at a lower concentration of ADP and with a reduced production of lactic acid.

Greater Fat Metabolism After Training

An additional adaptation to aerobic training that is observed during submaximal exercise is a greater use of fat for energy [8, 53]. Not only does training reduce respiratory exchange ratio (respiratory quotient) during exercise, but it also increases in muscles the rate of carbon dioxide production from radioactively labeled fatty acids [53]. Both of these results support the belief that trained muscles oxidize relatively more fat than untrained muscles. The mechanism responsible for this change in energy metabolism is not entirely clear, but may involve a greater mobilization of fatty acids from tissue stores into the blood. This adaptation in fat metabolism is important because the increased reliance on fat for energy allows muscle glycogen to be spared. Since muscle glycogen stores are directly related to endurance in moderately heavy work, a conservation of carbohydrates can extend performance time.

Cardiovascular Function at Rest

It is generally agreed that resting rates of oxygen consumption in trained persons do not differ significantly from those in untrained persons [8]. Also, resting cardiac output, regional blood flow, and arteriovenous oxygen difference are usually unchanged after training [8]. Resting heart rate is almost invariably reduced 5–10 beats per minute with at least a few weeks of aerobic endurance training [8, 70]. This training *bradycardia* is probably caused by increased activity of the parasympathetic nerves to the heart or by greater stores of acetylcholine in the heart itself, but some believe a decreased sensitivity to the sympathetic transmitters, epinephrine and norepinephrine, is also important [10]. However, there does not seem to be any substantial evidence that physical training causes a change in the number of receptors on the cardiac cell membranes or in their binding of drugs which mimic norepinephrine and acetylcholine [81]. Furthermore, there apparently is a reduction in heart rate that is independent of the autonomic nervous system [63]. Trained persons have lower heart rates when both sympathetic and parasympathetic nerve impulses are blocked. Thus, there may be some training-induced change in the electrical properties of the sinoatrial node that cause it to slow the heart rhythm both at rest and during exercise [63].

The bradycardia at rest and during submaximal exercise probably results in lower oxygen consumption by the heart, an adaptation that may help to explain the protective effect of exercise in minimizing the risk of early death from coronary artery disease [10].

If a normal resting cardiac output is to be maintained with a decreased heart rate, it is obvious that stroke volume must be greater at rest in trained individuals. This increased stroke volume, for example, from about 70 ml before training to perhaps 81 ml after training may be due to greater diastolic filling or to improved cardiac contractility [10].

Resting Blood Pressure. Any reduction in resting arterial blood pressure in trainees who begin training with blood pressures in the normal range is minimal and unpredictable [18, 70]. Exercise programs seem to have the greatest value in lowering blood pressure in older patients and in hypertensive patients [18, 70]. The effect of exercise training on reducing blood pressure in those with hypertension is not great enough to bring the pressure back to normal values; there are drugs which are much more effective in this regard than exercise. However, the exercise effect can lower the dosage of anti-hypertension drugs required to maintain a normal blood pressure. This can represent a substantial financial savings.

Pulmonary Function at Rest

In normal subjects little or no change in pulmonary function at rest is usually observed as a result of training. If subjects specifically improve the strength of their breathing musculature, they may experience some increase in vital capacity (especially in swimmers) and in maximal breathing capacity. Otherwise, only slight decreases in the breathing rate at rest and slight increases in tidal volume (depth of breathing) are sometimes reported [8, 73].

Other health-related adaptations to aerobic endurance training are described in Chapter 18.

Blood Characteristics

Aerobic training causes a number of changes in the characteristics of the blood at rest and during exercise. Many of these changes were described in Chapter 8. One explanation for the increased blood volume that often is associated with training involves the kidneys [14]. The explanation is as follows. The kidneys help regulate blood volume by excreting more fluid if blood volume is elevated and less fluid if the blood volume is diminished. The kidneys are stimulated to perform this function by stretch receptors located in the heart; as a greater blood volume stimulates the cardiac stretch receptors, they start a nerve reflex which causes the kidneys to excrete more fluid and bring the blood volume back toward a normal level. This reflex is triggered throughout the day as blood volume fluctuates with fluid intake, sweat loss, and fluid excretion. Apparently, one effect of training is to reduce the sensitivity of the cardiac stretch receptors to increased blood volume so that they allow blood volume to increase by 5–10 per cent without stimulating the kidneys to excrete more fluid [14]. We do not know how exercise training causes the cardiac stretch receptors to have a lessened sensitivity to increased blood volume.

Most of the changes in blood characteristics observed during *maximal* exercise, such as lower venous oxygen content, higher venous carbon dioxide content, and greater venous and arterial lactic acid concentration, are secondary effects of the greater aerobic and anaerobic capacity of the trained skeletal muscles and the greater capacity of the heart to deliver oxygen to these muscles.

As a rule, during *submaximal* exercise one would expect to observe less severe disturbances in blood values after training than before. This reflects the fact that the same exercise load after training is less stressful than before training because of improvements in cardiovascular function and muscular metabolism.

REVIEW QUESTIONS

1. Describe four principles of aerobic training.
2. What is the minimal exercise program that one could expect to cause an improvement in maximal oxygen uptake in young adults?
3. What are some ways of prescribing appropriate intensities of exercise on an individual basis?
4. How large a percentage of increase in maximal oxygen uptake could one expect to result from an endurance training program? What are some of the factors that contribute to differences in the magnitude of this adaptation?
5. Outline an interval training program designed to improve aerobic potential in a high school student who has a maximal heart rate of 200 beats per minute and a best time of 5 minutes for the mile run. Begin by listing the general principles that should underlie any such program. The program should encompass a 10-week period.
6. Describe and explain the cardiovascular adaptations to endurance training. Include in your discussion the possible role of altered mitochondrial function in contributing to a greater maximal arteriovenous oxygen difference.
7. What accounts for the improved tolerance to submaximal exercise observed in trained persons? What is the likely role of the skeletal muscle mitochondria in this adaptation?

REFERENCES

[1] Adams, G. M., and H. A. de Vries. Physiological effects of an exercise training regimen upon women aged 52–79. *Journal of Gerontology,* 1973, **28:**50–55.
[2] Adams, W. C., E. M. Bernauer, D. B. Dill, and J. B. Bomar, Jr. Effects of equivalent sea-level and altitude training on VO_2 max and running performance. *Journal of Applied Physiology,* 1975, **39:**262–266.
[3] Adolfsson, J., A. Ljungqvist, G. Tornling, and G. Unge. Capillary increase in the skeletal muscle of trained young and adult rats. *Journal of Physiology* (London), 1981, **310:**529–532.
[4] American College of Sports Medicine. *Guidelines for Graded Exercise Testing and Exercise Prescription,* 2nd ed. Philadelphia: Lea & Febiger, 1980.

[5] American College of Sports Medicine. Position statement on the recommended quantity and quality of exercise for developing and maintaining fitness in healthy adults. *Medicine and Science in Sports,* 1978, **10:**vii–x.

[6] American College of Sports Medicine. Opinion statement on the participation of the female athlete in long-distance running. *Medicine and Science in Sports,* 1979, **11:**vii–x.

[7] Applegate, V. W., and G. A. Stull. The effects of varied rest periods on cardiovascular endurance retention by college women. *American Corrective Therapy Journal,* 1969, **23:**3–6.

[8] Åstrand, P.-O., and K. Rodahl. *Textbook of Work Physiology,* 2nd ed., New York: McGraw-Hill, 1977.

[9] Barclay, J. K., and W. N. Stainsby. The role of blood flow in limiting maximal metabolic rate in muscle. *Medicine and Science in Sports,* 1975, **7:**116–119.

[10] Barnard, R. J. Long-term effects of exercise on cardiac function. *Exercise and Sport Sciences Reviews,* 1975, **3:**113–133.

[11] Barnard, R. J., H. W. Duncan, K. M. Baldwin, G. Grimditch, and G. D. Buckberg. Effects of intensive exercise training on myocardial performance and coronary blood flow. *Journal of Applied Physiology,* 1980, **49:**444–449.

[12] Bar-Or, O., and L. D. Zwiren. Physiological effects of increased frequency of physical education classes and of endurance conditioning on 9–10 year-old girls and boys. In O. Bar-Or, ed., *Pediatric Work Physiology—Proceedings of the Fourth International Symposium.* Wingate Post, Israel: Wingate Institute, 1972, pp. 183–198.

[13] Belcastro, A. N., and A. Bonen. Lactic acid removal rates during controlled and uncontrolled recovery exercise. *Journal of Applied Physiology,* 1975, **39:**932–936.

[14] Boning, D., and W. Skipka. Renal blood volume regulation in trained and untrained subjects during immersion. *European Journal of Applied Physiology,* **42:**247–254.

[15] Bouchard, C., W. Hollmann, H. Venrath, G. Herkenrath, and H. Schlussel. Minimal amount of physical training for the prevention of cardiovascular diseases. *Proceedings of the 16th World Congress of Sports Medicine, Hannover, Germany,* 1966, pp. 91–97.

[16] Brodal, P., F. Ingjer, and L. Hermansen. Capillary supply of skeletal muscle fibers in untrained and endurance-trained men. *American Journal of Physiology,* 1977, **232:**H705—H712.

[17] Brynteson, P., and W. E. Sinning. The effects of training frequencies on the retention of cardiovascular fitness. *Medicine and Science in Sports,* 1973, **5:**29–33.

[18] Choquette, G., and R. J. Ferguson. Blood pressure reduction in "borderline" hypertensives following physical training. *Canadian Medical Association Journal,* 1973, **108:**699—703.

[19] Clausen, J. P. Effect of physical training on cardiovascular adjustments to exercise in man. *Physiological Reviews,* 1977, **57:**779–815.

[20] Cooper, K. H. *The New Aerobics.* New York: Bantam Books, 1970.

[21] Cooper, M., and K. H. Cooper. *Aerobics for Women.* New York: M. Evans Co., 1972.

[22] Cunningham, D. A., D. McCrimmon, and L. F. Vlach. Cardiovascular response to interval and continuous training in women. *European Journal of Applied Physiology,* 1979, **41:**187–197.

[23] Daniels, J., and N. Oldridge. Changes in oxygen consumption of young boys during growth and running training. *Medicine and Science in Sports,* 1971, **3:**161–165.

[24] Daniels, J., and N. Oldridge. The effects of alternate exposure to altitude and sea level on world-class, middle-distance runners. *Medicine and Science in Sports,* 1970, **2:**107–112.

[25] Daniels, J., N. Oldridge, F. Nagle, and B. White. Differences and changes in VO_2 among young runners 10 to 18 years of age. *Medicine and Science in Sports,* 1978, **10:**200–203.

[26] Davies, K. J. A., L. Packer, and G. A. Brooks. Mitochondrial biogenesis and exercise energetics. *Medicine and Science in Sports and Exercise,* 1981, **13:**118.

[27] Davis, J. A., and V. A. Convertino. A comparison of heart rate methods for predicting endurance training intensity. *Medicine and Science in Sports,* 1975, **7:**295–298.

[28] deVries, H. A. Exercise intensity threshold for improvement of cardiovascular-respiratory function in older men. *Geriatrics,* 1971, **26:**94–101.

[29] deVries, H. A. Physiological effects of an exercise training regimen upon men aged 52 to 88. *Journal of Gerontology,* 1970, **25:**325–336.

[30] deVries, H. A. Tips on prescribing exercise regimens for your older patient. *Geriatrics,* 1979, **34:**75–81.

[31] Dill, D. B., and W. C. Adams. Maximal oxygen uptake at sea level and at 3,090-m. altitude in high school champion runners. *Journal of Applied Physiology,* 1971, **30:**854–859.

[32] Drinkwater, B. L., and S. M. Horvath. Detraining effects on young women. *Medicine and Science in Sports,* 1972, **4:**91–95.

[33] Durnin, J. V. G. A., J. M. Brockway, and H. W. Whitcher. Effect of a short period of training of varying severity on some measurements of physical fitness. *Journal of Applied Physiology,* 1960, **15:**161–165.

[34] Eddy, D. O., K. L. Sparks, and D. A. Adelizi. The effects of continuous and interval training in women and men. *European Journal of Applied Physiology,* 1977, **37:**83–92.

[35] Eisenman, P. A., and L. A. Golding. Comparisons of effects of training on VO_2 max in girls and young women. *Medicine and Science in Sports,* 1975, **7:** 136–138.

[36] Ekblom, B. Effect of physical training in adolescent boys. *Journal of Applied Physiology,* 1969, **27:**350–355.

[37] Ekblom, B., R. Huot, E. M. Stein, and A. T. Thorstenson. Effect of changes in arterial oxygen content on circulation and physical performance. *Journal of Applied Physiology,* 1975, **39:**71–75.

[38] Eriksson, B. O., and K. Gunter. Effect of physical training on hemodynamic response during submaximal and maximal exercise in 11–13 year old boys. *Acta Physiologica Scandinavica,* 1973, **87:**27–39.

[39] Flint, M. M., B. L. Drinkwater, and S. M. Horvath. Effects of training on women's response to submaximal exercise. *Medicine and Science in Sports,* 1974, **6:**89–94.

[40] Fox, E. L., R. L. Bartels, C. Billings, D. K. Mathews, R. Bason, and W. M. Webb. Intensity and distance of interval training programs and changes in aerobic power. *Medicine and Science in Sports,* 1973, **5:**18–22.

[41] Fox, E. L., and D. K. Mathews. *Interval Training: Conditioning for Sports and General Fitness.* Philadelphia: W. B. Saunders Company, 1974.

[42] Fringer, M. N., and G. A. Stull. Changes in cardiorespiratory parameters during periods of training and detraining in young adult females. *Medicine and Science in Sports,* 1974, **6:**20–25.

[43] Girandola, R. N., and F. I. Katch. Effects of physical conditioning on changes in exercise and recovery O_2 uptake and efficiency during constant-load ergometer exercise. *Medicine and Science in Sports,* 1973, **5:**242–247.

[44] Gollnick, P. D. Cellular adaptations to exercise. In R. J. Shephard, ed., *Frontiers of Fitness.* Springfield, Ill.: Charles C Thomas, Publisher, 1971, pp. 112–126.

[45] Guski, H. The effect of exercise on myocardial interstitium. An ultrastructural morphometric study. *Experimentelle Pathologie,* 1980, **18:**141–150.

[46] Hagberg, J. M., R. C. Hickson, A. A. Ehsani, and J. O. Holloszy. Faster adjustment to and recovery from submaximal exercise in the trained state. *Journal of Applied Physiology,* **48:**218–224.

[47] Hagberg, J. M., R. C. Hickson, J. A. McLane, A. A. Ehsani, and W. W. Winder. Disappearance of norepinephrine from the circulation following strenuous exercise. *Journal of Applied Physiology,* 1979, **47:**1311–1314.

[48] Hanson, J. S., and W. H. Nedde. Long-term physical training effect on sedentary females. *Journal of Applied Physiology,* 1974, **37:**112–116.

[49] Harri, M. N. E. Physical training under the influence of beta-blockade in rats. III. Effects on muscular metabolism. *European Journal of Applied Physiology,* 1980, **45:**25–31.

[50] Hellerstein, H. K., E. Z. Hirsch, R. Ader, N. Greenblott, and M. Siegel. Principles of exercise prescription for normals and cardiac subjects. In J. Naughton and H. K. Hellerstein, eds., *Exercise Testing and Exercise Training in Coronary Heart Disease.* New York: Academic Press, Inc., 1973, pp. 129–167.

[51] Hermansen, L. Anaerobic energy release. *Medicine and Science in Sports,* 1969, **1**:32–38.

[52] Hickson, R. C., and M. A. Rosenkoetter. Reduced training frequencies and maintenance of increased aerobic power. *Medicine and Science in Sports and Exercise,* 1981, **13**:13–16.

[53] Holloszy, J. O. Biochemical adaptations to exercise: aerobic metabolism. *Exercise and Sport Sciences Reviews,* 1973, **1**:45–71.

[54] Holloszy, J. O., and F. W. Booth. Biochemical adaptations to endurance exercise in muscle. *Annual Reviews of Physiology,* 1976, **38**:273–291.

[55] Holloszy, J. O., and W. W. Winder. Induction of δ-aminolevulinic acid synthetase in muscle by exercise or thyroxine. *American Journal of Physiology,* 1979, **236**:R180–R183.

[56] Hoppeler, H., P. Luthi, H. Claassen, E. R. Weibel, and H. Howald. The ultrastructure of the normal human skeletal muscle. *Pflügers Archiv,* 1973, **344**:217–232.

[57] Ingjer, F., and P. Brodal. Capillary supply of skeletal muscle fibers in untrained and endurance-trained women. *European Journal of Applied Physiology,* 1978, **38**:291–299.

[58] Kanakis, C., and R. C. Hickson. Left ventricular responses to a program of lower-limb strength training. *Chest,* 1980, **78**:618–621.

[59] Karvonen, M. J., E. Kentala, and O. Mustala. The effects of training on heart rate. A longitudinal study. *Annales Medicinae Experimentalis et Biologiae Fenniae,* 1957, **35**:305–315.

[60] Kearney, J. T., G. A. Stull, J. L. Ewing, Jr., and J. W. Strein. Cardiorespiratory responses of sedentary college women as a function of training intensity. *Journal of Applied Physiology,* 1976, **41**:822–825.

[61] Kilbom, A. Physical training in women. *Scandinavian Journal of Clinical and Laboratory Investigation,* 1971, **28**:(Supplementum 119).

[62] Knuttgen, H. G., L.-O. Nordesjo, B. Ollander, and B. Saltin. Physical conditioning through interval training with young male adults. *Medicine and Science in Sports,* 1973, **5**:220–226.

[63] Lewis, S. F., E. Nylander, P. Gad, and N.-H. Areskog. Non-autonomic component in bradycardia of endurance trained men at rest and during exercise. *Acta Physiologica Scandinavica,* 1979, **109**:297–305.

[64] Lewis, S., P. Thompson, N.-H. Areskog, P. Vodak, M. Marconyak, R. Debusk, S. Mellen, and W. Haskell. Transfer effects of endurance training to exercise with untrained limbs. *European Journal of Applied Physiology,* 1980, **44**:25–34.

[65] Martin, B. J., K. E. Sparks, C. W. Zwillich, and J. V. Weil. Low exercise ventilation in endurance athletes. *Medicine and Science in Sports,* 1979, **11**:181–185.

[66] Masicotte, D. R., and R. B. J. Macnab. Cardiorespiratory adaptations to training at specified intensities in children. *Medicine and Science in Sports,* 1974, **6**:242–246.

[67] Maxwell, L. C., T. P. White, and J. A. Faulkner. Oxidative capacity, blood flow, and capillarity of skeletal muscles. *Journal of Applied Physiology,* 1980, **49**:627–633.

[68] Michael, E., J. Evert, and K. Jeffers. Physiological changes of teenage girls during five months of detraining. *Medicine and Science in Sports,* 1972, **4**:214–218.

[69] Pechar, G. S., W. D. McArdle, F. I. Katch, J. R. Magel, and J. DeLuca. Specificity of cardiorespiratory adaptation to bicycle and treadmill training. *Journal of Applied Physiology,* 1974, **36**:753–756.

[70] Pollock, M. L. The quantification of endurance training programs. *Exercise and Sport Sciences Reviews,* 1973, **1**:155–188.

[71] Roskamm, E. Optimum patterns of exercise for healthy adults. *Canadian Medical Association Journal,* 1967, **96**:895–899.

[72] Rowell, L. B. Human cardiovascular adjustments to exercise and thermal stress. *Physiological Reviews,* 1975, **54**:75–159.

[73] Saltin, B. Physiological effects of physical conditioning. *Medicine and Science in Sports,* 1969, **1**:50–56.

[74] Schaible, T. F., and J. Scheuer. Effects of physical training by running or swimming on ventricular performance of rat hearts. *Journal of Applied Physiology,* 1979, **46**:854–860.

[75] Shephard, R. J. *Alive Man! The Physiology of Physical Activity.* Springfield, Ill.: Charles C Thomas, Publisher, 1972.

[76] Shephard, R. J. Intensity, duration, and frequency of exercise as determinants of the response to a training regimen. *International Zeitschrift fur Angewandte Physiologie,* 1968, **26**:272–278.

[77] Sjodin, B., and I. Jacobs. Onset of blood lactate accumulation and marathon running performance. *International Journal of Sports Medicine,* 1981, **2**:23–26.

[78] Stein, R. A., D. Michielli, J. Diamond, B. Horwitz, and N. Krasnow. The cardiac response to exercise training: echocardiographic analysis at rest and during exercise. *American Journal of Cardiology,* 1980, **46**:219–225.

[79] Stoedefalke, K. G. Physical fitness programs for adults. *American Journal of Cardiology,* 1974, **33**:787–790.

[80] Tibbits, G. F., R. J. Barnard, K. M. Baldwin, N. Cugalj, and N. K. Roberts. Influence of exercise on excitation-contraction coupling in rat myocardium. *American Journal of Physiology,* 1981, **240**:H472–H480.

[81] Williams, R. S. Physical conditioning and membrane receptors for cardioregulatory hormones. *Cardiovascular Research,* 1980, **14**:177–182.

[82] Wilmore, J. H. Individual exercise prescription. *American Journal of Cardiology,* 1974, **33**:757–759.

[83] Wilmore, J. H., and W. L. Haskell. Use of the heart rate-energy expenditure relationship in the individualized prescription of exercise. *The American Journal of Clinical Nutrition,* 1971, **24**:1186–1192.

[84] Wilmore, J. H., J. Royce, R. N. Girandola, F. I. Katch, and V. L. Katch. Physiological alterations resulting from a 10-week program of jogging. *Medicine and Science in Sports,* 1970, **1**:7–14.

[85] Winder, W. W., J. M. Hagberg, R. C. Hickson, A. A. Ehsani, and J. A. McLane. Time course of sympathoadrenal adaptation to endurance exercise training in man. *Journal of Applied Physiology,* 1978, **45**:370–374.

[86] Wolfe, L. A., D. A. Cunningham, P. A. Rechnitzer, and P. M. Nichol. Effects of endurance training on left ventricular dimensions in healthy men. *Journal of Applied Physiology,* 1979, **47**:207–212.

[87] Zeldis, S. M., J. Morganroth, and S. Rubler. Cardiac hypertrophy in response to dynamic conditioning in female athletes. *Journal of Applied Physiology,* 1978, **44**:849–852.

C H A P T E R

11

Temperature Regulation During Exercise

HEAT stroke or collapse from heat exhaustion may occur in one of every one hundred runners in mass road races of 10 kilometers or longer, and up to 20 per cent of distance runners may suffer less dangerous episodes of heat illness as a result of prolonged exercise in hot, humid conditions [14, 21]. This means that temperature regulation processes inadequately maintain body temperature at satisfactory levels in several hundred runners each summer. It is important, therefore, for everyone associated with prolonged exercise to have an adequate understanding of how the body responds to changes in its temperature and how these responses can be supported by appropriate human behaviors, such as increased fluid consumption and progressive warm-weather training.

The Range of Human Body Temperature

Under normal resting conditions, we are able to maintain our body temperatures within a very narrow range. However, under extreme environmental conditions, with fever, and with prolonged vigorous exercise, the body may be unable to regulate its temperature satisfactorily. When the body cools below 35.4°C (96°F), enzymes in the cells of the brain and other tissues become less active. Cellular metabolism will eventually become depressed so respiration and heart function slow and finally cease. Although there are exceptions, inner body (core) temperatures below 26°C (79°F) are usually fatal because of heart failure. Above temperatures of 43°C (109°F) death is also very likely (Fig. 11.1) [37]. Consequently, temperature regulation is a critically

221

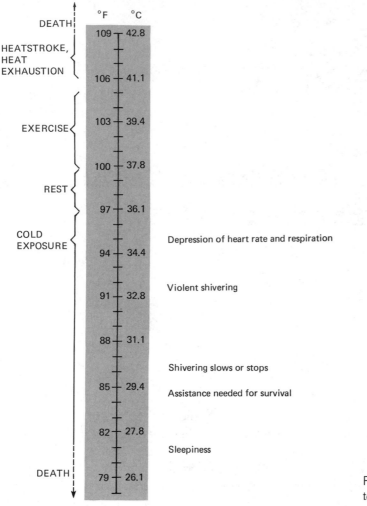

FIGURE 11.1. Range of oral body temperature.

important consideration in human physiology, particularly during prolonged exercise when the body core temperature can exceed 40.6°C (105°F).

Skin temperature is much more variable than that of the liver, heart, lungs, and other deep core tissues and is closely related to the environmental temperature. In a 20°C (68°F) room, average skin temperature may be 29°C (84°F), but it may fall below 20°C (68°F) in a cold environment and may rise to the same level as body core temperature in extremely hot, humid conditions.

Physical Mechanisms of Heat Transfer

The human body is constantly exchanging heat energy with its environment. Whether the body gains or loses heat depends upon the operation of four different mechanisms of heat transfer: 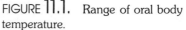 radiation, conduction, convection, and evaporation. *Radiation* is the transfer of heat energy as electromagnetic waves (similar to the transfer of radio waves or photons of light) through space from one object to another. All objects radiate heat to other objects in their environment. A person is warmed by radiation if objects in the environment (especially the sun) radiate more heat energy to him than he does to his surroundings. Conversely, if the surface of one's body is warmer than the surroundings, the body loses heat by radiation to its environment. Radiation does not require the presence of matter between the objects that are radiating heat to each other. Thus, on a cold day one can feel chilled in a well-warmed room if the body radiates heat to poorly insulated cold windows and walls.

The rate of heat loss or gain by radiation depends upon the temperature gradient between a person's skin and the environment. Therefore, if the skin temperature is 30°C (86°F) and the temperature of the gymnasium walls is 15°C (59°F), the body's rate of heat loss by radiation will be much greater than if the walls were at 25°C (77°F). (In general, the greater the difference between temperatures of objects, the greater the temperature gradient between those objects.)

Conduction is the process whereby heat energy is transferred from a warmer to a cooler object with which it has direct physical contact, such as the transfer of heat from hot water in a bathtub to a body immersed in the water. SWIMMING

Convection is the transfer of heat between the surface of the body and the air (or water, if one is swimming) because of the circulation of air or water molecules next to the skin. For example, if cool air around a person is completely still and the person is immobile, heat is transmitted by conduction to a thin shell of air molecules that make contact with the skin. But if a breeze blows, the warm air molecules are displaced by cooler molecules that can, then, pick up more heat energy by conduction. The greater the difference in temperature between the skin and the neighboring air or water molecules, the greater the heat transfer. In air, the loss of heat by convection is proportional to the square of the air velocity. Thus, if wind speed doubles, heat loss increases by four times.

Conduction and convection also occur between the warm core of the body and the cooler limbs and skin. There is some conduction of heat through the warmer inner tissues to the outer parts of the body, and the blood circulating from the warm core can carry heat to the skin by convection. For example, blood flow to the fingers can increase 90-fold to help carry away excess heat from the core.

Evaporation is the transfer of heat from the body surface through the change of liquid water on the skin to a gaseous water vapor in the environment. Just as one must impart heat energy to a kettle of water to make it turn into steam, body water must absorb heat from the body surface if it is to evaporate as water vapor. For every liter of sweat that is evaporated from the surface of the body, about 580 kilocalories of heat energy are removed from the body. Evaporation is vitally important to temperature regulation in a hot environment where heat is *gained* from the environment by radiation, convection, and conduction, leaving evaporation as the only avenue for heat loss. Because evaporation is the diffusion of water molecules from the skin to the air, no evaporation can occur if the air is saturated with water vapor. Accordingly, when the relative humidity is high on a hot day, temperature regulation may not be possible if one is producing heat at a high rate while exercising. It is under conditions of high heat and humidity that most cases of heat illness occur.

Physiological Control of Heat Transfer

1. blood flow

There are two principal mechanisms by which the body can control the transfer of heat by radiation, convection, conduction, and evaporation between the surface of the body and the environment. First, the body can alter the temperature of its surface by changing blood flow to the skin. If skin blood vessels are open, warm blood from the core of the body is brought to the surface where the heat is then more easily lost by radiation, conduction, and convection. On the other hand, if the blood vessels to the skin are constricted, heat will be conserved within the inner regions of the body, and less heat will be lost by radiation, convection, and conduction.

2. sweat

The second mechanism by which the body can control heat transfer between its surface and the environment is the control of sweat secretion by the sweat glands. Obviously, if more sweat is evaporated, there will be a greater loss of heat from the body.

Blood flow to the skin and sweat secretion are both governed by the activity of the hypothalamus at the base of the brain [3, 5]. The hypothalamus is responsive to changes in skin temperature, to changes in the temperature of the blood, and perhaps to temperature changes in other parts of the body. When the skin and/or blood are warmed, the hypothalamus generates nerve impulses which lead to the dilation of cutaneous (skin) blood vessels and the secretion of more sweat. Under cool conditions of the skin and blood, the hypothalamus brings about cutaneous vasoconstriction and diminished sweating. The temperature of the face is especially important in determining the subjective sensation of a hot or cold environment and determining sweat rate [10]. The thermal receptors in the skin of the face seem to be much more sensitive to temperature changes than those in other parts of the body. This accounts for the fact that a cool fan blowing on the face on a hot day is so pleasant, and for the common experience among distance runners that they would often rather pour water over their heads than drink it.

Temperature Regulation in a Cool, Dry Environment

Heat production in a resting person is about 75 kilocalories per hour. Exercise may increase caloric expenditure by 20-fold, that is, to 1,500 kilocalories per hour for short durations. Obviously, most of this extra heat must be dissipated, or body temperature will rapidly rise to a dangerous level. Some of this heat is not removed during exercise, however. The body stores some heat and simply carries on its functions at a higher temperature during work and for 30 minutes [29] to 11 hours [13] after the exercise is completed. It is as though the body's hypothalamic "thermostat" were reset at a higher level. This resetting of the hypothalamic thermostat may be caused by increased sodium or decreased calcium ion concentration in the extracellular fluid bathing the hypothalamus [27].

It has been shown that dynamic strength, maximal power produced during brief exercise, maximal oxygen uptake, and tolerance for severe exercise lasting about 8 minutes all are increased with greater muscle temperature up to about 39°C [4]. However, it usually takes longer than 30 minutes of heavy exercise to raise the body's core temperature to 39°C. This may explain why many athletes prefer to engage in vigorous warmup activities before competition; such preparation helps to increase their muscle temperatures to optimal values. It should be noted that prolonged endurance performance *declines* when core temperature rises above 39°C [30].

Relationships Among Body Temperatures, Sweat Rate, Exercise Loads, and Environmental Temperature

Under cool, dry conditions, it is possible for the body to stabilize its core temperature during exercise which can be continued for 60 minutes or longer. In this type of environment, *skin temperature is dependent in large measure upon the temperature of the air or water surrounding the skin and is relatively independent of exercise load.* However, once the skin temperature reaches about 35°C during exercise in dry air, the evaporation of sweat cools the skin and minimizes any further rise in skin temperature [6]. If conditions are such that skin temperature rises to about 38°C, widespread blood vessel dilation occurs throughout the body, and cardiovascular function is impaired. Such conditions include exercise in a hot, humid environment and exercise while wearing plastic or rubber suits which impede the evaporation of sweat. These conditions are avoided by knowledgeable persons. Unlike skin temperature, the rise in *core* temperature with exercise is quite *independent* of the ambient temperature. Rather, *core temperature is primarily dependent upon the relative exercise load* [3, 28]. This means that if two people of different maximal oxygen uptakes perform the same absolute exercise load, e.g., 200 watts on an ergometer, the person with the lower maximal oxygen uptake will have a greater rise in core temperature than the more fit person. Of course, this is true only under environmental situations that eventually allow sweating and vasodilation to stabilize core temperature. If the same two persons exercised at the *same percentage* of their maximal oxygen uptakes, on the other hand, one would predict that their core temperatures would rise similarly; in this situation the more fit person would be accomplishing a greater absolute exercise load.

In contrast to the rise in core temperature with exercise, *the increase in sweat rate is more closely related to the absolute exercise load than to the relative load* [6]. However, the sweat rate is also related to the core temperature, which has about a 10-fold greater effect on sweating than does skin temperature [25]. One important effect of skin temperature seems to be that higher skin temperatures in a given individual sensitize the hypothalamus to elevations in core temperature so that sweating starts more quickly as core temperature begins to rise [25].

In a cool, dry environment (for example, 70°F (21.1°C) and 50 per cent relative humidity), the body can increase cutaneous blood flow and increase sweating rate to help rid itself of excess heat during exercise. During movement, the hypothalamus responds not only to the temperature of the warmed blood but also to reflex impulses originating in working muscles and/or joints [29]. This is shown by the fact that if the skin and/or core is warm, sweating begins within a few seconds of the start of movement, long before any temperature rise of the blood or even muscles could be detected [12, 29]. The increased sweating during exercise is useless, of course, if evaporation is impeded because of high humidity, or because the individual wears clothing that does not allow the sweat to evaporate. Sweating is especially blocked by plastic or rubberized sweat suits, and the use of such clothing is dangerous if it causes the body temperature to rise to critical levels.

In some persons, if the increased evaporative cooling caused by sweating is sufficient to maintain body temperature below 39°C, there may be no increased blood flow to the skin to increase heat loss by radiation and convection [30]. In fact, some of the blood flow to the skin at rest may be shifted to the working muscles during exercise [30]. However, for work loads above about 1 liter of oxygen consumption per minute, there is usually an increased skin blood flow as the work progresses. Probably about 70 per cent of the heat lost during exercise in a cool, dry environment is due to evaporation of sweat, whereas about 15 per cent is lost as a result of radiation, and 15 per cent by convection [3]. Because of the cooling effect of the evaporation of sweat from the skin, skin temperature often decreases during exercise except under hot, humid conditions [29].

Exercise in the Cold

Because of the potential 20-fold increase in heat production during vigorous exercise, body temperature can be easily maintained, even in subzero conditions, as long as one continues to exercise. There is little danger of frostbite to fingers, toes, and ears as long as gloves, warm footwear, and a head covering are worn. (A tremendous loss of heat can occur from an uncovered head because of a poor vasoconstriction response of the blood vessels in the skin of the head.) It is better to wear mittens than gloves to keep the fingers warm. In bitterly cold conditions, males should wear an extra pair of athletic shorts or similar garments beneath their long pants to protect the penis from frostbite. This type of injury is becoming more common as more males participate in running in cold climates. Shoes should not fit too tightly, lest circulation to the feet be restricted and the danger of frostbite increased [23]. Long underwear is a good choice for insuring that the legs are warm so that arterial blood circulating to the feet is also warm.

If frostbite should occur, the affected part should not be rewarmed if it will freeze again before obtaining medical help; the limb is more likely to be permanently damaged if it is thawed and refrozen than if it is thawed only once [23]. To rewarm a frostbitten area, it should be bathed or immersed in hot water at 45°C (113°F) without massage. Although this rapid rewarming causes great pain, it has been found that this is the most effective procedure to prevent permanent damage [23].

Although there is little risk of frostbite or hypothermia (lowering of the core temperature) if one dresses warmly and exercises continuously at high rates of energy expenditure, prolonged exposure with intermittent exercise presents a greater danger. Thus, hikers, skiers, orienteers, and mountaineers are subject to a much greater risk of cold injury than are joggers or sledders. A particular problem is that of remaining warm during periods of rest or light exercise (below 133 W) when clothing is soaked with perspiration or wet from rain or snowfall [16]. Damp clothing carries heat away from the body 20 times faster than dry clothing. Therefore, it is important to wear a water repellent outer garment to prevent soaking from rain or snow and to wear inner clothing which will allow evaporation during exercise so that moisture does not accumulate in the garments. Wool is especially good among the natural fibers because it absorbs less water than many other fabrics and retains some of its insulating properties even when it is wet. Some synthetic fabrics also are designed to repel water molecules from the outside but allow water to evaporate from the body surface, thus allowing the fabric to "breathe."

Another discomfort associated with exercise in a dry, cold environment is that of a parched mouth and throat and chapped lips. These problems can usually be prevented by wearing scarves or face masks to retain some of the moisture in exhaled air near the sensitive membranes of the mouth and lips. There is no substantial evidence that lung tissue can be frostbitten in the cold, presumably because of the tremendous warmth brought to the lungs by the pulmonary blood supply.

Exercise in Hot, Humid Conditions

Even under conditions of rest, prolonged exposures to hot and humid environments can lead to profound disruptions in the body's ability to maintain a stable internal environment for its cells and tissues. Exercise, especially endurance exercise, can accelerate the appearance of these harmful effects of heat exposure, not only because working muscles produce heat and thereby add to the heat load of the organism, but also because changes in the circulation that are associated with heavy exercise tend to decrease the body's ability to rid itself of excess heat. Certain types of athletic performance are not apt to be hindered by heat and, indeed, are probably aided by an elevated body temperature. For example, a single 100-meter sprint, a put of the shot, or a single lift in weightlifting competition would not be adversely affected by heat. However, the *repetition* of these activities many times during a prolonged training session in hot, humid conditions could easily lead to a failure of the temperature regulating ability of the athlete. In fact, many of the most severe effects of prolonged exposure to heat are observed in football players during early season practice sessions, a time when the players rarely exert themselves strenuously for more than forty yards or a few seconds at a time. Unfortunately, the effects of heat on football players are aggravated by the helmets, heavy padding, and clothing they must wear to prevent injury. Such clothing obviously hinders heat loss.

Work Tolerance in the Heat

It is common knowledge that conditions of high heat and humidity can adversely affect performance in many athletic events. Some of this detrimental effect of heat on performance is undoubtedly due to motivational factors; that is, some persons are psychologically less tolerant of heat than others and fail to maintain high levels of performance even when there is little evidence of physiological impairment [30]. More often, however, the adverse effect of heat on performance is the result of the competing demands of the circulation to the working muscles and the circulation to the skin [18, 22]. Since the capacity of the heart to pump blood is less than the maximal rate of blood flow to working muscles plus skin, and since the total blood volume is less than the maximal volume capacity of the muscles and skin, either the muscles must be short-changed in their blood supply so that the muscles become fatigued or the skin receives less than the optimal amount of blood needed to cool the organism. Excess body heat will then cause discomfort and, perhaps, neurological malfunction. In either case, performance suffers. It should again be emphasized, however, that environmental heat and humidity have little effect on performance that is of short duration. It is only in events lasting more than 15 minutes or in situations of repeated short work bouts over a prolonged period that one must be concerned about performance detriments of physiological origin [30].

Sex Differences in Heat Tolerance. For a number of years it was thought that females were less tolerant to exercise in the heat than males, primarily because women performing the same absolute exercise load as men tended to have lower sweat rates and higher heart rates. However, the women in these studies usually were working relatively harder than the males because the women had lower maximal oxygen uptakes. When exercise loads are equated so that all subjects exercise at the same percentage of their maximal oxygen uptakes, women are able to maintain their core temperatures at least as well as men with less sweat loss [37]. In one sense, females are better suited for exercise in the heat because they sweat less and thus conserve more body water than males while maintaining the same body temperature.

Obesity and Heat Tolerance. Obese persons of either sex suffer more physiological strain while performing a standard task in the heat than do lean persons [17]. Perhaps the most logical explanation of this effect of obesity is that fat serves as insulation and thus hinders heat exchange by radiation and convection. Also, obese persons must work at a greater percentage of their maximal oxygen uptakes to accomplish a standard task; this produces a greater strain on the circulation and on temperature regulation [12].

Maximal Oxygen Uptake in the Heat

If athletic performance suffers in hot, humid environments, it might be supposed that maximal oxygen uptake might also suffer. This relationship does not necessarily hold true. Some persons perform less well in the heat even though maximal oxygen uptake remains the same as that observed in a cool environment [9, 30].

Brief Exercise. Ordinarily, maximal oxygen uptake does not fall with short-duration exercise unless body temperature rises considerably, perhaps to 40°C [30]. This condition can occur if persons are exposed to high temperature and humidity for some time before the maximal oxygen uptake test begins or if body temperature is elevated by prolonged submaximal work before the test. Although the fall of maximal oxygen uptake under circumstances of prior temperature elevation may be due to shifts of blood from working muscle to skin, it could also be the result of insufficient motivation to exercise maximally [30]. A third possibility is that cardiac output may be reduced under such conditions because of a reduction in stroke volume [30].

There are no conclusive studies to tell us which of these possibilities or combinations thereof explain the decline in maximal oxygen uptake that is observed in subjects preheated before short-duration, maximal exercise. Because of the subjective discomfort most persons experience in the heat, it seems very likely that at least some of this decrement in maximal oxygen uptake is due to motivational factors. This is probably especially true in those whose performance is of mediocre caliber.

Prolonged Exercise. After an hour or more of exercise in the heat a more consistent decline of 3–8 per cent in maximal oxygen uptake is observed. This reduction may be caused by a fall in cardiac output as venous return to the heart is reduced by a pooling of blood in dilated skin vessels. The fall in maximal oxygen uptake after prolonged exercise could also be the result of a decreased arterio-venous difference in oxygen content of the blood. Such a decrease occurs when blood is shifted from working muscles to the skin, where less oxygen uptake occurs.

Cardiovascular Function

For both short-duration (less than 15 min.) and long-duration, *mild* exercise in the heat, cardiac output often rises above that observed with the same work load in a cool environment. This increase in cardiac output is accomplished by an increase in heart rate, because stroke volume often is diminished in the heat.

The extra cardiac output with submaximal work is directed to the skin so that more heat can be lost by radiation and convection. Blood pressure during mild work in the heat is not noticeably different from that observed in cool conditions because the dilatation of skin vessels (which tends to lower blood pressure) is balanced by vasoconstriction in liver, kidney, and nonworking muscles [30].

Cardiac output at more *strenuous* work loads in the heat is maintained throughout the exercise if it is a single, short-duration bout, but the output may fall toward the end of prolonged, vigorous exercise or after many repeated bouts of short-duration activity [30]. Repeated windsprints in football practice could produce such falls in cardiac output. At the beginning of these strenuous exercise periods, cardiac output is maintained even with a reduced stroke volume by increases in heart rate, but as heart rate is increased to maximal levels, maximal cardiac output and maximal oxygen uptake must fall as a result of the decreased stroke volume [30]. With the fall in cardiac output and increased vasodilatation in the skin, blood pressure also falls, sometimes by as much as 40 mm Hg. It is at this point of reduced cardiac output and lowered blood pressure that the danger of severe circulatory collapse and heat exhaustion occurs. This danger is increased if blood volume is diminished as a result of dehydration.

Body Fluids

Those who exercise for prolonged periods in the heat can lose more than 2 liters of body fluids (sweat) per hour and experience a total weight loss of 7 or 8 per cent of body weight in the course of an endurance event such as a marathon race. The body contains a total of only about 40 liters of fluid, including intracellular and extracellular compartments, and of that total, only about 5 liters are in the form of blood (3 liters of plasma and 2 liters of blood cells.) Therefore, if a major portion of the fluid lost during prolonged exercise in the heat were derived from the blood, it is obvious that blood volume, cardiac output, and blood pressure would all fall precipitously. Fortunately, with severe dehydration (greater than 2.5 liters of water loss), much of the fluid lost in sweat seems to come from tissue fluids. There is usually no more than a 20 per cent fall in plasma volume, that is, less than 600 ml., occurring during heavy exercise [3, 15, 24, 33]. There is a great variability in the effect on plasma volume of exercise in the heat. Some reports show no change in plasma volume even with sweat losses greater than 2.5 liters [9], and others show relatively greater losses of plasma volume by females than males [33]. A fall in plasma volume contributes to the reduction in stroke volume, cardiac output, and blood pressure during prolonged, vigorous exercise in the heat.

A loss of 2–3 liters of body fluids during exercise reduces sweating and thereby increases body temperature [24, 25]. Therefore, it is important that body fluids be replenished to aid sweating and to help maintain body temperature at a lower level than would be the case in one who is badly dehydrated.

It is interesting that the thirst mechanism is inadequate to stimulate complete rehydration after heavy fluid losses due to exercise [9]. This means that those who exercise in the heat will not voluntarily drink enough water to replenish body fluid stores after exercise, and body fluids are only gradually reestablished over a period of one or two days. Thus, an endurance athlete should learn to drink fluids even before he feels thirsty in order to delay dehydration as long as possible. If distance runners and football players would learn to drink a quart of water before competition and a cup of water every 10–15 minutes when they are exercising in hot, humid conditions, many problems of heat stress could be avoided [6, 9]. As a check on fluid replacement, athletes should be weighed before and after practice to see that most of the sweat loss is replaced during the practice period. Coaches and physical educators should make certain that water is available at all times and should insist on regular water breaks in the heat. It should be noted that novice runners who are not acclimatized to hot-weather running are subject to serious heat illness even when they consume liquids before and during distance races [21]. Thus, it is important for such athletes to train at least one week in the heat prior to a distance run which takes place in hot, humid conditions.

Electrolyte Disturbances

During early season conditioning, a substantial amount of sodium chloride may be lost in the sweat [8]. If not replenished by extra salt in the diet or perhaps electrolyte drinks, this loss of body salt can result in "heat cramps," that is, muscle cramps resulting from disturbed concentrations of sodium, potassium, and chloride on either side of

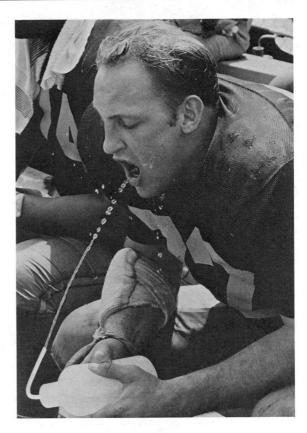

FIGURE 11.2. Fluid replenishment is important to maximize performance and minimize heat illness. (Courtesy of Office of Public Information, Purdue University, West Lafayette, Indiana.)

the muscle fiber membrane. Another adverse feature of this salt loss in the sweat is that as the water in the sweat evaporates, it leaves a coating of salt on the skin that increases the salt content of subsequent sweat secretions on the skin surface. As the salt concentration of sweat increases, it is more difficult to evaporate the sweat. (The heat required for vaporization of the sweat increases with increased salt concentration.) Therefore, it is probably beneficial to have some sweat drip off the body to carry excess salt with it and make evaporation more efficient. Although sweat that drips off the skin without evaporating does not directly contribute to cooling of the body, it indirectly helps by washing off salt that accumulates on the skin so that subsequent perspiration can evaporate more readily.

As training progresses, the sweat that is secreted has *less* salt than normal body fluids. Thus, loss of fluid by sweating tends to increase the concentration of salt in body fluids, and a large intake of salt before or after exercise is neither helpful nor desirable. Although consumption of several salt tablets per day is found to be beneficial for miners and others who labor in the heat for 6–10 hours daily, typical athletes should consume electrolyte drinks or simply sprinkle a total of 2–4 teaspoons more salt on their food each day than they normally would [9]. Excess ingestion of salt is not mandatory during prolonged exercise in trained individuals and may be more harmful than no salt at all.

If too much salt in the form of tablets or a salt solution is taken into the stomach, body fluids will be drawn by osmosis into the stomach. This will increase the state of dehydration of the cells and may cause stomach discomfort or vomiting [9].

Guidelines for Fluid Consumption in the Heat

The following guidelines for fluid consumption by those who exercise in hot environments are based on known changes in body fluids during exercise and on the effects of various protocols for replenishment [7, 8, 9, 19, 31, 38].

> 1) Consume approximately 600 milliliters (20 ounces) of a cold (10°C or 50°F) drink, preferably water, 20 to 30 minutes before exercise.

Too much salt or sugar in a drink will retard the emptying of the drink from the stomach. To speed stomach emptying, the osmolarity of solutions containing electrolytes and/or sugar should not be greater than that of the extracellular fluids of the body. Thus, if any sugar is added to the water, its concentration should be less than 5 per cent (less than 5 grams of sugar per 100 milliliters of water). Large volumes of cold solutions empty from the stomach and are absorbed into the blood more rapidly than smaller volumes of warm solutions. As long as the volumes consumed are within reason and the drink is not hypertonic to extracellular fluid, there is no need to be concerned about having stomach cramps or other discomfort while exercising.

> 2) Consume 100 to 200 milliliters of cold water or dilute glucose-electrolyte solution every 15 minutes during exercise.

Many athletes prefer to drink very little during exercise. They should be encouraged to drink fluids liberally because fluid intake during prolonged exercise in the heat reduces body temperature, reduces heart rate, usually enhances performance, and, most importantly, minimizes the risk of heat illness.

> 3) Record body weight daily before and after exercise in order to monitor fluid balance and minimize the potential for chronic dehydration.

Because many athletes do not voluntarily replenish the fluids they lose during prolonged exercise in the heat, they should keep records of weight changes to help them determine their state of hydration. If weight lost during exercise is not regained within 24 to 36 hours, the athlete should consume more fluids, even if this causes a sense of discomfort. Chronic dehydration can adversely affect exercise performance and subject the athlete to a greater risk of heat illness.

> 4) Replenish salt after exercise by salting more liberally or by consuming electrolyte drinks.

Sodium is the most important electrolyte that must be replenished. However, electrolyte replacement without adequate replenishment of water will increase the state of dehydration and may adversely affect performance.

Weight Loss in Wrestlers

It is common practice for wrestlers to attempt to gain advantages of leverage and maturity over their opponents by wrestling in a weight class lower than their normal body weights. Since wrestlers are very lean even before the training season [2, 36], much of the weight loss required to gain entrance to a lower weight classification tends to occur by voluntary dehydration a few days or hours before the weigh-in for certification. This rapid dehydration has both performance and health implications for the wrestler. Dehydration equivalent to 4–5 per cent of body weight usually does not markedly affect maximal oxygen uptake, maximal cardiac output, or stroke volume [3, 20, 38], but does markedly reduce endurance time and performance level for prolonged work [18, 19, 31, 38, 40]. However, dehydration usually causes small or insignificant decrements in strength or high-power exercise performance [2, 9, 19, 20, 38, 40]. It is suspected that the interaction of physiological and mental functions during a complex task such as wrestling is affected adversely by dehydration, but it is difficult to prove. Loss of 10 per cent of body weight by dehydration may lead to a dangerous reduction in blood volume and cardiac output [31].

Although dehydration may bring about severe changes in fluid volume, electrolyte balance, renal blood flow, and temperature regulation [2], there seems to be little conclusive evidence that these changes necessarily lead to heat illness, circulatory collapse, or diminished growth and development. However, it is important that the wrestler and the coach understand the harmful potential of repeated episodes of rapid weight loss by dehydration for both wrestling performance and for health. It is the position of the American College of Sports Medicine [2] that wrestlers whose fat content is less than 5 per cent of their certified body weights (as assessed several weeks in advance of the competitive season [36]) should receive medical clearance before they are allowed to compete. Also, wrestlers should be discouraged from consuming less food than required to meet their minimal needs (1,200–2,400 kilocalories per day) and should not be allowed to attempt weight loss through the use of rubber or plastic suits, steam rooms, saunas, laxatives or diuretics (substances taken to cause greater fluid loss through the kidneys) [2].

The complete position statement of the American College of Sports Medicine on weight loss in wrestlers is reprinted in the appendices.

Measurement of Heat Stress

It has been seen that prolonged or repeated short bouts of exercise in the heat are associated with a potential hazard to cardiovascular function and temperature regulation. Since the body receives and gives up heat by radiation, convection, and evaporation, a single measure of environmental temperature is not an *effective* means for evaluating heat stress on the organism. A better index of heat load is the interaction of dry bulb temperature and wet bulb temperature. A wet bulb thermometer is an ordinary dry bulb thermometer with the bulb encased in a wetted fabric wick. A *sling psychrometer* combines dry and wet bulb thermometer readings to measure relative humidity. When the environment is very humid the wet bulb thermometer reading will approach that of the dry bulb thermometer because little evaporative heat loss will occur from the wet wick. If the air is dry, the reading on the wet bulb thermometer will be much less than on the dry bulb thermometer. Therefore, a large difference between wet and dry bulb readings will be conducive to good performance in prolonged exercise. A small difference suggests a dangerous condition for prolonged exercise. Figure 11.3 illustrates various combinations of temperature and humidity that could lead to heat illness in athletes. Note that this chart does not include any correction for direct exposure to the sun or for clothing or protective pads which may impose an additional heat burden upon the athlete. Therefore, this chart should be conservatively interpreted under unusual conditions. When temperature and relative humidity intersect in the "Danger" zone of Fig. 11.3, athletes should take frequent rest- and water-breaks during prolonged exercise. Intersections of temperature and humidity in the "Cancel" zone suggests the need to cancel any prolonged activity such as a distance run or a football game that might lead to heat illness or even death.

Distance runners are especially susceptible to heat stress, and marathons should be run at dry bulb temperatures of about 40°F (4°C). Any time a marathon is run at dry bulb temperatures above 65°F (18°C), with more than 50 per cent relative humidity, many participants will be forced to stop because of heat stress. Distance runs on hot days should be conducted before 9:00 A.M. or after 4:00 P.M.

Adaptation to Exercise in the Heat

Enhanced Sweating Response. After as little as 4–14 days of training in the heat, both men and women are capable of exercising in hot, humid conditions with much less stress to the organism than prior to training [11, 30, 39]. One of the principal adaptations that is made is that the exerciser begins to sweat much more rapidly and profusely, and his sweat glands produce a more diluted and, therefore, more readily

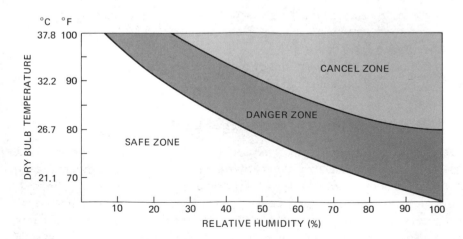

FIGURE 11.3. Exercise temperature and humidity guide.

evaporated sweat [1, 30]. Because of this sweating adaptation, one who has been trained in the heat can perform a standard, submaximal work task at a lower skin temperature, a lower rectal temperature and a lower heart rate than the untrained person [1, 30]. The reduction in heart rate seems to be a reflex response to decreased skin and/or core temperature.

The sweating adaptation is brought about by both an exercise effect and a heat effect [26]. The physical training somehow makes the sweat glands more sensitive to signals from the brain, whereas the heat acclimatization causes the brain to begin sending those signals to the sweat glands more rapidly, that is, at lower body temperatures [26]. The effect of training usually contributes about 50 per cent of the total adaptation to exercise in the heat, especially if the training elevates core temperature greatly and is pursued for about six months or more [11]. Ordinarily, training must be carried out in the heat for the greatest adaptation to heat to occur.

Increased Plasma Volume. A second important adaptation to exercise in the heat is an expansion of plasma volume [32]. This increase in plasma volume helps the exerciser to maintain adequate blood flow to the working muscles, the blood vessels in the skin, and other organs without overstressing the ability of the heart to pump blood. With training, there are more plasma proteins, and they hold water in the plasma by osmosis. Presumably, trained persons deliver less blood to the skin because their enhanced sweating response keeps them relatively cool. Since plasma proteins tend to leak out of the blood vessels in the skin, trained people lose less of their plasma proteins to the interstitial fluid than do untrained people. Also, trained persons seem to have a better return of proteins from the lymph to the blood plasma. The decreased loss of proteins from the skin vessels and the increased lymphatic contribution of proteins to the plasma helps to account for the greater plasma volume expansion in trained persons.

Increased Stroke Volume. Neither oxygen consumption nor cardiac output at submaximal loads commonly changes with heat acclimatization. Since cardiac output is unchanged and heart rate declines, it follows that stroke volume must rise in the acclimatized person. The increased stroke volume in acclimatized persons during exercise is still less than that seen in the same subjects working in a cool environment [30]. The exact reason for this rise in stroke volume is not known, but it may be a simple adjustment to lowered heart rate. There does not seem to be enough of a rise in venous return to the right side of the heart to account for the increased stroke volume [30]. Blood pressure during exercise is more stable after training in the heat, and during mild work there is a greater blood flow to the liver, kidneys, and other nonworking regions, with the exception of the skin [30]. The increased blood flow to the liver and kidneys is provided by a reduction in blood flow to the skin. Skin blood flow is less important for heat loss in the acclimatized person, who loses more heat by evaporation of sweat than the nonacclimatized person.

Heat Illness and Its Treatment

Some individuals tolerate heat poorly and experience a discomfort characterized by extreme fatigue, mental errors, and poor performance. These persons are suffering from *mild heat fatigue* and should rest in a cool place. A dramatic improvement in exercise performance has been observed when cold air is blown over a subject who seems to be approaching exhaustion from the heat. Heart rate falls dramatically, and the performer can continue a task that moments before had seemed too difficult. Indoors or outdoors, if electrical outlets are available on the playing field, a large fan would give welcome relief to athletes on a rest-break or water-break.

Simple heat exhaustion (*heat syncope*) results from diminished venous return to the heart as a consequence of increased blood flow to muscles and skin, and may result in a feeling of dizziness or actual fainting (syncope) accompanied by a rapid pulse and often cool skin. Syncope is most apt to occur in those who must stand in an upright posture in the heat for prolonged periods (such as Buckingham Palace Guards) or in persons who discontinue exercising in the heat and stand at rest. Because muscle contractions cease propelling blood back to the heart from the legs after exercise, the sudden reduction in venous return leads to a reduced cardiac output, a diminished flow of blood to the brain, and sometimes fainting. Such victims should be placed in a comfortable reclining position in a cool location and given fluids to replenish body fluids lost through sweating.

Heat cramps may occur in those who lose excessive amounts of fluids and salts during prolonged exercise. This condition may be alleviated by giving the victim commercial electrolyte drinks or several glasses of water, each containing a half teaspoon of dissolved table salt.

Heat stroke happens only rarely but is the most severe of the heat illnesses; victims of heat stroke often die. The symptoms of heat stroke include a high temperature (106°F, 41°C), a hot, dry, or moist skin, and sometimes mental confusion, convulsions, or loss of consciousness. These symptoms arise because the temperature-regulating nerve cells of the brain succumb to the high body temperature and fail to regulate the sweating response. The body temperature must be immediately lowered with any means available, and a physician's assistance should be sought. Early warning signs that heat illness is impending include a sensation of chilling, nausea, a throbbing head, weakness, and sometimes a dry skin.

It should be emphasized at this point that there should be no need to *treat* heat illness if proper precautions, as described in this chapter, are taken to *prevent* heat illness. If the athlete, coach, and physical educator will insist on frequent rest- and water-breaks under conditions of moderately high heat and humidity, and will not participate in or allow prolonged endurance activities or football contests to continue under severe weather conditions, there should be a minimal incidence of severe heat illness.

REVIEW QUESTIONS

1. Explain the various ways by which the body can conserve or rid itself of heat energy.
2. Describe the evidence that supports the idea that sweating is partly controlled by reflexes originating in working muscles and joints during exercise.
3. Why does skin temperature sometimes decline during exercise in the heat?
4. Describe the precautions one should take when exercising in the cold.
5. Explain why there is much greater risk of heat illness in humid weather than in dry weather.
6. Describe the changes in cardiovascular function that occur in the heat under exercise conditions.

7. Describe the responses of body fluids when one exercises for prolonged periods in hot, humid conditions. What precautions should be taken with respect to fluid and salt replenishment before, during, and after prolonged exercise in the heat?

8. Why is repeated rapid weight loss by dehydration in wrestlers frowned upon by medical authorities?

9. Describe the adaptations to exercise in the heat which occur with repeated exposures to exercise and thermal stress.

10. Describe the common forms of heat illness and their treatment.

REFERENCES

[1] Adams, W. C., R. H. Fox, A. J. Fry, and I. C. MacDonald. Thermoregulation during marathon running in cool, moderate, and hot environments. *Journal of Applied Physiology,* 1975, **39:**1,030–1,037.

[2] American College of Sports Medicine. Position stand on weight loss in wrestlers. *Medicine and Science in Sports,* 1976, **8:**xi–xiii.

[3] Åstrand, P.-O., and K. Rodahl. *Textbook of Work Physiology,* 2nd ed. New York: McGraw-Hill Book Company, 1977.

[4] Bergh, U. Human power at subnormal body temperatures. *Acta Physiologica Scandinavica,* 1980, (Suppl. 478).

[5] Boulant, J. A. Hypothalamic mechanisms in thermoregulation. *Federation Proceedings,* 1981, **40:**2843–2850.

[6] Buskirk, E. R. Temperature regulation with exercise. *Exercise and Sport Sciences Reviews,* 1977, **5:**45–88.

[7] Costill, D. L. Muscle water and electrolytes during acute and repeated bouts of dehydration. In J. Parizkova and V. A. Rogozkin, eds., *Nutrition, Physical Fitness, and Health.* Baltimore: University Park Press, 1978, pp. 98–116.

[8] Costill, D. L. Sweating: its composition and effects on body fluids. *Annals of The New York Academy of Sciences,* 1977, **301:**160–174.

[9] Costill, D. L. Water and electrolytes. In W. P. Morgan, ed., *Ergogenic Aids and Muscular Performance.* New York: Academic Press, Inc., 1972, pp. 292–320.

[10] Crawshaw, L. I., E. R. Nadel, J. A. J. Stolwijk, and B. A. Stamford. Effect of local cooling on sweating rate and cold sensation. *Pflügers Archives,* 1975, **354:**19–27.

[11] Gisolfi, C. V., and J. Cohen. Relationships among training, heat acclimation, and heat tolerance in men and women: the controversy revisited. *Medicine and Science in Sports,* 1979, **11:**56–59.

[12] Gisolfi, C. V., and S. Robinson. Central and peripheral stimuli regulating sweating during intermittent work in men. *Journal of Applied Physiology,* 1970, **29:**761–768.

[13] Haight, J. S. J., and W. R. Keatinge. Elevation in set point for body temperature regulation after prolonged exercise. *Journal of Physiology* (London), 1973, **229:**77–85.

[14] Hanson, P. G. Heat injury in runners. *Physician and Sportsmedicine,* 1979, **7:**91–96.

[15] Harrison, M. H., R. J. Edwards, and D. R. Leitch. Effect of exercise and thermal stress on plasma volume. *Journal of Applied Physiology,* 1975, **39:**925–931.

[16] Haymes, E. M. Physiological effects of a cold environment upon physical performance. In G. A. Stull, ed., *Encyclopedia of Physical Education, Fitness, and Sports,* Vol. 2. Salt Lake City: Brighton Publishing Co., 1980, pp. 161–168.

[17] Haymes, E. M., R. J. McCormick, and E. R. Buskirk. Heat tolerance of exercising lean and obese prepubertal boys. *Journal of Applied Physiology,* **39:**457–461.

[18] Henschel, A. The environment and performance. In E. Simonson, ed., *Physiology of Work Capacity and Fatigue.* Springfield, Ill.: Charles C Thomas, Publisher, 1971, 325–347.

[19] Herbert, W. G. Water and physical performance. In G. A. Stull, ed., *Encyclopedia of Physical Education, Fitness, and Sports,* Vol. 2. Salt Lake City: Brighton Publishing Co., 1980, pp. 151–160.

[20] Houston, M. E., D. A. Marrin, H. J. Green, and J. A. Thomson. The effect of rapid weight

loss on physiological functions in wrestlers. *Physician and Sportsmedicine*, 1981, **9**:73–78.

[21] Hughson, R. L., H. J. Green, M. E. Houston, J. A. Thomson, D. R. MacLean, and J. R. Sutton. Heat injuries in Canadian mass participation runs. *Canadian Medical Association Journal*, 1980, **122**:1141–1144.

[22] Johnson, J. M., and L. B. Rowell. Forearm skin and muscle vascular responses to prolonged leg exercise in man. *Journal of Applied Physiology*, 1975, **39**:920–924.

[23] Kinnear, G. R. Cold weather injuries: hypothermia and frostbite. In G. A. Stull, ed., *Encyclopedia of Physical Education, Fitness, and Sports*, Vol. 2. Salt Lake City: Brighton Publishing Co., 1980, pp. 169–176.

[24] Ladell, W. S. S. Terrestrial animals in humid heat: man. In D. B. Dill, ed., *Handbook of Physiology: Adaptation to the Environment*. Washington, D.C.: American Physiological Society, 1964, pp. 625–659.

[25] Nadel, E. R. Control of sweating rate while exercising in the heat. *Medicine and Science in Sports*, 1979, **11**:31–35.

[26] Nadel, E. R., K. B. Pandolf, M. F. Roberts, and J. A. J. Stolwijk. Mechanisms of thermal acclimation to exercise and heat. *Journal of Applied Physiology*, 1974, **7**:515–520.

[27] Nielsen, B. Effect of changes in plasma Na+ and Ca++ ion concentration on body temperature during exercise. *Acta Physiologica Scandinavica*, 1974, **91**:123–129.

[28] Nielsen, B., and C. T. M. Davies. Temperature regulation during exercise in water and air. *Acta Physiologica Scandinavica*, 1976, **98**:500–508.

[29] Robinson, S. Physiology of muscular exercise. In V. B. Mountcastle, ed., *Medical Physiology*, 13th ed. St. Louis, Mo.: The C. V. Mosby Company, 1974, pp. 1,273–1,304.

[30] Rowell, L. B. Human cardiovascular adjustments to exercise and thermal stress. *Physiological Reviews*, 1974, **51**:75–159.

[31] Saltin, B. Fluid, electrolyte, and energy losses and their replenishment in prolonged exercise. In J. Parizkova and V. A. Rogozkin, eds., *Nutrition, Physical Fitness, and Health*. Baltimore: University Park Press, 1978, pp. 76–97.

[32] Senay, Jr., L. C. Effects of exercise in the heat on body fluid distribution. *Medicine and Science in Sports*, 1979, **11**:42–48.

[33] Senay, Jr., L. C., and S. Fortney. Untrained females: effects of submaximal exercise and heat on body fluids. *Journal of Applied Physiology*, 1975, **39**:643–647.

[34] Simonson, E. Physiochemical changes. In E. Simonson, ed., *Physiology of Work Capacity and Fatigue*. Springfield, Ill.: Charles C Thomas, Publisher, 1971, pp. 71–82.

[35] Staff. Weight reduction in wrestling. *Physician and Sportsmedicine*, 1981, **9**:79–96.

[36] Tcheng, T., and C. M. Tipton. Iowa Wrestling Study: anthropometric measurements and the prediction of a minimal body weight for high school wrestlers. *Medicine and Science in Sports*, 1973, **5**:1–10.

[37] Wells, C. L. Physiological effects of a hot environment upon physical performance. In G. A. Stull, ed., *Encyclopedia of Physical Education, Fitness, and Sports*, Vol. 2. Salt Lake City: Brighton Publishing Co., 1980, pp. 123–139.

[38] Williams, M. H. *Nutritional Aspects of Human Physical and Athletic Performance*. Springfield, Ill.: Charles C Thomas, Publisher, 1976, pp. 169–207.

[39] Wyndham, C. H., N. B. Strydom, A. J. S. Benade, and A. J. Van Rensburg. Limiting rates of work for acclimatization at high wet-bulb temperatures. *Journal of Applied Physiology*, 1973, **35**:454–458.

[40] Zambraski, E. J. Weight loss for sports competition. In G. A. Stull, ed., *Encyclopedia of Physical Education, Fitness, and Sports*, Vol. 2. Salt Lake City: Brighton Publishing Co., 1980, pp. 369–376.

C H A P T E R
12

The Physiological Basis of Muscular Strength

THE ability of skeletal muscles to produce force not only enables us to move about in search of food, shelter, and companionship but also allows us to express our human uniqueness. Without muscular force we are unable to express our thoughts and emotions in speech, writing, painting, dance, and other forms of artistic endeavor. Muscular contraction produces the force called "strength."

What Is Strength?

The word "strength" has at least 12 definitions in the dictionary and many uses in the English language. Unfortunately, this has led to rather careless usage of the term in physical education and athletics. Thus, we have all heard the phrases "strong runner" and "strong swimmer" used to describe a distance runner or swimmer with great endurance, "strong fullback" to describe a football player who is difficult to tackle, and "strongman" to describe one who can lift heavy weights. *Muscular strength is best defined operationally as the greatest amount of force that muscles can produce in a single maximal effort.* Therefore, a person who can lift a greater weight than another in a single lift is stronger than the second person, even though the second person may be able to lift more total weight for perhaps ten repetitions.

   In earlier chapters we learned some important details about the structure of skeletal muscle, the way it contracts, and the different means muscles can use to obtain energy to sustain contractions. We will now investigate how the body controls the degree of force produced by muscle contraction and how maximal force can be increased by appropriate overload training. These topics will be taken up in this and the following chapter.

Types of Contraction

Static (isometric), isotonic, and isokinetic types of strength are produced by static, isotonic, and isokinetic contractions, respectively. A *static contraction* is one in which minimal muscle fiber shortening produces force with no change in the angle of a joint. *Isotonic contractions* result from muscle fiber shortening that causes a joint to move through some range of motion against a constant resistance. *Isokinetic contractions* occur as muscle fibers shorten to counteract an "accommodating" resistance developed by a device that allows only a constant rate of movement regardless of the force exerted by contracting muscle.

Examples of Static, Isotonic, and Isokinetic Contractions

An example of a *static* or *isometric* contraction is the carrying of a heavy bag of groceries with the arms or a single sheet of paper with the thumb and forefinger. In these activities little or no joint motion occurs as the muscles exert the required force. Also, there are brief isometric phases to many common athletic events; the weight of the body is supported isometrically during the early swing phase of the pole vault and during many gymnastic routines on apparatus such as the still rings and parallel bars.

Common examples of *isotonic* contractions are pushups, situps, pullups, the high jump, the lifting of dumbbells or barbells, and most aspects of swimming and running. In these examples note that a standard load (the weight of the body, of dumbbells, or of barbells) is moved through some range of motion against the action of gravity or the resistance of water. The word *isotonic* means "equal tension," but typically the muscle exerts varying amounts of tension at different angles of the involved joints to move the same fixed external load. What is "equal" throughout the range of motion is the exter-

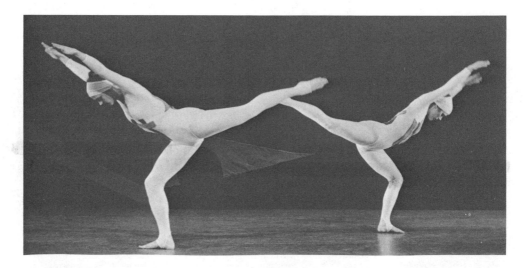

FIGURE 12.1. Static muscular contractions are common in dance. (Courtesy of Office of Public Information, Purdue University, West Lafayette, Indiana.)

nal load, not the muscular tension. For example, in elbow flexion the flexor muscles of the arm must create much more tension at an elbow angle of 170 degrees to lift a 20 kg dumbbell than at an angle of 115 degrees. Therefore, the tension in the muscles changes throughout the range of motion of elbow flexion to move a 20 kg dumbbell.

Isokinetic means "equal motion" and is construed to mean "equal rate of motion" or "equal speed." Thus, in a true *isokinetic* contraction, the joint angle changes at a constant rate—for example, 300 degrees per second, 180 degrees per second, or 60 degrees per second. To achieve a constant speed of movement, the load or resistance to the movement must change at different joint angles to accommodate the changing ability of the muscle(s) to produce force at those joint angles. This can only be accomplished with expensive mechanical equipment such as a Cybex dynamometer (Lumex, Bayshore, NY). However, there are other devices available that are designed to stabilize the speed of movement by providing greater external loads at joint angles where the muscles can produce greater tension and lesser loads at weaker joint angles. Typically these devices use cams or clutches to adjust the resistance. To the extent that such devices approach a constant speed throughout a range of motion they produce a more nearly isokinetic movement.

It should be pointed out that "isometric," "isotonic," and "isokinetic" contractions are far more important concepts to those engaged in research on muscle function than to those who wish to design strength development programs. The scientist must be able to state the exact nature of the contractions being investigated; the athlete, trainer or coach, on the other hand, will find that small deviations from true isometric, isotonic, or isokinetic conditions will have little effect on the outcomes of strength training. Our discussion will center on the three well-defined types of contraction, but it should be clear that forms of training which result in some sort of hybrid contractions may be very effective in strength training.

Concentric and Eccentric Contractions

Isotonic, isokinetic, and other types of *dynamic* contractions (as opposed to static contractions) may also be classified as *concentric* or *eccentric* contractions, depending upon whether the whole active muscles shorten or lengthen, respectively, during the movement. For example, in the upward phase of a pullup or "chin," the elbow flexors (biceps brachii, for example) are shortening and the angle of the elbow joint is decreasing from 180 degrees to perhaps 15 degrees. Since the active muscles are shortening, this is a *concentric* contraction. On the other hand, during the downward phase of a pullup, elbow flexors lengthen as progressively fewer muscle fibers are activated. This contraction causes a gradual increase in the angle of the elbow joint until it is once again 180 degrees. Therefore, the downward phase of a pullup is an example of an *eccentric* contraction.

Although during this type of *isotonic, eccentric* contraction each elbow flexor muscle as a whole is lengthening, remember that some fibers must be attempting to shorten or the subject would drop immediately from the pullup bar. The amount of shortening of any given fiber, however, becomes increasingly less as the muscle is lengthened and fewer fibers are activated. For example, a fiber of the biceps brachii may contract to perhaps 50 per cent of its resting length when it is activated by nerve stimuli near the top of a pullup, but when activated from a lengthened state near the bottom of the "letdown" phase, this same fiber may shorten by only 5 per cent of its resting length. Eventually, the number of active muscle fibers is so small that total contractile force just equals the force required to stretch the connective tissues of the muscle and tendon, but it is not great enough to raise the body from the straight hang position. These few fibers at this time are contracting "isometrically."

In an *isokinetic, eccentric* contraction, a mechanical device or a human assistant gradually overcomes the contractile force of a muscle group to cause a joint angle to increase at a constant rate. In this instance, muscle fiber shortening is overcome by a more powerful mechanical force which gradually inhibits or stretches more and more fibers. It appears that either muscle fibers are inhibited from contracting by a nerve reflex triggered by the great tension on the muscle (described later in this chapter), or some sacromeres in the active fibers are being stretched as they attempt to shorten, while others are simultaneously contracting. Exactly how this phenomenon might occur is unknown. Intuitively, it seems that cross bridges in some sarcomeres may be more susceptible to disruption by mechanical forces than others.

Neural Control of Muscular Strength: Graded Contractions

The body has an amazing ability to call forth just the right amount of muscular force to perform an endless variety of tasks—from drawing a fine line on a sheet of paper to lifting a 90-pound barbell. If it were not for this ability to control contractile force, it would be common to see ice cream cones plastered to their owner's foreheads and seamstresses going berserk while attempting to thread needles. There are two ways by which the organism can vary the strength of a muscle contraction: it can vary the *total number* of motor units recruited in a muscle, or it can vary the *frequency* with which a *given number* of motor units is activated.

Motor Units

A motor unit consists of a motor nerve cell (neuron) that originates in the spinal cord and all of the muscle fibers that are supplied by that neuron (Fig. 12.2). The number of muscle fibers innervated by a single motor nerve fiber varies from as few as 5 in some eye muscles, which require fine control, to as many as 1,000 or more in large muscles (such as the gastrocnemius), which do not require a high degree of control. All of the muscle fibers within a given motor unit are of the same fiber type, that is, either slow twitch (Type I), fast twitch with both aerobic and anaerobic capacities (Type IIA), or fast twitch with anaerobic capacity (Type IIB). The muscle fibers of a given motor unit are usually located throughout the muscle and are not found close together. The motor neuron that supplies a unit of muscle fibers determines to a great extent the fiber type of those fibers. There are chemicals (*neurotrophic substances*) which flow in the nerve axon from the spinal cord to the muscle fibers. These substances seem to cause the muscle fibers to take on their particular fiber type characteristics [9]. There

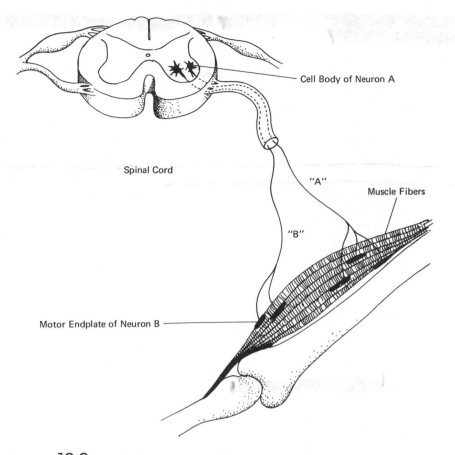

FIGURE 12.2. Sketch of two motor units. Neuron "A" innervates three muscle fibers, neuron "B" only two.

are also substances which travel from the muscle to the motor nerve and help determine the nerve's firing characteristics [16]. Thus, the nerve and muscle fibers within a motor unit are interdependent; changes in one can affect the other. As described in the chapter on muscle contraction, the slow twitch units are ordinarily recruited before the fast twitch units because the motor nerves to the slow units are smaller and more easily activated. However, in some circumstances the order of recruitment can be reversed [13].

The All or None Law. As the name "motor unit" implies, all the muscle fibers within a given motor unit contract or relax nearly simultaneously: that is, it is not possible for some of the muscle fibers of a motor unit to relax while others contract. Also, if the muscle fibers of a motor unit are activated sufficiently by the nerve to contract, those fibers will contract maximally. This is the so-called "all or none" law; under a given set of conditions muscle fibers in a motor unit either contract maximally or they do not contract at all. This is an important concept for understanding graded muscle contractions. Remember that this "all or none" law applies to the muscle fibers of a given motor unit and not to an entire muscle. This application of the law is explained in the following paragraph.

Let us assume that a gastrocnemius muscle is innervated by 300 neurons that are contained in a branch of the sciatic nerve and that each of those 300 neurons supplies from 50 to 2,000 muscle fibers. Thus, this muscle has 300 motor units, each consisting of a neuron and 50–2,000 muscle fibers. Since all the muscle fibers of each of these motor units will contract maximally if the motor units are adequately stimulated, the smallest number of muscle fibers that can contract is 50, the size of the smallest motor unit. If each muscle fiber produces a force of 0.01 newton[1], the *minimum* force that this muscle can produce is 50 × 0.01 = 0.5 newton. The *maximum* amount of force that could be exerted depends on the total number of muscle fibers in the muscle. If we suppose that the average motor unit has 400 muscle fibers, then a total of *300 motor units ×400 fibers per unit ×0.01 newton force per fiber =1,200 newtons* of force could be produced by our hypothetical gastrocnemius muscle. Therefore, the muscle could produce almost any degree of force between 0.5 and 1,200 newtons, depending on how many motor units were called into play at one time.

Frequency of Stimulation of Motor Units. All motor units do not fire in unison except under conditions of maximal stimulation. For submaximal contractions some motor units are at rest, while others produce the required force. But the resting and active motor units exchange roles frequently so that fatigue of any one motor unit is avoided. This *asynchronous* contraction of motor units is also responsible for the smooth, nonjerky nature of voluntary contractions. By increasing the frequency with which a given number of motor units is fired (so that rest pauses are shorter), more of these motor units can be active at any given time to give a greater strength of contraction. An exaggerated example of the effect a change in rate of stimulation can have on total muscle force is shown in Fig. 12.3. In Fig. 12.3 it is assumed that the muscle is composed of three motor units, each capable of generating 0.01 newton of force when activated. When each unit fires asynchronously *every 3 milliseconds*, only one unit is active at any given millisecond, and the *total* muscle force is 0.01 newton. If the units begin to fire *every millisecond*, their contractions will occur at essentially the same instant, and the total muscle force will be about .03 newtons. The example is exaggerated because no muscle contains only three motor units, the frequency of contraction is far too great, and it would be rare to have all units active simultaneously.

As another example, assume that each of 100 motor units, each having an equal number of muscle fibers, fires every 0.01 second and that, at any one time, there are about 60 motor units active and 40 at rest. Next, assume that each motor unit begins to fire more frequently so that there are 90 active motor units at a given instant with only 10 at rest. According to the "all or none" law, the force exerted when 90 of the motor units are simultaneously active is 50 per cent greater than when only 60 are active. Thus, the same 100 motor units can produce a stronger or weaker contraction when their rate of firing is either increased or decreased, respectively.

Varied Patterns of Motor Unit Activation. There is evidence that certain patterns of activation of motor units are preferred in certain types of muscular contrac-

[1] A newton (N) is the force that confers an acceleration of 1 m s^{-2} on a mass of 1 kg.

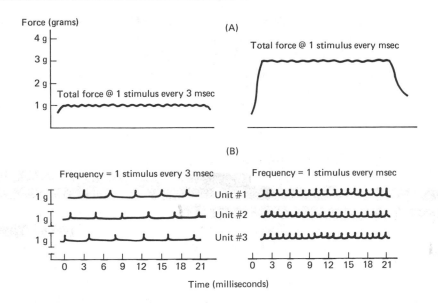

FIGURE 12.3. Example of how increasing the frequency of stimulation of the same three individual motor units from once every three milliseconds to once every millisecond can increase the force produced by the total muscle. As shown in (A), the total force at any given instant when the motor units are stimulated asynchronously at a frequency of once per 3 msec is much less than when the frequency of stimulation is once per millisecond. The stimulation patterns for the individual motor units are shown in (B).

tions [21, 33]. In other words, repetitive stimulation of motor units at a constant rate is not always the most efficient way to produce force. For example, in isometric contractions and in rapid, forceful limb movements such as those in running and throwing, optimal force production may be achieved when two rapid nerve impulses are followed by volleys of slower impulses. With regard to whether the body prefers to recruit *more* motor units or stimulate the *same* units *more frequently* to generate additional muscular force, it appears that recruitment of additional units is usually the first approach for maximal, brief contractions. Increasing frequency of activation probably plays a greater role as the duration of contraction increases. Our knowledge of patterns of motor unit activation is rudimentary, but it is clear that different patterns are optimal for different activities.

Smooth, Voluntary Contractions. When skeletal muscles are stimulated briefly with a massive electric shock, they "twitch" or produce a rapid maximal contraction for a brief instant before returning to the rested state. This sort of contraction is not of much use in most physical activity; instead, a much smoother, longer acting type of contraction is needed. The smooth contractions that are typical of human movements result from the fusion of asynchronous twitches of fibers from different motor units so that, at any given instant, only the appropriate amount of force is produced.

As a rough illustration of the fusion of asynchronously twitching fibers to produce a smooth movement, assume that a slow, continuous flexion of the index finger requires the force of contraction of 100 muscle fibers (but not the same 100 fibers) during the entire movement. This contractile force could be accomplished by activating different groups of 10 motor units, each with 10 muscle fibers, every 20 milliseconds. Accordingly, twitch contractions of 100 fibers would start the movement and would be immediately succeeded by the twitching of another 100 fibers, which would be followed by twitches of another 100 fibers, and so on. The twitches of the first group of 100 fibers would be smoothly fused into the twitches of successive batches of 100 fibers until the movement was completed.

Tetanic Contractions of Motor Units. It is possible to produce greater force in a smooth voluntary movement by the high frequency stimulation of individual motor units, so that twitches of muscle fibers in these units fuse into a constant, steady contraction for as long as these motor units are active (only a fraction of a second, except during maximal contractions). These steady contractions are called *tetanic contractions;* and the muscle fibers involved are said to be in a state of tetanus (Fig. 12.4). Tetanus of a certain number of motor units at any one time does not, of course, mean that an entire muscle is in a state of rigid contraction. As more or fewer motor units fire tetanically, a greater or lesser contraction will result, so that a movement such as a pullup can be completed smoothly.

As inspection of Fig. 12.4 shows, a tetanic contraction produces more force than a single twitch. The explanation given for this phenomenon is that during a *twitch* contraction, part of the contractile energy is used to overcome the resistance to change of length of the connective tissue and other components of the muscle. However, in *tetanus,* the muscle is not allowed to return to its resting length, so that resistance of the tissue need not be repeatedly overcome (2). Thus, the contractile energy normally expended in overcoming internal muscle resistance in a twitch can be used to do work in a tetanic contraction. The fact that tetanic contractions produce more force than twitch contractions is not a violation of the "all or none" law because the conditions (length, temperature, etc.) of the muscle fibers prior to stimulation are dissimilar.

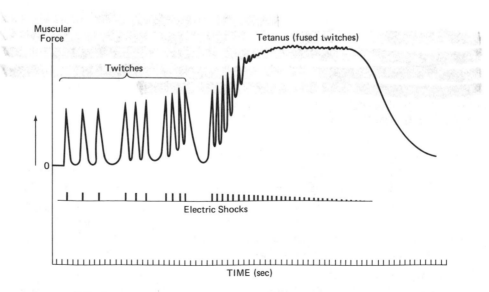

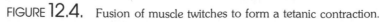

FIGURE 12.4. Fusion of muscle twitches to form a tetanic contraction.

Neural Control of Muscular Force: Excitatory and Inhibitory Neurons

In the previous portions of this chapter, reference has often been made to the role of the motor neuron in the activation of muscle fibers. The motor neuron is influenced by stimuli from other neurons that reach the cell body of the motor neuron as it lies in the anterior part of the gray matter of the spinal cord (Fig. 12.5). The biceps muscle of the upper arm will not contract maximally, for example, until the brain sends thousands of stimuli down to the spinal cord to stimulate (facilitate) all the motor neurons of the biceps. In addition to stimuli from the motor areas of the cortex of the brain and from other lower brain areas (such as the basal ganglia, the reticular formation, and the cerebellum), reflex stimuli from higher and lower levels of the spinal cord, and from peripheral organs such as muscle spindles, modify the activity of anterior motor neurons and, consequently, are involved in the control of muscle strength [19]. A basic understanding of how the activity of the motor neurons is affected by other parts of the nervous system is helpful in determining how strength is affected by psychological, emotional, environmental, and training phenomena.

Excitatory and Inhibitory Stimuli to Motor Neurons

All neurons send signals to other neurons by transmitting small amounts of chemicals (*neurotransmitters*) to the other neurons. Some of these neurotransmitters excite a neuron and tend to make it fire, whereas others inhibit the neuron and keep it quies-

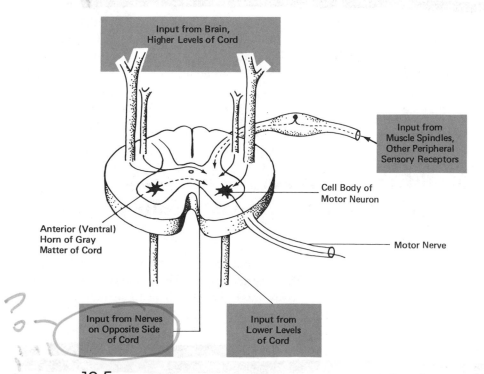

FIGURE 12.5. Schematic diagram of some of the many types of nerve fibers that affect the activity of the lower motor neuron.

cent. These neurotransmitters are called *excitatory (facilitory)* and *inhibitory* neuro-transmitters, respectively. Any given neuron secretes either an excitatory or an inhibitory substance, not both, and is therefore known either as an excitatory neuron or an inhibitory neuron.

Whether or not a motor neuron fires or becomes quiet depends upon the *net* effect of all the excitatory and inhibitory stimuli that arrive at the motor neuron at any instant. Let us assume for illustration purposes that a motor neuron will fire if it has a *net* of 100 *excitatory* neurotransmitter molecules on its cell body at any given time. Now suppose that we measure all the molecules of excitatory and inhibitory chemicals that are on this neuron at time X and find 200 excitatory molecules and 150 inhibitory molecules. The net result of these stimuli is $200 - 150 = 50$ excitatory molecules; the motor neuron will not fire because its threshold of a net 100 excitatory molecules has not been met. Next, suppose that 150 excitatory molecules and 20 inhibitory molecules are present at a given moment. In this situation a net of $150 - 20 = 130$ excitatory molecules surpasses the firing threshold of 100, and the nerve will now fire. Therefore, there are three ways in which a quiet motor neuron can be stimulated to fire: by increasing the excitatory stimuli while the inhibitory stimuli remain constant, by decreasing the inhibitory stimuli while the excitatory stimuli remain constant, and by a combination of increasing the excitatory and decreasing the inhibitory stimuli. The last method is probably the most common.

There are both excitatory and inhibitory stimuli that descend from lower parts of the brain to the spinal motor nerves. The inhibitory impulses are important in helping man avoid spastic, painful contractions of muscles whenever a violent burst of excitatory impulses reaches the motor neuron from other parts of the nervous system. However, when a person wishes to exert a maximal strength effort, the inhibitory influences from the brain stem may interfere with the ability to activate all motor units at once. One explanation of individual differences in strength is that a stronger individual is the one who is capable of blocking more of the inhibitory neurons so that more motor units can reach their firing thresholds [4]. Perhaps through strength training, one can learn to reduce the inhibitory output of the brain to the lower motor neurons.

Central Modifiers of Muscular Force — The Cortex, Cerebellum, Lower Brain Centers, and Spinal Cord

It is now clear that the motor unit activation patterns for common movements such as walking can be generated by neurons in the spinal cord. This is shown by the fact that animals can walk on a treadmill after having the bulk of their brains removed surgically. However, it is also clear that the movement patterns generated by the spinal cord are affected by information descending from the brain [14, 21, 28]. The *idea* for a complex movement originates in the *association areas* of the cerebral cortex. The *planning* of the pattern of stimulation of motor units involves not only the association areas of the cortex, but also clusters of brain cells known as the *basal ganglia* (caudate

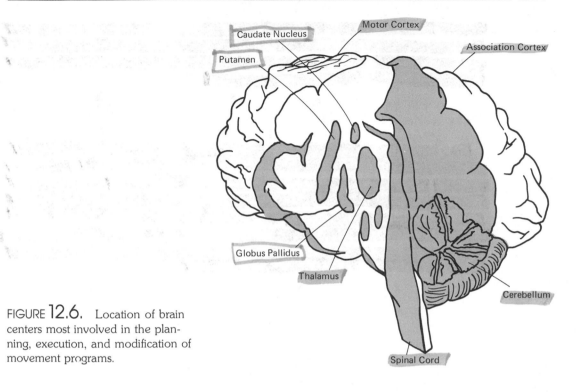

FIGURE 12.6. Location of brain centers most involved in the planning, execution, and modification of movement programs.

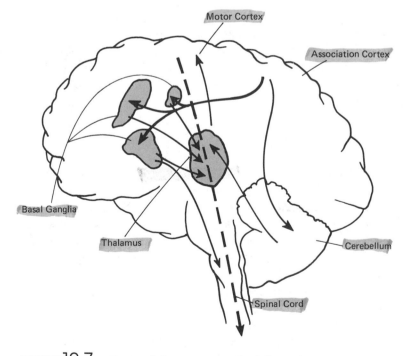

FIGURE 12.7. Some of the many complex relationships among areas of the brain involved in development of a motor response.

nucleus, putamen, and globus pallidus) and the *cerebellum* [14, 28] (Fig. 12.6, 12.7). Once the movement pattern has been programmed, the *motor area* of the cerebral cortex receives the appropriate information to *execute the program* by stimulation of the appropriate motor neurons in the spinal cord. Throughout the entire process of movement planning and execution, the cerebellum and other areas of the brain monitor information arriving from the muscles, skin, and joints, process the information, and bring about the appropriate movement corrections by the motor cortex.

It is also apparent that other groups of brain cells can generate stimuli which influence the final pattern of movement and force generation by the muscles. The *vestibular nuclei* report information on balance as sensed by the inner ear, and the *auditory* and *visual areas* of the cerebral cortex relay information sensed by the ears and eyes which can alter movement patterns. In addition, emotional activity arising in the *limbic lobe* of the cortex and in the *hypothalamus* can have an important influence on motor activity, including a complete cessation of movement after overwhelming fear or shock and uncontrollable movements associated with rage. A coach must understand the powerful impact that emotions have on individuals and avoid fostering inappropriate emotions which could result in physical or psychological injury to sport participants.

Peripheral Modifiers of Muscular Force— Joint Receptors, Muscle Spindles, and Tendon Organs

It would be convenient if there were located in moving limbs some sensors that could 1) determine the extent to which a movement initiated by the brain were accomplishing its goal and 2) report that information back to the brain and spinal cord so that any necessary corrections in the movement could be made. Fortunately, such a movement feedback system is present in muscles and joints. It can report to the brain and cord the status of joint movements, limb positions, muscle force, muscle stretch and speed of muscle stretch.

The ability to judge the appropriateness of a muscle contraction, to judge where limbs are in space in relation to each other, and to know how fast and to what extent joint angles are changing is called the *kinesthetic sense.* This sense is obviously of vital importance in all human movements, but especially those involved in skills such as tumbling, diving, and pole vaulting where a failure of kinesthetic sense could easily result in severe injury or death. The nerve endings or receptors that sense limb and joint *position* lie in the connective tissues around joint capsules and in ligaments; they are extremely sensitive and conduct their information back to the spinal cord and brain very rapidly so that corrections in movements may likewise be made quickly [35].

The role of joint receptors in modifying muscular force can be illustrated as follows. In executing a pole vault, the joint receptors feed back information on how the body parts are aligned just prior to the "handstand" at the peak of the vault. If the vaulter senses from this information that he must bring himself closer to the pole, he exerts more arm strength to accomplish that goal. If, on the other hand, the vaulter senses that his body is too far ahead of the pole, he can decrease the strength of his arm contractions to correct the faulty position. As another example, consider a weightlifter who, while completing a press, senses that his extended arms are moving behind his head and makes a rapid decision about what to do with the 200-pound barbell supported above his head by his rapidly tiring arms! Kinesthetic sense has doubtless saved many weightlifters embarrassing falls and serious injuries.

Muscle Spindles, the Stretch Reflex, and the Gamma Motor System

Changes in the length of muscles and the *rate of changes in muscle length* are sensed by receptors called *muscle spindles* that are buried in the muscles themselves (Fig. 12.8) [7, 20, 35]. These spindles are covered by connective tissue that is interwoven with that surrounding the regular (*extrafusal*) muscle fibers, so that anytime the whole muscle is stretched or shortened, the spindle is also stretched or shortened. The interior of the muscle spindle usually contains 2–12 small, peculiar muscle fibers called *intrafusal fibers* because of their location inside the *fusiform* (tapering from the middle toward each end) spindle (Fig. 12.8). The larger, extrafusal muscle fibers that surround the spindles are innervated by large *alpha motor neurons* with cell bodies located in the spinal cord (Fig. 12.9).

The middle portion of an intrafusal fiber does not contract; this portion of the fiber is stretched whenever the contractile ends of the intrafusal fiber are stimulated to contract by their motor nerves, the small *gamma motor neurons* (Fig. 12.9). Thus, *there are two ways in which the middle, noncontractile part of the intrafusal fibers can be stretched.* First, when the whole muscle (extrafusal fibers) is stretched, the stretch is transmitted through the connective tissue to the muscle spindle, which then is also stretched. Second, if a motor impulse comes from the spinal cord down the gamma

FIGURE 12.8. Schematic diagram illustrating location of muscle spindles and tendon organs.

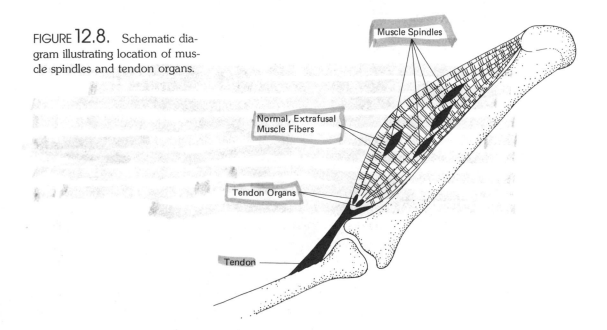

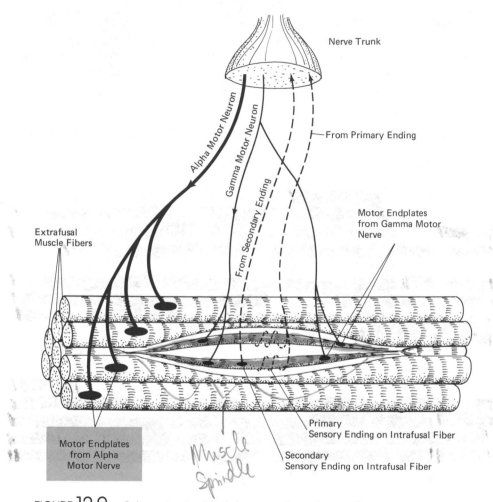

FIGURE 12.9. Schematic simplified diagram of muscle spindle anatomy.

motor nerve, the outer two thirds of the intrafusal fibers contract and pull on the non-contractile middle third of the fibers thereby causing them to be stretched.

Once the middle portion of an intrafusal fiber is stretched, the stretch is sensed by one or both of two sensory nerve endings attached to this middle part of the intrafusal fiber (Fig. 12.9). The *primary* ending senses not only the stretch of the intrafusal fiber, *but also the velocity* of the stretch and feeds this information back to the spinal cord and on up to the cerebral cortex and cerebellum, so that any necessary adjustments can be made in muscle contraction, as will be described in the next section [32]. The *secondary* endings sense only the stretch of the intrafusal fibers. The muscle spindles are responsible for the myotatic or stretch reflex, an important spinal reflex that is involved in many human movements.

The Stretch Reflex. If a muscle is suddenly stretched, for example by a wrestler who forcefully pulls his opponent's arm in an attempted takedown, the muscle almost instantaneously contracts to resist that stretch. This reflex operates at the level of the spinal cord; that is, it does not require conscious thought by the brain. A simple example of the stretch (myotatic) reflex is the knee jerk reflex that is diagrammed in Fig. 12.10. As the reflex hammer strikes the patellar tendon, the quadriceps muscles are rapidly stretched. This stretch of extrafusal fibers is transmitted via connective tissue to the muscle spindle and its intrafusal fibers. As the central portions of the intrafusal fibers are stretched, the primary and secondary sensory endings are stimulated to send an excitatory impulse to the *alpha motor neurons* in the spinal cord. These large alpha motor neurons then stimulate the extrafusal fibers of the same muscle to contract, thereby relieving the stretch. At the same time inhibitory impulses are transmitted to the antagonistic muscles to cause them to relax (reciprocal inhibition).

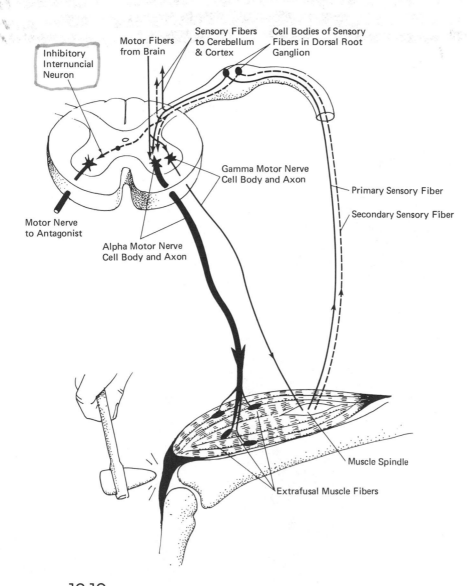

FIGURE **12.10.** Schematic illustration of stretch reflex.

Whenever muscle length changes, the muscle spindles report the changing conditions back to the brain and spinal cord so that appropriate adjustments in muscle contraction can be made. Note, however, that a muscle jerk does not always occur when a muscle is stretched. Ordinarily, muscle stretch is less rapid than when caused by a tap of the tendon hammer. Also, other stimuli from the brain act to modify the reflex activity so that a more mild contraction, not a muscle jerk, results.

Until quite recently it was thought that the stretch reflex was primarily responsible for the maintenance of standing posture. It was thought, for example, that a forward sway caused stretching of the muscles at the back of the leg and that this then triggered a stretch reflex and contraction of those muscles to help regain a vertical position. It now appears that the reflex activity does not originate in the muscle spindles, but rather in disturbances in equilibrium which activate higher centers in the brain, presumably including the vestibular center [8]. However, the muscle spindles are probably involved in fine control of these reflex contractions once the contractile activity has begun.

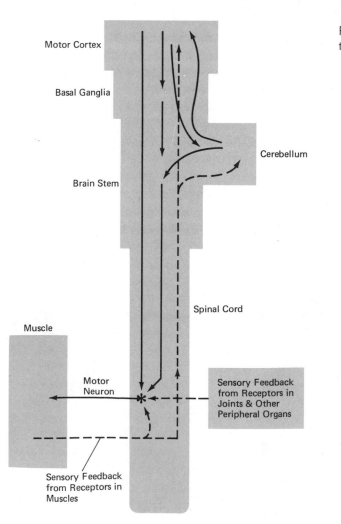

FIGURE 12.11. Schematic diagram illustrating some modifiers of motor stimuli.

Motor Cortex

Basal Ganglia

Cerebellum

Brain Stem

Spinal Cord

Muscle

Motor Neuron

Sensory Feedback from Receptors in Joints & Other Peripheral Organs

Sensory Feedback from Receptors in Muscles

It is important to think of the information that comes to the alpha motor neurons from the muscle spindles as only one of many types of information that the motor neurons receive. These neurons are constantly being bombarded with information from the muscles, joints, ligaments, and tendons; from other neurons at the same and different levels of the spinal cord; and from various parts of the brain (Fig. 12.11). Muscle spindles are, however, one of the more important sources of information for movement because of their ability to sense muscle length and speed of length change. That is not to say that no movements can be carried out satisfactorily without feedback from joints and muscles. Monkeys and other laboratory animals can perform many tasks adequately after total loss of sensory feedback from the limbs [34]. However, such movements tend to be performed in a rather clumsy manner, and the timing of such movements is not precise. Therefore, it is clear that highly skilled athletic performance would be impossible without peripheral feedback.

The Gamma Motor System and Muscle Force. The small motor neurons which cause the intrafusal fibers to shorten are the *gamma* motor neurons. If these neurons fire, the shortening of the ends of the intrafusal fibers causes stretch of the middle portion of the fibers. This stretch stimulates the primary and secondary sensory endings. The increased firing of these sensory neurons feeds back to the spinal cord and triggers a reflex excitation of the alpha motor neurons. This excitation causes more forceful contraction of the extrafusal muscle fibers that surround the muscle spindles. In other words, if the gamma motor system is activated during contraction of the extrafusal fibers, the afferent feedback from the muscle spindles can help produce more powerful contractions.

There are, in fact, several pathways from the motor cortex, other brain centers, and the spinal cord which do activate the gamma system at the same time that the alpha motor neurons to the extrafusal fibers are activated [32]. This dual activation of both alpha and gamma motor systems is called "alpha-gamma coactivation" or "alpha-gamma" linkage. It appears to be a regular feature of isometric contractions, of slow, forceful dynamic contractions, and of the initial contractions which begin rapid movements such as kicking, throwing, and striking [7, 32]. However, during most phases of rapid movements there appears to be only a minor contribution of muscle spindle feedback to muscular force [7]. It has been suggested that spindle feedback is most important in the early stages of learning of skills, when the movements tend to be relatively slow; once the skill has been learned and can be performed "automatically," the gamma system may become unimportant [7].

The gamma system sometimes operates during movements of the limbs to "reset" muscle spindles that have been shortened by movements of surrounding extrafusal fibers; the spindles are then able to respond to stretch of the now shortened extrafusal fibers (Fig. 12.12) [17]. As an illustration of this complex phenomenon, let us imagine that a wrestler is about to contract his gastrocnemius muscle by plantar flexion of the ankle, in order to escape from a particularly troublesome hold by his opponent. Upon shortening the gastrocnemius during plantar flexion, the intrafusal fibers would go slack with little tension at the ends of the fibers were there no gamma activity (Fig. 12.12b). If this should happen, any lengthening or stretch of the gastrocnemius from its newly shortened position could not be sensed by the spindles until after the intrafu-

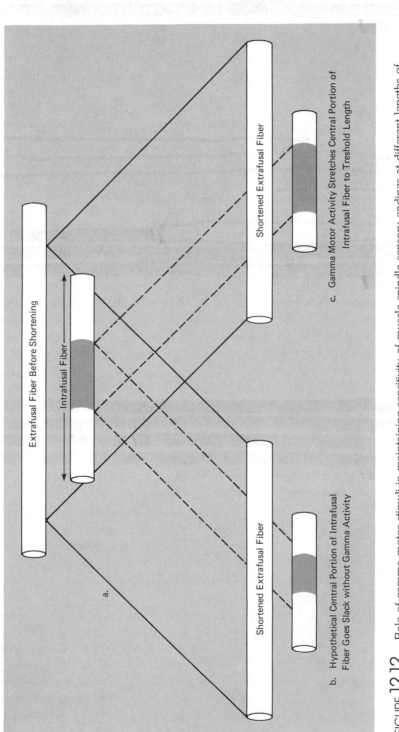

a.

Extrafusal Fiber Before Shortening

Intrafusal Fiber

Shortened Extrafusal Fiber

c. Gamma Motor Activity Stretches Central Portion of
Intrafusal Fiber to Treshold Length

Shortened Extrafusal Fiber

b. Hypothetical Central Portion of Intrafusal
Fiber Goes Slack without Gamma Activity

FIGURE 12.12. Role of gamma motor stimuli in maintaining sensitivity of muscle spindle sensory endings at different lengths of
extrafusal muscle fibers. See text for discussion.

sal fibers had been stretched past their original positions. Thus, without gamma motor activity, the wrestler would be unable to sense muscle stretch until his gastrocnemius had returned to its original length; he might, therefore, be unable to rapidly counteract a move by his opponent that would stretch the gastrocnemius.

This example is similar to that shown in Fig. 12.12. In Fig. 12.12a the relative lengths of intrafusal and extrafusal fibers are shown before contraction of the muscle. In Fig. 12.12b, the diagram shows what might occur if there were *no* tonic gamma motor nerve stimuli to reset the central portions of the intrafusal fibers to their initial stretch-sensitive lengths. Fig. 12.12c shows the effect of gamma activity on maintaining the central portions of the intrafusal fibers at their sensitive lengths, that is, the lengths shown in Fig. 12.12a. Note that in Fig. 12.12c, the *total* intrafusal fiber length is the same as that shown in Fig. 12.12b, but the gamma activity in Fig. 12.12c has shortened the outer contractile portions while stretching the central portions to reset them to their stretch-sensitive lengths.

Tendon Organ Reflexes and Muscular Force. In previous paragraphs, we have discussed how stimuli from sensory endings in muscle spindles might increase strength by exciting alpha motor nerves in the spinal cord. We should also consider the possibility that *fewer inhibitory impulses* delivered to the alpha motor nerves would also tend to increase muscle force. In an earlier section it was suggested that with strength training, inhibitory influences from the brain may be reduced. We shall now show that peripheral reflexes called tendon organ reflexes also inhibit alpha motor neuron activ-

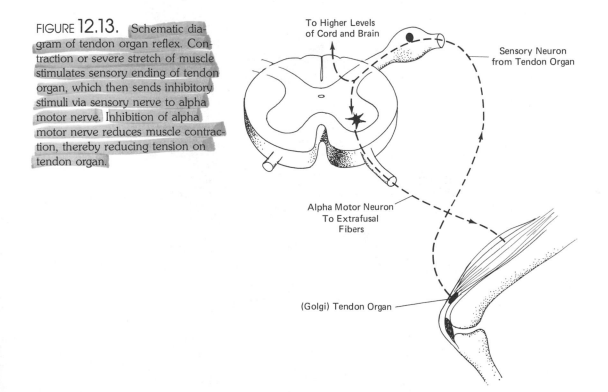

FIGURE 12.13. Schematic diagram of tendon organ reflex. Contraction or severe stretch of muscle stimulates sensory ending of tendon organ, which then sends inhibitory stimuli via sensory nerve to alpha motor nerve. Inhibition of alpha motor nerve reduces muscle contraction, thereby reducing tension on tendon organ.

To Higher Levels of Cord and Brain

Sensory Neuron from Tendon Organ

Alpha Motor Neuron To Extrafusal Fibers

(Golgi) Tendon Organ

ity as the force of muscle contraction increases. It may be that strength training also leads to a reduction of these inhibitory impulses.

Tendon organs (Golgi tendon organs) are located at the junctions of muscle and tendon (Fig. 12.8) and are sensitive mostly to contractile force, although extreme stretch of a muscle can also cause these receptors to fire. These tendon organs, consequently, report the level of muscle tension being exerted back to the spinal cord and the brain so that any necessary corrections in force can be made (Fig. 12.13). The tendon organ reflex is inhibitory: that is, greater amounts of tension in the muscle cause proportionate increases in inhibitory stimuli to flow from the tendon organ receptors to the alpha motor neurons so that even greater contraction tends to be inhibited.

Although some authorities see the tendon organ reflex as a safety mechanism that prevents separation of tendon from bone when a contraction becomes too strong, it probably serves primarily to feed back data about force levels in the muscle to the central nervous system [19]. Regardless of its primary function, its role in the expression of muscular strength is obviously an inhibitory one. Any involvement of this reflex in strength training must include an adaptation whereby the sensitivity of the organ to high levels of tension is reduced, or reaches a plateau. Such an involvement is highly

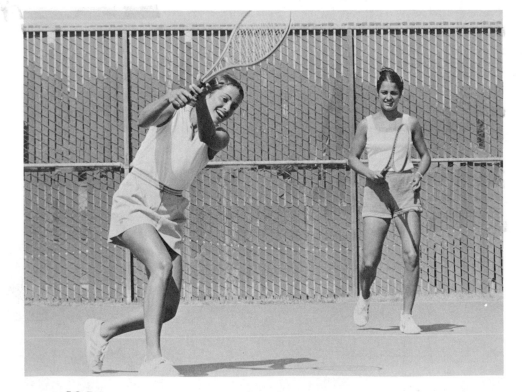

FIGURE 12.14.   For tennis and other sports activities, feedback from visual and vestibular areas of the brain and from spindles and tendon organs in the muscles is crucial to making appropriate adjustments in movement patterns and force generation. (Courtesy of Office of Public Information, Purdue University, West Lafayette, Indiana.)

speculative, and strength improvements may in fact proceed in spite of increased inhibition by tendon organ reflexes.

Can All Motor Units Be Activated During Maximal Effort?

There has long been controversy over the possibility of voluntary activation of all motor units during maximal exertion. Typically, investigators have compared force production during maximal voluntary efforts with force production during strong electrical shocks of the motor nerve that supplies the muscle being tested. It now appears that some muscles can be maximally activated during voluntary effort, whereas others cannot [5]. It is not clear why muscles differ in this respect, but it may be that those muscles which can be more fully activated voluntarily are stimulated by input from the brain to a greater extent. It is technically difficult to determine which muscle groups can be fully activated by voluntary commands, so we may never be certain about the extent of activation of muscles used in most sports skills.

There are suggestions in the research literature that physical training causes adaptations in the structure and function of the brain and spinal cord. Such adaptations could

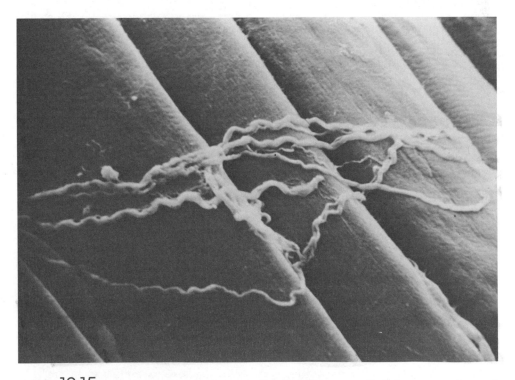

FIGURE 12.15. Stereo electron micrograph showing white nerve fibrils lying on surfaces of four muscle fibers. (Courtesy of R. E. Carrow, W. W. Heusner and W. D. Van Huss, Michigan State University, E. Lansing, Michigan.)

help explain how motor skills are learned and how more motor units may be activated after training [22, 30]. For example, physical activity at an early age causes significant changes in the structure of nerve cells of the cerebellum in mice [30], and the ability of human subjects to recruit more motor units simultaneously seems to increase with training [22].

Strength and Muscle Cross-Sectional Area

There is a nearly perfect relationship between the cross-sectional area of an isolated muscle from an animal and the maximal force that muscle can produce [24]. For each square centimeter of cross-sectional area, various muscles can produce about 10–20 newtons of measured force [36]. In the intact human being, this relationship between cross-sectional area and muscular strength is still very strong. However, increases in strength caused by training are often proportionately greater than increases in muscle size, so that the relationship between muscle size and strength is somewhat weaker in the whole organism than in the isolated muscle preparation. Nevertheless, the single best predictor of the strength of a person's muscles is the cross-sectional area of those muscles.

Cross-sectional area of muscles is, of course, only roughly estimated by measuring the circumference or girth of a limb. Girth measurements include not only muscle, but fat and bone as well. Also, they do not take into account differences in the spatial arrangements of muscle fibers, that is, whether the fibers run parallel or at angles to the long axis of the muscle. Consequently, limb girth is even less closely related to muscle strength than muscle cross-sectional area. Nevertheless, a significant linear relationship does exist between limb girth and strength.

From the physiological standpoint, why should bigger muscles generally be stronger? The answer seems to be that larger muscles have greater quantities of actin and myosin and, therefore, greater numbers of cross bridges that can be activated to produce muscular force during contraction. The only reason someone with relatively small muscles might possess greater strength than a larger person is that the smaller individual may be able to activate more motor units.

Strength and Muscle Fiber Types

Strength is related to cross-sectional area of muscle fibers, and fast twitch fibers produce greater force than slow twitch fibers. Therefore, it seems logical to predict that subjects with a greater cross-sectional area of fast twitch fibers should be able to generate more force with their muscles. Indeed, most studies do show such a relationship, although the relationship between fast twitch area and strength is quite modest [18, 26]. Thus, fast twitch fiber area is only one of many factors which determine strength. The relationship between strength and simple percentage distribution of fast twitch fibers is weaker than that between strength and fast twitch area [18, 26].

Strength and Angle of Muscle Pull on Bone

A second important factor in determining the measured strength of a muscle contraction in man is the angle at which the muscle must exert tension on the bone. For elbow flexion, as an illustration, more vertical force is transmitted to the lower part of the arm at about 115 degrees of flexion than at either greater or lesser angles (Fig. 12.16). Therefore, a muscle has its optimal strength (when measured in humans) at or near its optimal angle of pull on the bone where resistance is being applied. (Note that the angle of pull of the muscle on the bone is of major importance; the joint angle often, but not always, reflects this angle.) This fact should be remembered when reading the following paragraphs and when developing technique in a particular athletic skill. For example, at the start of a 100 meter dash, the best combination of hip, knee and ankle joint angles should be selected to provide the most explosive first stride away from the starting blocks. Studies of mechanical analysis and applied anatomy are helpful in developing such techniques.

Strength and Muscle Length

According to the sliding filament theory of muscle contraction there should be an optimal length of a muscle at which the greatest number of cross bridges can be activated to generate force. If a muscle was stretched too far, thin filaments would tend to be pulled away from thick filaments and cross bridge attachments, whereas if a muscle was shortened too much, it appears that thin filaments might interfere with each other in making cross bridges effective for contraction (Fig. 12.17) [36]. These concepts seem to be borne out in electron micrographs of stretched and shortened muscles.

The relationship between the length of a given muscle and the *active* force that muscle can produce is shown in Fig. 12.18. By "active" force we mean the force caused by the interaction of myosin and actin in the contractile process. If a muscle is stretched while it is contracting, there is also "passive" force produced. Such a stretch

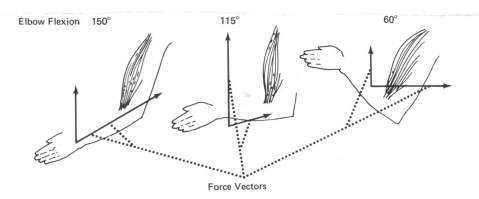

FIGURE 12.16. Effectiveness of angle of biceps pull on radius during elbow flexion at various elbow angles.

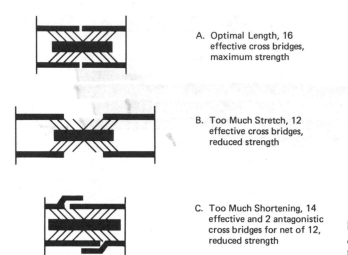

A. Optimal Length, 16
   effective cross bridges,
   maximum strength

B. Too Much Stretch, 12
   effective cross bridges,
   reduced strength

C. Too Much Shortening, 14
   effective and 2 antagonistic
   cross bridges for net of 12,
   reduced strength

FIGURE 12.17. Effect of muscle length on number of potentially active cross bridges.

would occur, for example, in the gastrocnemius and other plantar flexors during the foot strike while sprinting or hurdling. Passive force is caused by the resistance to stretch of connective tissue and other elastic elements of the muscle; it increases dramatically as muscle is stretched forcefully.

As can be seen in Fig. 12.18, muscles are generally their strongest at lengths slightly longer than their normal resting lengths in the fully extended position of the joint(s) they serve. The muscles are weaker at shorter and longer lengths than the optimum. Part of the explanation for the relationship between muscle length and force is that the optimal overlap between thick and thin filaments occurs at lengths just greater than maximal resting lengths [24, 36]. It has also been suggested that too much shortening of a muscle reduces muscle force by decreasing the calcium activation of cross bridges [31]. Also, when a muscle is stretched, the stretch reflex will contribute to the force of contraction by facilitating the alpha motor neurons of the stretched muscle [25, 32].

The principle that a muscle produces its greatest force at a length slightly longer than its maximal resting length is always true when a muscle is isolated from the rest of the body in the laboratory. However, in the living human being, this principle is valid

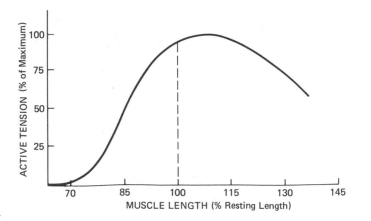

FIGURE 12.18. Relationship between muscle length and active tension.

only for certain muscles and movements because of the more dramatic effect of the angle of pull of muscle on bone. To illustrate the effectiveness of the principle that muscles produce their greatest force at greater lengths, it is necessary to select a muscle that, when stretched, will not be at an ineffective angle of pull. The gastrocnemius is such a muscle; it should contract somewhat more forcefully when the ankle is first dorsiflexed so that the gastrocnemius is stretched just beyond its normal resting length. Thus, a high jumper could expect to get a stronger plantar flexion on takeoff with a shoe that had a thick sole and a low heel that would place the plantar flexor muscles, including the gastrocnemius, on stretch. Alas, after such a shoe was used successfully by Soviet high jumpers in the early 1960's, it was banned from competition.

There are, however, other examples in athletics where muscles stretched just prior to contraction produce the greatest force. To achieve the greatest distance, the discus thrower must allow his outstretched throwing arm to follow his trunk as he spins around the throwing circle prior to the final release of the discus. Likewise, the weight-lifter stretches hip and knee extensors as he squats to raise a heavy barbell, and the canoeist stretches his elbow extensors prior to initiating a stroke of his paddle.

As was cautioned in the previous section, one must always consider the most effective angle of pull of a muscle before deciding whether or not a muscle should be stretched prior to contraction. Consider the biceps of the arm, for example. If the biceps were placed on stretch, the elbow would be extended maximally, and most of the contractile force of the biceps would be directed toward pulling the head of the radius toward the humerus at the elbow. As shown in Fig. 12.16, the elbow flexors give maximal force at about 115 degrees of elbow flexion, not at 180 degrees or more. Thus, one must consider many factors when developing techniques in athletics; initial muscle length and angle of muscle pull must be considered together as only two of those factors. In measuring isometric muscular strength one should always document the joint angle at which the measurement is taken.

FIGURE 12.19. Increasing force in the discus throw by stretching shoulder and arm muscles prior to contraction. (Courtesy of Office of Public Information, University of Toledo, Toledo, Ohio.)

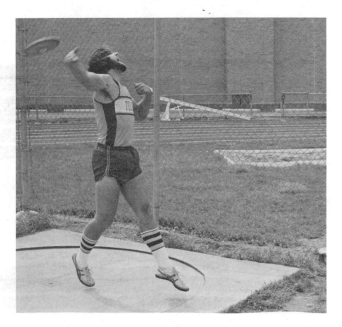

Strength and Pre-Exertion Countermovement (Windup)

In the previous section it was stated that placing the biceps muscle on stretch would not be effective in increasing strength because of the inefficient angle of attachment of the muscle to the bone when the elbow is extended. This is true when strength is measured isometrically, but if elbow flexion *through the complete range of motion* of the elbow joint is to be made, one can exert a greater force on a dynamometer or lift a heavier weight by first making and then braking a rapid countermovement (in this case, elbow extension) with a resistance such as the weight of the dumbbell to be lifted during the subsequent elbow flexion [1, 3]. This countermovement or windup causes the biceps to be stretched as it contracts eccentrically to brake the downward movement of the dumbbell. Thereafter an immediate high level of force is generated during the rapidly ensuing elbow flexion movement. A similar sort of positive effect of countermovement is sought whenever one winds up prior to throwing a javelin, baseball, football, or discus; when one winds up with a sledge hammer as he tries to ring the gong at a carnival; or when a woodsman winds up with his ax prior to chopping a tree. The apparent reason why a windup or countermovement aids the expression of strength is that by stretching the elastic muscle and connective tissue during the eccentric contraction phase, energy is stored in these tissues that is immediately released during the first part of the subsequent concentric contraction [3, 11]. This stored energy is somewhat similar to that observed when a rubber band is first stretched and then released. When measuring strength, precautions should be taken to either eliminate or standardize windup movements because there will be differences in subjects' skills in performing them.

Muscular Force and Speed of Contraction

It is common knowledge that greater muscular force is produced at slower movement speeds than at faster speeds, but the physiological explanation for this phenomenon is not entirely clear. The relationship between movement speed and the force that can be produced by contraction is shown in Fig. 12.20 [10, 29]. It seems that more time must be required to activate the extra cross bridges that are required to produce greater and greater force, but exactly why this should be is unknown [19].

Notice in Fig. 12.20 that at 100 per cent of maximum tension, the muscle is in a state of isometric contraction, that is, it cannot move the load. Therefore, maximum isometric strength at any joint angle is always greater than dynamic concentric strength at that angle. This does not seem to be the case for eccentric contractions, however. Maximum strength at a given joint angle is greater when the muscle is lengthening (as it attempts to overcome too great a load) than when it is concentrically or isometrically contracting [2]. The explanation for the greater strength of eccentric contractions is also not known, but is probably due in part to the lack of muscle force needed to overcome internal resistance of muscle and connective tissue during an eccentric con-

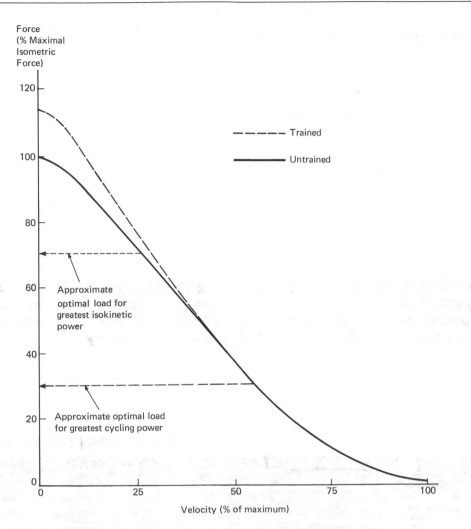

FIGURE 12.20. Relationship between force and speed of contraction.

traction. The "wasted" force that is used to overcome internal resistance during concentric and isometric contractions can be used to help overcome external resistance in eccentric contractions.

The relationship between load and speed of contraction suggests that there must be an optimal combination of speed and force required to provide the greatest possible muscular *power, which is defined as the product of force and speed,* that is, Power = Force × Speed or Force × Distance/Time. Power is particularly important in athletic events such as the shot put, discus throw, high jump, long jump, and pole vault. In the shot put and discus throw, muscular strength (force) can be improved to a much greater extent than speed. Since there is no evidence that increases in strength cause decreases in speed (in fact, speed of loaded movements such as a shot put will improve), the athlete simply applies maximum strength with all the speed that can be mustered. In the jumps and vaults, on the other hand, some optimal body weight will result in the greatest strength and speed combination. If the jumper loses too much

$$F \cdot \vec{V} = F \cdot \frac{s}{t}$$

weight, strength may be lost, but should the jumper get too heavy, extra strength will be of no value.

In an industrial situation an efficiency expert may determine that packages weighing about 30 per cent of one's maximal isometric strength will be optimal for the most rapid loading of a truck. Packages heavier or lighter than this would require too long a time to lift the same total weight of the product onto the truck. Of course, other factors such as fatigue and package bulk would have to be considered. It is known that humans produce maximum bicycling power when pedaling at about 30 per cent of leg extensor maximal strength (4). On the other hand, maximal power with isokinetic knee extensions occurs at about 67 per cent of maximal isometric strength [29].

Strength and Warmup

When an isolated muscle in the laboratory is cooled, its strength and speed of contraction and relaxation are reduced, whereas heat increases contractile strength and speed. Nerves also conduct impulses more rapidly, and connective tissues such as ligaments and tendons become more pliable with greater temperature. These enhanced functions are probably the result of greater enzyme activity and less resistance to change of length (lower "viscosity") in the heated tissues. If such effects of warming occur in man, then maximal strength should be somewhat improved by warmup of the muscle prior to exertion.

There are many types of warmup that different performers have tried in hopes of increasing strength [15]. These can be classified as *passive warmup, active general warmup,* and *active practice warmup*. Passive warmup includes massage and the local or general application of heat by means of infrared lamps, ultrasound, diathermy, steam baths, sauna baths, hot water baths, hot showers, and hot packs. Active general warmup is the use of physical activity such as running or calisthenics to raise body temperature, and active practice warmup is the practice of all or parts of a movement prior to measurement or competition in that same movement.

Most research on passive warmup has shown that it is not particularly helpful in the expression of muscular strength, perhaps because many of the warmup techniques were applied too briefly or without enough intensity to change deep muscle temperature [15]. As an example, several studies included the use of hot showers for only a few minutes, probably because of the discomfort of the subjects. Although a brief shower may warm the skin, this warmth is transmitted slowly to the muscles, and the important factor is that muscle temperature must be elevated. Similarly, when only a portion of the body such as an arm or leg is heated, the body very effectively rids itself of the extra heat load by evaporative heat loss through increased sweating, and by greater radiation of heat from the rest of the body surface, so that muscle temperature, even of the heated arm, is little changed; the blood cools the muscle faster than the environment heats it. Massage does not change muscle temperature, and it is therefore not surprising that massage does not affect muscle strength [15].

On the other hand, dynamic (but not isometric) strength is usually somewhat benefitted by active general warmup and active practice warmup [6, 15]. Running, stair stepping, and cycling for 5–30 minutes prior to strength or vertical jump measurements usually improve performance. Similarly, repeated trials with the shot, discus or javelin prior to competition improve performance by 5–50 per cent over the no-warmup condition. Active warmup appears to be most effective if practiced for 5 to 30 minutes and should usually precede testing or competition by no more than 15 minutes [15].

Some or most of the effectiveness of active practice warmup such as skill practice is thought to be due to an activation of the appropriate nerve pathways so that more motor units can be brought into play. One must also consider the likelihood that for some individuals the warm-up effect is partly psychological because most performers have been taught to believe in the value of warmup. Since there is no evidence that active warmup of a reasonable duration is detrimental to performance, such warmup routines should be recommended with a view toward not only an enhancement of strength performance, but also toward the possibility of preventing injury to "cold" muscles and joints. This last assumption on injury prevention is unsupported by experimental research, but it is warranted on the basis of the experiences of many athletes and coaches.

Strength, Age, and Sex

Prior to puberty, boys and girls are quite similar in strength. At puberty, however, males begin a much more rapid increase in absolute strength, presumably because of increased levels of testosterone, the male sex hormone. Testosterone promotes muscular hypertrophy. If strength is expressed on a relative basis—that is, per kilogram of body weight—the strength of leg muscles in females after puberty is similar to that in males, but arm and shoulder muscles are about half as strong [18, 27].

There is undoubtedly a cultural effect that also plays some role in determining sex differences in strength. Young girls in general have been taught that forceful physical exertion is unfeminine, and consequently, after puberty they usually shy away from activities that would have a training effect on strength. Therefore, comparisons in strength between males and females may be somewhat unfair, since males are likely to be in a more "trained" state than females. In this light, it is interesting that leg muscle strength is very similar in girls and boys. Perhaps the explanation for this is that young boys and girls tend to have similar amounts of training of these leg muscles because they do similar amounts of walking and running. For muscles of the arms and shoulders, though, boys usually have more training from rope climbing, wrestling, throwing, and other "masculine" activities.

Figs. 12.21 and 12.22 show the relationship between age and absolute or relative knee extension strength in males [26]. The changes in strength with age are probably caused not only by changes in muscle mass with growth (in youth) and atrophy (in older persons), but also by changes in the central nervous system [26]. This role of the nervous system becomes apparent when one considers that increases in strength with age are greater than the corresponding increases in muscle mass. Therefore, it appears that the maturation of the nervous system in young persons allows the simultaneous

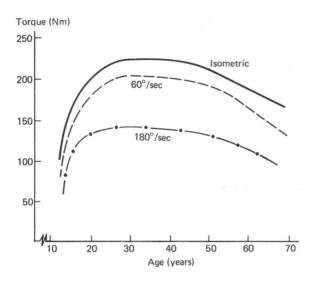

FIGURE 12.21. Approximate relationship between age and strength in males. Curves shown are for isometric strength and for isokinetic strength at 60°/sec. and 180°/sec. Strength is expressed in Newton meters (Nm). (Modified from reference 27.)

recruitment of more motor units; this phenomenon may be reversed with advancing age.

Variation in Strength within Sexes and Age Groups

Although a definite effect of age and sex on muscular strength can be shown if large numbers of subjects are tested, one must not expect every 10-year-old to be stronger than every 8-year-old, or every 15-year-old girl to be weaker than every 15-year-old boy. There is a wide range of strength at a given age or in a given sex. One of the reasons for strength differences within an age group, especially before age 18, is that children mature at different rates, so that it is possible to find two 12-year-olds whose biological or maturation age as determined by x-ray measurements of bones are 10 and 15, respectively [1]. The 12-year-old who has not matured as rapidly will probably have smaller muscles, a less highly developed nervous system, and, if males are

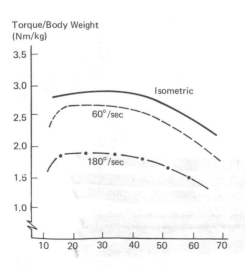

FIGURE 12.22. Approximate relationship between age and strength per kilogram of body weight in males. Curves shown are for isometric strength and for isokinetic strength at 60°/sec. and 180°/sec. Strength is expressed in Newton meters/kilogram of body weight (Nm/kg). (Modified from reference 27).

compared, a lower secretion of male sex hormones. All of these factors will tend to make the less mature person less strong than his more mature counterpart. In the physical education class, therefore, instructors should compare strength performances of children classified according to height or some other estimate of biological age rather than according to chronological age. In like manner, a small, immature boy should not be expected to be stronger than larger girls his same age. The physical educator who recognizes the impact of age, sex, maturity, and muscle size on strength is better prepared to help reduce potentially harmful peer pressures among children who, in the case of boys, think that weaker classmates are "sissies" or, in the case of girls, think that stronger classmates are "Amazons."

REVIEW QUESTIONS

1. Define the following terms: maximal strength, isotonic contraction, isometric contraction, isokinetic contraction, motor unit, tetanic contraction.
2. Explain how the nervous system governs the amount of force generated by skeletal muscles so that the same muscles are capable of smoothly lifting both a piece of paper and a heavy tire. Include in your explanation a discussion of asynchronous twitches of muscle fibers from different motor units.
3. Describe how excitatory and inhibitory stimuli from the central nervous system, and from peripheral receptors, modify the output of the lower motor neurons and thereby modify the contractions of muscles.
4. Diagram and describe the stretch reflex.
5. Define: intrafusal fibers, extrafusal fibers, primary and secondary endings of muscle spindles, the gamma motor system, and alpha motor neuron.
6. Explain how muscle spindles can remain sensitive to stretch of a muscle while the muscle is undergoing changes in length.
7. What is the function of the Golgi tendon organs?
8. Describe and explain the relationships between muscle strength and the following: cross-sectional area of the muscle, angle of muscle pull on bone, muscle length, windup, speed of contraction, warmup, age, and sex.

REFERENCES

[1] Asmussen, E. Growth in muscular strength and power. In G. L. Rarick, ed., *Physical Activity: Human Growth and Development.* New York: Academic Press, Inc., 1973, pp. 60–79.
[2] Asmussen, E. The neuromuscular system and exercise. In H. B. Falls, ed., *Exercise Physiology.* New York: Academic Press, Inc., 1968, pp. 3–42.
[3] Asmussen, E., and F. Bonde-Petersen. Storage of elastic energy in skeletal muscles in man. *Acta Physiologica Scandinavica,* 1974, **91:**385–392.
[4] Åstrand, P.-O, and K. Rodahl. Textbook of Work Physiology, 2nd ed. New York: McGraw-Hill Book Company, 1977.
[5] Belanger, A. Y., and A. J. McComas. Extent of motor unit activation during effort. *Journal of Applied Physiology,* 1981, **51:**1131–1135.
[6] Bergh, U., and B. Ekblom. Influence of muscle temperature on maximal muscle strength and power output in human muscles. *Acta Physiologica Scandinavica,* 1979, **107:**33–37.
[7] Burke, D. Muscle spindle function during movement. *Trends in NeuroSciences,* 1980, **3:**251–253.
[8] Burke, D., and G. Eklund. Muscle spindle activity in man during standing. *Acta Physiologica Scandinavica,* 1977, **100:**187–199.

[9] Burke, R. E., and V. R. Edgerton. Motor unit properties and selective involvement in movement. *Exercise and Sport Sciences Reviews,* 1975, **3:**31–81.

[10] Caiozzo, V. J., J. J. Perrine, and V. R. Edgerton. Training-induced alterations of the in vivo force-velocity relationship of human muscle. *Journal of Applied Physiology,* 1981, **51:**750–754.

[11] Cavagna, G. A. Storage and utilization of elastic energy in skeletal muscle. *Exercise and Sport Sciences Reviews,* 1977, **5:**89–129.

[12] Coyle, E. F., D. C. Feiring, R. C. Rotkis, R. W. Cote III, F. B. Roby, W. Lee, and J. H. Wilmore. Specificity of power improvements through slow and fast isokinetic training. *Journal of Applied Physiology,* 1981, **51:**1437–1442.

[13] Desmedt, J. E., E. Godaux. Spinal motoneuron recruitment in man: rank deordering with direction but not with speed of voluntary movement. *Science,* 1981, **214:**933–936.

[14] Evarts, E. V. Brain mechanisms of movement. *Scientific American,* 1979, **241:**164–179.

[15] Franks, B. E. Physical warm-up. In W. P. Morgan, ed., *Ergogenic Aids and Muscular Performance.* New York: Academic Press, Inc., 1972, pp. 159–191.

[16] Gallego, R., M. Kuno, R. Nunez, and W. D. Snider. Dependence of motoneurone properties on the length of immobilized muscle. *Journal of Physiology,* 1979, **291:**179–189.

[17] Granit, R. Linkage of alpha and gamma motoneurones in voluntary movement. *Nature New Biology,* 1973, **243:**52–53.

[18] Gregor, R. J., V. R. Edgerton, J. J. Perrine, D. S. Campion, and C. Debus. Torque-velocity relationships and muscle fiber composition in elite female athletes. *Journal of Applied Physiology,* 1979, **47:**388–392.

[19] Henneman, E. Peripheral mechanisms involved in the control of muscle. In V. B. Mountcastle, ed., *Medical Physiology,* 13th ed. St. Louis: The C. V. Mosby Co., 1974, pp. 617–635.

[20] Hettinger, T. *Physiology of Strength.* Springfield, Ill.: Charles C Thomas, Publisher, 1961.

[21] Hoffer, J. A., M. J. O'Donovan, C. A. Pratt, and G. E. Loeb. Discharge patterns of hindlimb motoneurons during normal cat locomotion. *Science,* 1981, **213:**466–468.

[22] Hutton, R. S. Central and peripheral neural adaptations with use-disuse. In B. Wolman, ed., *International Encyclopedia of Psychiatry, Psychology, Psychoanalysis and Neurology.* New York: Aesculapius Publishers, Inc. (In press).

[23] Ikai, M., and A. H. Steinhaus. Some factors modifying the expression of human strength. *Journal of Applied Physiology,* 1961, **16:**157–163.

[24] Josephson, R. K. Extensive and intensive factors determining the performance of striated muscle. *Journal of Experimental Zoology,* 1975, **194:**135–154.

[25] Kamen, G. Serial isometric contractions under imposed myotatic stretch conditions in high-strength and low-strength men. *European Journal of Applied Physiology,* **41:**73–82.

[26] Larsson, L., G. Grimby, and J. Karlsson. Muscle strength and speed of movement in relation to age and muscle morphology. *Journal of Applied Physiology,* 1979, **46:**451–456.

[27] Malina, R. M. Adolescent changes in size, build, composition and performance. *Human Biology,* 1974, **46:**117–131.

[28] McGeer, P. L., and E. G. McGeer. The control of movement by the brain. *Trends in NeuroSciences,* 1980, **3:**III–IV.

[29] Perrine, J. J., and V. R. Edgerton. Muscle force-velocity relationships under isokinetic loading. *Medicine and Science in Sports and Exercise,* 1978, **10:**159–166.

[30] Pysh, J. J., and G. M. Weiss. Exercise during development induces an increase in Purkinje cell dendritic tree size. *Science,* 1979, **206:**230–232.

[31] Ridgeway, E. B., and A. M. Gordon. Muscle activation: effects of small length changes on calcium release in single fibers. *Science,* 1975, **189:**881–884.

[32] Smith, J. L. Fusimotor loop properties and involvement during voluntary movement. *Exercise and Sport Sciences Reviews,* 1976, **4:**297–333.

[33] Stein, R. B., and E. Parmiggiani. Optimal motor patterns for activating mammalian muscle. *Brain Research,* 1975, **175:**372–376.

[34] Taub, E. Movement in nonhuman primates deprived of somatosensory feedback. *Exercise and Sport Sciences Reviews,* 1976, **4:**335–374.

[35] Tracey, D. J. Joint receptors and the control of movement. *Trends in NeuroSciences,* 1980, **3:**253–255.

[36] Zierler, K. L. Mechanism of muscle contraction and its energetics. In V. B. Mountcastle, ed., *Medical Physiology,* 13th ed. St. Louis: The C. V. Mosby Company, 1974, pp. 77–120.

CHAPTER
13

Training for Improved Muscular Strength

ANYONE who has read popular magazines on strength fitness or has visited a weight training room in a school or in a commercial health salon knows that every weight training devotee has unique ideas about the best ways to gain strength. These ideas include strange dietary concoctions, synthetic hormone shots, special breathing routines, and gorilla-like shouts during a lift. Since gains in strength can be brought about by "psychological/emotional" techniques [25, 36], it is likely that any technique that the trainee firmly believes in will have some beneficial effect on strength. However, if one analyzes the research on principles for strength training and on various training methods, it becomes apparent that for most individuals certain principles and techniques lead to greater gains in strength than others. These research-based principles and techniques are described in this chapter and should serve as the basis of strength training programs.

General Principles of Strength Training

Regardless of whether one trains by isometric, isotonic, or isokinetic methods, there are four general principles that should be followed to insure that the greatest possible training adaptation and strength gains will occur. These principles are discussed in the following paragraphs.

Principle 1: The training program should provide a progressive heavy overload of the specific muscle groups that are to be strengthened [9]. The determination of the specific muscle groups that are to be strengthened can be made in either a simple or a sophisticated manner. Simply, one needs only to perform slowly a movement one

272

wishes to strengthen and to squeeze or palpate muscles on each side of the joint(s) involved until one finds those muscle groups that become tense and hard to the touch during the movement. The muscles that become tense are the muscles that are responsible for the movement, and these muscles must be trained with heavy resistance if the movement is to be strengthened. For example, if one wishes to improve vertical jumping ability, one must overload primarily the hip and knee extensors and ankle plantar flexors that become tense and cause the jumping movement. To train these muscles one need only to perform movements of the joints that mimic the joint movements during jumping and to overload those movements with isometric, isotonic or isokinetic resistance. Such activities would include overloaded squats and toe raises. With this simple system of determining the specific muscle groups to be overloaded, one need not know the names of muscles or the names of strength-training exercises; one need only find out by trial and error which muscles become tense during a movement that is to be strengthened and then, again somewhat by trial and error, one must decide how to perform similar movements against heavy resistance.

A more sophisticated approach to the determination of muscle groups that should be overloaded would include the use of mechanical analysis of the movement with cinematography, the use of electromyography, and the application of knowledge gained from a study of applied anatomy. Such sophisticated procedures are beyond the scope of this text, but they are usually described in applied anatomy, kinesiology, and biomechanics books. *When in doubt one must remember that one should overload movements that are as similar as possible to those movements that are to be strengthened.*

Once the muscles to be strengthened have been determined and appropriate resistive exercises, either isometric, isotonic, or isokinetic, have been selected, one must perform those exercises with maximal or near maximal resistance to bring forth the greatest strength increments. The muscles will adapt only to the load placed upon them; a minimal overload will bring about a minimal strength gain, whereas a maximal overload will bring about a maximal strength gain. To gain the greatest strength one must exercise with few repetitions and heavy resistance.

Not only must heavy loads be placed on the muscles at the start of a strength-training program, but the loads must be progressively increased to keep pace with newly won increments in strength. Thus, heavy resistance is relative to the capacity of the muscle and must increase as the muscle improves its capacity.

Principle 2: Make the training as interesting as possible. One of the chief problems of all physical fitness training programs is simply to maintain the enthusiasm of the trainee so that he or she does not drop out of the program. A poorly designed strength-training program can be unrelentingly boring. No matter how great a program is in theory, it is useless if no one can stick to it. The maintenance of interest is particularly important in physical training programs for children of elementary school age who have a difficult time understanding the need for fitness programs. If those programs can be disguised as gamelike activities, young children will enjoy becoming fit without having to appreciate fitness intellectually. With older persons, it is important to vary the training routines by rotating the use of isometric, isotonic, and isokinetic programs and by varying to some extent the progression of the prescribed exercises.

Principle 3: Exercise large muscle groups before smaller ones. As muscles become fatigued, further training during that period becomes less and less effective and eventually impossible. Most movements become fatiguing as smaller muscle groups involved in those movements are fatigued. Therefore, it is important to exercise the larger muscles involved in the movement first so that the capacities of those muscles can be overloaded before the smaller muscles become fatigued. For example, if one wished to improve his ability to lift a heavy barbell from the floor to a position overhead with elbows extended, he should exercise large leg muscles early in his routines and the smaller elbow extensors later.

Principle 4: Allow adequate recovery of the muscles between individual exercises and between exercise periods. This principle is related to the previous one because underlying it is the idea that strenuous overload of muscles is difficult to achieve when the muscles are tired, sore, or generally have not recovered from previous activity. According to this principle, it is important to arrange a strength-training routine so that successive exercises only minimally involve the same muscle groups. For example, it would not make sense to follow pushups with dips on the parallel bars because both these activities overload the elbow extensors, and relatively few dips could be done immediately after the pushups. A better idea would be to follow the pushups with weighted situps and then perhaps squats before performing the dips. In this way abdominal and thigh muscles would be exercised before returning to the elbow extensors.

This principle also suggests that there is some minimal time period that should intervene between training sessions. Studies have shown that it sometimes takes many hours before muscles respond to exhaustive exercise by increasing their energy reserves and their protein contents to greater than pre-exercise values. It is only logical that the greatest training adaptation should occur when the muscle is best prepared to tolerate the greatest overload, that is, when it has almost fully recovered from a previous training session. From a practical standpoint, most weight trainers find that isotonic workouts about three times per week allow the greatest training adaptation with the least soreness.

Isometric Training: General Principles

Systematic research on different methods of improving muscular strength with isometric exercise routines received its greatest impetus in the 1950's with the publication of numerous studies in Germany. Isometric exercise programs were hailed as the "quick and easy" way to enhanced muscular strength because these studies had effectively demonstrated that very little time was needed to develop substantial levels of strength. Later experience and further research soon showed that isometric strength training was not without its drawbacks, however. Some of these drawbacks will be discussed in later paragraphs, but let us now consider the basic principles of isometric training that most authorities agree will maximize the value of this particular training method [9, 22].

Isometric training should be practiced at several different joint angles because the training effect tends to occur mostly at the angle selected for training [15]. If elbow flexion is overloaded at 90 degrees, for example, most of the strength gain will occur at that angle with little or no improvement at angles other than 90 degrees. If a recognized "weak spot" in a particular movement needs specific training, isometric exercise at that angle of the joint(s) involved in the movement may be in order. Otherwise, angles throughout the range of motion of the joint(s) should be selected for training. It often makes sense to concentrate on angles at the extremes of the joint range of motion because the extreme portions of the range of motion are usually the weakest and, therefore, the limiting phases of the movement.

Each contraction should be a maximal voluntary contraction. Although several studies indicate that maximal strength gains can occur with contractions of about 50 per cent of maximum, it is usually not feasible to measure the strength of each contraction to make certain that 50 per cent of maximal force is being applied. Also, since some do not respond to this lower level of exertion, a maximal effort should insure that all trainees get a training benefit [22]. Finally, by always applying a maximum effort as strength improves, a progressive increase in the training stimulus is assured.

Each maximal contraction should be held for 2–5 seconds. The maximal contraction does not usually fatigue a person until after about 10 seconds, but research has shown that holding the contraction longer than 2–5 seconds does not increase the training effect [22]. Since fatigue is usually associated with pain and soreness, there seems to be no good reason to hold the contraction for longer than a few seconds.

The isometric contractions should be repeated one to five times during each training session. The training sessions should be held daily unless unusual soreness occurs. Muscles should be allowed 2–3 minutes recovery between maximal efforts. During this recovery period, other muscles can be trained. Because isometric training sessions are usually of brief duration, there is less depletion of energy stores, and usually less soreness than with isotonic or isokinetic exercise. Consequently, the muscles seem to need less time to recover from previous exercise than with other training methods. Training three or four times per week will eventually lead to the same strength gains as the daily routines, but progress will be slower [22].

Strength gains achieved with isometric training can be maintained with the normal training session conducted once per week. All categories of physical fitness improvements are more difficult to achieve than to maintain; strength improvements are no exception. Maintenance training once per week is a somewhat conservative suggestion since some authorities have found that a single maximal contraction held for 2 seconds once every 2 weeks is sufficient to maintain strength gains [22]. Once again, it seems prudent to provide a somewhat greater than minimal maintenance program to insure that all trainees respond maximally. Without maintenance programs, improved isometric strength regresses toward starting strength levels. Although perhaps 40 per cent of strength gains may be lost in a month or two without a strength maintenance program, some of the strength gain—up to 40 per cent in some studies—seems to be retained for a year or more [9, 22].

Isometric contractions produce extreme rises in blood pressure if held more than a second or two and should be avoided by those afflicted with cardiovascular disease. Although there is a paucity of evidence that patients have actually suffered physical harm with isometrics, the potential for such harm certainly exists, and the prudent course of action is to prohibit cardiac patients from using isometrics until it is demonstrated that isometric exercise is not harmful to those with atherosclerosis, high blood pressure, and other cardiovascular diseases [35].

As with other training programs, isometric training should be made as interesting as possible by varying the routines. Also, large muscle groups should be exercised before smaller ones to minimize early fatigue of the small muscles.

Isotonic Training: General Principles

Isotonic weight training programs have stood the test of time not only in the training of most champion weightlifters, but also in the rehabilitation of muscles grown weak by immobilization in plaster casts or by neuromuscular disease. Any overload of the muscles beyond their normal daily activities will improve muscular strength, but systematic experimentation has shown that certain general principles of isotonic training should be followed if the greatest gains possible with this method are to be achieved.

During each training session, three or four sets of each exercise should be performed with the heaviest weight that can be correctly lifted one to six times during each set. Another way to express this degree of overload is in terms of *repetitions maximum* (R.M.). One R.M. is the maximum weight that can be lifted correctly one time, 2 R.M. is the maximum weight that can be lifted twice, and so forth. Obviously, the greater the number of R.M., the lighter is the weight that can be lifted. Research suggests that a few repetitions with near maximal weights produce the greatest strength gains [9]. The stated principle of three or four sets of 1–6 R.M. is broad enough to

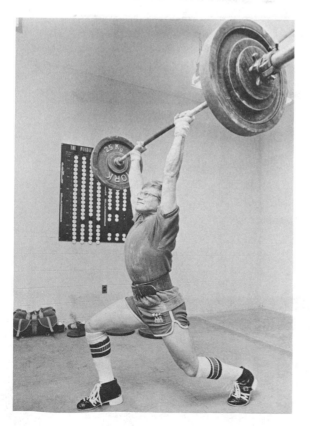

FIGURE 13.1. Isotonic training with the aid of a barbell. (Courtesy of Office of Public Information, Purdue University, West Lafayette, Indiana.)

satisfy the recommendations of most well-conducted research studies. As training goes beyond the level of 6 R.M., it becomes progressively less effective for training muscular strength and better for improving anaerobic muscular endurance.

A person who just begins a weight training program is wise to use a load equivalent to about 12 R.M. for three sets rather than 1–6 R.M. This will minimize the risk of injury from tissue strains and will give time to build up the neuromuscular coordination required to handle heavier weights in exercises which may be novel to the trainee. The initial 12 R.M. load should be progressively increased to 8 R.M. during the first few weeks of training. After a month or so, the 1–6 R.M. protocol can be safely followed.

The determination of how much weight can be correctly lifted through a range of motion for a given number of repetitions is made on a trial-and-error basis. To provide for a progressive increase in the overload to the muscle, the determination of 1–6 R.M. should be made about once every two weeks of training. It is important to perform the exercises correctly, without excessive jerking or the use of extra muscle groups. When a trainee lifts improperly as a result of attempting to lift too much, he is in danger of injuring himself.

2. During an isotonic training session, allow about 5–10 minutes for recovery between sets of the same exercise. Training sessions should be held three or four times per week [9]. Heavy isotonic training can be extremely fatiguing and may result in a great deal of soreness if adequate recovery time between exercise sets and between training sessions is not allowed. Because isotonic workouts are usually longer than isometric sessions, greater depletion of energy reserves and greater production of lactic acid occurs. Accordingly, somewhat longer recovery periods are needed after isotonic exercise. Depending upon one's training goals, isotonic training sessions normally last 1–2 hours, whereas isometric routines are often completed in 30 minutes or less.

3. Exercise large muscle groups first. Most weight lifting exercises are primarily designed to overload large muscle groups and only secondarily to overload smaller, supporting muscles. If the small muscle groups are fatigued early, it may be impossible to adequately overload the large muscles. The bench press, for example, is primarily used to strengthen muscles of the chest and upper arms, but one must be able to grip the barbell adequately with the hands while performing the movement. If the hands are fatigued by previous dumbbell curls or wrist exercises, they may be unable to support adequate weight on the barbell for optimal loads in the bench press. Consequently, exercises such as the bench press, the inclined press, or the full- or half-squat should be performed prior to dumbbell curls, wrist and forearm exercises, or toe raises so that fatigue of relatively small muscle groups does not interfere with adequate stress on the large muscles [38]. Presses and squats stress larger muscle groups than the other exercises.

4. Strengthening of muscles responsible for a complex movement should be accomplished with exercises designed to incorporate or mimic that movement. Because complex movements such as a baseball throw or a dolphin kick in swimming are acutely dependent upon the nervous system for accuracy, weight training for such movements should simulate as closely as possible the actual movements. This can usually be accomplished fairly satisfactorily with the help of weighted baseballs and bats, and with weights suspended from pulleys anchored to walls, ceilings and floors.

5. Maintain isotonic strength with two normal workouts per week. With fewer than

two workouts per week most trainees find that strength gains are lost after a few months. Two training sessions per week, on the other hand, are usually adequate to maintain, but not to increase, strength gained during prior training [9].

Eccentric versus Concentric Contractions. There seems to be no particular advantage to exercising with eccentric rather than concentric contractions during isotonic training [27]. Although eccentric routines subjectively seem easier to accomplish, this benefit may be offset by the greater soreness usually reported with eccentric contractions.

Isokinetic Training: General Principles

Isokinetic strength training programs combine the features of both isometric and isotonic programs in the sense that isokinetic training should be done with maximal exertions (as in isometric training) throughout a complete range of motion (as in isotonic training). In the absence of comprehensive research, the following principles for isokinetic training are recommended:

For the improvement of strength 30–75 maximal isokinetic contractions should be performed at speeds of 60–300 degrees per second during four or five training sessions per week. (More contractions can be performed at the faster speeds.) For the improvement of strength in a complex rapid movement, each maximal contraction should be completed at a speed as similar as possible to that achieved in the normal unloaded movement.

The contractions should be performed in sets of five to ten with five to ten minutes of recovery between sets. The longer recovery periods should follow the slower contractions.

Brief movements in throwing, kicking, and striking activities may be faster than 5,000 degrees per second. When muscles are trained isokinetically at speeds ranging from 60 to 300 degrees per second, improvements in maximal force tend to be quite specific. That is, if one trains at higher velocities, improvements in strength are greatest at high velocities, whereas training at slower velocities usually produces the greatest strength increments at the slower velocities [7, 10]. It has been suggested that strength improvements at slower velocities are primarily due to neural adaptations [7, 10], whereas improvements after high velocity training may also be a function of hypertrophy of fast twitch fibers [10].

Adequate maintenance of isokinetic strength gains can probably be achieved with one or two normal training sessions per week. This recommendation is a compromise between the suggested maintenance programs for isometric and isotonic strength.

Choice of Training Methods

As is perhaps obvious by now, each method of strength training has its advantages and drawbacks. It should be emphasized that *any method of training that overloads the muscles will result in strength gains.* It is extremely important that the trainee use a method in which he or she has confidence and which will maintain the trainee's interest for the months required to develop substantial strength. Rigorous adherence to a particular type of program is probably far more important than the type of program selected.

Isometric

There are several advantages often ascribed to isometric training. It takes little time, requires no expensive equipment, can be performed anywhere, usually causes little soreness, and is easy to maintain. Disadvantages of this technique are that 1) strength is not developed well throughout the range of motion unless so many angles within the range are strengthened that the time advantage is lost, 2) training of the nervous system in a movement does not occur, 3) progress is difficult to assess without a tensiometer or dynamometer so that the training becomes boring, 4) isometric contractions produce high systolic and diastolic blood pressure, and 5) isotonic or isokinetic methods generally seem to produce greater strength gains than isometric training [9]. Isometric training is generally not very popular with serious devotees of strength. However, it does have some merit in rehabilitation programs, particularly in situations where plaster casts, injuries, or disease prevent use of a limb through a full range of motion.

Isotonic

Isotonic training is the most common method of strength training used by specialists in the strength business—weightlifters. Isotonic training builds strength throughout a range of motion and provides some training of the nervous system as well as the muscles. Progress is easy to follow as more weight is added with newly gained strength, so isotonic training tends to be less boring than isometric training. This type of training can be adapted to many different kinds of athletic movements with the aid of weighted implements (balls, disci, shots, and so on) and pulleys. However, isotonic training can be relatively expensive, depending on the sophistication of equipment desired. It also often results in soreness and injury due to the possibility of selecting a weight that is too heavy for the lifter's capacity. If this weight cannot be handled in a weak part of the range of motion, the lifter must either risk muscle injury by excessive straining or risk injury from a falling barbell. Isotonic training takes 1–2 hours per session, and it becomes frustrating to continually have to change weights on barbells and dumbbells for different exercises unless several bars and extra weight discs are purchased. Finally, most of the strength gained in isotonic training occurs at the weakest points of the range of motion so that the entire range is not maximally trained.

Isokinetic

Isokinetic training is a relatively new system and has not been as thoroughly tested as the other techniques. It does seem to provide a good combination of the attributes of both isometric and isotonic training with few of their disadvantages. Isokinetic training provides maximal resistance to the muscles at all points in the range of motion, requires less time than isotonic programs, can be performed at different speeds, and is said to cause less injury and soreness than isotonic training [16, 38]. A few "isokinetic" devices are similar in cost to a good set of barbells and dumbbells and offer the advantage that no changes of weights or turning of knobs is required to switch from one exercise to another or from one trainee to another; the same device can be used to train the little finger or the powerful leg muscles. Isokinetic devices that provide a force readout or recorder can be used to provide motivation and to assess whether or not the trainee is giving the effort required for best results.

Most of the isokinetic training equipment, however, tends to be very expensive and more suitable for a physical rehabilitation ward in a hospital than for the high school gymnasium or for the home. Also, some believe that a scale reading on an isokinetic training device does not provide as good a motivation as the weight added to a barbell as strength improves.

One factor that should not be overlooked when comparing strength training methods is the procedure used to evaluate strength. If isometric contractions are used to test strength, isometric training is likely to provide the best training stimulus. Isotonic training should provide the best results when strength is tested isotonically, because isotonic training provides heavy overload to the weakest point in the range of motion of the tested movement. Likewise, it seems logical that isokinetic training would be the best method to use if isokinetic evaluation were employed, because only isokinetic training can provide maximal resistance through the entire range of motion [16].

A summary of the relative advantages of isokinetic, isotonic, and isometric training is shown in Table 13.1.

TABLE 13.1

Summary of Advantages of Isokinetic, Isotonic, and Isometric Training Methods. A Rating of 1 Is Superior; 2, Intermediate; and 3, Inferior

	Type of Training		
Criterion	**Isokinetic**	**Isotonic**	**Isometric**
Rate of Strength Gain	1	1	2
Strength Gain Throughout Range of Motion	Excellent	Good	Poor
Time per Training Session	2	3	1
Expense	3	2	1
Ease of Performance	2	3	1
Ease of Progress Assessment	Expensive Equipment Required	Excellent	Dynamometer Required
Adaptability to Specific Movement	1	2	3
Probability of Soreness	Little Soreness	Much Soreness	Little Soreness
Probability of Musculo-skeletal Injury	Slight	Moderate	Slight
Cardiac Risk	Some	Slight	Moderate
Skill Improvement	Some	Some	None

Strength Trainability: Effects of Age, Sex, and Previous Training

The extent to which training will produce improvements in strength depends on how much the cross-sectional area of the muscles can be increased and how much improvement can be made in the ability of the body to activate more motor units through changes in the nervous system. These two factors are in turn influenced by the age, sex, and previous training experience of the trainee.

Muscle Cross-sectional Area and Trainability

It is known that large muscles ordinarily have a greater ability to increase their size and *absolute* strength than smaller muscles [22, 43]. As an illustration, one may perhaps gain 100 kilograms (220 pounds) in strength of the large leg muscles, but only 4 kilograms (8.8 pounds) in forearm strength. Consequently, persons younger than about 20 years of age and older than 35 tend to increase their absolute strength less than those in the 20–35 age bracket because the muscle mass is smaller in the earlier and later years. Males at puberty have a relatively great strength trainability because of a rapid increase of muscle mass associated with high levels of male sex hormone (Fig. 13.2). On the other extreme, males 60 years of age and older may not exhibit any noticeable hypertrophy after strength training [37].

The *percentage* of strength increase in a muscle relative to pretraining values is not necessarily less for smaller muscles. In other words, a forearm muscle may improve its relative strength by 7 per cent, the same as a large thigh muscle, even though the absolute strength of the thigh muscle improves by many more kilograms [38]. This is

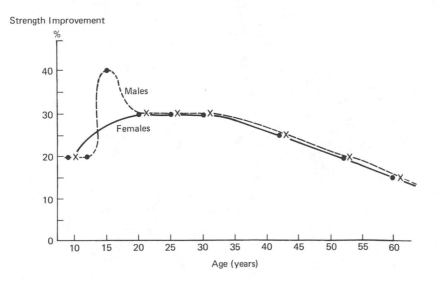

FIGURE 13.2. Hypothetical adaptations of males and females to 10 weeks of strength training. Note the effect of pubertal changes in both males and females.

demonstrated in part by the fact that untrained college-age females, who generally have smaller muscles than males, may increase their strength by roughly the same *percentage* (but somewhat less in *absolute* units) as untrained males after a 10-week training program [43]. It is clear that females who train for power lifting competition can lift at least as great a proportion of their body weights in the various lifts as can males. Therefore, it appears that females are not different from males in the trainability of their muscles for strength performance; they usually start at lower absolute levels and may improve less on an absolute basis, but the percentage gains are similar for both sexes.

Most females do not exhibit as great a degree of muscle hypertrophy after weight training as do males. This lesser hypertrophic effect compared to most males is probably related to lower levels of testosterone in females. Nevertheless, female body builders can show excellent definition of muscles, partly by decreasing the amount of subcutaneous fat tissue that normally obscures the muscles (Figs. 13.3, 13.4).

There obviously is a plateau for increases in muscle size as an adaptation to strength training; muscles do not continue to enlarge indefinitely. Therefore, the rate of strength gain will also be reduced as training progresses. If the first 10 weeks brings about a 25 per cent increase in strength, the next 10 weeks may add only another 5 per cent. If a person has been regularly engaged in a previous serious strength training program, improvements in that person's strength should not be expected to be as great as those in an untrained person.

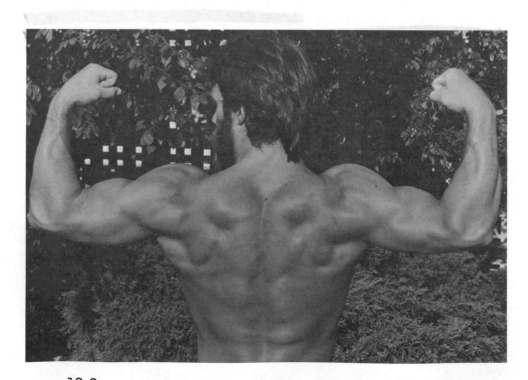

FIGURE 13.3. Muscle hypertrophy exhibited by a male body builder. Note especially the definition of the deltoid muscles of the shoulders. (Photo by Dean F. Connors.)

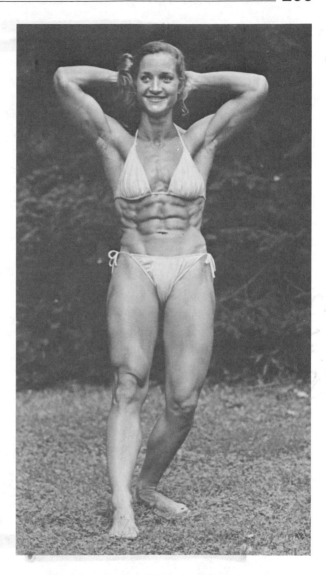

FIGURE 13.4. Muscle hypertrophy exhibited by a female body builder. Note that the extreme definition of the abdominal musculature is made possible by the relatively slight subcutaneous fat layer. (Photo by Kathy Tuite.)

Nervous System Adaptability and Strength Training

Children do not adapt to strength training as well as young adults. In addition to their smaller muscle mass, children do not have the mature nervous systems apparently required to bring about great improvements in strength through greater recruitment of motor units. This phenomenon may also apply to elderly persons, whose nervous systems begin to show the effects of the aging process. However, it is clear that elderly persons can make small but significant strength gains with training, mostly by virtue of nervous system adaptations [37].

As with muscle size improvements, increases in motor unit recruitment by nervous system adaptations are progressively more difficult to achieve as training progresses. However, it seems likely that continued improvement in strength with long term training is more a function of better motor unit recruitment than it is a function of increased muscle mass. This conclusion is based on the fact that increases in muscle mass are far less than improvements in strength, especially during the first 2–3 weeks [37] and after the first few months of training.

There are no apparent sex-related differences in the ability to cause adaptations in motor unit recruitment ability. If anything, the observation that females gain strength to about the same relative extent as males but exhibit smaller increases in muscle mass suggests that females may be superior in adaptability for motor unit recruitment.

Figure 13.2 illustrates hypothetical adaptations in the percentage of strength improvement in males and females at different ages after a 10-week strength training program. Although there is an approximate equality in the *relative* strength trainability of males and females (except at puberty), the *absolute* gains in strength for males are usually greater than for females.

Examples of Training Effects on Muscular Strength

With isometric training of nonathletic adult males for about 10 weeks, strength of the wrist flexors (handgrip muscles) might increase by about 9 per cent, the elbow flexors by about 18 per cent, elbow extensors by 2 per cent, hip extensors by 35 per cent, and plantar flexors of the lower leg by 50 per cent [22]. With isotonic weightlifting routines for 10 weeks, the elbow extensor and chest muscles used in the bench press may improve their maximum strength by 7–29 per cent, and the hip and knee extensors used in the squat or leg press may gain 4–40 per cent in strength [16, 38, 43]. After isokinetic training, it has been shown that 15–45 per cent gains in strength of knee extensor muscles might be expected [8].

It should also be pointed out that with large muscle groups, strength increases are usually slow to begin but then accelerate rapidly for a few weeks and reach a plateau or slow down their rates of gain after the muscles have become quite strong. In other words, a greater percentage of improvements in strength should be expected in persons who begin with very low levels of strength. Although strength gains are more difficult to obtain as training progresses, serious weightlifters can keep improving strength significantly for several years.

Physical educators and coaches should become familiar with the differences in strength trainability among age groups, so that they do not expect the same responses of all ages. Once again it should be emphasized that there is a great variability in responsiveness within sexes and age groups. The wise physical education instructor or coach is the one who can detect these individual differences and adapt his programs to best suit the individuals whom he is trying to develop.

Physiological Mechanisms Underlying Strength Improvement

There are two basic ways in which training with overload could enhance the maximal strength of muscles—more motor units could be called into action, or individual motor units could exert more force. The first of these possibilities would implicate the nervous system in the strength adaptation, whereas the second would involve an adaptation in the muscles themselves.

Adaptations of the Nervous System to Strength Training

Although the precise nature of neural adaptations to strength training is obscure, there is substantial evidence that such adaptations do occur.

One line of evidence that links nervous system changes to strength increases is that strength in a limb can be increased even when the limb on the opposite side of the body is the only one to undergo training [9, 28]. For example, suppose that both right and left maximal knee-extension strengths were found to be 50 newtons prior to training. After training with the right leg only, the right leg strength might increase by 20 per cent, but the left leg might also gain strength, perhaps by 10 per cent, with no increase in size [28]. Most authorities conclude that the nervous system must somehow be able to transfer some of the effect of training of the right limb to the left, perhaps by way of neurons in the spinal cord.

A second type of experiment also implicates the central nervous system in muscle strength changes. In these experiments strength increases are shown when a subject shouts during exertion, or when a pistol shot is fired near the subject a few seconds before strength testing [25]. Similar strength increases are sometimes found when a subject is given hypnotic suggestions of increased strength, whereas strength decrements are often shown after hypnotic suggestion of decreased strength [36]. The strength enhancement results are usually interpreted to mean that the brain under hypnosis has either increased its flow of excitatory stimuli or decreased the flow of inhibitory stimuli to the motor neurons of the spinal cord.

A third argument in support of nervous system involvement in the expression of strength includes evidence from electrical stimulation experiments; this evidence usually shows that a voluntary maximal contraction in man is not as forceful as a contraction brought on by electrical stimulation of the muscles in question [26, 40]. The interpretation given to these results is that one does not voluntarily send enough excitatory stimuli from the brain to the motor neurons of the spinal cord to counteract inhibitory stimuli sufficiently for excitation of all motor units. The extended logic is that by training, one can "learn" to either increase excitatory output from the brain or decrease inhibitory output and thereby increase strength.

Although electrical stimulation usually causes a greater expression of strength than does a maximal voluntary exertion, muscular *training* by electrical stimulation of the nerve supplying a muscle does *not* result in as great a strength increase as does training by voluntary contractions of the same muscle [33]. Again, this fourth kind of evidence supports the idea that some of the strength increments brought on by voluntary training must rely on changes in the nervous system that do not occur when the muscles are stimulated electrically.

There is a fifth type of evidence which suggests that changes in the nervous system are responsible for a large portion of the increase in strength that accompanies training. This evidence is that the electrical activity of the muscles (integrated electromyogram) during maximal contraction increases substantially as a result of strength training [28, 37]. These results suggest that more motor units are recruited or that motor units are recruited more frequently after training than before.

Finally, it is widely accepted that the increase of muscle size that accompanies regular strength training for many months is not proportionately as great as the increase in ability to produce force [12]. A muscle such as the gastrocnemius in man can increase its strength greatly with training and yet change very little in size. Unless some undiscovered changes are occurring in the muscles, it appears that a portion of the strength gain with training is caused by a nervous system adaptation. Assuming this to be true, it is unfortunate that nothing is yet known about the precise location within the nervous system where this adaptation occurs (that is, whether in the motor cortex, reticular formation, spinal cord, muscle spindles, tendon organs, or some other part of the nervous system) or the physical or chemical changes responsible for the adaptation.

Changes in Muscle Cross-sectional Area after Training

Only slightly more is known about the mechanism by which individual motor units exert more force after training. It seems apparent that a nerve stimulus causes the activation of more actin-myosin cross bridges with maximal efforts after training. Such a change could occur if there were more muscle fibers (hyperplasia) in the trained muscle or if individual fibers increased in size (hypertrophy) because of a greater number of actin and myosin filaments after training.

Hypertrophy versus Hyperplasia. As long ago as 1879 it was demonstrated that the growth of skeletal muscle that accompanies physical training is caused by hypertrophy of individual fibers and not by an increase in the number of fibers. More recently, however, a number of studies suggested the possibility that muscle fibers split longitudinally during training with a resultant increase in fiber number [20, 24]. The fiber number in these studies was analyzed by cutting thin cross-sections of the muscles and counting the number of fibers. This procedure is satisfactory if all fibers run parallel to the long axis of the muscle for the entire muscle length. However, it has been shown to give erroneous results in other types of muscles, namely, those in which an increased number of fibers was claimed [19]. A more direct and valid approach, albeit very tedious, is to separate the individual fibers in a muscle and count them one by one. Using this approach, it has been shown that there is no increase in fiber number caused by training [19]. Other approaches have also confirmed that muscle overload does not result in hyperplasia [2, 3]. It now appears that the concept of muscle fiber hyperplasia is down for the count!

Adaptations in Protein Synthesis and Degradation. Research has demonstrated that heavy overload training somehow stimulates the production of greater amounts of actin, myosin, and other myofibrillar proteins, so that more cross bridges are available to produce force during a maximal strength effort [13, 18, 21]. In contrast, endurance training tends to increase the production of enzymes involved in providing energy for aerobic metabolism, namely, the enzymes of the mitochondria [21]. The increase in myofibrillar protein that is brought about as a result of heavy resistance exercise could conceivably be the result of an increased rate of buildup (synthesis) of proteins from amino acids delivered to the muscle, a decreased rate of breakdown (degradation) of proteins to amino acids, or a combination of increased synthesis and decreased degradation of proteins. It is difficult to precisely determine rates of skeletal muscle protein synthesis and degradation in humans. Consequently, most studies have used laboratory animal models. The best evidence from these experiments suggests that the rates of both synthesis and degradation are increased during exercise [29]. The increase in the rate of *synthesis* is greater than the increase in the rate of *degradation;* therefore, the *net concentration* of myofibrillar protein increases.

Exactly what transpires between strenuous muscle contractions and greater protein synthesis is unknown. Although the effect of male sex hormone (testosterone) on strength seems apparent when observing strength differences between males and females, efforts to find consistently higher plasma levels of testosterone in trained subjects, or higher uptakes of testosterone into trained muscle where the hormone works to promote protein synthesis, have not been encouraging. Since muscle hypertrophy occurs in animals that are diabetic and in animals that have had their pituitaries removed, it seems unlikely that either insulin or growth hormone (secreted from the pancreas and pituitary, respectively) is required for the hypertrophy associated with strength training in man [17].

Although the uptake of amino acids from the blood into muscles is depressed *during* exercise, it is increased above resting values for some time *after* exercise [32, 44, 45]. Perhaps there is some local change in the muscle membrane brought about by strenuous contractions that makes the membrane more permeable to amino acids so that they may more readily diffuse from the tissue fluids into the muscle cells to serve as building blocks for protein synthesis. A mechanical change in the shape of molecules in the muscle membrane because of tension on the membrane during contraction could be the critical initiating factor in stimulating amino acid uptake into muscle fibers and incorporation into myofibrillar proteins. Such a mechanism is highly speculative, but has been suggested because stretching muscle fibers results in enhanced protein synthesis in those fibers [6, 17, 29, 31].

It has recently been shown that hypertrophied muscles contain more somatomedin-like activity than control muscles [41]. *Somatomedins* are hormone-like substances in the body which increase growth, amino acid uptake, and glucose uptake in skeletal muscle. Therefore, increased production or release of somatomedins may explain muscle hypertrophy. Confirmation of this concept by additional experiments is needed.

Regardless of the precise physiological mechanism involved, it is now widely accepted that the greater size of trained muscle fibers results in part from greater amounts of actin, myosin, and other intracellular proteins. In addition, muscle connective tissue, tendons, and ligaments are strengthened by heavy exercise [5]. Adaptations such as these would seem to be important in making trained muscles less susceptible to injury. These adaptations are, consequently, good justification for rigorous strength training programs prior to the initiation of seasonal athletic activities such as snow skiing, water skiing, football, and wrestling.

Strength Training and Muscle Fiber Types

There is no consistent evidence that strenuous strength training selectively causes hypertrophy of one fiber type to the exclusion of the other [12, 30, 42]. One experiment with isokinetic training of the elbow flexors showed a 39 per cent increase in fast twitch fiber area compared to a 31 per cent increase in slow twitch fiber area [30].

Effect of Improved Strength on Athletic Skills

Common sense suggests that greater muscular strength is more important for some athletic events than others. Performance in those events which rely on power (force × distance/time) logically should be enhanced by strength training more than performance in events which are governed more by endurance, and available research bears out this rationale. Performance is especially improved in events that involve less complex movements of one or two limbs. For example, research literature supports the conclusion that strength training improves performance in vertical jump, standing long-jump, softball, basketball, and medicine ball throws for distance, baseball throwing speed, and speed of limited arm and leg movements, such as arm movement in a horizontal plane from the side of the body to the front [4, 9, 38]. Mixed results have been reported for the effectiveness of strength training on track and swimming sprints that involve more coordinated movements of all limbs, and insignificant effects of strength training are usually found for events such as distance running or swimming [9].

Let us consider the basis for improvements in athletic power, that is, the ability to move the body or some implement such as a shot or discus rapidly through space. Increased arm strength or leg strength would be of no use in improving power unless that strength somehow enabled the movement to be completed more rapidly. If movement speed with the same load were improved by training, it should be apparent on a graph of speed plotted against load [1]. In Fig. 13.5, two plots of movement speed versus load are shown on the same set of axes; curve A is the pretraining curve, and curve B is the posttraining curve. It is obvious that strength training resulted in an improved speed of movement for all loads. The mechanism underlying this improved speed is not known, but it seems that only a certain percentage of the potential cross bridges in a muscle can be activated quickly [11]; if one increases the number of cross bridges in a muscle with strength training, one increases the number that can be activated rapidly.

As an example of this highly speculative explanation, consider the case of that famous shot putter, Klaus Carbuncle, who, prior to training, had exactly 1,000 potentially active cross bridges in his shot putting muscles. Of these 1,000 force-generating sites in his muscles, 40 per cent or 400 could be quickly activated, with the remainder more slowly entering into the contractile effort. After training, by lifting a hippopotamus every day from birth until it weighed 5,000 pounds, Klaus had increased the number of potentially active actin-myosin cross bridges in his muscles to 2,000 and the number of rapidly activated cross bridges to 800 (40 per cent of 2,000). Small wonder

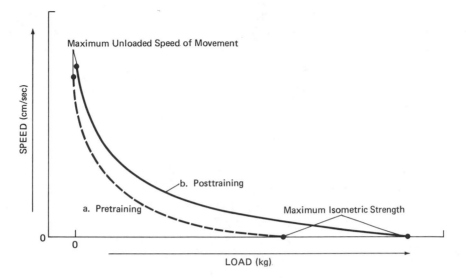

FIGURE 13.5. Approximate effects of strength training on muscle force-velocity curves.

then that Mr. Carbuncle improved his putting speed (and, therefore, power) so that his shot put distance improved, according to legend, from 70 to 140 feet. It is not quite clear why other sons of hippopotamus trainers have not also become outstanding shot putters.

Whatever the actual explanation is for the improved speed of loaded movements that accompanies improved strength, it appears that, at least within a certain range of the force-velocity curve, speed must increase with greater strength. This increase in speed seems to be especially true for slower, more heavily loaded movements, perhaps because as the muscles are freed from loads, nerve coordination of progressively faster movements becomes relatively more important than muscle strength. This dominance of nerve coordination may account for the reported failure of strength training programs to improve speed in more complex movements such as sprinting.

Strength Training and Muscular Hypertrophy

Two of the most common questions a physical educator or coach is faced with are: "How can I build up my muscles so I don't look so skinny?" and "How can I avoid getting big, ugly muscles when I start exercising?" The first question is usually asked by males, and the second, by females; the correct answers are not easy to give. The enhancement of muscular bulk or hypertrophy should accompany any type of overload training, but it is highly variable both in terms of which muscles increase in size and in terms of how great those size changes are. Three general principles pertaining to muscular hypertrophy can be gleaned from the research literature and from observing the effects of strength training programs on various groups of people.

First, there are tremendous individual differences in the adaptation of muscles to training, with females usually demonstrating less hypertrophy than males, probably due to differences in male sex hormones. Thus, most females need not worry about their muscles getting disproportionately large, and some males will gain very little muscle bulk, regardless of the type or amount of strength training they undergo. It is extremely difficult to predict which few females will adapt to training by developing knotty muscles, but experience suggests that girls and women who already are beginning to develop such muscles are probably the only females who should be concerned. Likewise, one who attempts to guess which males will fail to develop with training is likely to be incorrect many times. Usually it is the thin, ascetic type who will probably remain relatively thin and ascetic after training, and the heavily muscled individual who will show dramatic increases in muscle growth.

Second, the greatest hypertrophy usually is shown by those muscles which in everyday life do the least work in relation to their genetic potential. Some of the fastest gains in muscle size have been reported in persons whose muscles have wasted away (atrophied) because of prolonged hospitalization. Accordingly, those whose lives have been relatively sheltered from physical work often show great increases in muscle bulk after a period of overload training. Also, larger muscles such as the pectoralis major and quadriceps femoris usually show greater size changes than smaller muscles such as those of the forearm. However, well-defined appearance of muscular hypertrophy (often called "definition") can be obscured by subcutaneous fat tissue; consequently, this hypertrophic definition is also highly variable and dependent upon inherited patterns of localized fat deposition. This effect of fat on obscuring muscle definition probably also partly explains why females, who have more subcutaneous fat, are less apt than males to demonstrate enlarged muscles after training.

Third, the extent to which a muscle in any given individual gains in bulk depends not only on the severity of overload, but also on the total duration of the overload. Thus, most studies of the problem show that isometric training, which supposedly gives the maximal severity of overload, is not as effective in producing muscular hypertrophy as isotonic training. Isotonic training is usually less severe but has a longer total duration of contraction time. Even within the isotonic category of training, it appears that for most persons, sets of about 10–20 R.M. are better for developing bulk than are sets of 1–6 R.M. [12]. Again, however, it should be noted that individuals vary in their adaptations to these programs and that there are many exceptions to these principles. Although it is inefficient, the trial-and-error method of choosing a muscle bulking program is often useful.

When designing a program to enhance body contours, it is important to include activities for all major muscle groups so that a pleasing body symmetry is achieved. The development of the male upper body to the exclusion of the legs, for example, is not uncommon among "Adonis" types, but it leads to a total appearance that suggests both physical and mental imbalance.

Finally, for those who wish to add pounds to a lanky frame, dietary advice is often essential. High calorie meals are usually recommended for those who would build muscle rapidly. There is little evidence that extra protein will be used for muscle growth. Young people should remember that bulk often comes with maturation, so that a little patience will be well rewarded. The majority of adults in Western countries

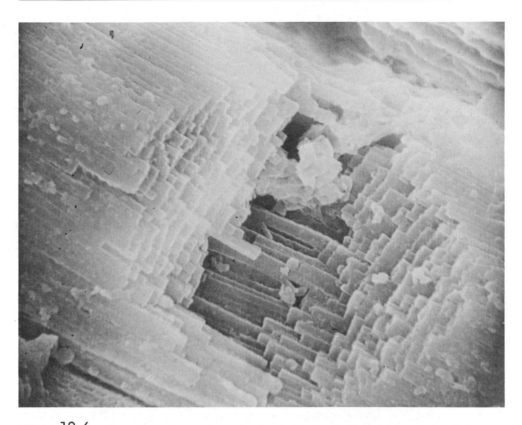

FIGURE 13.6. Stereo electron micrograph of a single muscle fiber. A section of the fiber has been removed to show internal arrangement of myofibrils. (Courtesy of R. E. Carrow, W. W. Heusner and W. D. Van Huss, Michigan State University, E. Lansing, Michigan.)

are victims of too much body tissue, not too little. Slender individuals should perhaps be grateful for their appearance because they are given the best chance to avoid early death from obesity-related cardiovascular disease and other degenerative diseases.

REVIEW QUESTIONS

1. What is meant by "progressive overload" when applied to strength training?
2. List the advantages and disadvantages of isometric, isotonic, and isokinetic strength training programs.
3. Why should strenuous isometric contractions be avoided by those afflicted with cardiovascular disease?
4. Explain why age and sex are important variables in determining responses to strength training.
5. What are the two general mechanisms underlying adaptations to strength training?
6. Describe some of the evidence that the nervous system is involved in adaptations to strength training.
7. Why should protein synthesis be related to strength improvement?
8. What types of athletic activities are most apt to be affected by improved muscular strength?
9. Explain why some persons do not exhibit substantial muscular hypertrophy as a result of strength training.

REFERENCES

[1] Asmussen, E. Growth in muscular strength and power. In G. L. Rarick, ed., *Physical Activity: Human Growth and Development.* New York: Academic Press, Inc., 1973, pp. 60–79.

[2] Atherton, G. W., N. T. James, and M. Mahon. Studies on muscle fibre splitting in skeletal muscle. *Experientia,* 1981, **37:**308–310.

[3] Barnett, J. G., R. G. Holly, and C. R. Ashmore. Stretch-induced growth in chicken wing muscles: biochemical and morphological characterization. *American Journal of Physiology,* 1980, **239:**C39–C46.

[4] Berger, R. A. Effects of dynamic and static training on vertical jump ability. *Research Quarterly,* 1963, **34:**419.

[5] Booth, F. W., and E. W. Gould. Effects of training and disuse on connective tissue. *Exercise and Sport Sciences Reviews,* 1975, **3:**83–112.

[6] Buresova, M., E. Gutmann, and M. Klicpera. Effect of tension upon the rate of incorporation of amino acids into proteins of cross-striated muscle. *Experientia,* 1969, **25:**144–145.

[7] Caiozzo, V. J., J. J. Perrine, and V. R. Edgerton. Training-induced alterations of the in vivo force-velocity relationship of human muscle. *Journal of Applied Physiology,* 1981, **51:**750–754.

[8] Carr, L. S., R. K. Conlee, and A. G. Fisher. Effects of fast and slow isokinetic weight training on strength and endurance. *Medicine and Science in Sports and Exercise* (abstract), 1981, **13:**108.

[9] Clarke, D. H. Adaptations in strength and muscular endurance resulting from exercise. *Exercise and Sport Sciences Reviews,* 1973, **1:**73–102.

[10] Coyle, E. F., D. C. Feiring, R. C. Rotkis, R. W. Cote III, F. B. Roby, W. Lee, and J. H. Wilmore. Specificity of power improvements through slow and fast isokinetic training. *Journal of Applied Physiology,* 1981, **51:**1437–1442.

[11] Davies, R. E. The dynamics of the energy-rich phosphates. In J. Keul, ed., *Limiting Factors of Physical Performance.* Stuttgart: Georg Thieme Publishers, 1973, pp. 56–62.

[12] Dons, B., K. Bollerup, F. Bonde-Petersen, and S. Hancke. The effect of weight-lifting exercise related to muscle fiber composition and muscle cross-sectional area in humans. *European Journal of Applied Physiology,* 1979, **40:**95–106.

[13] Edgerton, V. R. Exercise and the growth and development of muscle tissue. In G. L. Rarick, ed., *Physical Activity: Human Growth and Development.* New York: Academic Press, Inc., 1973, pp. 1–31.

[14] Faulkner, J. A., L. C. Maxwell, D. A. Brook, and D. A. Lieberman. Adaptation of guinea pig plantaris muscle fibers to endurance training. *American Journal of Physiology,* 1971, **221:**291–297.

[15] Gardner, G. W. Specificity of strength changes of the exercised and nonexercised limb following isometric training. *Research Quarterly,* 1963, **34:**98–101.

[16] Gettman, L. R., and M. L. Pollock. Circuit weight training: a critical review of its physiological benefits. *Physician and Sportsmedicine,* 1981, **9:**44–60.

[17] Goldberg, A. L., J. D. Etlinger, D. F. Goldspink, and C. Jablecki. Mechanism of work-induced hypertrophy of skeletal muscle. *Medicine and Science in Sports,* 1975, **7:**248–261.

[18] Goldspink, G., and K. F. Howells. Work-induced hypertrophy in exercised normal muscles of different ages and the reversibility of hypertrophy after cessation of exercise. *Journal of Physiology* (London), 1974, **239:**179–193.

[19] Gollnick, P. D., B. F. Timson, R. L. Moore, and M. Riedy. Muscular enlargement and number of fibers in skeletal muscles of rats. *Journal of Applied Physiology,* 1981, **50:**936–943.

[20] Gonyea, W. J. Muscle fiber splitting in trained and untrained animals. *Exercise and Sport Sciences Reviews,* 1980, 19–40.

[21] Gordon, E. E., K. Kowalski, and M. Fritts. Adaptations of muscle to various exercises. *Journal of the American Medical Association,* 1967, **199:**103–108.

[22] Hettinger, T. *Physiology of Strength.* Springfield, Ill.: Charles C Thomas, Publisher, 1961.

[23] Hickson, R. C. Interference of strength development by simultaneously training for strength and endurance. *European Journal of Applied Physiology,* 1980, **45:**255–263.

[24] Ho, K. W., R. R. Roy, C. D. Tweedle, W. W. Heusner, W. D. van Huss, and R. E. Carrow. Skeletal muscle fiber splitting with weight-lifting exercise in rats. *American Journal of Anatomy,* 1980, **157:**433–440.

[25] Ikai, M., and A. H. Steinhaus. Some factors modifying the expression of human strength. *Journal of Applied Physiology,* 1961, **16:**157–163.

[26] Ikai, M., and K. Yabe. Training effect of muscular endurance by means of voluntary and electrical stimulation. *European Journal of Applied Physiology,* 1969, **28:**55–60.

[27] Johnson, B. I., J. W. Adamczyk, K. O. Tennoe, and S. B. Stromme. A comparison of concentric and eccentric muscle training. *Medicine and Science in Sports,* 1976, **8:**35–38.

[28] Komi, P. V., J. T. Viitasalo, R. Rauramaa, and V. Vihko. Effect of isometric strength training on mechanical, electrical, and metabolic aspects of muscle function. *European Journal of Applied Physiology,* 1978, **40:**45–55.

[29] Laurent, G. J., and D. J. Millward. Protein turnover in skeletal muscle hypertrophy. *Federation Proceedings,* 1980, **39:**42–47.

[30] MacDougall, J. D., G. C. B. Elder, D. G. Sale, J. R. Moroz, and J. R. Sutton. Effects of strength training and immobilization on human muscle fibres. *European Journal of Applied Physiology,* 1980, **43:**25–34.

[31] Mackova, E., and P. Hnik. Compensatory muscle hypertrophy is not true working hypertrophy. *Physiologia Bohemoslovaca,* 1973, **22:**43–44.

[32] Makarova, A. F. Biochemical changes in animal muscles in experimental training of various kinds. *Ukrainian Biochemical Journal,* 1958, **30:**903–910.

[33] Massey, B. H., R. C. Nelson, B. J. Sharkey, and T. Comden. Effects of high-frequency electrical stimulation on the size and strength of skeletal muscle. *Journal of Sports Medicine,* 1973, **5:**136–144.

[34] McManus, B. M., D. R. Lamb, J. J. Judis, and J. Scala. Skeletal muscle leucine incorporation and testosterone uptake in exercised guinea pigs. *European Journal of Applied Physiology,* 1975, **34:**149–156.

[35] Mitchell, J. H., and K. Wildenthal. Static (isometric) exercise and the heart: physiological and clinical considerations. *Annual Review of Medicine,* 1974, **25:**369–381.

[36] Morgan, W. P. Hypnosis and muscular performance. In W. P. Morgan, ed., *Ergogenic Aids and Muscular Performance.* New York: Academic Press, Inc., 1972, pp. 193–233.

[37] Moritani, T. Electromyographic analysis of muscle strength gains: neural and hypertrophic effects. *National Strength Coaches Journal,* 1980, **1:**32–37.

[38] O'Shea, J. P. *Scientific Principles and Methods of Strength Fitness,* 2nd ed. Reading, Mass.: Addison-Wesley Publishing Co., Inc., 1976.

[39] Schiaffino, S., and V. Hanzlikova. On the mechanisms of compensatory hypertrophy in skeletal muscle. *Experientia,* 1970, **26:**152–153.

[40] Stephens, J. A., and A. Taylor. Fatigue of maintained voluntary muscle contraction in man. *Journal of Physiology* (London), 1972, **220:**1–18.

[41] Sturek, M. S., D. R. Lamb, and A. C. Synder. Somatomedin-like activity and muscle hypertrophy. *IRCS Medical Science: Physiology,* 1981, **9:**760.

[42] Thorstensson, A. Muscle strength, fibre types and enzyme activities in man. *Acta Physiologica Scandinavica,* 1976, Supplementum 443.

[43] Wilmore, J. H. Alterations in strength, body composition and anthropometric measurements consequent to a 10-week weight training program. *Medicine and Science in Sports,* 1974, **6:**133.

[44] Yakovlev, N. N., A. F. Krasnova, and N. R. Chagovets. The influence of muscle activity on muscle proteins. In E. Gutmann and P. Hnik, eds., *The Effect of Use and Disuse on Neuromuscular Functions.* Prague: Publishing House of the Czechoslovak Academy of Sciences, 1963, pp. 461–473.

[45] Zimmer, H.-G., and E. Gerlach. Protein synthesis in heart and skeletal muscle of rats during and subsequent to exercise. In J. Keul, ed., *Limiting Factors of Physical Performance.* Stuttgart: Georg Thieme, Publishers, 1973, pp. 102–109.

CHAPTER

14

Anaerobic Power and Capacity

MANY sporting and everyday activities have energy demands which must be met through the anaerobic breakdown of ATP, creatine phosphate, and muscle glycogen.

Anaerobic power is the maximal rate at which energy can be produced or work can be done without a significant contribution of aerobic (mitochondrial) energy production.

Anaerobic capacity is the ability to persist at the maintenance or repetition of strenuous muscular contractions that rely upon anaerobic mechanisms of energy supply.

Anaerobic activities include the sprint events in track, in cycling, and in swimming; vigorous wrestling competition; carrying heavy luggage or bags of groceries; vigorous shoveling of snow; and the rapid manual sawing of wood. Anaerobic activities may be dynamic, as in the case of sawing wood or sprinting, or static, as exemplified by carrying heavy loads, but all are characterized by intense muscular contractions that demand substantially greater rates of energy (ATP) production that can be provided by aerobic metabolism alone. For most persons, this class of activities includes all those that, by reason of their high intensities, can be sustained for less than 1 or 2 minutes [2]. Activities that can be sustained for longer than 1 or 2 minutes demand a substantial rate of oxygen delivery by the cardiovascular system and are designated aerobic endurance activities in this text. Accordingly, anaerobic power and capacity require a type of physical fitness lying in the center of a continuum between strength fitness and aerobic endurance fitness. Remember that this sort of classification of the characteristics of physical fitness is arbitrary and that the boundaries separating the various categories are not precisely defined. For example, an activity that was originally classified in the anaerobic category for an untrained individual may be reclassified after a period of training as the person increases the ability to persist in that activity beyond the arbitrary 2-minute limit. These arbitrary classifications, although imprecise, serve a useful

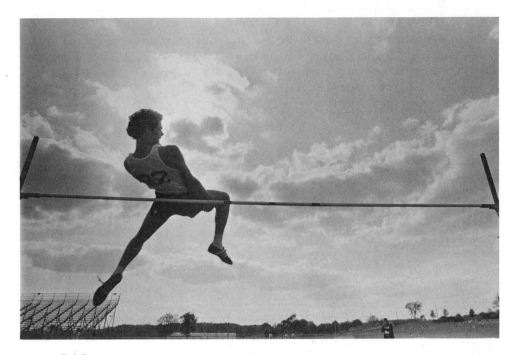

FIGURE 14.1. Successful high jumping requires great anaerobic power. (Courtesy of Office of Public Information, Purdue University, West Lafayette, Indiana.)

function by drawing our attention to the principal physiological mechanisms underlying various types of activities.

Tests of Maximal Anaerobic Power and Capacity

A person can maintain the greatest muscular force for only a few seconds. If this force is allowed to move a mass some distance, the maximal rate of performing work can be computed. Since the rate of performing work is defined as *power,* and since work at the maximal rate is performed at the expense of the anaerobic splitting of ATP and creatine phosphate, a measure of this maximal work rate is also a measure of maximal anaerobic power. If an athletic event or some industrial task can be completed in 5–10 seconds, a measure of maximal anaerobic power might pove valuable in the assessment of a candidate's ability to perform such a task. Short sprints and jumps are some of the athletic events that are obviously dependent upon maximal anaerobic power.

Maximal Stair Climb

A rather simple test of anaerobic power consists of a fast run up a flight of stairs [10]. The subject stands 6 meters in front of the stairs and runs up the stairs, two or three at a time, as fast as possible. On the third stair the subject steps on a switchmat that starts a timer, and on the ninth stair the subject stops the timer by stepping on a second switchmat. Time elapsed between the third and ninth stairs is recorded to the nearest hundredth of a second. Since power = (mass × distance)/time, one must know the weight (mass) of the subject in kilograms, the vertical height in meters between the third and ninth stairs, and the elapsed time between the third and ninth stairs in seconds to calculate power in kilogram-meters per second. For example, if the vertical distance between two steps is 16.9 cm., the total vertical distance between stairs three and nine is 6 × 16.9 = 101 cm. = 1.01 m. If the subject weighs 70 kg. and the elapsed time between the two switchmats is 0.50 sec., power (kgm/sec) = (70 × 1.01)/0.50 = 141.4 kgm/sec. Conversion of kgm/sec to watts is accomplished by multiplying kgm/sec by 9.8. (The watt is the preferred unit of power.)

If a staircase or timing apparatus is unavailable, another estimate of anaerobic power can be obtained by timing a subject in a 50-yard dash with a 15-yard running start. Table 14.1 shows a classification scheme for maximal anaerobic power based on the staircase or 50-yard dash scores [10, 22].

Sprinters, ice hockey players, and speed skaters have about 35 per cent greater anaerobic power than distance runners and cross-country skiers and 15–20 per cent greater values than 800-meter runners, ski jumpers, downhill skiers, and non-athletes [22]. About 90 per cent of the variability in maximal anaerobic power as measured by the stair climb test is explained by heredity, and the scores of persons at age 60 are about 60 per cent of the values at age 20 [7]. The scores are increased by any extra load (up to 29.2 kg) supported by the subject [3]. Some persons are fearful of tripping on the steps, and those with short legs may have difficulty taking two or three steps at a time. On the whole, however, the maximal stair climb test is quite useful in measuring the power generated by the splitting of ATP and creatine phosphate.

TABLE 14.1
Classification of Anaerobic Power Scores (10, 22)

Male Classification	Stair Climb (kg-m/sec) Age in Years	50 Yard Dash (sec) Age in Years	
	18–35	15–20	20–30
Poor	Under 70	Over 7.1	Over 7.8
Fair	71–94	7.1–6.8	7.8–7.5
Average	95–105		
Good	106–120	6.7–6.5	7.4–7.1
Excellent	Over 120	Under 6.5	Under 7.1

Female Classification	Age in Years	Age in Years	
	18–35	15–20	20–30
Poor	Under 60	Over 9.1	Over 10.0
Fair	61–84	9.1–8.4	10.0–9.2
Average	85–95		
Good	96–110	8.3–7.9	9.1–8.7
Excellent	Over 110	Under 7.9	Under 8.7

The Wingate Anaerobic Cycling Test

Scientists at the Wingate Institute in Israel have developed a 30-second all-out cycling test to determine maximal anaerobic power (maximal rate of work production at the expense of ATP and creatine phosphate breakdown) and maximal anaerobic capacity (average rate of work production in 30 seconds, presumably at the expense of ATP, creatine phosphate, and anaerobic glycolysis) [28]. The test can be performed with either legs or arms, and the protocol is as follows:

1. *Warmup.* The subject cycles 2–4 minutes at an intensity sufficient to cause the heart to beat at 150–160 beats per minute. The cycling should be interspersed with two or three all-out bursts of cycling for 4–8 seconds each.
2. *Rest Interval.* A 3–5 minute rest interval follows the warmup before the test begins.
3. *The Test.* On command the subject pedals the ergometer as fast as possible to overcome inertia of the flywheel. At the same time the resistance is progressively increased to a predetermined load by a tester so that the final load (Table 14.2) is reached within 2–4 seconds. At the moment the final load has been reached, a count of the pedal revolutions begins and continues for 30 seconds as the subject continues to pedal as fast as possible. Pedal count must be recorded every 5 seconds, either electronically or by a reliable pair of observers, one of whom counts out the revolutions while the other records the appropriate count every 5 seconds.
4. *Cool-down.* To minimize the risk of a subject fainting after completing this arduous task, the subject should be encouraged to continue pedaling at a light load for 2–3 minutes after the test. Forty-five to sixty minutes should be allowed for recovery before the test is repeated.
5. *Reporting of test results.* Results for each 5-second period are recorded in watts according to the following equation:

$$Watts = load \ (kg) \times revolutions \times 11.765$$

(This equation is used for a Monark ergometer. Other types of ergometers will require different equations.)

The greatest power in a 5-second period (usually the first period) is the *peak anaerobic power.* Presumably, this represents the power created by the splitting of ATP and creatine phosphate.

The *average (mean) power* for the six periods of 5 seconds each presumably represents the maximal capacity to produce energy anaerobically by breaking

TABLE 14.2

Optimal Loads (kilograms per kg body weight)

Leg Test		Arm Test	
Children & Women	Men	Women	Men
0.075	0.083–0.092	0.050–0.058	0.058–0.067

down ATP, creatine phosphate, and glycogen. This measure represents anaerobic capacity.

Power decline is an index of fatigue rate and is calculated as a percentage of peak power by subtracting the lowest power in 5 seconds from the peak power score, dividing by peak power, and multiplying by 100. For example, if peak power were 800 W and the lowest power were 400 W, the power decline would be:

$$100 \times (800 - 400)/800 = 50\%.$$

The Wingate test has a test-retest reliability coefficient of 0.95, and performance on the test is not impaired by a body weight loss of up to 5 per cent caused by rapid dehydration in the heat [20]. Norms for the test were not available in early 1982, but mean values for 11 college wrestlers were 859 W for peak power and 639 W for mean power [20].

Oxygen Debt As a Measure of Anaerobic Capacity

Oxygen debt is defined as the excess oxygen uptake during recovery from exercise, that is, the oxygen uptake above and beyond what would have occurred in the same time period had the subject remained at rest. Oxygen debt capacity is the greatest oxygen debt one can accumulate and is ordinarily achieved with exercise that can be sustained for 1–3 minutes [15]. The reason that oxygen debt capacity has sometimes been used to estimate anaerobic capacity is that some of the excess oxygen consumed after exercise is used by the mitochondria for replenishing the stores of ATP, creatine phosphate, and glycogen that were depleted anaerobically during the exercise period. Thus, if there were a perfect relationship between oxygen debt capacity and anaerobic ATP production, oxygen debt capacity would obviously be a useful measure of anaerobic potential.

However, oxygen debt capacity is not solely related to the production of ATP anaerobically. It is thought, for example, that such factors as high epinephrine levels, elevated body temperature, and increased oxygen uptake by the rapidly beating heart and by the respiratory muscles all contribute to the elevated rate of oxygen uptake during recovery from vigorous activity [15]. Because of the above considerations, it is apparent that there is only a limited association between oxygen debt capacity and anaerobic capacity. Nonetheless, oxygen debt capacities have been successfully used to distinguish between athletes and untrained persons by some [15], but not all, investigators [13]. Athletes' oxygen debt capacities average about 10.5 liters (139 ml/kg) and 5.9 liters (95 ml/kg) for males and females, respectively, whereas corresponding values for untrained subjects are 5.0 liters (68 ml/kg) and 3.1 liters (50 ml/kg) [15]. The variability of oxygen debt measurements for a given individual is large [13]. Also, in a group of subjects having similar physical characteristics, oxygen debt capacity cannot be used to accurately predict performance in short-duration activities [21].

Other Tests of Anaerobic Capacity

In the physical education setting, it is common to assess anaerobic capacity as the number of squat-thrusts, pullups, pushups, or dips on parallel bars one can perform at a rapid cadence. However, such measurements tend to favor lighter students because the greater muscular strength of heavier students does not adequately compensate for their greater body weights [2]. This is particularly true in the case of pullups. Therefore, if these activities are used to evaluate anaerobic capacity, normal values should be established for different body weight classifications.

Static endurance of the elbow flexors could be measured as the time one can hold a 50-pound dumbbell at 90 degrees of elbow flexion. Common measures of anaerobic capacity of various muscle groups would be the number of repeated knee extensions one can perform at a given rate with a given load, the time one can persist at strenuous exercise on a bicycle ergometer or a treadmill, or the time one can maintain a given static force on a dynamometer.

Measurements of anaerobic capacity are much less reproducible than strength measurements, probably because of variability in motivation for maintaining painful muscle contractions [4].

Anaerobic Power, Anaerobic Capacity, and Muscle Fiber Type

Those with higher percentages of fast twitch muscle fibers tend to produce greater anaerobic power during brief tests such as the stair climb [22] and the Wingate anaerobic test [20]. This is to be expected since fast twitch motor units produce greater force than slow units. However, fast twitch motor units are quick to fatigue. Therefore, as the contribution of aerobic metabolism increases with progressively less intense contractions, the importance to anaerobic capacity of fast twitch units decreases. In other words, for very intense contractions which demand extremely high rates of anaerobic metabolism, the fast twitch units will play a large role in anaerobic power and capacity; for contractions of lesser intensity there will be greater blood flow and a lesser contribution of fast twitch motor units to anaerobic capacity [19].

Strength and Anaerobic Capacity

Anaerobic capacity for simple, submaximally loaded movements is directly related to maximal muscle strength. Thus, one whose elbow flexors can support a maximal load of 48 kilograms at a joint angle of 90 degrees could expect to hold a 16 kilogram dumbbell at 90 degrees for twice as long as one who can support a maximal load of only 24 kilograms [5, 27]. For submaximal, static contractions at less than 60–70 percent of maximal strength, there are at least two reasons for this relationship. First, the stronger person can support a load of 16 kilograms with fewer motor units than the weaker person. Consequently, more motor units can be resting at any one time in the muscles of the stronger individual so that it will take longer to fatigue all the motor units. Second, in the case of static contractions, bloodflow is reduced in proportion to the relative severity of the muscle contraction. If the stronger person is contracting at only one-third of his maximal strength, blood flow to the elbow flexors will be much less restricted than that to the muscles of the weaker subject, who must produce two-thirds of his maximal force.

For static contractions with loads *greater than* 60–70 per cent of maximal strength, blood flow is totally cut off [11]. For such contractions, the relationship between maximal strength and anaerobic capacity exists solely because of differences in the number of motor units that must be recruited to maintain the contraction for weaker and stronger persons. With *maximal* contractions, both static and dynamic, presumably the same total number of motor units must be recruited for both weak and strong persons so that there is little relationship between absolute strength and endurance with maximal loads [5]. In other words, the weaker person will be able to exert less force for about the same time that the strong person exerts a greater force.

For submaximal *dynamic* contractions, stronger persons have greater anaerobic capacity because they need to recruit fewer motor units to exert the same force. The reason for this is that the individual muscle fibers within each motor unit of the stronger person have more actin-myosin cross bridges to produce greater force.

Strength and Relative Anaerobic Capacity

Just as contractions of 100 per cent of maximal strength can be held by the weaker person for about as long as the stronger one, so, too, a weaker person can persist at any given percentage of maximal strength, whether it be 30, 50, or 70 per cent, for about the same time as a stronger individual. Another way of stating this is that *there is not a direct relationship between maximal strength and the time one can persist at producing force equal to any standard percentage of that maximal strength*.

[handwritten margin note: confusing]

Age, Sex, and Anaerobic Capacity

Because there is a direct relationship between strength and anaerobic capacity at submaximal loads, and because strength increases with age until about 30, before beginning a gradual decline, *both strength and anaerobic capacity are affected in a similar fashion by age.* Likewise, *because males have greater maximal strength than females, they also have greater anaerobic capacity for submaximal loads*. The age range of 12–15 years seems to be optimal for improving anaerobic capacity in simple movements [1]. The underlying physiological mechanism for this phenomenon is not clear, although it may be explained by the fact that motivational levels are often high in young adolescents.

Training for Improved Anaerobic Capacity

As was seen in Chapter 13 regarding strength training, an important factor in establishing a training routine is to try to develop exercises that will train the body in a highly specific manner, improving its response to the precise demands that will be placed upon it in competition, manual labor, or daily life. In other words, *the exercises used to improve anaerobic capacity should mimic the actual task performance that the trainee is attempting to improve.* If one wishes to have better capacity for swinging a heavy ax, one should train with movements similar to, if not identical to, that task; but if one wishes to improve the ability to engage in a highly isometric type of performance such as moving furniture, one should probably train isometrically. By training in a specific manner, it is thought that the appropriate adaptations in the nervous system are more effectively brought about. Thus, if one is training to improve an isokinetic or isotonic type of performance, it is probably best to design a program that emphasizes isokinetic or isotonic exercises.

Anaerobic Training for Dynamic Activities

As was described in the introduction of this chapter, there is a wide range of physical activities that might be classified as anaerobic. Dynamic anaerobic capacity is needed for such activities as chopping wood at a fast rate; sprinting for up to 1–2 minutes in track, swimming, or cycling; wrestling; and the prolonged sprinting phases of such sports as basketball, soccer, field hockey, canoe racing, and football. Also, although running, swimming, and cycling over long distances depend much more on the cardiovascular system's delivery of oxygen, champions in these activities also have the capacity to sustain anaerobic sprints at the finish of their events. Consequently, distance performers must not overlook the anaerobic aspects of their training.

Because of the varied nature of these dynamic anaerobic activities, it is impossible to give specific training programs for each of them. The physiological principles for the development of specific programs are, however, similar for all types of dynamic anaerobic events. It is these principles, with some examples, that will be described in the following discussion.

Interval Training. The body adapts to repeated exercise sessions so that subsequent exercise of a similar nature is tolerated more easily. Therefore, *it is important in training sessions to produce as much high quality work* as is feasible.* This means that the type of movement, the strength of the muscle contractions, and the speed of movement must be similar to what one is striving to accomplish as a training goal. Accordingly, if a beginning high school runner is trying to achieve a time of 2 minutes in an 800 meter competition, most of the training should be at that pace or faster; that is, the athlete should run repeat 100's in less than 15 seconds, 200's in 30 seconds, and 400's in 60 seconds or faster. Likewise, a wrestler whose goal is to wrestle intensely for three 3-minute periods should practice intensely for repeated bouts of less than 3 minutes in length.

The use of repeated work periods interspersed with recovery periods to help adapt the body to stressful demands placed upon it is known as *interval training.* In interval training the exercise periods are commonly called *work intervals* and the rest periods, *recovery intervals.* Although it is true that some championship performers have

---

* "Work" is used as a synonym for "exercise" and not in the sense of physics.

achieved greatness by training only at a slow pace for long durations, it is likely that many who train at a slow pace become better equipped to perform at that slow pace.

Because very little work can be performed at a *fast pace* when a continuous long-duration type of training is used, it is important to use repeated work intervals of rather short duration for the bulk of the training sessions. (Remember, though, that such training is extremely exhausting and must occasionally be interrupted by other types of training for the sake of variety; any method, no matter how grand in theory, is useless if the exerciser drops out of the training program.)

Duration of Work and Recovery Intervals. *Because energy for anaerobic activities is mostly provided by anaerobic mechanisms, training programs should be designed to stress or overload the cellular machinery responsible for producing ATP anaerobically.* This means that the exercise periods must be very intense to place the greatest possible demands on the enzymes involved in anaerobic energy production, namely, the enzymes used to break down creatine phosphate and muscle glycogen. *Accordingly, work intervals should last no longer than 1–2 minutes.* Work intervals longer than 1–2 minutes do not increase the load on anaerobic capacity, but rather begin to rely more on aerobic energy supply [12]. Since only a few long-duration work intervals can be tolerated in any given training session, it is important to keep the exercise periods under 1–2 minutes to maximize the total amount of work at the greatest anaerobic loads.

Also, it has been demonstrated that work intervals shorter than about 20 seconds do not bring about the maximal amount of anaerobic energy production if interspersed with recovery intervals of similar length [2, 12]. This may be due to the ability of oxygen stored in muscles to promote aerobic ATP replenishment during the recovery intervals [2]. Oxygen is stored in the muscles by being bound to *myoglobin,* which may release its oxygen to the mitochondria during periods of great oxygen demand [2]. With interval training that includes very short work intervals, it is thought that myoglobin-bound oxygen is used during the work intervals, but can be rapidly replenished during rest intervals of similar length, so that anaerobic energy reserves such as creatine phosphate and glycogen are conserved [2]. Consequently, *if work intervals of less than 20 seconds are used, recovery intervals should be limited to about 10–15 seconds so that myoglobin cannot be fully recharged with oxygen during the recovery intervals.* After a few repeats of such intervals, a more complete recovery period (15–20 minutes, for example) is required before beginning another set of work intervals.

Recovery intervals following work intervals longer than 20 seconds must be long enough to allow substantial recovery of the muscles. With adequate recovery, an adequate number of high quality work intervals can be completed during a training session. But recovery must not be so long that subsequent work intervals are not somewhat more stressful than the preceding ones. *Therefore, recovery intervals following short work intervals (20–30 seconds) should be about 1–2 minutes long, and longer work intervals should be followed by more complete recovery periods of 2–15 minutes.* The longer recovery intervals for a given work interval are needed for younger athletes or those with poor anaerobic capacities. Since lactic acid is removed more rapidly when mild exercise is performed during recovery than with complete inactivity [12, 29], slow jogging, swimming, and so on during recovery are often prescribed.

Intensity of Work Intervals. The exercise performed during work intervals designed to improve dynamic anaerobic capacity must be at maximal or near-maximal intensities. A commonly used rule of thumb suggests that anaerobic capacity begins to be taxed at about 80 per cent of one's maximal effort for a given duration of exercise [2]. To insure a near maximal reliance on anaerobic capacity, therefore, it would be wise to exercise at no less than 90 per cent of maximal effort in longer duration activities (1–2 minutes), and to exercise maximally for shorter work intervals. Thus, if a runner's best 400 meter run time is 60 seconds (6.67 meters/second), he could run 400 meter intervals in 66.7 seconds (400/(6.67 × 0.90)), or he could run 360 meters in 60 seconds (90 per cent of 400 = 360) to insure that he would stress his anaerobic capacity.

The number of training sessions per week needed to cause the greatest improvement in anaerobic capacity is not well established, but some evidence indicates that three or four training sessions per week may be optimal, at least with unconditioned college males [10].

Table 14.3 summarizes information on interval training for improving anaerobic endurance. The suggested scheme in Table 14.3 should be useful in devising appropriate training procedures for any type of activity, especially when the work is performed at maximal intensity. It should be noted that a training program could include more repetitions with shorter recovery intervals than are shown in Table 14.3, but the work done then would be of relatively poor quality.

There are many combinations of work and recovery intervals that could be used during any training session. One might wish to combine 10-second work intervals and 2-minute work intervals in the same session. This could be done by completing perhaps 12 repetitions of the suggested routine with 10-second work intervals and then four or five repetitions of the 2-minute work and recovery intervals. It bears repeating that the suggestions presented in Table 14.3 are meant to serve only as rough guidelines for training. Younger or less capable performers may not be able to complete as many repetitions or recover adequately with the recovery intervals suggested, and better performers may not be adequately stressed with these routines.

TABLE 14.3

Suggested Scheme of Interval Training for Improving Anaerobic Capacity and Dynamic Local Muscular Endurance

Length of Work Interval	Percent of Intensity of Effort	Length of Recovery Interval	Number of Work Intervals Per Session	Training Sessions Per Week
10 sec	100	10 sec	20–30	3–4
20 sec	100	15 sec	10–20	3–4
30 sec	100	1–2 min	8–18	3–4
1 min	95–100	3–5 min	5–15	3–4
2 min	90–100	5–15 min	4–10	3–4

Responses to Interval Training for Improved Anaerobic Capacity. Do the interval-training programs described in this chapter actually overload the biochemical mechanisms responsible for the anaerobic replenishment of ATP in skeletal muscles? Evidence obtained from analysis of blood and muscle tissue supports an affirmative answer to this question [12, 14, 15, 18, 24, 25]. In Fig. 14.2, there are illustrated the idealized changes in the muscle stores of glycogen and creatine phosphate, the accumulation of lactic acid in blood and muscle, and the repeated attainment of maximal capacity for oxygen deficit as the result of an interval-training session. As this illustration reveals, near maximal or maximal oxygen deficit is reached during each of the eight work intervals. This shows indirectly that anaerobic mechanisms for supplying ATP are being heavily stressed. The other data shown in Fig. 14.2 give direct evidence

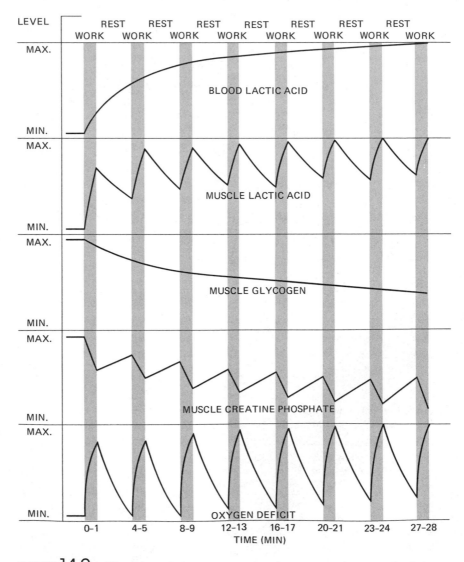

FIGURE 14.2. Physiological changes occurring during interval training session.

that anaerobic events are occurring in the muscle: Creatine phosphate is gradually depleted during work and only partially replenished during each recovery period; glycogen is broken down; and extremely high levels of muscle and blood lactic acid progressively accumulate. Other evidence that interval training can be an effective means of stressing anaerobic capacity is that such training leads to adaptations in anaerobic enzymes and to improved oxygen debt capacity [12, 15].

Maintenance of dynamic anaerobic capacity can be accomplished with one or two training sessions per week [10].

Improving Dynamic Anaerobic Capacity for Simple Movements. For anaerobic training of simple dynamic movements, such as repeated elbow flexions, most authorities conclude that repetition of movements is far more important than is true for strength training. Thus, *for dynamic anaerobic capacity in simple movements, one should train with relatively light resistance and many repetitions.* However, it should be emphasized that strength improvement should probably be the most important secondary goal of any such anaerobic training program. Strength improvement in this context has such importance because of the strong relationship between strength and anaerobic capacity. Accordingly, one should not stress repetitions over load until one has established a sound foundation of muscular strength [4]. For most kinds of anaerobic training of a dynamic type (4–5 sets of 10–20 repetitions maximum) performed 3 or 4 days per week will approach the optimal general pattern of training. *Maintenance programs* for anaerobic endurance gained by training can be reduced to performance of the usual training routine once or twice per week.

Anaerobic Training for Static Activities

To improve anaerobic capacity for static activities one should perform many static contractions in each training session with a load greater than what will be faced in competition, on the job, or in daily life. One should start with intensive, short-duration contractions performed 10–20 times each session, 3–4 times per week. As strength improves, the program should be altered to include 5–10 long-duration contractions, with loads just above those to be faced after training. In this way the organism can adapt to stress by improving not only strength, but also the ability of anaerobic metabolic systems to produce ATP under endurance conditions. Maintenance of anaerobic capacity for static activities can probably be achieved by repetition of the normal training session once per week.

Other Considerations

As with strength training and other types of fitness training, *it is important to vary the approach to anaerobic training so that boredom does not cause one to drop out of the training program.* An occasional training session of exercises that may not be ideal for improving anaerobic capacity but that is interesting to the trainee is better than no training at all. One must not become too rigid in designing training programs lest no one be willing to become trained.

When designing training programs for the improvement of anaerobic capacity in physical education classes, many exercises can be accomplished in the form of sports activities or games, so that most students can better enjoy their fitness training. Rope climbs and "tugs of war" are good examples of activities that improve anaerobic capacity for static activities, whereas hopping races and relays in which participants must move on all four limbs can be used to improve dynamic anaerobic capacity. As was mentioned earlier in this chapter, excessive emphasis on pullups and rope climbs as tests of anaerobic capacity penalizes heavier students whose greater strengths do not compensate for their heavier body weights. Therefore, scoring on any such tests should be based on normative data for various weight classifications.

Duration of Training Effects on Anaerobic Capacity

As with gains in strength, improvements in anaerobic capacity for simple movements begin to be lost after about a month of inactivity. Much of the gains, up to 80 per cent in many cases, are retained for as long as 6 months, however [4]. It seems likely that most of the retention of endurance gains for simple movements is caused by retention of strength improvements. The duration of training effects for activities such as swimming have not been adequately studied, but limited evidence suggests that a 2-month period of inactivity may completely obliterate any training effects [10].

Physiological Mechanisms Underlying Improvements in Anaerobic Capacity

In any attempt to assess the relative importance of possible mechanisms that could explain how a training program could enhance anaerobic capacity, one must consider the nature of the various types of anaerobic capacity, such as the extent of static contractions, the degree of aerobic involvement, and the relative intensity of the work, because it seems probable that different mechanisms may underlie gains in different activities. With simple movements, the only common factor that can help explain improvements in capacity brought about by training is a gain in muscular strength. However, strength gains cannot be the sole mechanism underlying gains in anaerobic capacity because strength rarely improves by as much as 100 per cent after a few months of training, whereas anaerobic capacity may increase by more than 5,000 per cent for submaximal loads [2]. Some of the other mechanisms that may be responsible for endurance improvements are described in the following paragraphs.

Intense Static Contractions

Assume that one maintained a severe static contraction of the knee extensor muscles at a joint angle of 90 degrees for as long as possible. Next, he undertook an intensive training program to improve the strength of the knee extensors. A posttraining test at the pretraining load would show a gain in holding time from a pretraining time of about 10 seconds to a posttraining time of perhaps 20–30 seconds. Because any static contraction at a load greater than 60–70 per cent of maximal strength causes complete compression of the arteries, so that no blood enters the muscles, the contraction must be maintained almost totally anaerobically, and improvements in circulation do not enter into the explanation of endurance gains. Also, muscle pain is not usually a major factor in limiting such brief contractions. Therefore, the mechanism responsible for these gains could involve two factors—a reduction in the number of motor units recruited to perform the task (because the trained muscle fibers in each motor unit can produce more force) and an increase in the capacity of the muscle to supply ATP anaerobically.

Regarding this latter possibility, some studies have shown increased muscle stores of ATP and creatine phosphate and a slight improvement in the capacity of the muscle to break down glycogen [12, 18]. However, most of the increased ATP content of the muscles after training is thought to reflect a greater storage of ATP in the mitochondria. This mitochondrial ATP is not useful for intensive static contractions. Accordingly, it appears that most, if not all, of the improvement in holding time for a very intense static contraction is caused by gains in strength that allow the muscle to rest some motor units that would have been recruited immediately to maintain the contraction prior to training. Since gains in holding time for such intense static contractions are rather modest, there is little reason to believe that factors other than strength improvements are involved in these gains in anaerobic capacity.

Moderate Static Contractions

For static contractions held at less than 60 per cent of maximal strength, substantial training effects can be shown. Much of this gain in anaerobic capacity is undoubtedly caused by a greater strength of individual motor units, so that fewer need to be recruited at any one time after training. But other factors also probably play a role. These factors include a greater potential of the trained muscle to produce energy, an improved blood supply, a reduced production of lactic acid early in the work, and perhaps a greater tolerance to the fatiguing effects of lactic acid later in the effort.

Little direct evidence is available, but it seems likely that muscles trained for anaerobic endurance have greater stores of glycogen and creatine phosphate which can be heavily used if the contraction is greater than about 20 per cent of the maximal strength (the level at which arterial blood flow begins to be reduced). Thus, trained muscles probably are better equipped to provide energy for sustained contractions than are untrained muscles.

For static workloads up to about 60 per cent of maximum strength, an improved circulation of blood to working muscles may contribute to enhanced endurance performance if the relative intensity of the contraction is less after training because of improved strength. In other words, prior to training, maintenance of a 15 kilogram load may have required 50 per cent of one's maximal strength, whereas after training the same load may demand only 30 per cent of a maximal contraction. Thus, a corresponding lesser restriction of blood flow to the working muscles would have been accomplished.

Assuming that trained muscles have a greater oxygen supply during heavy work, less demand is placed upon the anaerobic breakdown of muscle glycogen to lactic acid for energy supply. Consequently, the trained individual produces less lactic acid for a static contraction that produces a given force. If lactic acid limited performance prior to training [16], it is then less apt to cause fatigue after training. With heavier static work that eventually does lead to a buildup of lactic acid, the trained person may not tire until he has a greater level of acid in his tissues than the untrained has. This may indicate a better ability to tolerate the lactic acid, or it may reflect a greater muscle glycogen store and improved capacity to break down glycogen to form lactic acid.

Dynamic Contractions

An enhanced anaerobic capacity for dynamic contractions after training is brought about by most of the mechanisms described for improvements in static endurance. Improved strength of individual motor units will allow the same force to be exerted by fewer motor units contracting at one time. Both a greater capacity to produce energy and a greater tolerance to lactic acid or greater capacity to produce lactic acid could contribute to improved capacity for both moderate and heavy dynamic contractions. There is evidence that training can increase both total [15] and alactic oxygen debt capacities (9). Enhancements have also been shown in the capacity to store glycogen (2, 31) and to catabolize it to lactic acid [27]. These changes are sometimes associated with alterations in the activities of enzymes responsible for glycogen synthesis and degradation [12, 26, 30, 31].

In addition, better circulation is probably important in bringing more oxygen to, and removing more metabolic "waste" products from, muscles that are performing heavy (but not lighter) dynamic contractions. For lighter contractions a somewhat reduced blood supply after training has been reported; trained muscle apparently can extract a greater percentage of the oxygen delivered. Thus, more ATP is produced by aerobic metabolism, so that less lactic acid has to be produced by anaerobic glycolysis.

For skilled movements that require a substantial amount of neuromuscular coordination, an additional mechanism is a major factor in improved endurance. That factor is the elimination of unnecessary contractions by muscles that are not required to perform the movement under the newly acquired skill pattern. For example, a beginning swimmer uses many unnecessary muscles as he begins to develop skill. Those extraneous muscle contractions are gradually eliminated as the swimmer learns to use only the muscles actually required. As the swimmer's skill develops, he finds that his endurance improves, too. Part of that improved endurance can be attributed to the fact that extraneous muscle contractions have been eliminated. Thus, there is less oxygen uptake and less of a demand for blood flow to serve the unneeded muscle fibers. More oxygen and blood are then available for the fibers that are required for performance.

REVIEW QUESTIONS

1. List five athletic events and three daily activities that rely heavily on anaerobic metabolism for energy supply.
2. Briefly describe the techniques which can be used in the laboratory and in the school setting to evaluate one's potential for performing anaerobic exercise.
3. Explain how interval training can be used to maintain the quality of work performed in a training session. What implications does this maintenance of quality have for any neural adaptations that may occur with training?

4. Explain why a stronger child has greater endurance in sawing wood than a weaker child. ✔
5. List the principles of training for anaerobic endurance and explain each one.
6. Based on appropriate physiological principles, design an interval training program for an anaerobic activity of your choice. Design the program for one week in the middle of the training season.

REFERENCES

[1] Asmussen, E. Growth in muscular strength and power. In G. L. Rarick, ed., *Physical Activity—Human Growth and Development.* New York: Academic Press, Inc., 1973, pp. 60–79.

[2] Åstrand, P.-O., and K. Rodahl. *Textbook of Work Physiology,* 2nd ed. New York: McGraw-Hill Book Company, 1977.

[3] Caizzo, V. J., and C. R. Kyle. The effect of external loading upon power output in stair climbing. *European Journal of Applied Physiology,* 1980, **44:**217–222.

[4] Clark, D. H. Adaptations in strength and muscular endurance resulting from exercise. *Exercise and Sport Sciences Reviews,* 1973, **1:**73–102.

[5] deVries, H. A. *Physiology of Exercise for Physical Education and Athletics,* 3rd ed. Dubuque, Iowa: William C Brown Company, Publishers, 1980.

[6] di Prampero, P. E. The alactic oxygen debt: its power, capacity, and efficiency. In B. Pernow and B. Saltin, eds., *Muscle Metabolism During Exercise.* New York: Plenum Publishing Corporation, 1971, pp. 371–382.

[7] di Prampero, P. E., and P. Mognoni. Maximal anaerobic power in man. In E. Jokl, ed., *Medicine and Sport,* Vol. 13. Basel: S. Karger, 1981, pp. 38–44.

[8] di Prampero, P. E., L. Peeters, and R. Margaria. Alactic oxygen debt and lactic acid production after exhausting exercise in man. *Journal of Applied Physiology,* 1973, **34:**628–632.

[9] Fox, E. L. Differences in metabolic alterations with sprint versus endurance interval training programs. In H. Howald and J. R. Poortmans, eds., *Metabolic Adaptation to Prolonged Physical Exercise.* Basel: Birkhauser Verlag, 1975, pp. 119–126.

[10] Fox, E. L., and D. K. Mathews. *Interval Training*—Conditioning for Sports and General Fitness. Philadelphia: W. B. Saunders Company, 1974.

[11] Funderburk, C. F., S. G. Hipskind, R. C. Welton, and A. R. Lind. Development of, and recovery from fatigue induced by static effort at various tensions. *Journal of Applied Physiology,* 1974, **37:**392–396.

[12] Gollnick, P. D., and L. Hermansen. Biochemical Adaptations to exercise: anaerobic metabolism. *Exercise and Sport Sciences Reviews,* 1973, **1:**1–43.

[13] Graham, T. E., and G. M. Andrew. The variability of repeated measurements of oxygen debt in man following a maximal treadmill exercise. *Medicine and Science in Sports,* 1973, **5:**73–78.

[14] Henriksson, J., and J. S. Reitman. Quantitative measures of enzyme activities in type I and type II muscle fibres of man after training. *Acta Physiologica Scandinavica,* 1976, **97:**392–397.

[15] Hermansen, L. Anaerobic energy release. *Medicine and Science in Sports,* 1969, **1:**32–38.

[16] Hermansen, L. Muscular fatigue during maximal exercise of short duration. In E. Jokl, ed., *Medicine and Sport.* Basel: S. Karger, 1981, pp. 45–52.

[17] Hermansen, L., and O. Vaage. Lactate disappearace and glycogen synthesis in human muscle after maximal exercise. *American Journal of Physiology,* 1977, **233:**E422–E429.

[18] Houston, M. E., and J. A. Thomson. The response of endurance-adapted adults to intense anaerobic training. *European Journal of Applied Physiology,* 1977, **36:**207–213.

[19] Hudlicka, O. Differences in development of fatigue in slow and fast muscles. In J. Keul, ed., *Limiting Factors of Physical Performance.* Stuttgart: Georg Thieme, Publishers, 1973, pp. 36–41.

[20] Jacobs, I. The effects of thermal dehydration on performance of the Wingate anaerobic test. *International Journal of Sports Medicine,* 1980, **1:**21–24.

[21] Katch, V., and F. M. Henry. Prediction of running performance from maximal oxygen debt and intake. *Medicine and Science in Sports,* 1972, **4:**187–191.

[22] Komi, P. V., H. Rusko, J. Vos, and V. Vihko. Anaerobic performance capacity in athletes. *Acta Physiologica Scandinavica,* 1977, **100:**107–114.

[23] Margaria, R., P. Cerretelli, P. E. di Prampero, C. Massari, and G. Torelli. Kinetics and mechanism of oxygen debt contraction in man. *Journal of Applied Physiology,* 1963, **18:**371–377.

[24] Pendergast, D., P. Cerretelli, and D. W. Rennie. Aerobic and glycolytic metabolism in arm exercise. *Journal of Applied Physiology,* 1979, **47:**754–760.

[25] Saltin, B., and B. Essen. Muscle glycogen, lactate, ATP, and CP in intermittent exercise. In B. Pernow and B. Saltin, eds., *Muscle Metabolism During Exercise.* New York: Plenum Publishing Corporation, 1971, pp. 419–424.

[26] Saubert IV, C. W., R. B. Armstrong, R. E. Shepherd, and P. D. Gollnick. Anaerobic enzyme adaptations to sprint training in rats. *Pflügers Archiv,* 1973, **341:**305–312.

[27] Simonsen, E., ed. *Physiology of Work Capacity and Fatigue.* Springfield, Ill.: Charles C Thomas, Publisher, 1971.

[28] Staff. The Wingate anaerobic test—general description. (Unpublished manuscript.) *Department of Research and Sports Medicine,* Wingate Institute, Israel, 1981.

[29] Stamford, B. A., A. Weltman, R. Moffatt, and S. Sady. Exercise recovery above and below anaerobic threshold following maximal work. *Journal of Applied Physiology,* 1981, **51:**840–844.

[30] Staudte, H. W., G. U. Exner, and D. Pette. Effects of short-term, high intensity (sprint) training on some contractile and metabolic characteristics of fast and slow muscle of the rat. *Pflügers Archiv,* 1973, **344:**159–168.

[31] Taylor, A. W. The effects of exercise and training on the activities of human skeletal-muscle, glycogen-cycle enzymes. In H. Howald and J. R. Poortmans, eds., *Metabolic Adaptation to Prolonged Physical Exercise.* Basel: Birkhauser Verlag, 1975, pp. 451–462.

[32] Tesch, P. A., D. S. Sharp, and W. L. Daniels. Influence of fiber type composition and capillary density on onset of blood lactate accumulation. *International Journal of Sports Medicine,* 1981, **2:**252–255.

[33] Wasserman, K., B. J. Whipp, S. N. Koyal, and W. L. Beaver. Anaerobic threshold and respiratory gas exchange during exercise. *Journal of Applied Physiology,* 1973, **35:**236–243.

CHAPTER
15

Neuromuscular Fatigue and Delayed Muscular Soreness After Exercise

MUSCULAR fatigue is the inability to maintain or repeat the production of a given force by muscular contraction. Fatigue of muscles during physical exercise has been experienced by everyone. Its rate of onset often determines who will be a champion athlete, who will be the most productive laborer, and who will become the most easily frustrated when attempting to become physically fit. Accordingly, an examination of some of the possible mechanisms of fatigue is warranted in a text on exercise physiology. Because muscular fatigue is often studied under relatively anaerobic conditions of exercise, it seems especially appropriate to consider fatigue in a chapter following the analysis of anaerobic capacity.

Anatomical Site of Fatigue

The limitation on one's ability to maintain muscular contractions at a given level of force conceivably could lie in 1) *the central nervous system,* 2) *the final motor neuron,* 3) *the neuromuscular junction,* or 4) *the muscle.* (See Fig. 15.1.) Much of the material in this chapter describes the evidence for and against each of these structures as potential sites of neuromuscular fatigue. It is clear that we do not presently know enough about fatigue to state that any one site or mechanism can account for fatigue in all types of exercise. The reader should keep in mind that fatigue is a complex phenomenon that may have many different causes [42].

311

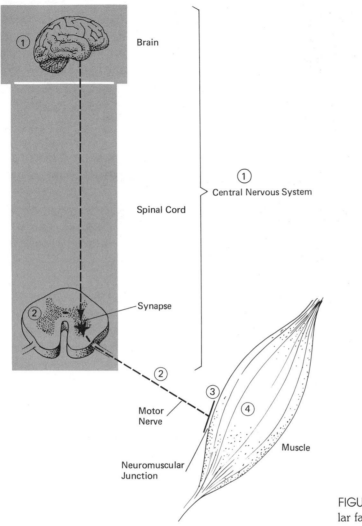

FIGURE 15.1. Possible sites of muscular fatigue.

Evidence That the Central Nervous System May Be a Site of Neuromuscular Fatigue

Effects of Electrical Stimulation after Voluntary Fatigue. An experiment used to show that the fatigue mechanism is located in the brain or spinal cord involves exhausting a muscle with voluntary isometric contractions and then restoring the contractile force of the muscle by electrically stimulating the motor nerve to the muscle [9, 31]. This restoration of force demonstrates that the "fatigued" muscle, the motor nerve, and the neuromuscular junction are able to function if stimulated by an adequate signal. Therefore, it must have been a weakened signal from the central nervous system that caused the voluntary fatigue. Such experiments provide evidence that at least certain types of fatigue involve functional defects in the central nervous system.

Effects of Mental Activity on Fatigue.   Another experiment performed to demonstrate a central nervous system component of fatigue is one in which mental activity is manipulated during sustained exercise. If a change in fatigue pattern occurs after a change in mental activity, it is considered evidence that central nervous system function influences fatigue. In one such case, subjects improved their endurance to repeated isometric contractions by 46 per cent when they performed mental arithmetic during the exercise [39]. On the other hand, contrary to what might be expected, encouragement by cheering hastened the onset of fatigue [44]. In each of these examples, it is presumed that activity in higher centers of the brain somehow enhances or interferes with the signals delivered by the motor nerves to the contracting muscles.

Evidence from Electromyography (EMG).   The electromyogram (EMG) is a record of the electrical activity (action potentials) in contracting motor units. Totally inactive muscles are electrically silent. The EMG activity is monitored by electrodes placed on the skin above a muscle or inserted directly into muscle fibers. Reduced EMG activity suggests that fewer or weaker nerve signals have been delivered to the muscle to stimulate contraction; greater EMG activity is a sign that the muscle has been excited by more frequent or stronger nerve signals.

The EMG can give some clues about the site of fatigue. Generally, if EMG activity is progressively reduced as muscle fatigue develops, less stimulation must be reaching the muscle fibers (Fig. 15.2 A). In this case, it may be assumed that the site of fatigue is in the neuromuscular junction or the nervous system because the nerve signal is not getting to the muscle. On the other hand, if the EMG is not reduced with declining muscular force, it might be concluded that the fatigue site is in the muscle (Fig. 15.2 B). If the *total* EMG activity is unchanged but the *pattern* of EMG activity changes, perhaps to a lower frequency, it would appear that the neuromuscular junction continues to function but that the central nervous system output has been altered [8, 36, 38, 54].

Evidence That the Motor Nerve Is Not a Site of Fatigue

The only potential fatigue site that scientific experiments seem to have ruled out is the motor nerve that conducts the stimulus from the spinal cord to the muscle. It is exceedingly difficult to stimulate this nerve to the point where it fails to conduct an impulse; muscular fatigue always precedes nerve fatigue, even at high rates of stimulation [50]:

Evidence That the Neuromuscular Junction May Be a Site of Fatigue

There is evidence that the site of fatigue in some circumstances is located either in the neuromuscular junction, in the coupling of the action potential to contraction (presumably by affecting calcium release from the sarcoplasmic reticulum), or in the contractile process itself [51]. It was shown that EMG activity declined with the onset of fatigue, whether that fatigue was caused by *maximal* sustained voluntary contractions or by *electrical stimulation* of the nerve. This implicates the neuromuscular junction in the

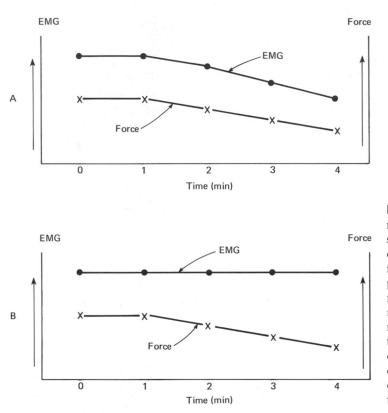

FIGURE 15.2. Schematic representation of possible record of surface electromyogram (EMG) during development of muscular fatigue. A. EMG activity declines progressively with decline in force, suggesting failure of the nervous system or the neuromuscular junction. B. EMG activity remains steady as force declines, suggesting failure of contractile process or failure of coupling of action potential to the contractile process.

fatigue process because the EMG activity of the muscle should not have been diminished during electrical stimulation if the neuromuscular junction was still functioning properly. However, a second phase of the fatigue process was shown where the continued decline in contractile force occurred more rapidly than the decrement in EMG. Accordingly, this phase of the fatigue process seems to rest in the muscle and not in the neuromuscular junction. Supposedly, higher threshold motor units consisting of fast twitch muscle fibers are more susceptible to junctional fatigue, whereas lower threshold slow twitch fibers eventually succumb to fatigue processes in the muscle fibers themselves. The neuromuscular junction failure is thought to be due to a diminished release of the chemical transmitter acetylcholine from the nerve ending. Possibilities for failure in the muscle are discussed in the following section.

Evidence That the Muscle May Be a Site of Fatigue

If an exercise physiologist were asked to pick the most likely single site of fatigue, he or she would probably choose the contractile process in the muscle. There are many experimental studies that demonstrate a rather straightforward relationship between the depletion of energy sources such as creatine phosphate and glycogen and the progression of fatigue [6, 30, 35, 36, 37, 49]. These relationships suggest, but do not prove, that fatigue is caused by a lack of energy stores to replenish the ATP needed for continued muscle contraction. It is also possible, of course, that the relationship be-

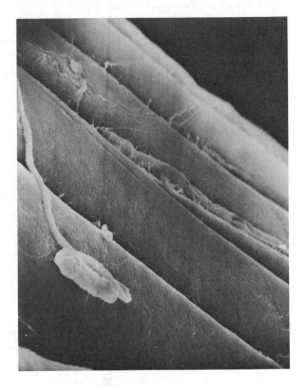

FIGURE 15.3. Stereo electron micrograph showing surfaces of four muscle fibers with white nerve fibril and large motor end-plate on lowest muscle fiber. (Courtesy of R. E. Carrow, W. W. Heusner and W. D. Van Huss, Michigan State University, E. Lansing, Michigan.)

tween energy store depletion and fatigue is merely associative and not causative. Nevertheless, because this relationship is so consistent, and because there are so few other reproducibly demonstrated relationships with fatigue, the depletion of energy stores remains one of the most accepted explanations for fatigue. Another commonly accepted explanation for fatigue is the accumulation of lactic acid in the muscle. Again, there is a large body of evidence to support this notion [32, 46].

Fatigue in Activities That Can Be Sustained Less Than 10 Seconds. For maximal or near-maximal exercise that can be sustained less than 10 seconds, oxygen delivery to the muscles is of limited importance. This is so because the rate of energy expenditure is too high to be met aerobically or because in static contractions above 60–70 per cent of maximal strength, blood flow is shut off by the strongly contracted muscles [22]. What is important in these strenuous contractions is the rate at which ATP can be replenished by anaerobic metabolism, that is, by the anaerobic breakdown of creatine phosphate and muscle glycogen.

When energy stores in muscles are measured after contractions that can be maintained for less than 10 seconds, it is unusual to find a severe depletion of muscle glycogen, and only 20–50 per cent of the ATP and creatine phosphate stores may be depleted [6]. Therefore, it seems likely that the *rate* of ATP utilization during severe muscle contractions is simply too great to be met by resupply from muscle stores of ATP and creatine phosphate [16]. In other words, the making and breaking of actin-myosin cross bridges is happening too rapidly for the transfer of energy from stored ATP and creatine phosphate to keep pace. The work must slow down or stop so that ATP can move to the cross bridges from nearby storage sites.

Fatigue in Activities That Can Be Sustained Between 10 Seconds and 2–3 Minutes. For exercise that can be sustained for longer than 10 seconds but less than about 2–3 minutes, a substantial drop in creatine phosphate stores (perhaps greater than 90 per cent) can be measured along with a 30–40 per cent decrease in ATP [6, 23, 35]. Because much of the ATP seems to be stored in the mitochondria, the sarcoplasmic reticulum, and in other compartments, a rather small fraction of the ATP is available for muscle contraction. Therefore, it appears that creatine phosphate depletion may limit the ability of the muscles to sustain contractions at these high loads. Another factor to consider is that lactic acid accumulates rapidly during intensive exercise of short duration and may contribute to fatigue. As lactic acid is produced in anaerobic glycolysis, it causes a reduction in the intracellular pH of the muscle to values as low as 6.4, compared to an intracellular pH at rest of about 7.0 [46]. At such a low pH, the activity of phosphofructokinase, an important enzyme in glycolysis, is markedly reduced. Therefore, the replenishment of ATP by glycolysis may also be reduced when lactic acid builds up with strenuous exercise. Thus, for exhaustive exercise sustained between 10 seconds and 2–3 minutes, the likely causes of fatigue are creatine phosphate depletion and lactic acid accumulation.

Fatigue in Activities That Can Be Sustained Between 3 and 15 Minutes— The Case for Lactic Acid as a Fatigue Factor. Physical exercise that can be sustained for 3–15 minutes does not seem to be limited by depletion of either ATP, creatine phosphate, or glycogen. Although there is a large fall in creatine phosphate levels in the muscles, this reduction is similar for exercise that can be sustained for 6–7 minutes and for exercise lasting 20–25 minutes [35]. (See Fig. 15.4.) Accordingly, if creatine phosphate depletion were the limiting factor for this type of exercise, it should be impossible to continue working beyond 6–7 minutes. Muscle glycogen falls by only 10–30 per cent in work of less than 15 minutes' duration [49]. Therefore, since it is widely agreed that neither fat nor blood glucose makes a significant contribution to activity that leads to exhaustion in less than 15 minutes, it seems that some factor other than depletion of energy reserves limits exercise of 3–15 minutes' duration. Perhaps lactic acid accumulation is that factor.

Lactic Acid Accumulation in Muscles. The theory that lactic acid accumulation in the muscles limits muscular performance has been widely held since at least 1935 [50]. There are several reasons why this idea has achieved such popularity. With

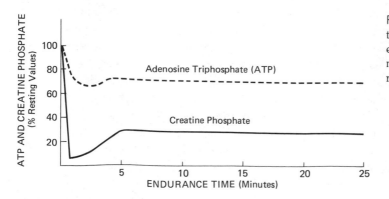

FIGURE 15.4. ATP and creatine phosphate depletion with exercise sustained for 1–25 minutes. Data primarily from reference 35.

most types of heavy exercise, fatigue is associated with high levels of lactic acid, and the *rate* of lactic and pyruvic acid accumulation in the working muscles is very closely related to the intensity of contractions [2]. This relationship is shown in Fig. 15.5; it demonstrates that the time one can hold an isometric contraction decreases with increasing load and increasing *rate* of acid accumulation in the muscle. Other evidence which supports the idea that the accumulation of lactic acid leads to fatigue is the strong relationship between the concentration of lactic acid in muscle and the time course of fatigue development and recovery [19, 20, 36]. As illustrated in Fig. 15.6, the force produced by a muscle progressively decreases as lactic acid concentration increases; also, the force generated progressively recovers as lactic acid concentration is reduced. It has also been shown that fatigue with the legs occurs earlier if previous exercise with the arms has raised the circulating lactic acid level in the blood [52].

The effect of lactic acid on promoting early fatigue is probably the result of the accumulation of hydrogen ions (H+), which lowers the pH of the muscle [19, 46, 47, 48]. One of the effects of such a reduction in pH is a decrease in the binding of calcium to troponin, thereby reducing the activation of actin-myosin cross bridges in muscle contraction [7, 11, 19, 23]. Also, several key enzymes of glycolysis, including glycogen phosphorylase and phosphofructokinase, are inhibited by excess acidity [6, 23, 46]. This means that less ATP can be replenished by glycogen breakdown when lactic acid levels are high. Finally, it has been shown that if body fluid pH is made more acidic by the consumption of ammonium chloride capsules before exercise, exercise endurance is markedly diminished; however, upon administration of sodium bicarbonate (an alkaline substance), endurance is increased [33]. Thus, there is a large body of evidence that lactic acid accumulation is causally related to fatigue in exercise of 3–15 minutes' duration.

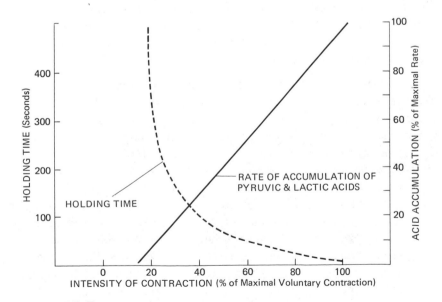

FIGURE 15.5. Isometric contraction holding times and rates of accumulation of lactic and pyruvic acids at various intensities of muscular contraction. Data from reference 2.

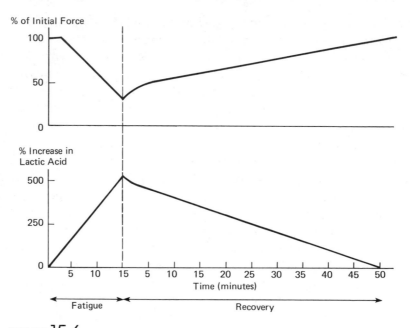

FIGURE 15.6. The relationship between lactic acid concentration in muscle and the time course of fatigue and recovery. Data from reference 19.

Fatigue in Activities That Can Be Sustained Between 15 and 60 Minutes. There does not seem to be a single factor that is strongly associated with the onset of fatigue in exhaustive exercise of 15–60 minutes' duration. Lactic acid accumulation and glycogen depletion are less than maximal in this type of exercise [36]. It has been suggested that some combination of a modest increase in lactic acid, a modest depletion of muscle glycogen, and an increase in body temperature may be sufficient to cause fatigue in these case [36].

Fatigue in Activities That Can Be Sustained Between 1 and 4 Hours. It is very likely that exercise which leads to exhaustion in 1–4 hours is limited by the stores of glycogen in the exercising muscles [36, 49]. This type of activity typically requires an oxygen cost equivalent to 70–90 per cent of one's maximal oxygen uptake. Numerous studies have shown that manipulation of glycogen stores by diet and exercise can have a substantial effect on endurance [4, 29]. The association between endurance time and glycogen stores in exercising muscles is shown in Fig. 15.7. It should be noted that glycogen is likely to be depleted earlier in untrained persons, who obtain more of their energy from carbohydrate and less from fatty acids, compared to those who are trained. Also, activities (such as cycling) that require more intensive contractions of a particular muscle (such as the vastus lateralis) lead to earlier glycogen depletion in that muscle than activities (such as running) that require less intensive localized muscular contractions.

In situations where a person becomes dehydrated during prolonged exercise in the heat, a failure of temperature regulation may bring on fatigue by heat exhaustion before glycogen depletion is severe.

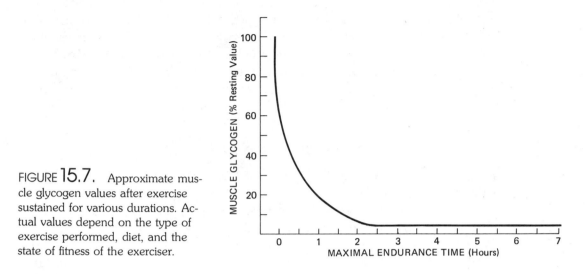

FIGURE 15.7. Approximate muscle glycogen values after exercise sustained for various durations. Actual values depend on the type of exercise performed, diet, and the state of fitness of the exerciser.

Fatigue in Activities That Can Be Sustained More Than 4 Hours. If exercise leads to exhaustion after 4 hours, it is possible that fatigue may be caused by muscle glycogen depletion, by liver glycogen depletion and inadequate delivery of blood glucose to the nervous system [30], and/or by failure of temperature regulation. Blood glucose is usually maintained at relatively normal levels up to 90–120 minutes of exercise at 65 per cent of maximal oxygen uptake.

Other Factors Associated with Neuromuscular Fatigue

Muscle Fiber Type Distribution and Fatigue

Fast twitch motor units are easily fatigued compared to slow twitch units [36, 38, 54]. Persons with high percentages of slow twitch fibers tend to have low maximal strength, but they can reproduce maximal contractions after brief rest periods for a long time compared to stronger persons with higher proportions of fast twitch fibers. Some authorities believe that the changes in EMG activity which occur early in the development of fatigue, especially in subjects with greater percentages of fast twitch fibers, may be a reflection of the early fatigue of the fast twitch motor units [54].

Calcium Accumulation by Transverse Tubules

The transverse tubules (T-tubules) of skeletal muscle are the channels which conduct action potentials from the sarcolemma to the sarcoplasmic reticulum. The action potentials trigger the release of calcium ions from the sarcoplasmic reticulum; the calcium in turn binds with troponin to start the contractile process. As fatigue develops in stimulated muscles, it has been shown that calcium progressively accumulates in the transverse tubules [7]. This means that less calcium is then available for release from the sarcoplasmic reticulum to initiate further muscle contraction. Therefore, it is possible that fatigue may ultimately be caused by insufficient calcium to initiate contraction. Increased lactic acid, depletion of creatine phosphate, depletion of glycogen, increased temperature, and other factors may simply accelerate the accumulation of calcium by the transverse tubules.

Ischemia and Hypoxia

Ischemia is the condition of diminished blood supply to a tissue because of some obstruction of arterial blood flow, whereas *hypoxia* is a deficiency of oxygen that can be caused either by ischemia, by breathing air low in oxygen content, or by other factors. Both ischemia and hypoxia can hasten the onset of fatigue, but their relative importance under normal exercise conditions is not fully established [5]. Ischemia produced by the inflation of a blood pressure cuff around a limb decreases endurance time in all but very brief, near-maximal dynamic contractions and in all static contractions that require less than about 60–70 per cent of one's maximal strength to maintain. These exceptions are the types of contractions that are maintained without a major contribution of aerobic energy metabolism. Dynamic contractions lasting only a few seconds obtain energy at the expense of ATP and creatine phosphate, and static contractions held at greater than 60–70 per cent of one's maximal strength completely block the flow of blood to the muscles by compressing the arteries so that the blood pressure cuff has no additional effect [22].

Likewise, if persons breathe a gas mixture that has an abnormally low content of oxygen while performing exercise, endurance time will decrease except in anaerobic activities [34]. Accordingly, because ischemia produces hypoxia, it is usually assumed that ischemia reduces endurance time by causing a state of hypoxia in the exercising muscles. However, some workers suggest that the adverse effect of ischemia on endurance is not caused by hypoxia but, rather, by a distruption of afferent nerve impulses from the working muscles or a failure of the circulation to remove lactic acid and other "waste" products of metabolism. Experiments that have manipulated the amount of oxygen delivered to the working muscles have, in fact, led some to the conclusion that hypoxia does not limit the endurance of muscles under normal exercise conditions where the exerciser breathes normal concentrations of oxygen [34]. These experiments have mainly been concerned with *dynamic* work. In this type of work, hypoxia may not develop because blood flow is not drastically reduced as in intense static contractions. The bulk of the evidence points to ischemic hypoxia as a main cause of fatigue in strenuous *isometric* contractions.

Temperature

The temperature of working muscles has a somewhat variable effect on the onset of fatigue. Thus, warmup seems to prolong *brief,* strenuous exercise on a treadmill, probably because the increased body temperature is associated with increased blood flow to the muscles and because the enzymes of energy metabolism are somewhat more active at higher temperatures.

An adverse effect of increased body temperature as far as *prolonged* exercise is concerned is that blood must be diverted from working muscles to the skin for purposes of cooling the body. Accordingly, after a muscle reaches about 38° or 39°C., additional heat is detrimental because it leads to a greater shift of blood away from the working muscles to the skin [50]. As the blood is diverted to skin, the working muscles are deprived of some of the oxygen needed for aerobic energy metabolism, and more lactic acid is produced as anaerobic glycolysis contributes increasingly to ATP replenishment. This lactic acid, in turn, may further accelerate the development of fatigue.

Pain and Motivation

Finally, sustained work can produce discomfort and sometimes pain that causes the exerciser to cease working before there is any evidence that the muscles themselves could no longer be stimulated to contract. The pain limitation to endurance is especially apparent in sustained static contractions. For example, when one attempts to hang from a horizontal bar for as long as possible, excruciating pain of the forearms and hands forces one to give up before there is any sign of muscle fatigue [18]. It is as though the motor nerves to the active muscles are receiving intensive volleys of inhibiting stimuli from the pain-sensing areas of the brain, so that no matter how greatly the subject wants to keep on hanging, he must ultimately drop from the bar. The exact cause of this type of pain is unknown.

There are, of course, great differences in the motivation levels of individuals, so that perseverance in an activity such as a "bar-hang" also varies greatly. Although there is no totally accurate method to test one's motivation to persevere in endurance exercise, physiologists sometimes check blood lactic acid levels after exertion to determine whether the subject persevered long enough to significantly elevate lactic acid levels.

In summary, muscular fatigue may have many causes depending upon the type of physical activity in question and upon individual factors such as motivation. Because it seems logical to expect that a specific malfunction in the contractile process or in nerve transmission should be a common cause of fatigue in all types of exercise, many have attempted to pinpoint a unique cause of fatigue that is applicable to all forms of physical activity. As we have seen, such attempts have not met with great success. Therefore, until some research breakthrough is made, we are forced to the intellectually unsatisfying conclusion that muscular fatigue is a phenomenon that may be caused by several different factors, and that some of these factors may bring about fatigue only when they act in concert with each other.

Muscle Soreness Caused by Exercise

Although certain kinds of strenuous efforts are associated with muscle pain *during* the exercise period, muscle soreness often develops some hours or even days *after* exertion. The soreness that begins as fatigue approaches during heavy contractions, especially those that have a large static component, is thought to be caused by an inadequate blood flow to the working muscles. This deprives the muscles of oxygen and fails to wash "pain substances" out of the muscles. There are several products of contraction that could build up in the muscles or tissue fluid surrounding the muscles and cause pain by stimulating nerve endings in the muscle or connective tissue within the muscle. Lactic acid and potassium, for example, can cause local pain when they are injected into a muscle. A lack of oxygen by itself does not cause muscular pain, but hypoxia does have an indirect effect by increasing the diffusion of substances out of capillaries into tissue fluid. This fluid accumulates in the tissue spaces, leading to swelling and consequent stimulation of pain nerve endings in the area of the swelling.

Delayed Soreness After Unaccustomed Exercise—The Role of Eccentric Contractions

It is curious that the greatest delayed soreness in muscles occurs in response to eccentric (lengthening) contractions, which are less difficult to perform with the same load than concentric contractions [3]. In a bench press, for example, soreness is much more likely to occur in a person who repeats only the lowering (eccentric) phase of the movement than in one who only raises the load, even though it is much more difficult to raise than to lower a given load. Because there is less electromyographic activity and less oxygen uptake with eccentric exercise [10], it appears that fewer (or different) motor units are activated or there is a lower frequency of motor unit recruitment during eccentric contractions than during concentric contractions. Therefore, each individual muscle fiber may produce greater force while lengthening than while shortening. If this is so, it seems probable that the individual fibers and their connective tissue attachments are under greater stress during the eccentric exercise and are thus more subject to disruption [3].

Possible Causes of Delayed Muscle Soreness

There are three common hypothetical explanations of the soreness that occurs usually a day or two after strenuous exercise—the lactic acid accumulation hypothesis, the muscle spasm hypothesis, and the tissue damage hypothesis.

The Lactic Acid Accumulation Hypothesis. It is well established that lactic acid accumulates to a greater extent in more intensive types of exercise and that more intensive exercise generally causes the greatest delayed muscle soreness. However, there are several lines of evidence which suggest that lactic acid has little to do with delayed soreness. *First,* lactic acid does not remain elevated above resting values more than 15–30 minutes after exercise [35], yet soreness typically is delayed until 24–48 hours following exercise. The onset of soreness is so far removed from the period of elevated lactic acid that it is difficult to believe that lactic acid could cause the soreness. *Second,* the greatest soreness accompanies eccentric contractions, which are associated with relatively slight lactic acid accumulation. *Third,* there are some activities which produce much soreness but essentially no lactic acid. As an example, consider an overweight, middle-aged, unfit person who begins a training program with a few vigorous straight-legged toe touching exercises. Within a day after the stretching, which causes little or no lactic acid production, the backs of the trainee's legs would be very sore. *Finally,* patients who have a hereditary absence of phosphorylase, an enzyme required for breaking down glycogen to lactic acid, still experience great muscle pain after strenuous contractions, in spite of a lack of lactic acid accumulation. Accordingly, it seems extremely unlikely that lactic acid accumulation can explain delayed muscular soreness after unaccustomed exercise.

The Muscle Spasm Hypothesis. Those who believe in the muscle spasm hypothesis say: a) that strenuous contractions cause a reduction in blood flow (ischemia) to the working muscles, b) that this ischemia in turn triggers the release of pain substances out of the muscle fibers into the tissue fluid where the pain substances stimulate nerve endings, and c) that the pain receptors cause reflex spastic contractions of the painful muscle fibers to produce further ischemia and continued release of pain substances to renew the pain cycle [15]. This hypothesis is sometimes [15], but not always [1], supported by electromyographic evidence that under some circumstances fatigued muscles may indeed continue to contract after exercise. Also, stretching of the muscles may reduce the contractile activity and the associated pain. However, it seems very unlikely that ischemia and postexercise spasms occur after all types of exercise that can result in pain. For example, in untrained persons the mere act of stretching in limbering-up exercises surely does not cause ischemia but can result in pain the next day. Therefore, the spasm-pain substance hypothesis is not a completely satisfactory explanation of all muscle pain caused by exercise.

The Tissue Damage Hypothesis. A more persuasive hypothesis is that free nerve endings are stimulated by swelling (edema) of muscle tissue after microscopic damage to a relatively few muscle fibers or their surrounding connective tissue. There are several reasons for believing that strenuous, unaccustomed exercise may cause some minor damage to muscle tissue. *First,* microscopic disruptions of myofibrils, especially of the Z-lines, have been observed in biopsy specimens from the calf muscles of men who ran down 10 flights of stairs 10 times [21]. (Note that running down stairs requires eccentric contractions of the calf muscles.) All of the subjects in this experiment suffered intense muscle discomfort, especially 2–3 days following the exercise. In addition, animal studies have shown evidence of muscle fiber damage after exhaustive exercise [53].

Second, myoglobin appears in the blood [43] and urine [1] of subjects who participate in strenuous activity. Since myoglobin is a large protein found only in muscle, its appearance in blood and urine suggests muscle damage. After training, there is less exercise-induced soreness; there is also less myoglobin released into the blood [43].

Third, large enzyme molecules such as lactic acid dehydrogenase and creatine phosphokinase leak out of the muscles into the blood to a much greater extent after eccentric exercise than after concentric exercise at the same absolute load. The appearance of these enzymes in the blood is widely viewed as an index of muscle fiber damage. Since delayed soreness is also much greater after the eccentric exercise, it therefore seems likely that tissue damage is a precursor to delayed soreness after exercise.

Fourth, there is substantial evidence that muscle protein degradation is accelerated for at least 6 hours after treadmill running or weight lifting [17]. This increased degradation of muscle protein may be a reflection of increased activity of *lysozymes,* enzymes which become especially active in response to cellular damage [53]).

Finally, it has been reported that connective tissue in skeletal muscle may be degraded by exercise that produces soreness [1]. This may be especially important in view of the suggestion that eccentric exercise (which causes the greatest soreness) places more stress on connective tissue than does concentric exercise [3].

Summary. There is little evidence to support the view that lactic acid accumulation is causally related to delayed muscle soreness. Muscle spasms may accompany soreness after certain types of exercise, but it is unlikely that ischemia and spasms occur in mild eccentric exercise which produces soreness. Such spasms may be a result of tissue damage and not the direct cause of soreness. Most of the evidence suggests that minor damage to muscle and/or connective tissue causes a gradual increase (over 12–48 hours) in the leakage of chemicals into the extracellular spaces of the muscle. These chemicals may directly stimulate free nerve endings in the tissues or cause a progressive swelling of the tissues that places pressure on the nerve endings and causes the discomfort reported as "stiffness," "soreness," or "pain."

Minimizing Muscle Soreness

Whatever the exact mechanism underlying muscle soreness may be, there are enough facts known about soreness to enable us to minimize its development. It is known that soreness is more apt to occur with relatively intense, phasic, or jerking movements which involve strenuous eccentric contractions. Also, soreness is more common in those who are undertaking an exercise program after a long period of inactive living. Therefore, a rational approach to the initiation of a fitness program is: Begin with *extremely* light activity that does not require any lunging or thrusting movements, conduct the exercise periods for only 15–20 minutes during the first few sessions, and progressively and slowly increase both the intensity and duration of the exercise sessions. This will allow the muscle fibers and the connective tissue in the muscle to have a chance to become toughened as an adaptive response to the training. Older trainees, especially, should be made aware of those activities that increase the risk of becoming sore. Vigorous attempts to bob down and touch the toes, all-out efforts to perform as many situps as possible, and repetitions of deep knee bends with a barbell on the shoulders are all the kinds of activities that new trainees should avoid in the early course of a fitness program. Slow, easy movements should be the rule at this stage of fitness improvement.

Muscle Cramps and Pain in the Side

There are many different origins of muscle cramps. These origins range from a central nervous system imbalance to a hypersensitive muscle membrane. Most cramps associated with extreme athletic exertion are probably caused by salt imbalances in the fluids surrounding the muscle fibers. A disruption in the normal relationships between sodium, potassium, and chloride concentrations inside and outside the muscle fiber can cause spastic contractions, as can a failure in the ability of the muscle to withdraw calcium from the myofibrils back into the sarcoplasmic reticulum so that the muscle can relax. Unfortunately, by the time one can begin to measure all these factors in the tissues, a cramp has usually passed away.

The same problem besets any research into the mechanism underlying the pain or stitch in the side that often is experienced during distance running. Because it is difficult to produce pain in the side with any reliability, it is almost impossible to measure any of the possible disruptions in function that may cause this pain. There seems to be no good reason to believe one of the commonly offered explanations of pain in the side over any of the others. Explanations that have been presented, often by word of mouth, from one generation of athletes to the next include: spasm of the diaphragm, spasm of the intercostal muscles of the ribcage, ischemic pain of abdominal organs because of reduced blood flow, swelling of the liver, stomach spasm, swelling of the spleen, and jouncing of abdominal organs during activity. Jouncing supposedly causes tension on nerves in the connective tissue that maintains the position of the abdominal organs in the abdominal cavity. Because there is so little objective evidence to support any of these proposed causes of pain in the side, one should pick one cause that is most attractive to him or contribute another. In the author's view, the "jouncing" explanation has some merit solely because pain in the side seems to be more common in distance running and even in motorcross competition than in other activities that are of a less "jouncing" nature. Also, this pain is felt more often when exercising soon after eating with extra weight in the stomach and intestines to intensify the "jouncing" phenomenon. However, there is no experimental evidence to support this opinion.

REVIEW QUESTIONS

1. Outline the possible sites of fatigue and describe the evidence that supports each of these possibilities.
2. Defend the statement that lactic acid accumulation is not the sole cause of fatigue in all types of exercise.
3. State your opinion about the cause of exercise-induced muscle soreness and support your opinion with evidence from the text, from your personal experiences, and from other sources available to you.
4. Poll the members of your class to determine by recall a) the nature of pain in the side they have experienced, b) whether there was "jouncing" associated with the pain or not, c) whether they probably had food in their stomachs during the activity, and d) whether they have discovered any way to relieve the pain. See if this information can lead the class to an alternate hypothesis about the cause of pain in the side.
5. Outline the possible mechanisms of fatigue described in this chapter.

REFERENCES

[1] Abraham, W. M. Factors in delayed muscle soreness. *Medicine and Science in Sports,* 1977, **9**:11–20
[2] Ahlborg, B., J. Bergstrom, L.-G. Ekelund, G. Guarnieri, R. C. Harris, E. Hultman, and L.-O. Nordesjo. Muscle metabolism during isometric exercise performed at constant force. *Journal of Applied Physiology,* 1972, **33**:224–228.

[3] Asmussen, E. Observations on experimental muscular soreness. *Acta Rheumatologica Scandinavica,* 1956, **2:** 109–116.

[4] Åstrand, P.-O., and K. Rodahl. *Textbook of Work Physiology,* 2nd ed., New York: McGraw-Hill, 1977.

[5] Barclay, J. K., and W. N. Stainsby. The role of blood flow in limiting maximal metabolic rate in muscle. *Medicine and Science in Sports,* 1975, **7:**116–119.

[6] Bergstrom, J., R. C. Harris, E. Hultman, and L.-O. Nordesjo. Energy-rich phosphagens in dynamic and static work. In B. Pernow and B. Saltin, eds., *Muscle Metabolism During Exercise.* New York: Plenum Press, 1971, pp. 341–355.

[7] Bianchi, C. P., and S. Narayan. Muscle fatigue and the role of transverse tubules. *Science,* 1982, **215:**295–296.

[8] Bigland-Ritchie, B., E. F. Donovan, and C. S. Roussos. Conduction velocity and EMG power spectrum changes in fatigue of sustained maximal efforts. *Journal of Applied Physiology,* 1981, **51:**1300–1305.

[9] Bigland-Ritchie, B., D.A. Jones, G. P. Hosking, and R. H. T. Edwards. Central and peripheral fatigue in sustained maximum voluntary contractions of human quadriceps. *Clinical Science and Molecular Medicine,* 1978, **54:**609–614.

[10] Bigland-Ritchie, B., and J. J. Woods. Integrated electromyogram and oxygen uptake during positive and negative work. *Journal of Physiology* (London), 1976, **260:**267–277.

[11] Bolitho Donaldson, S. K., and L. Hermansen. Differential, direct effects of H^+ on Ca^{++}-activated force of skinned fibers from the soleus, cardiac and adductor magnus muscles of rabbits. *Pflügers Archiv,* 1978, **376:**55–65.

[12] Ceretilli, P., and G. Ambrosoli, Limiting factors of anaerobic performance in man. In J. Keul, ed., *Limiting Factors of Physical Performance.* Stuttgart: Georg Thieme, Publishers, 1973, pp. 157–165.

[13] Clarkson, P. M., W. Kroll, and T. C. McBride. Plantar flexion fatigue and muscle fiber type in power and endurance athletes. *Medicine and Science in Sports and Exercise,* 1980, **12:**262–267.

[14] Davies, K. J. A., L. Packer, and G. A. Brooks. Biochemical adaptation of mitochondria, muscle, and whole-animal respiration to endurance training. *Archives of Biochemistry and Biophysics,* 1981, **209:**539–554.

[15] deVries, H. A. *Physiology of Exercise for Physical Education and Athletics,* 3rd Ed., Dubuque, Iowa: W. C. Brown, 1980.

[16] di Prampero, P. E. The alactic oxygen debt: Its power, capacity, and efficiency. In B. Pernow and B. Saltin, eds., *Muscle Metabolism During Exercise.* New York: Plenum Press, 1971, pp. 371–382.

[17] Dohm, G. L., R. T. Williams, G. J. Kasperek, and A. M. van Rij. Increased excretion of urea and N^r-methylhistidine by rats and humans after a bout of exercise. *Journal of Applied Physiology,* 1982, **52:**27–33.

[18] Elkus, R., and J. V. Basmajian. Endurance in hanging by the hands. *American Journal of Physical Medicine,* 1973, **52:**124–127.

[19] Fitts, R. H., and J. O. Holloszy. Lactate and contractile force in frog muscle during development of fatigue and recovery. *American Journal of Physiology,* 1976, **231:**430–433.

[20] Fitts, R. H., and J. O. Holloszy. Effects of fatigue and recovery on contractile properties of frog muscle. *Journal of Applied Physiology,* 1978, **45:**899–902.

[21] Friden, J., M. Sjostrom, and B. Ekblom. A morphological study of delayed muscle soreness. *Experientia,* 1981, **37:**506–507.

[22] Funderburk, C. F., S. G. Hipskind, R. C. Welton, and A. R. Lind. Development of and recovery from fatigue induced by static effort at various tensions. *Journal of Applied Physiology,* 1974, **37:**392–396.

[23] Gollnick, P. D., and L. Hermansen. Biochemical adaptations to exercise: anaerobic metabolism. *Exercise and Sport Sciences Reviews,* 1973, **1:**1–43.

[24] Haralambie, G. Importance of humoral changes to physical performance. In J. Keul, ed., *Limiting Factors of Physical Performance.* Stuttgart: Georg Thieme Publishers, 1973, pp. 189–200.

[25] Harris, R. C., E. Hultman, and K. Sahlin. Glycolytic intermediates in human muscle after isometric contraction. *Pflügers Archiv,* 1981, **389:**277–282.

[26] Hermansen, L. Anaerobic energy release. *Medicine and Science in Sports,* 1969, **1:** 32–38.

[27] Hermansen, L. Lactate disappearance and glycogen synthesis in human muscle after maximal exercise. *American Journal of Physiology,* 1977, **233:**E422–E429.

[28] Heuer, H. Selective fatigue in the human motor system. *Psychological Research,* 1980, **41:**345–354.

[29] Hultman, E., and J. Bergstrom. Local energy-supplying substrates as limiting factors in different types of leg muscle work in normal man. In J. Keul, ed., *Limiting Factors of Physical Performance.* Stuttgart: Georg Thieme, Publishers, 1973, pp. 113–125.

[30] Hultman, E., and L. Nilsson. Liver glycogen as a glucose-supplying source during exercise. In J. Keul, ed., *Limiting Factors in Physical Performance.* Stuttgart: George Thieme, Publishers, 1973, pp. 179–189.

[31] Ikai, M., and K. Yabe. Training effect of muscular endurance by means of voluntary and electrical stimulation. *European Journal of Applied Physiology,* 1969, **28:**55–60.

[32] Jacobs, I. Lactate, muscle glycogen and exercise performance in man. *Acta Physiologica Scandinavica,* Supplementum 495, 1981, 1–35.

[33] Jones, N. L., J. R. Sutton, R. Taylor, and C. J. Toews. Effect of pH on cardiorespiratory and metabolic responses to exercise. *Journal of Applied Physiology,* 1977, **43:**959–964.

[34] Kaijser, L. Oxygen supply as a limiting factor in physical performance. In J. Keul, ed., *Limiting Factors of Physical Performance.* Stuttgart: Georg Thieme, Publishers, 1973, pp. 145–156.

[35] Karlsson, J. Muscle ATP, CP, and lactate in submaximal and maximal exercise. In B. Pernow and B. Saltin, eds., *Muscle Metabolism During Exercise.* New York: Plenum Press, 1971, pp. 383–395.

[36] Karlsson, J. Localized muscular fatigue: role of muscle metabolism and substrate depletion. *Exercise and Sport Sciences Reviews,* 1979, **7:**1–42.

[37] Karlsson, J., L.-O. Nordesjo, L. Jorfeldt, and B. Saltin. Muscle lactate, ATP, and CP levels during exercise after physical training in man. *Journal of Applied Physiology,* 1972, **33:**199–203.

[38] Komi, P. V., and P. Tesch. EMG frequency spectrum, muscle structure, and fatigue during dynamic contractions in man. *European Journal of Applied Physiology,* 1979, **42:**41–50.

[39] Kotz, Y. M., I. M. Rodionov, B. F. Sitnikov, V. I. Tkhorevsky, and O. L. Vinogradova. On the mechanism of an increase of muscle performance and of vasodilation during emotional stress in man. *Pflügers Archiv,* 1978, **373:**211–218.

[40] Kurihara, T., and J. E. Brooks. The mechanism of neuromuscular fatigue. *Archives of Neurology,* 1975, **32:**168–174.

[41] Nilsson, J., P. Tesch, and A. Thorstensson. Fatigue and EMG of repeated fast voluntary contractions in man. *Acta Physiologica Scandinavica,* 1977, **101:**194–198.

[42] Porter, R., and J. Whelan, eds., *Human Muscle Fatigue: Physiological Mechanisms,* Ciba Foundation symposium 82. London: Pitman Medical Limited, 1981.

[43] Ritter, W. S., M. J. Stone, and J. T. Willerson. Reduction in exertional myoglobinemia after physical conditioning. *Archives of Internal Medicine,* 1979, **139:**644–647.

[44] Rube, N., and N. H. Secher. Paradoxical influence of encouragement on muscle fatigue. *European Journal of Applied Physiology,* 1981, **46:**1–7.

[45] Ruegg, J. C. Mechanochemical energy coupling. In J. Keul, ed., *Limiting Factors of Physical Performance.* Stuttgart: Georg Thieme, Publishers, 1973, pp. 63–66.

[46] Sahlin, K. Intracellular pH and energy metabolism in skeletal muscle of man. *Acta Physiologica Scandinavica,* Supplementum 455, 1978, pp. 1–56.

[47] Sahlin, K., R. C. Harris, and E. Hultman. Resynthesis of creatine phosphate in human muscle after exercise in relation to intramuscular pH and availability of oxygen. *Scandinavian Journal of Clinical and Laboratory Investigation,* 1979, **39:**551–558.

[48] Sahlin, K., R. C. Harris, B. Nylind, and E. Hultman. Lactate content and pH in muscle samples obtained after dynamic exercise. *Pflügers Archiv,* 1976, **367:**143–149.

[49] Saltin, B., and J. Karlsson. Muscle glycogen utilization during work of different intensities. In B. Pernow and B. Saltin, eds., *Muscle Metabolism During Exercise.* New York: Plenum Press, 1971, pp. 289–299.

[50] Simonsen, E. (ed.), *Physiology of Work Capacity and Fatigue.* Springfield, Ill.: C. C. Thomas, Publisher, 1971.

[51] Stephens, J. A., and A. Taylor. Fatigue of maintained voluntary muscle contraction in man. *Journal of Physiology* (London), 1973, **220:**1–18.

[52] Tesch, P. Muscle fatigue in man. *Acta Physiologica Scandinavica,* Supplementum 480, 1980, pp. 1–40.

[53] Vihko, V., A. Salminen, and J. Rantamaki. Exhaustive exercise, endurance training, and acid hydrolase activity in skeletal muscle. *Journal of Applied Physiology,* 1979, **47:**43–50.

[54] Vitasalo, J. T., and P. V. Komi. EMG, reflex and reaction time components, muscle structure and fatigue during intermittent isometric contractions in man. *International Journal of Sports Medicine,* 1980, **1:**185–190.

CHAPTER
16

Kidney and Gastrointestinal Responses and Adaptations to Exercise

IN previous chapters of this book, it has been emphasized that the nature of physiological responses and adaptations to exercise is dependent in large measure upon the specific character of the exercise stimulus, that is, its intensity, duration, frequency and specific muscular involvement. This fact is perhaps best illustrated by the complex nature of the changes in kidney and gastrointestinal functions during exercise. Compared to our knowledge of such systems as the cardiovascular and respiratory systems, our understanding of kidney and gastrointestinal responses and adaptations to exercise is rudimentary. Both the complex nature of the responses and a lack of research contribute to our poor understanding of the function of these systems under exercise conditions. Accordingly, our treatment of this subject will be brief and undoubtedly oversimplified.

The Kidney at Rest—A Brief Review

Within each kidney are located a million or more compact tubules (the *nephrons*) and their associated blood vessels. A diagrammatic sketch of one such nephron and its blood supply is shown in Fig. 16.1. Nephrons such as this are responsible for the functions of the kidney, that is, filtration of blood plasma, reabsorption and retention of useful materials in the filtered liquid, and excretion of a small volume of excess water, salt, and potentially harmful substances such as ammonia and hydrogen ions (acid). Blood plasma is filtered out of the capillaries (glomerulus) into Bowman's capsule, the first part of the tubule (Fig. 16.1). The kidneys receive about 25 per cent of the total cardiac output at rest; therefore, the renal blood flow is about 1.25 liters per minute or 1,800 liters per day. From the 1,800 liters of blood that pass into the glomerular capil-

329

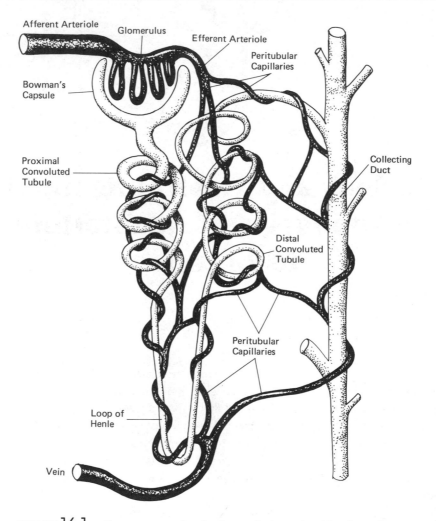

FIGURE **16.1.** Diagrammatic sketch of a nephron and its blood supply.

laries of the kidneys each day, only about 180 liters of fluid (glomerular filtrate) are filtered into the tubules (7.5 liters per hour). This rate at which fluid is filtered out of the plasma into the nephrons is called the *glomerular filtration rate*. It is obvious that all of the 180 liters of glomerular filtrate that enter the kidney tubules are not excreted into the urine each day—only about 1–2 liters achieve this end. The remainder of the glomerular filtrate, that is, 178–179 liters, is reabsorbed from the tubules and diffuses through the interstitial fluid into the peritubular capillaries, which deliver the retained fluid back to the main circulation by way of the renal veins (Figs. 16.1, 16.2).

There are two principal mechanisms by which substances in the glomerular filtrate are reabsorbed and retained by the body—*active reabsorption* and *passive reabsorption*. Active reabsorption is a process by which the cells of the tubules move dissolved material such as sodium, potassium, glucose and amino acids out of the tubules by expending chemical energy (ATP). Passive reabsorption does not require ATP breakdown and consists of: 1) simple diffusion of molecules such as urea from an area of

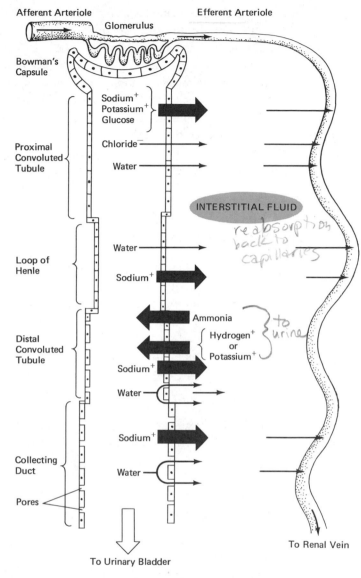

FIGURE 16.2. Schematic diagram illustrating transport processes in the kidney. Heavy arrows represent active reabsorption from tubule to interstitial fluid or active secretion into the tubule. Light arrows show passive reabsorption by osmosis (water), by electrical attraction (chloride) and by simple diffusion into peritubular capillary.

higher concentration inside the tubules to lower concentrations in the interstitial fluid, 2) movement by the attraction of oppositely charged ions (for example, negatively charged chloride ions following positively charged sodium ions out of the tubule as the sodium ions are actively reabsorbed), and 3) osmosis of water out of the tubule because of the attraction of osmotically active substances such as sodium ions, which were previously actively reabsorbed into the interstitial fluid. Thus, passive reabsorption of water by osmosis is made possible chiefly by the active reabsorption of sodium and other osmotically active particles.

Two hormones that enhance the rate of reabsorption of materials in the glomerular filtrate are aldosterone and antidiuretic hormone (vasopressin). Aldosterone is secreted by the adrenal gland and primarily accelerates the active reabsorption of sodium; it secondarily increases the passive reabsorption of chloride, bicarbonate

(HCO_3^-) and water. Antidiuretic hormone from the posterior pituitary gland seems to enlarge the pores of the distal convoluted tubules and collecting ducts, allowing water molecules to be passively reabsorbed by osmosis at a faster rate. In the absence of antidiuretic hormone, much more urine than normal is excreted.

Sometimes substances that may be toxic or are in excess of the body's needs accumulate in the interstitial fluid and are actively transported from the interstitial fluid through the walls of the tubules to the interior of the tubules. These potentially harmful substances are then excreted from the body by way of the urine. The movement of materials such as ammonia, hydrogen ions, and potassium from the exterior to the interior of the tubules is known as *active secretion* and is illustrated in Fig. 16.2.

Kidney Responses to Exercise

The alterations in kidney function brought on by a single exercise session are highly variable from day to day for an individual and also between individuals. Part of this variability is a result of 1) the technical difficulties inherent in evaluating renal function and in precisely controlling fluid intake and excretion so that rest and exercise periods are strictly comparable, 2) differences in the severity and duration of the exercise, and 3) variations in temperature and physical fitness [8, 14]. For example, to assure that there will be enough urine formed during a brief exercise period to make measurements of kidney function possible, it is not unusual for investigators to give subjects extra water and even tea to stimulate urine formation. But this fluid loading may create changes in kidney function that are not strictly related to the exercise itself. Similarly, brief, mild exercise by fit subjects in a cool environment is less apt to alter kidney function than vigorous, long-duration work by unfit persons. Therefore, although it is tempting to generalize about the effects of exercise on kidney function, one should always consider the several factors described here when assessing the probable responses of the kidneys to exercise.

Renal Blood Flow

Because kidney function obviously depends upon the amount of blood delivered to the nephrons, any change in renal blood flow during exercise must have profound effects on the operation of the kidneys—for example, upon glomerular filtration rate, reabsorption and secretion, and ultimately upon urine volume. Thus, one should note that during heavy exercise, renal blood flow may be reduced by 65 per cent or more from the value found at rest [6, 8]. This reduction in renal blood flow is apparently not substantial until the exercise intensity is sufficient to increase heart rate to about 135–140 beats per minute or to elevate oxygen uptake to about 50 per cent of one's maximal oxygen uptake (Fig. 16.3), [6, 8]. After this threshold is reached, the reduction in blood flow to the kidneys increases in unison with further increases in workload; that is, *renal blood flow during heavy exercise is inversely related to the intensity of exercise expressed as a percentage of one's maximal oxygen uptake* [6, 8]. Therefore, during a run or swim that requires an oxygen uptake of 3.0 liters per minute, renal

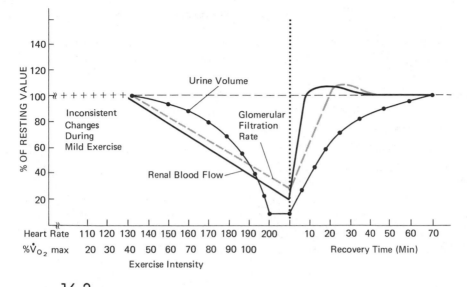

FIGURE 16.3. Schematic illustration of changes in renal blood flow, glomerular filtration rate and urine volume during exercise and recovery.

blood flow might be reduced by 70 per cent in an untrained person who has a maximal oxygen uptake of 3.1 liters per minute, but by only 40 per cent in an athlete who has a maximal oxygen uptake of 5.0 liters per minute.

Even during heavy exercise rather minor decreases in renal blood flow are sometimes observed if the exercise period is of short duration, that is, 15 minutes or less [8]. Accordingly, the changes in blood flow to the kidneys are related not only to the *intensity* of the exercise, but also to its *duration,* and are probably physiologically significant only in aerobic endurance exercises such as distance running or swimming. It seems that the reduction of blood flow to the kidneys serves the purposes of shifting blood to the working muscles for energy and to the skin for cooling.

Renal blood flow during severe exercise is reduced to a large extent when a subject is hypohydrated because of inadequate water intake or excessive water loss and when a subject exercises in a hot environment [8]. The kidneys behave as if they knew when more water loss could be harmful to the body, but the exact mechanisms by which a hot environment and hypohydration cause reductions in renal blood flow are not clear.

Likewise, the mechanism underlying the exercise effect on renal blood flow has not been precisely determined. Blood flow to the kidneys can be diminished 1) by sympathetic nervous system activity, which constricts the afferent and/or efferent arterioles to the nephrons, 2) by greater levels of epinephrine and norepinephrine secreted by the adrenals, and 3) by increased levels of angiotensin, a potent vasoconstrictor which circulates in the blood [14]. It seems likely that the sympathetic nerves are responsible for renal vasoconstriction during relatively short-duration intense exercise but that the circulating adrenal hormones and angiotensin, all of which are elevated substantially, account for more of this vasoconstriction response during prolonged activity.

Glomerular Filtration Rate

As would be expected, the glomerular filtration rate during heavy exercise decreases as a function of the decreased renal blood flow but shows highly variable changes with lighter work loads. However, the reduction in the glomerular filtration rate during severe physical activity is usually observed at slightly greater work intensities and is not as marked as the reduction in renal blood flow, that is, a greater fraction of the blood flowing into the glomerular capillaries is filtered into Bowman's capsule during severe exercise (Fig. 16.3). The explanation offered for this greater *filtration fraction* during severe exercise is that the efferent arterioles are constricted to a greater extent than the afferent arterioles; this causes a pressure rise within the glomeruli to force more fluid into Bowman's capsule [3, 8, 14]. The effects of environmental temperature, exercise duration, physical fitness, and the exerciser's hydration state on glomerular filtration rate during exercise are similar to those described for renal blood flow and are probably direct reflections of changes in blood flow.

Urine Volume

It is not unusual for persons who have undergone prolonged heavy exercise to be unable to produce any urine whatsoever shortly after exercise [8]. Part of this *anuria* is probably associated with hypohydration, but even in well-hydrated subjects, a decline in urine formation during heavy exercise is to be expected [8]. This reduced urine production with severe work is mostly a function of the diminished renal blood flow, which results in decreased glomerular filtration; that is, a reduction in glomerular filtration is usually associated with a reduction in urine volume. However, in exercisers who are also hypohydrated, it is thought that greater secretion of antidiuretic hormone increases the reabsorption of what little water is formed in the tubules [14].

Poor physical condition, hypohydration, long exercise duration, and a hot environment—all enhance the *antidiuretic* effects of heavy exercise because of the role these factors play in reducing renal blood flow.

In contrast to the effects of *strenuous* exercise, mild walking has been reported to cause increased urine production [8, 9]. This diuretic effect (greater urine volume) of mild exercise may be the result of a greater excretion of solutes in the urine during *mild* activity. These solutes could exert an osmotic effect to hold water in the tubules for excretion that normally would have been reabsorbed had exercise not taken place. Why the solute load is greater in urine from subjects who have exercised mildly is not known.

Excretion of Urinary Solutes

Since the volume of urine produced during heavy exercise is less than during rest or mild exercise, one might expect that the concentration of dissolved substances in this small volume of urine would be greater, so that the total amount of excreted solutes would be at least as great as the amount during rest. An *increase* in the concentration of dissolved substances does occur if one undergoes *thermal dehydration,* that is, prolonged exposure to heat in a desert environment, a sauna, or an environmental chamber. However, the reverse of this phenomenon occurs during heavy exercise; that is, the concentration of urinary solutes such as sodium and chloride is *less* during heavy exercise [8]. Consequently, urinary specific gravity, which reflects the concentration of dissolved substances in urine, usually *decreases* after severe exercise.

One reason why the excretion of substances such as sodium, chloride, magnesium, and creatinine decreases during heavy exercise is that the reduced glomerular filtration of these substances means that there are fewer ions and molecules in the tubules to be excreted [4, 7, 8]. But sodium and chloride and perhaps other substances are excreted at a rate lower than would be predicted by the decreased glomerular filtration rate. Accordingly, it seems that these substances must be reabsorbed from the tubules and retained by the body at a greater rate than at rest [14]. It seems likely that increased aldosterone secretion during heavy exercise serves to enhance the active reabsorption of sodium from the tubules, and that chloride ions follow the sodium out of the tubules by electrical attraction [21]. The aldosterone output by the adrenal gland is apparently stimulated by the renin-angiotensin system as follows:

Renin-Angiotensin Cycle

1. Decreased renal blood flow stimulates specialized cells of the nephrons (juxta-glomerular apparatus) to secrete an enzyme, *renin,* into the bloodstream.
2. Renin catalyzes the transformation of an inactive plasma protein, *angiotensinogen,* into *angiotensin I.*
3. Angiotensin I undergoes a further enzyme-catalyzed change into *angiotensin II,* which, in turn, stimulates the adrenal gland to release aldosterone.

Potassium excretion may be decreased, remain the same, or increase after exercise [7, 14]. On the one hand, serum potassium usually rises during exercise, and one might predict that this would lead to a greater filtration and excretion of potassium in the urine. On the other hand, the rise in serum potassium might often be offset by the decreased renal blood flow observed during heavy exercise. There is at present no adequate explanation for the contradictory results achieved with similar exercise programs.

Phosphate excretion usually is diminished during exercise but rises during 30–40 minutes of recovery [23]. The decrease during exercise is probably a function of the reduced glomerular filtration rate, whereas the rebound during recovery results not only from elevated glomerular filtration but also from reduced reabsorption by the kidney tubules [23].

Ammonia. Blood levels of ammonia (NH_3) increase during severe exercise in proportion to exercise intensity and remain high for about 30 minutes of recovery [13, 23]. Part of this increase may be explained by a greater synthesis of ammonia from amino (NH_2) groups split from intramuscular adenosine monophosphate or amino acids in exercising muscle, and part may be explained by a reduced blood flow to the liver, where ammonia molecules are combined to form urea. Whatever the reason for elevated ammonia levels in the blood during exercise, this increase leads to a greater excretion of ammonia or ammonium ions (NH_4^+) into the urine during strenuous work. However, much of the increased urinary ammonia comes from the kidney tubule cells themselves. Kidney cells have a large capacity to form ammonia from amino acids. This ammonia can be actively secreted into the tubules to help carry away hydrogen ions (H^+) by forming ammonium salts such as ammonium chloride (ammonia + lactic acid + sodium chloride → ammonium chloride + sodium lactate). In this way, ammonia can help decrease the acidity of the urine by combining with the hydrogen ions of lactic acid to form ammonium ions, which, in turn, combine with negative chloride ions to form neutral salts of ammonium chloride.

In excessive amounts, ammonia in the blood can be toxic to the brain, but it has not been conclusively shown that increases in blood ammonia during exercise contribute to fatigue.

Acid Excretion.　During aerobic exercise of a mild to moderate nature the excretion of acids in the urine is not consistently altered from resting conditions [8]. But during anaerobic exercise, which is associated with the production of lactic acid, there is a marked increase in the excretion of acid in the urine, with a concomitant decrease in pH during exercise and for 30 minutes or longer during recovery [23]. The absolute pH value of urine from exercised subjects depends upon the pre-exercise control value, but may be 1.0–1.5 units lower than at rest in previously hyperhydrated subjects [23]. The excretion of more acid is obviously related to the elevated lactic acid levels in the extracellular fluids; that is, more acid is filtered out of the glomeruli into the tubules and more acid is actively secreted by the kidney cells into the tubules.

Protein Excretion and "Athletic Pseudonephritis".　Nephritis is a disease of the kidney tubules characterized by a marked urinary loss of proteins, blood cells, and substances from the tubular structures. Ordinarily these materials do not appear or appear only in minute amounts in the urine of normal persons at rest. During and after exercise, especially with prolonged, heavy exercise, an increase in proteins, cells, and other abnormal substances can be observed in 80 per cent or more of healthy individuals [10, 17]. Because these changes in excretion are similar to those seen in nephritis, but do not persist, the term "athletic pseudonephritis" has been used to describe this apparently benign effect of exercise. The total amount of protein lost in the urine during exercise is small. In fact, the chemically treated paper strips commonly used for detecting urinary proteins in kidney disease often show no increase in proteins after exercise. More sophisticated tests show that some types of proteins may be elevated up to 100 times their levels at rest [14, 16], but the total lost is still quite small. Myoglobin, a protein found in skeletal muscle, may appear in the urine 24–48 hours after strenuous exercise and is thought to reflect damage to muscle fibers during exercise [14].

The mechanism underlying "athletic pseudonephritis" has not been conclusively determined but may include an increased permeability of the glomerular capillary membrane to large molecules resulting from hypoxia caused by reduced renal blood flow [8]. Another possibility that has been considered is that higher levels of plasma proteins during exercise result in the filtration of a greater amount of proteins into the tubules; in some subjects these extra proteins cannot be reabsorbed rapidly enough by the tubular cells. Finally, it may be that the reduced rate of renal blood flow through the glomerular capillaries during exercise simply allows large molecules more time to filter through pores in the capillary membrane; perhaps there is no actual change in the membrane structure during exercise [1, 8, 14, 15].

Kidney Function During Recovery from Exercise

After exercise has ceased, most kidney functions return to normal resting values within an hour of recovery [23], but prolonged exercise may cause changes lasting up to 10 hours after exercise [3]. Most of those substances which were excreted at reduced rates during exercise—for example, sodium, chloride, magnesium, and creatine—show an initial increase in excretion for 30 minutes after exercise before resting excretion rates are re-established. This effect can be accounted for by the increased glomerular filtration of such substances following the rapid resumption of normal renal blood flow after exercise. Urine volume will also increase following the rise in the glomerular filtration rate and rehydration if the exerciser had been severely hypohydrated. Acid and ammonia excretion remain elevated after heavy exercise for 30 minutes or longer until the lactic acid levels in the body are returned to normal levels [23].

Value of Renal Responses to Exercise

The responses of the kidneys to heavy exercise are important because of their contributions to: 1) the maintenance of adequate blood flow to the working skeletal muscles, 2) the conservation of body fluids needed for evaporative cooling, and 3) the control of pH in body fluids.

The kidneys at rest receive about 1.0–1.5 liters of cardiac output per minute, and about 65 per cent of that value or 650–975 milliliters of blood per minute can be shifted from the kidneys to the skeletal muscles during heavy exercise [8, 18]. This obviously can be important to the supply of oxygen and nutrients to the muscles, and also to the maintenance of adequate blood pressure, by helping to maintain venous return to the right side of the heart.

During heavy, prolonged work, particularly in a hot environment, the body can lose 1–2 liters of body water per hour by sweating. As the body becomes progressively hypohydrated under these conditions, sweat production may be retarded and evaporative cooling less effective. This diminished effectiveness of the sweating mechanism would be even more severe if the kidneys produced their normal volume of urine and contributed to greater hypohydration. Fortunately, the reduction of urine formation during heavy work tends to conserve body fluids.

Finally, although the respiratory system probably is more important quantitatively [8], the kidneys do help rid the body of excess acid and ammonia and, thus, prolong the time one can exercise without a debilitating accumulation of acid. In addition to excreting acidic hydrogen ions, the kidneys take up lactic acid and convert it to glucose, which can be released to the blood for transport to the working muscles [14]. The contribution of the kidneys to the maintenance of fuel homeostasis is small, but it may be significant in prolonged work.

Renal Adaptations to Training

Little is known about the effects of habitual exercise on kidney function, and even less is understood about the mechanisms responsible for training effects. It does appear, however, that trained persons exhibit fewer and less marked renal responses to a standard exercise bout than do untrained persons. For example, lesser reductions in renal blood flow, glomerular filtration rate, and urine formation are observed in well-conditioned subjects [8, 14]. These adaptations are probably the result of a less marked vasoconstriction of afferent and efferent arterioles in the trained persons so that renal blood flow is reduced to a lesser degree. Because of these adaptations in renal blood flow, it would also be expected that trained subjects would have less marked changes in excretion rates of solutes that are primarily affected by alterations in renal blood flow and glomerular filtration rate. Thus, trained subjects excrete less ammonia and protein during severe exercise than do untrained subjects [13]. Also, at moderately heavy work loads trained individuals produce a greater percentage of their energy aerobically and, therefore, rely less on anaerobic glycolysis. Accordingly, less lactic acid will be excreted in the urine of the trained subjects if the exercise has become more aerobic in nature as a result of training.

Gastrointestinal Responses and Adaptations to Exercise

Investigations of the effects of exercise on gastrointestinal function are technically even more difficult than studies of kidney function. Consequently, it is not surprising that our knowledge of such effects is meager. Reports of gastrointestinal responses to exercise in human beings and laboratory animals can be summarized with the following conclusions: 1) *mild* exertion either slightly enhances or has no effect on gastric (stomach) emptying and acid secretion, 2) increasing rates of *heavy* work cause progressively decreasing rates of both gastric emptying and acid secretion, 3) recovery of normal gastric function after *severe* exercise occurs within about 1–2 hours, and 4) there is inadequate evidence that exercise has any meaningful effects on the small or large intestines [11, 17, 20]. There is evidence that patients with duodenal ulcers who undertake mild exercise have an increased secretion of acid and an increased volume of stomach fluid after exercise [11]. This difference in the response of the ulcer patients has not been explained, but it would appear that mild exercise may be harmful to these patients.

The fact that there is a progressive decrease in gastric movements and secretion with increasing intensities of exercise is reminiscent of the relationship between kidney function and exercise rate; this suggests that changes in the sympathetic and parasympathetic nervous system may be important mediators of the effects of exercise on the stomach. Since splanchnic blood flow, which includes gastrointestinal blood flow, is progressively diminished with increasing work loads [18], it seems probable that increased sympathetic activity and decreased parasympathetic activity are responsible for much of the reduced motility and secretion of the stomach during heavy exercise.

(In the gastrointestinal tract, parasympathetic (vagus) activity stimulates and sympathetic activity depresses function.) However, because blood transfusions from exercised to rested dogs cause depression of stomach secretion in the rested dogs, it appears that some circulating factor may also play a role in the responses of the stomach to exercise [20].

Exercise and Bile Secretion

Bile is produced by the liver, stored in the gall bladder, and transported to the intestine to help digest fat. Bile contains highly concentrated cholesterol. The excretion of bile from the intestine is the major pathway for cholesterol excretion from the body. If exercise accelerates the output of bile into the intestine, this could help to reduce the cholesterol level in the blood. It has been found that mild exercise does stimulate bile and cholesterol output into the intestine [19]. However, more often than not, exercise training does not lead to an overall reduction in blood cholesterol. Therefore, the importance of the stimulated bile secretion is unknown.

Gastrointestinal Adaptations to Training

Training probably reduces the depression of gastric function with any standard work task because the task after training requires a smaller percentage of the exerciser's maximal oxygen uptake. Accordingly, a smaller increase in sympathetic activity and a smaller decrease in parasympathetic activity would be expected. Thus, trained persons have a greater splanchnic blood flow during a standard exercise test than do untrained subjects [18].

Whether physical training has a protective effect on the appearance of stomach ulcers after different types of stress remains controversial [22]. Studies of this question have been conducted with rats, but results have been contradictory.

In other rat studies, training caused a reduction in cholesterol concentration in the bile of the rested animals [19]. The extent to which this adaptation is useful for reducing cholesterol stores in the body and the extent to which the adaptation occurs in humans are unclear.

REVIEW QUESTIONS

1. Describe the effects of light and severe exercise on renal blood flow, glomerular filtration rate, and urine volume.
2. Discuss the apparent involvement of renal blood flow changes in the mechanisms of other kidney responses to exercise.
3. What role does aldosterone seem to play in mediating the effect of severe exercise on renal excretion of sodium and chloride?
4. What effect does exercise have on protein excretion in the urine? Explain a likely mechanism underlying this effect.
5. Does the effect of exercise on excretion of proteins, red blood cells, and so on, have pathological overtones? What is meant by "athletic pseudonephritis"?
6. List some of the potential benefits of the exercise response in the kidneys.
7. Describe the probable adaptations in kidney function that follow exercise training.
8. Describe and explain the effects of exercise on gastrointestinal function.

REFERENCES

[1] Bohrer, M. P., W. M. Deen, C. R. Robertson, and B. M. Brenner. Mechanism of angiotensin II-induced proteinuria in the rat. *American Journal of Physiology,* 1977, **233:**F13–F21.

[2] Boning, D., and W. Skipka. Renal blood volume regulation in trained and untrained subjects during immersion. *European Journal of Applied Physiology,* 1979, **42:**247–254.

[3] Castenfors, J. Renal function during prolonged exercise. *Annals of the New York Academy of Sciences,* 1977, **301:**151–159.

[4] Cerny, F. Protein metabolism during two hour ergometer exercise. In H. Howald and J. R. Poortmans, eds., *Metabolic Adaptation to Prolonged Physical Exercise.* Basel: Birkhauser Verlag, 1975, pp. 232–237.

[5] Decombaz, J., P. Reinhardt, K. Anantharaman, G. von Glutz, and J. R. Poortmans. Biochemical changes in a 100 km run: free amino acids, urea, and creatine. *European Journal of Applied Physiology,* 1979, **41:**61–72.

[6] Grimby, G. Renal clearances during prolonged supine exercise at different loads. *Journal of Applied Physiology,* 1965, **20:**1294–1298.

[7] Haralambie, G. Changes in electrolytes and trace elements during long-lasting exercise. In H. Howald and J. R. Poortmans, eds., *Metabolic Adaptation to Prolonged Physical Exercise.* Basel: Birkhauser Verlag, 1975, pp. 340–351.

[8] Kachadorian, W. A. The effects of activity on renal function. In J. F. Alexander, ed., *Physiology of Fitness and Exercise.* Chicago: Athletic Institute, 1972, pp. 97–116.

[9] Kachadorian, W. A., and R. E. Johnson. Renal responses to various rates of exercise. *Journal of Applied Physiology,* 1970, **28:**748–752.

[10] Kachadorian, W. A., R. E. Johnson, R. E. Buffington, L. Lawler, J. J. Serbin, and T. Woodall. The regularity of Athletic Pseudonephritis after heavy exercise. *Medicine and Science in Sports,* 1970, **2:**142–145.

[11] Markiewicz, K., M. Cholewa, and M. Lukin. Gastric basal secretion during exercise and restitution in patients with chronic duodenal ulcer. *Acta Hepato-Gastroenterologica,* 1979, **26:**160–165.

[12] Millard, R. W., C. B. Higgins, D. Franklin, and S. F. Vatner. Regulation of the renal circulation during severe exercise in normal dogs and dogs with experimental heart failure. *Circulation Research,* 1972, **31:**881–888.

[13] Poortmans, J. R. Effects of exercise and training on protein metabolism. In H. Howald and J. R. Poortmans, eds., *Metabolic Adaptation to Prolonged Physical Exercise.* Basel: Birkhauser Verlag, 1975, pp. 212–228.

[14] Poortmans, J. R. Exercise and renal function. *Exercise and Sport Sciences Reviews,* 1977, **5:**255–294.

[15] Poortmans, J. R., and G. Haralambie. Biochemical changes in a 100-km run: proteins in serum and urine. *European Journal of Applied Physiology,* 1979, **40:**245–254.

[16] Poortmans, J. R., and R. W. Jeanloz. Quantitative immunological determination of 12 plasma proteins excreted in human urine collected before and after exercise. *Journal of Clinical Investigation,* 1968, **47:**386–393.

[17] Rasch, P. J., and I. D. Wilson. Other body systems and exercise. In H. B. Falls, ed., *Exercise Physiology.* New York: Academic Press, Inc., 1968, pp. 129–151.

[18] Rowell, L. B. Human cardiovascular adjustments to exercise and thermal stress. *Physiological Reviews,* 1974, **51:**75–159.

[19] Simko, V., and R. E. Kelley. Effect of physical exercise on bile and red blood cell lipids in humans. *Atherosclerosis,* 1979, **32:**423–434.

[20] Stickney, J. C., and E. J. Van Liere. The effects of exercise upon the function of the gastrointestinal tract. In W. R. Johnson, ed., *Science and Medicine of Exercise and Sports.* New York: Harper & Row, Publishers, 1960, pp. 236–250.

[21] Sundsfjord, J. A., S. B. Stromme, and A. Aakvaag. Plasma aldosterone (PA), plasma renin activity (PRA) and cortisol (PF) during exercise. In H. Howald and J. R. Poortmans, eds.,

Metabolic Adaptation to Prolonged Physical Exercise. Basel: Birkhauser Verlag, 1975, pp. 308–314.

[22] Tharp, G. D., and J. L. Jackson. The effect of exercise training on restraint ulcers in rats. *European Journal of Applied Physiology,* 1974, **33:**285–292.

[23] Wesson, L. G., Jr. Kidney function in exercise. In W. R. Johnson, ed., *Science and Medicine of Exercise and Sports.* New York: Harper & Row, Publishers, 1960, pp. 270–284.

C H A P T E R
17

Endocrine Responses and Adaptations to Exercise

Two organ systems, the nervous system and the endocrine system, are primarily involved in regulating the rates at which the cells of various tissues carry on their chemical activities. The nervous system is characterized by a rapid response to disturbances in cellular homeostasis, to changes in the external environment, and to changing emotional circumstances. The endocrine system, on the other hand, although usually responding more slowly, often has a more profound and prolonged effect on cellular activities. Because of the widespread effects of endocrine regulation on cellular function, it is probable that changes in endocrine function are responsible for many of the physiological responses and adaptations to exercise. However, our knowledge of endocrine changes with exercise is so limited that there is little consensus concerning exactly how the endocrine system is involved in these responses and adaptations. In this chapter, therefore, we will describe what is known about the endocrine responses and adaptations to exercise and speculate on how these endocrine changes might play a role in the overall bodily reactions brought on by single or repeated bouts of exercise.

Review of Endocrine Secretions

An endocrine organ is imprecisely defined as a gland that secretes, directly into the bloodstream, small amounts of a substance which has specific effects on tissues somewhat distant from the endocrine gland. By this definition, a substance such as carbon dioxide is not considered an endocrine (hormone) because it is secreted in large amounts from muscles and other tissues. However, the releasing factors of the hypothalamus are generally classified as hormones, even though these substances have

342

their effects on the pituitary gland at a distance of only a few millimeters from the hypothalamus. Table 17.1 lists some of the hormones that may be involved, at least indirectly, in one or more of the functional changes resulting from exercise.

Mechanisms of Endocrine Action

Endocrines do not bring about *new* cellular activities but, rather, act to change the *rates* of specific activities already present in the cells. Endocrines are usually presumed to act in one or more of the following three ways: 1) by altering the rate of synthesis of enzyme proteins, 2) by altering the rate of synthesis of molecules such as cyclic AMP (a special type of adenosine monophosphate) or prostaglandins, which, in turn, bring about changes in enzyme activity or permeability of cell membranes to important substances, and 3) by directly altering the permeability of cell membranes. Endocrinologists are making progress in gradually specifying which types of action are most important for a given hormone, but conclusive evidence demonstrating the primary effect of most hormones is still lacking.

Methods of Research in Endocrinology

To determine whether a given hormonal substance is involved in the responses or adaptations to exercise, physiologists use several procedures. One approach is to surgically remove the endocrine gland that is the source of the hormone and to compare the responses of such operated animals with those of unoperated control animals. A second approach is to compare the responses not only of control animals and operated animals, but also of operated animals that receive hormone injections to replace the hormone lost by the removal of the endocrine gland. A third method often used to study the importance of endocrines in exercise is to measure the levels of those hormones in urine, blood, muscle, and other tissues. If the concentrations of hormones change in response to exercise, it is often assumed that the hormones must be involved in helping the body respond or adapt to the exercise. This is not necessarily so, as the discussion in the next paragraph explains.

Difficulties in Interpretation of Altered Hormone Concentration

Studies of changes in hormone levels in urine, blood, and tissue in response to exercise may produce some misleading results. This is so because the concentration of a hormone at any moment in time is affected by several variables. For example, the concentration of hormone is obviously dependent upon *the rate at which the endocrine gland is producing the hormone,* but the hormone concentration is also dependent upon *the rate of hormone destruction* by enzymes in the liver, kidney, and other tissues. In addition, the concentration of hormone in blood and urine is also depen-

TABLE 17.1

Endocrines Possibly Involved in Responses and Adaptations to Exercise*

Endocrines	Some Functions
Produced by Hypothalamus	
Growth Hormone Releasing Hormone *GHRH* (Somatoliberin)	Stimulates release of growth hormone from anterior pituitary
Somatostatin *GHRIH* (Growth Hormone Release Inhibiting Hormone)	Inhibits release of growth hormone from anterior pituitary
Thyrotropin Releasing Hormone *TRH* (Thyroliberin)	Stimulates release of thyrotropin (TSH) from anterior pituitary
Corticotropin Releasing Factor *CRF* (Corticoliberin)	Stimulates release of corticotropin (ACTH) from anterior pituitary
Follicle Stimulating Hormone Releasing Hormone *FSHRH* (Folliberin) (Gonadotropin Releasing Hormone)	Stimulates release of follicle stimulating hormone (FSH) from anterior pituitary; helps regulate menstrual cycle
Luteinizing Hormone Releasing Hormone *LHRH* (Luliberin) (Gonadotropin Releasing Hormone)	Stimulates release of luteinizing hormone from anterior pituitary; helps regulate menstrual cycle
Prolactin Releasing Factor *PRF* (Prolactoliberin)	Stimulates release of prolactin (PRL) from anterior pituitary
Prolactin Inhibiting Factor *PIF* (Prolactostatin)	Inhibits release of prolactin (PRL) from anterior pituitary
Vasopressin (Antidiuretic Hormone) *ADH*	Released from posterior pituitary; increases water retention by kidneys
Produced by Anterior Pituitary	
Growth Hormone *GH* (Somatotropin)	Stimulates growth of body tissues; aids in mobilization of fatty acids for energy
Thyrotropin *TSH* (Thyroid Stimulating Hormone)	Stimulates production & release of thyroid hormones from thyroid gland
Corticotropin *ACTH* (Adrenocorticotropic Hormone)	Stimulates production & release of cortisol, aldosterone & other hormones by adrenal cortex
Follicle Stimulating Hormone *FSH* (Follitropin)	Works with LH; stimulates production of estrogen by ovaries
Luteinizing Hormone *LH* (Lutropin)	Works with FSH; stimulates production of estrogen, progestin by ovaries; testosterone by testes
Prolactin *PRL*	Inhibits testosterone secretion by testes; mobilizes fatty acids
Endorphins (Dynorphin, Beta Endorphin, Beta Lipotropin)	Stimulate feeding; may cause euphoria, may block pain
Produced by Thyroid Gland	
Thyroxine T_4, Triiodothyronine T_3	Stimulates mitochondrial function; promotes cell growth
Calcitonin	Lowers blood calcium
Produced by Parathyroid Glands	
Parathyroid Hormone *PTH*	Raises blood calcium; lowers phosphate in blood
Produced by Adrenal Cortex	
Cortisol and Others	Promote use of fatty acids for energy; conserve blood glucose; reduce inflammation
Aldosterone and Others	Promote retention of sodium and water by the kidneys
Produced by Adrenal Medulla	
Epinephrine, Norepinephrine (Adrenaline, Noradrenaline)	Increase cardiac output; regulate blood vessels; increase glycogen breakdown & fatty acid release

(continued)

TABLE 17.1
Endocrines Possibly Involved [*Cont.*]

Endocrines	Some Functions
Produced by Pancreas	
Insulin	Promotes uptake of blood glucose by cell; promotes glycogen storage
Glucagon	Promotes release of glucose from liver to blood; mobilizes fat for energy
Produced by Testes	
Testosterone	Increases muscle mass; increases red blood cell production; decreases body fat; promotes male secondary sex characteristics
Produced by Ovaries	
Estradiol, Progesterone	Control menstrual cycle (with FSH & LH); increase fat deposits; promote female sex characteristics
Produced by Blood Vessels, Muscles, and Other Tissues	
Prostaglandins *PG*	Promote vasodilation; regulate heart rate; regulate blood clotting
Produced by Liver and Other Tissues	
Somatomedins and Other Growth Factors	Promote growth of muscle, cartilage, and other tissues

* Abbreviations are italicized; alternate nomenclature is shown in parentheses.

dent upon *the rate at which the hormone is taken up into the tissues* in which the hormone has its effect and upon *the extent to which any changes in blood volume occur.* Finally, it is important to know how long any change in hormone level persists after exercise; some hormones are broken down in as little as a few seconds after they are produced and have only brief effects, whereas others last for several hours and may produce effects lasting several days.

Accordingly, a rise in hormone concentration in the blood during exercise could be interpreted as an increased output of the hormone by its endocrine gland source, a decreased destruction of the hormone (perhaps because of reduced blood flow to the liver or kidneys), or a decreased uptake of the hormone by its target tissues. Even if it was demonstrated that the rise in hormone concentration was caused by increased production, the total adaptive effect of this increased hormone production may be insignificant if the production rate does not remain elevated long enough to allow the greater hormone levels to have any substantial effects on the target tissues. Thus, one must use great caution in the interpretation of changes in blood or urine levels of hormones with exercise. Such changes may indeed reflect some important alteration in endocrine function, or they may only reflect changes in blood flow either to target organs or to sites of hormone degradation. Unfortunately, most of the available data on endocrine changes with exercise consists only of reports of changes in blood or urine levels of the hormones in question. Until more complete information on other aspects of the metabolism of such hormones is available, one is probably wise not to place too much importance on observed changes in hormone concentrations in blood or urine.

Hypothalamic and Pituitary Hormones and Exercise

With the exception of somatostatin (GHRIH) there is no direct evidence that exercise causes a change in the rates of secretion of any of the liberins (releasing hormones) or statins (release inhibiting hormones) from the hypothalamus (Table 17.1). Logically, though, it seems that some of these hormones ought to be secreted in greater quantities to account for apparent changes in the rates of hormone secretion by the anterior pituitary and by glands such as the thyroid and adrenals. For example, exercise is generally accepted to be a stimulator of growth hormone release from the anterior pituitary. If growth hormone release is stimulated by hypothalamic somatoliberin (GHRH), then it follows that a rise in growth hormone is preceded by a rise in somatoliberin and followed by a later rise in somatostatin, which would prevent too great a rise in growth hormone. There are no reports of changes in somatoliberin levels with exercise, but there is some evidence that somatostatin increases with prolonged mild exercise [17]. (Somatostatin is also secreted by the pancreas.) Similarly, since both ACTH (corticotropin) and TSH (thyrotropin) are increased in response to certain types of exercise, it might be predicted that both corticotropin releasing factor (CRF) and thyrotropin releasing hormone (TRH) would be released in greater amounts to stimulate the release of more ACTH and TSH.

Two explanations may account for the apparent discrepancy between the presumed need for greater secretion rates of hypothalamic releasing factors and the lack of evidence that enhanced secretion does occur. First, until recently no simple reliable methods for quantifying the secretion rates of the hypothalamic hormones existed. Accordingly, physiologists have been unable to measure any changes in these hormones that might occur during exercise. Second, although higher blood levels of ACTH, TSH, and GH *seem* to implicate the hypothalamic hormones, it must be remembered that these higher blood levels may be partly accounted for by lesser rates of destruction rather than by greater rates of secretion. Thus, it may be that there is no real need for greater secretion of releasing hormones from the hypothalamus because there is no genuine increase in the rates of secretion of pituitary hormones such as ACTH, TSH, and GH.

Antidiuretic Hormone (Vasopressin)

A greater secretion of antidiuretic hormone from the hypothalamus and a greater release of this hormone from the posterior pituitary may explain some of the increased retention of water by the kidneys during severe exercise, especially when the exerciser is dehydrated. (See Chapter 16). Such an increased secretion of antidiuretic hormone would be a useful response to help conserve body water during exercise. There is evi-

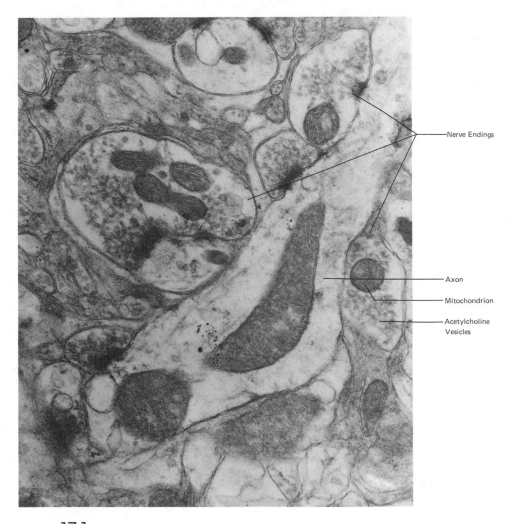

FIGURE 17.1. Electron micrograph of hypothalamus (magnification ×5,300). Large irregular shaped central structure is a nerve axon, and smaller, globular shaped structures in contact with the axon are nerve endings containing dark mitochondria and many small vesicles of acetylcholine. (Courtesy of G. Colin Budd, Physiology Department, Medical College of Ohio, Toledo, Ohio.)

dence that exercise does cause a 30–800 per cent increase in plasma concentrations of antidiuretic hormone [9, 10, 14, 17, 21, 38, 54]. The levels of antidiuretic hormone appear to increase progressively with greater exercise loads [9, 10, 54], and a threshold may occur at about 40 per cent of maximal oxygen uptake [10]. This means that reproducible changes in the hormone level may not occur below this intensity of exercise. One half of any newly secreted antidiuretic hormone is degraded in 5–20 minutes, and the levels of the hormone reattain resting values about 1 hour after exercise [9].

The mechanism responsible for the increased antidiuretic hormone concentration with exercise is unknown, but it is related to the increased osmotic activity of the blood that occurs as plasma volume is decreased during exercise [10]. There is some controversy over whether or not the increased antidiuretic hormone levels are responsible for the decreased water excretion which accompanies exercise [10, 54].

Adaptation to Training. Training does not change values of antidiuretic hormone in rested subjects [9, 21], but the increase in hormone concentration with the same absolute exercise load is less in trained subjects [21, 38]. Also, the increase with exercise is less in subjects who consume water just prior to exercise [54].

Growth Hormone

Growth hormone elevations with exercise would seem to be useful because of the beneficial effect of growth hormone on connective tissue and muscular growth; this effect could partly account for the greater strength of tendons, ligaments, and muscles, and for the greater bone thickness observed in those who are physically trained. Also, growth hormone helps to mobilize fatty acids from adipose tissue stores and to increase the fatty acid levels in the blood. This could be a useful response during exercise to help provide fuel for working muscles. Half of the newly secreted growth hormone is degraded by the liver in about 17–45 minutes, so a substantial portion of the hormone persists in the blood long enough to have significant effects on tissue growth and fatty acid mobilization. Since there is a lag period of about one hour before any effect of growth hormone on fat mobilization is observed [45], such an effect would seem important only in prolonged exercise.

Response to Exercise. Most investigations of the effects of a single bout of exercise on growth hormone levels in human blood have revealed a substantial rise that often is not seen for the first 15–20 minutes of the exercise. (See Fig. 17.2 and Refs. 23, 24,

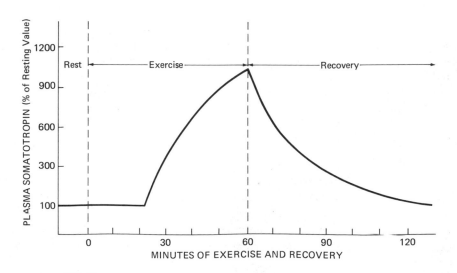

FIGURE 17.2. Diagram of growth hormone concentration in blood plasma during exercise and recovery.

35, 40, 45.) Incidentally, this response also occurs in pigs and monkeys, but not in rats. Usually the increase in growth hormone is greater with a longer duration and greater intensity of exercise [45], but even short-term, submaximal work can result in somatotropin increases in the blood [40].

The increase in growth hormone concentration in plasma as a response to exercise is so great that it is not likely to be totally a function of decreased hormone degradation or hormone uptake into tissues, and more probably results from an increased rate of secretion of growth hormone from the anterior pituitary [45]. Although there is an association between body temperature and plasma growth hormone levels [6], there does not seem to be a strong cause-and-effect relationship between these two variables [45]. It is widely recognized that growth hormone levels in blood increase in response to psychological stress, but exercise raises growth hormone concentrations even when precautions are taken to minimize psychological effects [23, 24]. There have been other factors proposed as possible stimulants for growth hormone release during exercise, but the mechanism underlying this hormonal response is still unknown [45].

Adaptation to Training. There is no reproducible effect of physical training on growth hormone levels in the blood under resting conditions, but there are several reports that those who are trained tend to have less dramatic rises in blood growth hormone during exercise [24, 45]. Such an adaptation is perhaps in part a result of the reduced psychological stress of exercise in trained persons.

Thyrotropin (Thyroid Stimulating Hormone)

There is reason to believe that the rate of thyrotropin secretion should be elevated during exercise because there seems to be an increased secretion of thyroxine with exercise; secretion of thyroxine by the thyroid gland is stimulated by thyrotropin released from the pituitary. Most authors report no change in thyrotropin concentrations in blood in response to exercise [14, 20, 50, 51], but studies using progressive treadmill exercise suggest that very intense exercise does elevate TSH levels [17, 19].

Corticotropin (Adrenocorticotropic Hormone)(ACTH)

Both marathon running and cycling cause elevated concentrations of blood corticotropin [7, 14, 17]. It is generally assumed that this response is triggered by a greater secretion of corticotropin from the pituitary. Corticotropin (ACTH) is a potent stimulator of adrenal hormone secretion. Corticotropin also directly enhances fat mobilization from fat stores, and this could be deemed a useful response in long duration exercise. Physical training does not alter ACTH levels in rested subjects but may cause a greater increase in ACTH concentration in blood plasma after exercise at the same relative intensity [7]. However, this training effect may only reflect the fact that subjects performed at greater absolute intensities after training to achieve the same relative intensity.

Corticotropin has a half-life of 4–18 minutes. (The half-life of a hormone is the time elapsed before one half of a given amount of the hormone is destroyed by the body.) Corticotropin stimulates cortisol secretion from the adrenal glands within 1–2 minutes, and this cortisol is only slowly degraded, with a half-life of 4 hours [45]. Therefore, an increase in ACTH secretion could have an important influence on cortisol and cortisol-related effects.

Follicle Stimulating Hormone (FSH) and Luteinizing Hormone (LH)

Since a number of studies have shown small increases in the plasma concentrations of sex hormones from the ovaries and testes, it might be expected that levels of follicle stimulating hormone and luteinizing hormone would also rise during exercise. However, the dominant finding in the literature is that FSH and LH do not change during exercise, regardless of whether the exerciser is a male or a female [4, 20, 28, 33, 47]. In fact, both FSH and LH showed a small decline in both males and females after a marathon run [13].

Prolactin (PRL)

Prolactin secretion during exercise could be useful both in conserving water through its antidiuretic effect on the kidneys and in mobilizing fat for energy. Some studies have shown increased prolactin levels in blood following exercise [17, 20]. Half of any newly secreted prolactin is destroyed in 15–30 minutes. This half-life should allow time for a significant effect of any increased secretion of prolactin during exercise. The increased prolactin release during exercise is presumably caused by activation of the sympathetic nervous system; when receptors for epinephrine and norepinephrine are blocked by drugs, the prolactin response to exercise is diminished [17].

Endorphins

Endorphins are compounds produced by the pituitary that have actions similar to morphine. The name *endorphins* stems from the terms "endogenous" (produced within the body) and "morphine." Many of these compounds have been discovered in the last few years. In particular, *beta-endorphin, beta-lipotropin* and *dynorphin* seem to have potent effects on relief of pain and stimulation of food intake, among many other actions. Most of the effects of these chemicals take place in the brain, and it is difficult to interpret the relationship between any changes in blood levels of endorphins and the possible changes that might occur in the brain. It may even be premature to classify these substances as endocrines or hormones.

Nevertheless, there are studies which suggest that a single strenuous exercise bout increases the concentration of beta-endorphin and/or beta-lipotropin in the blood [7, 8]. In one study, a period of training seemed to result in an increased level of these substances after exercise, but the exercise was probably of greater absolute intensity after training than before [7]. Enhanced levels of endorphins conceivably could explain the increased tolerance to the discomfort of exercise which occurs in trained persons or the so-called "runner's high," a pleasant feeling experienced by some distance runners during long runs.

Thyroxine and Triiodothyronine

The endocrine secretions of the thyroid gland are thyroxine (T_4) and triiodothyronine (T_3), collectively called "thyroid hormone." Thyroid hormone can mobilize fatty acids from adipose tissue stores and can promote cardiac hypertrophy. Both of these actions might help the body become better able to withstand the rigors of prolonged exercise, and it is, therefore, not surprising that several studies of thyroid responses to exercise have been undertaken. Thyroxine is especially interesting as a possible agent for adapting to exercise stress because it has a half-life of 6–7 days and produces effects that may be noticeable for 2 weeks or longer. Accordingly, a very small change in thyroxine availability as a result of exercise could have profound and long lasting effects, especially on tissue growth.

Response to Exercise

The total concentrations of thyroxine and triiodothyronine do not change with a single session of exercise [13, 14, 19, 50, 51], but the concentration of *free* thyroxine may increase by about 35 per cent during an exercise session [51]. About 99.96 per cent of all thyroxine is bound to proteins in the blood plasma and is not available for quick exchange with the tissues. It is the 0.04 per cent that represents the free thyroxine which is the metabolically active form of the hormone. Thus, an increase in the free fraction may have some importance. The increase in the free thyroxine is caused by a decreased binding of the plasma proteins to the thyroxine, perhaps because increased fatty acid levels during exercise make the proteins less apt to bind thyroxine [51].

It has been shown that there is no increase in the uptake of the free hormone by skeletal muscles during exercise. On the other hand, the liver, where most of the breakdown of thyroxine occurs, does increase its uptake of free thyroxine during exercise [51]. Thus, the increased free thyroxine, which is no longer protected from degradation by the liver when separated from the binding proteins in the blood, may have no important physiological effect and may simply be more susceptible to degradation by the liver.

Adaptation to Training

At rest, trained persons have slightly reduced concentrations of *total* thyroxine and slightly increased concentrations of *free* thyroxine. They also are characterized by higher rates of both secretion and degradation, with degradation rates being enhanced more than secretion rates [51].

There is no conclusive evidence that elevated concentrations of free thyroxine in the blood of trained animals have any beneficial effects. For example, most studies show no effect of physical training on basal metabolic rate, the rate at which a resting organism consumes oxygen [51]. Since thyroxine is the most potent stimulus to basal metabolism, one might expect that trained animals would have greater metabolic rates, but this is not the case.

Calcitonin and Parathyroid Hormone

Calcitonin (thyrocalcitonin) from the thyroid gland and parathyroid hormone are potent regulators of calcium and phosphate levels in the blood. Since both these minerals play important roles in muscle contraction and perhaps fatigue, it might seem reasonable to expect some changes in their hormonal regulation during exercise. One investigation showed that plasma levels of parathyroid hormone did not change after one hour of exercise at 50 per cent of maximal oxygen uptake [11]. No reports of calcitonin studies related to exercise were discovered.

Hormones of the Adrenal Cortex

The adrenal cortex is stimulated by corticotropin (ACTH) from the pituitary to produce and secrete three general classes of hormones: glucocorticoids, mineralocorticoids, and sex hormones. The sex hormones are of minor significance in persons with normal testicular or ovarian functions, but the glucocorticoids and mineralocorticoids are necessary for survival in a normal stressful environment. Each of these two classes of hormones contains some 20 individual hormones, but only one in each class is of major physiological significance; cortisol represents about 95 per cent of all glucocorticoid activity, and aldosterone about 95 per cent of all mineralocorticoid activity. The half-lives of cortisol and aldosterone are about 240 and 30 minutes, respectively, so any increase of blood concentrations during exercise could have a prolonged effect.

Cortisol and the other glucocorticoids promote fat utilization in tissues by mobilizing fats and proteins and conserving carbohydrates. Under the influence of cortisol, blood glucose tends to be elevated. This conservation of blood glucose could conceivably be of some importance in helping provide the brain with adequate nutrients during prolonged exercise, because nerve tissue depends heavily on glucose for energy. The mobilization of fatty acids for energy could also be useful in long duration work.

The glucocorticoids are also essential for organisms to resist stressful situations, including the stress of severe exercise training. Adrenalectomized animals are much less able to endure exercise than are normal animals [52].

The mineralocorticoids, of which aldosterone is the major representative, are involved primarily in the regulation of water, sodium, and potassium retention by the kidney. The maintenance of appropriate levels of sodium and potassium in the body fluids is vital to nerve and muscle functions because of the involvement of sodium and potassium in maintaining membrane potentials—without them nerves could not conduct impulses, and muscles could not contract. Also, aldosterone works in the kidney in cooperation with antidiuretic hormone to conserve body water, an especially important function during prolonged exercise in the heat.

Cortisol Response to Exercise

There is substantial controversy in the research literature about the effect of a single exposure to exercise on cortisol levels in the blood [45, 50, 52]. Thus, at light and moderate levels of exercise, there have been reports of increases, decreases, and no change in blood cortisol concentration. However, there is agreement that plasma cortisol concentrations and urinary excretion rates of free cortisol are enhanced by heavy, prolonged exercise [7, 14, 33, 39, 45, 52]. Accordingly, it appears that the exercise must be relatively intense for a given person and must be of long duration in order to achieve reliable increases in plasma cortisol levels and excretion rates [3, 45]. Increases in plasma cortisol caused by exercise may persist for as long as 2 hours after exercise.

The mechanism underlying elevations in plasma cortisol probably involves increased secretion under the influence of corticotropin and is not thought to result from decreased rates of degradation or decreased uptake by tissues [45].

Cortisol Adaptation to Training

In rats, the major glucocorticoid is corticosterone rather than cortisol. The concentration of corticosterone in plasma is enhanced both at rest and after exercise in animals trained for 3–4 weeks, but these levels are returned to normal after 6 weeks of training [53]. Also, the adrenals of trained rats release progressively less corticosterone upon stimulation by a standard amount of corticotropin as training progresses from 6 weeks onward. This decreased release of corticosterone has been shown to be caused by a decreased sensitivity of the adrenals to corticotropin [53].

In man, there does not seem to be any reliable effect of training on cortisol values in plasma, either at rest or after exercise [24, 45, 50]. Whether more discrete changes in adrenal glucocorticoid physiology follow physical training remains to be elucidated.

Aldosterone Response to Exercise

Plasma aldosterone concentrations rise progressively during exercise of increasing intensity with peak aldosterone levels of up to 6 times the resting value having been reported [12, 21, 37, 38, 39]. This rise in aldosterone concentration may persist for 6–12 hours after completion of the exercise [12].

The mechanism underlying the aldosterone response to exercise apparently involves the renin-angiotensin system (Chapter 16), because the concentrations of both renin and angiotensin II also show substantial rises in plasma with exercise [37]. Thus, sympathetic nervous system activity during exercise reduces renal blood flow which, in turn, stimulates the kidney to release renin into the blood. The elevated renin activity increases the production of angiotensin, which then stimulates the adrenal cortex to release aldosterone [36]. Renin activity increases progressively with increased exercise loads [10, 54]. However, the increased plasma renin activity is not necessarily correlated with the increased aldosterone levels, and the changes in aldosterone are not highly correlated with changes in plasma sodium or potassium [38].

Aldosterone Adaptation to Training

Training does not affect resting levels of aldosterone or the aldosterone response to a bout of exercise [21, 38]. One study suggests that plasma renin activity at rest is lower in trained subjects, but the increase in renin activity in response to exercise is unaffected by training [21].

Sympathoadrenal Hormones

All sympathetic nerve endings, including those to the adrenal glands, secrete both epinephrine (adrenaline) and norepinephrine (noradrenaline). Therefore, it is usually difficult to separate the effect of adrenal output from that of the secretion of sympathetic nerves in general when a change in plasma epinephrine or norepinephrine is observed. That is why in this discussion reference will be made to the sympathoadrenal system rather than to the adrenal glands only.

Sympathetic stimulation of blood vessels and of cardiac output is obviously important for exercise. Also sympathetic hormones increase circulating fatty acids and raise blood glucose; these effects could likewise be useful during prolonged exercise. Epinephrine and norepinephrine are quickly destroyed after their release and would not be expected to have any prolonged effects on the organism. Plasma epinephrine and norepinephrine return to resting values within 6 minutes after the end of exercise [1]. About 75 per cent of the secretion of the adrenal medulla is epinephrine, whereas the sympathetic nerve endings in blood vessels and other tissues secrete mostly norepinephrine.

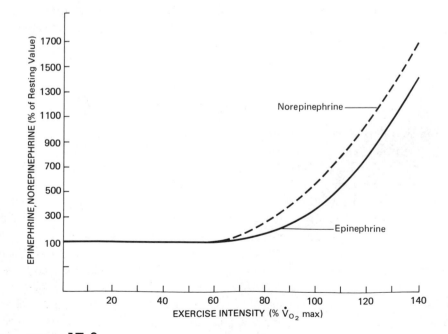

FIGURE 17.3. Diagram depicting rise in epinephrine and norepinephrine with various intensities of exercise.

Response to Exercise

Ordinarily, one does not observe a rise in either epinephrine or norepinephrine in the blood with *mild* exercise unless that exercise is accompanied by unusual psychological stress. But as soon as the exercise intensity is great enough to elicit an oxygen uptake of more than about 60 per cent of one's maximal rate of consuming oxygen, a rise in plasma levels of both epinephrine and norepinephrine occurs [1, 15, 18, 23, 24, 41, 56]. As exercise intensity progressively increases, so do the concentrations of these two hormones in the blood (Fig. 17.3). The fact that more norepinephrine than epinephrine is released during exercise has led some to conclude that the sympathetic nerves to blood vessels and other tissues are more important sources of these hormones than are the adrenal glands [24].

The mechanisms triggering the greater secretion of epinephrine and norepinephrine during exercise are not clear, but they probably include nerve reflexes originating in the cardiovascular system plus psychological effects.

FIGURE 17.4. Epinephrine flows in both participants and spectators. (Courtesy of Office of Public Information, University of Toledo, Toledo, Ohio.)

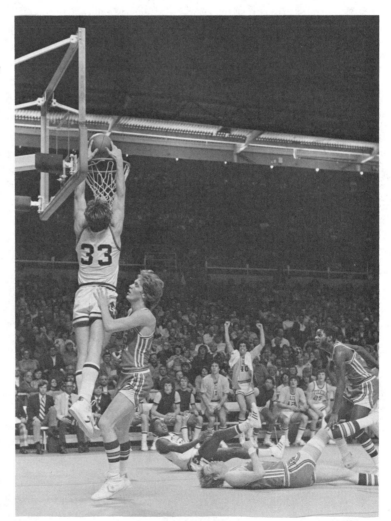

Adaptation to Training

Most workers have found that with the same submaximal workload there is a somewhat lesser elevation of sympathoadrenal hormones in the blood after training [24, 41, 56]. However, postexercise hormone excretion in the urine of trained persons is not necessarily different from that found before training [5]. Any reduction in hormone elevations with submaximal exercise after training might be accounted for by the diminished psychological and physiological stresses associated with a standard exercise load after training. Levels of epinephrine and norepinephrine in plasma of rested subjects are not changed by physical training [41, 56].

Hormones of the Pancreas

Insulin and glucagon are both involved in the regulation of blood glucose levels. On the one hand, insulin tends to lower blood glucose by causing more glucose to be taken up out of the blood and across cell membranes into tissues such as skeletal muscle. On the other hand, glucagon tends to raise blood glucose by activating an enzyme that breaks down liver glycogen into glucose, which is then released into the blood. Glucagon also stimulates the heart to beat more forcefully and activates an enzyme that releases fatty acids into the blood from fat stores throughout the body. All of these hormonal actions could be important during prolonged exercise. In addition, insulin has a powerful effect on increasing glycogen stores in skeletal muscle and could conceivably be involved in the supercompensation of muscle glycogen that follows severe exercise. The half-lives of glucagon and insulin are 5–10 minutes and 40 minutes, respectively.

Insulin Response to Exercise

Plasma insulin concentrations after exercise may decline to less than 50 per cent of levels observed in resting subjects [18, 22, 24, 42, 56, 57]. As with other hormonal changes during exercise, responses are apt to be greater with exercise regimens of greater intensity and greater duration [18, 24]. Accordingly, one might not expect a significant fall in insulin after 5 minutes of jogging, but would be very likely to find a large decrease in plasma insulin after an exhaustive run of 2 or 3 hours. The plasma insulin concentration may not return to pre-exercise values for an hour or more after exercise [24].

It appears that the reduction in insulin found in the blood during exercise results both from a decreased secretion of insulin by the pancreas and from an increased uptake of insulin by working skeletal muscles.

The working muscles can get along nicely with a reduced concentration of insulin in the blood because more blood is circulating through those muscles during exercise. At the same time, blood flow to the liver is reduced so that there is less insulin circulating through the liver where insulin tends to block glucose delivery from the liver to the blood. Thus, the liver is free to supply additional glucose to the blood as the muscles use up glucose during exercise. The decreased secretion of insulin by the pancreas during exercise is caused by increased activity of the sympathetic nervous system [24, 26, 42]. The fact that plasma insulin falls by 50 per cent during exercise in patients who have no adrenal glands [26] suggests that the sympathetic nerve supply to the pancreas is more important in the depression of insulin than circulating epinephrine and norepinephrine from the adrenal glands. Since there is no reliable fall in blood glucose with many types of exercise which trigger a fall in insulin, the decline in insulin is not caused by changes in blood glucose levels.

Insulin Adaptation to Training

The effect of physical training on concentrations of insulin in the blood at rest is the subject of some controversy. In comparisons of well-trained groups with untrained groups, the trained groups generally have lower resting levels of insulin [2, 32, 50, 57]. However, when untrained subjects are placed on a training program, no change in resting insulin concentrations is noted [22, 56]. Many [2, 22, 24, 50], but not all [56, 57], reports show that trained subjects have less of a decline in plasma insulin with the same absolute exercise load. This muted depression of insulin with exercise is probably caused by the lower levels of epinephrine and norepinephrine that are present in trained individuals during exercise [24].

Training also increases one's sensitivity to insulin [2]. This means that less insulin is required to handle the same rise in blood glucose after training than before. The explanation for this increased insulin sensitivity is that the binding of insulin to the body's cells, especially the muscles, increases after training [2, 32]. This increased sensitivity may only hold true for the resting state; one report suggests that insulin binding during exercise is decreased in trained subjects [32]. A decrease in insulin sensitivity during exercise could explain the fact that less glucose and more fatty acids are used for energy in trained persons [32].

Exercise and Diabetes. Insulin-dependent diabetics (about 10 per cent of all diabetics) must receive insulin injections to compensate for low levels of natural insulin secretion by the pancreas. The insulin allows the cells to use glucose from the blood. Without adequate insulin, the blood glucose levels rise; with too much insulin, blood glucose levels fall. For the diabetic, both sharp increases and sharp decreases in blood glucose must be avoided. If the diabetic person has adequate levels of insulin during exercise, regular exercise can be beneficial because blood glucose is taken up by the muscles more rapidly during exercise than at rest. Less insulin therapy is needed in diabetics who exercise regularly [31]. On the other hand, if the diabetic has inadequate insulin therapy, exercise can result in an increase in blood glucose because the liver produces more glucose than the muscles can use up. In this case, exercise is not beneficial to the diabetic.

The anatomical site of insulin injection is an important consideration if a diabetic is to exercise. If the insulin is injected into the leg prior to leg exercise, the diabetic can become hypoglycemic. The insulin is absorbed into the bloodstream too rapidly if it is injected near the working muscle [31]. Usually, the abdomen is the best site for injection if one is going to exercise, unless abdominal exercise is to be stressed.

If the physically trained diabetic becomes more sensitive to insulin, less insulin therapy will be required to manage the diabetic state. Also, training has beneficial effects on blood fats (Chapter 18) that should improve the health of the diabetic in the long term. Therefore, physical training is often useful therapy for diabetic persons [31].

Glucagon Response to Exercise

Glucagon from the pancreas can accelerate the release of glucose to the blood from stored glycogen in the liver. Glucagon can also activate the lipase enzymes which release fatty acids from stored fat supplies. Therefore, it would be logical to predict that glucagon levels in the blood might be elevated with prolonged exercise, and this is exactly what happens. Short duration exercise causes either no change or even a slight decrease in glucagon concentrations in the blood [17, 18]. With an hour or more of exercise at 50 per cent of maximal oxygen uptake, however, glucagon levels can increase from 30 per cent to 300 per cent [22, 40, 56].

In rats, the increase in glucagon secretion is caused by increased levels of epinephrine and norepinephrine [50], but in man the mechanism is apparently different. In man, the glucagon response to exercise is blocked if glucose feedings are provided [50]. Therefore, it appears that the pancreas becomes very sensitive to slight reductions in blood glucose as exercise continues beyond one hour and secretes more glucagon in response to these minor reductions in glucose [17, 50].

Glucagon Adaptation to Training

As little as three weeks of training produces a noticeable blunting of the glucagon response to exercise [22, 56]. There is a much smaller increase in glucagon levels during exercise both at the same absolute exercise load and at the same relative load [56]. It is tempting to speculate that the cause of this reduced glucagon response to exercise is the reduced levels of epinephrine and norepinephrine in trained persons, but the fact that drug blockade of the effects of these hormones does not alter the glucagon response to exercise speaks against this hypothesis [17, 50]. There are no major changes in blood glucose with training that appear related to the reduced glucagon response to exercise.

Testosterone

Prior to puberty there is little difference in muscular strength between males and females. But as males begin to develop into sexual adulthood, they rapidly become stronger than females. This increased strength gives the male an advantage in many athletic events, so one might ask whether the greater strength results from the principal male sex hormone, testosterone, and whether stronger, more athletically successful males have more circulating testosterone than their weaker counterparts. A corollary question has been whether synthetic testosterone-like compounds can be administered to athletes to cause significant gains in muscular mass and strength.

Besides its relationship to muscular strength, testosterone has been implicated in the enhancement of aggressive behavior, red blood cell production, bone thickness, muscle glycogen storage, and muscle protein synthesis—all of which could theoretically be beneficial to athletic performance of various types [34]. The half-life of testosterone is up to 3.4 hours, so any changes in plasma testosterone during exercise could exert effects over a considerable time.

Testosterone Response to Exercise

The responses of plasma testosterone to exercise are quite variable. For example, in response to weight lifting exercise, both increases [16] and no change [16, 46] in testosterone levels have been reported. Slight increases are commonly [19, 20, 55], but not always [33, 34], shown with short duration, high intensity exercise. Similar discrepancies occur in reports of testosterone responses to prolonged exercise. For example, there is a report of a modest increase in testosterone concentration in the blood after an intense training session of swimming and rowing, but not after a submaximal session of comparable activities [49]. Similarly, there is a small increase in testosterone after a marathon [13], no change during a 90 minute run [33], and an increase after a 40 minute run [19].

Because there usually is no increase in luteinizing hormone with exercise, it appears that the modest increases in testosterone commonly observed may be related to other factors. It has been suggested that many of the reported changes can be explained by the hemoconcentration effect of exercise—that is, as muscle contraction forces water from the blood plasma and into the tissues, the concentration of testosterone in the blood naturally rises [55]. Another hypothesis is that the increased concentrations of testosterone are caused by a decreased rate of degradation of the hormone because of a decreased blood flow to the liver during strenuous exercise [50]. The fact that any increase in testosterone concentration is usually small and variable plus the fact that luteinizing hormone is not increased during exercise suggests that any increase in testosterone with exercise is probably physiologically insignificant.

Testosterone Adaptation to Training

Strength training does not change the levels of circulating testosterone [25]. There is, therefore, no evidence that training causes an increase in testosterone secretion. Also, luteinizing hormone concentrations are unaffected by eight weeks of strength training [47].

Estradiol and Progesterone

Estradiol and progesterone, the most important hormones of the ovaries, may increase glycogen storage at rest and minimize glycogen breakdown to lactic acid during exercise [27]. Also, these hormones are vital in the regulation of the menstrual cycle. Their structures are very similar to that of the male sex hormone, testosterone. Therefore, one might expect that responses of the female sex hormones to exercise might be similar to those of testosterone in men.

Response to Exercise

When tested during the latter (luteal) phase of the menstrual cycle, after ovulation has occurred, both estradiol and progesterone concentrations in the blood increase by about 15–50 per cent with exercise [4, 28]. It is more difficult to detect any rise in estradiol during exercise in the early part of the menstrual cycle, but the increases in progesterone concentrations continue to be significant in this *follicular* phase [4, 28]. The increases in these hormones are greater with progressively more intensive exercise loads [28]. There is good evidence that the cause of the increase in hormone concentrations is a reduced rate of degradation of the hormones in the liver as blood flow to that organ decreases during exercise [29].

Cardiovascular function and aerobic exercise performance are unaffected by the phases of the menstrual cycle, but there may be an increased endurance to brief (1–3 minute), intensive exercise during the luteal phase, when both progesterone and estradiol levels are high [27]. One possible explanation for this increased endurance is that the exercise is associated with lower lactic acid levels in the blood during the luteal phase [27]. This reduction in acid may slow the development of fatigue. It is conceivable that the increased levels of estradiol and progesterone slow the breakdown of glycogen to lactic acid during exercise in the luteal phase [27].

Adaptation to Training

At the same absolute exercise load, trained subjects do not exhibit the increased blood levels of estradiol and progesterone which occur before training [4]. This finding fits in well with the notion that the increase in hormone concentrations before training is caused by reduced blood flow to the liver. At the same absolute load after training, there is less sympathetic vasoconstriction in the liver. Therefore, liver blood flow will be greater after training, and the rate of degradation of the hormones will not be reduced.

Menstrual Cycle Disturbances with Physical Training

There is a high incidence of amenorrhea (absence of menstrual cycles) and of oligomenorrhea (highly irregular menstrual cycles) in women who are engaged in strenuous athletic training [44]. These menstrual cycle disturbances are especially prevalent among distance runners and dancers but also occur in athletes engaged in many other sport activities. The cause of these changes in the menstrual cycle is unknown, but the disturbances have been related to decreased body weight, decreased body fat, increased lean body mass, decreased intake of protein as a per cent of all calories, and increased psychological stress [44]. Upon cessation of strenuous training, body fat increases and normal menstrual function usually resumes. Although it is possible that prolonged disturbances in hormone levels could be harmful over a period of years, there is presently no solid evidence that these menstrual cycle alterations are hazardous to a woman's health.

Prostaglandins

Prostaglandins are biologically active substances that are produced from polyunsaturated fatty acids. The name "prostaglandin" refers to the fact that these compounds were first found in extracts of prostate glands, but research has since shown that prostaglandins are produced in many tissues throughout the body. There are many different types of prostaglandins, each producing somewhat different actions from the others. Some are vasodilators, some, vasoconstrictors; some raise blood pressure, others lower it; some increase cardiac contractility, and some decrease fat breakdown. Thus, changes in the levels of prostaglandins or their breakdown products could be involved in some of the physiological responses and adaptations to exercise.

Response to Exercise

After a marathon race, the blood concentrations of two prostaglandins and a breakdown product of a third increased significantly [13]. The concentration of prostaglandin E increased by about 48 per cent, prostaglandin $F_{2\alpha}$ by about 55 per cent, and the metabolite of prostaglandin I_2 (prostacyclin) by more than 100 per cent. Similarly, a progressive cycling task to exhaustion, using both arms and legs, caused a modest rise in prostaglandin E [30]. The mechanism for the increase in prostaglandin levels is unknown but could involve decreased degradation of these chemicals in the liver and other tissues.

Adaptation to Training

No comprehensive studies of training effects on prostaglandin levels have been completed, but one study suggested that marathon runners had higher values at rest than normal untrained persons [13].

Somatomedins

Somatomedins are chains of amino acids produced by the liver and other tissues, often in response to growth hormone release. Some of their properties include the stimulation of protein synthesis, ribonucleic acid synthesis, amino acid uptake, cartilage growth, and muscle growth. Some authorities refer to the somatomedins as "growth factors" and have not yet labeled them as endocrines. No studies of somatomedin responses to exercise have been reported, but one study in rats showed a marked increase in somatomedin-like activity of hypertrophied, overloaded muscles compared to normal muscles [48]. It remains to be seen if this adaptation can be verified in other models of muscle hypertrophy.

TABLE 17.2
**Summary of Most Commonly Observed Endocrine Changes
with Exercise and Training**

Endocrine	Exercise Response	Training Adaptation
Somatostatin	Increase	No evidence
Vasopressin (ADH)	Increase	Less increase with exercise; no change at rest
Growth Hormone	Increase	Less increase with exercise; no change at rest
Thyrotropin (TSH)	No change	No evidence
Corticotropin (ACTH)	Increase	No change at rest; possible greater increase with exercise
FSH and LH	No change	No evidence
Prolactin	Increase	No evidence
Endorphins	Increase	Possible greater increase with exercise
Thyroid Hormones (T_4 and T_3)	No change in total; increase in free T_4	Slight decrease in total; increase in free T_4
Parathyroid Hormone	No change	No evidence
Calcitonin	No evidence	No evidence
Cortisol	Increase if exercise is prolonged	No reliable change
Aldosterone	Increase	No change
Epinephrine and Norepinephrine	Increase	No change at rest; lesser increase with same absolute exercise load
Insulin	Decrease	Possible decrease at rest; lesser decrease with same absolute exercise load
Glucagon	Increase if exercise is prolonged	No change at rest; lesser increase with exercise at any load, including maximal
Testosterone	Slight increase	No change
Estradiol and Progesterone	Increase	Lesser increase at same absolute load during exercise
Prostaglandins	Increase	No evidence
Somatomedins	No evidence	Possible increase

Summary

The study of endocrine responses and adaptations to exercise is of recent origin, but is rapidly expanding. There are many reports which describe changes in concentrations of hormones in the blood during exercise and as a result of training. Unfortunately, there have been few comprehensive studies of changes in secretion rates, degradation rates, and rates of hormone uptake. Therefore, we cannot always be certain of the correct interpretation of changes in hormone concentration. Table 17.2 summarizes the general trends of hormone changes with exercise and training.

REVIEW QUESTIONS

1. Review the relationships between the hypothalamic releasing hormones (liberins), the release inhibiting hormones (statins), and the hormone secretions of the anterior pituitary. Make certain you can follow the logic of assuming that more releasing hormone is secreted if the concentration of a hormone from the anterior pituitary is increased with exercise.
2. Speculate on the possible value of a decreased concentration of insulin in the blood during prolonged exercise. Remember that insulin inhibits fatty acid mobilization from fat stores.

3. Explain how changes in blood flow through the liver during exercise may account for some of the increased concentrations of hormones observed.
4. How can hemoconcentration explain some of the small increases in concentration observed in some hormones?
5. For each hormone discussed in the text, make certain you understand how its function might be important to exercise or training. Also, review the description of changes in hormone levels caused by exercise and training and the mechanisms proposed to explain those changes. Be prepared to discuss these points in class or in an oral or written examination.

REFERENCES

[1] Banister, E. W., and J. Griffiths. Blood levels of adrenergic amines during exercise. *Journal of Applied Physiology,* 1972, **33**:674–676.
[2] Bjorntorp, P. The effects of exercise on plasma insulin. *International Journal of Sports Medicine,* 1981, **2**:125–129.
[3] Bonen, A. Effects of exercise on excretion rates of urinary free cortisol. *Journal of Applied Physiology,* 1976, **40**:155–158.
[4] Bonen, A., W. Y. Ling, K. P. MacIntyre, R. Neil, J. C. McGrail, and A. N. Belcastro. Effects of exercise on the serum concentrations of FSH, LH, progesterone, and estradiol. *European Journal of Applied Physiology,* 1979, **42**:15–23.
[5] Brundin, T., and C. Cernigliaro. The effect of physical training on the sympathoadrenal response to exercise. *Scandinavian Journal of Clinical and Laboratory Investigation,* 1975, **35**:525–530.
[6] Buckler, J. M. H. The relationship between changes in plasma growth hormone levels and body temperature occurring with exercise in man. *Biomedicine,* 1973, **19**:193–197.
[7] Carr, D. B., B. A. Bullen, G. S. Skrinar, M. A. Arnold, M. Rosenblatt, I. Z. Beitins, J. B. Martin, and J. W. McArthur. Physical conditioning facilitates the exercise-induced secretion of β-endorphin and β-lipotropin in women. *New England Journal of Medicine,* 1981, 560–563.
[8] Colt, E. W. D., S. L. Wardlaw, and A. G. Frantz. The effect of running on plasma beta-endorphin. *Life Sciences,* 1981, **28**:1637–1640.
[9] Convertino, V. A., P. J. Brock, L. C. Keil, E. M. Bernauer, and J. E. Greenleaf. Exercise training-induced hypervolemia: role of plasma albumin, renin, and vasopressin. *Journal of Applied Physiology,* 1980, **48**:665–669.
[10] Convertino, V. A., L. C. Keil, E. M. Bernauer, and J. E. Greenleaf. Plasma volume, osmolality, vasopressin, and renin activity during graded exercise in man *Journal of Applied Physiology,* 1981, **50**:123–128.
[11] Cornet, F., G. Heynen, A. Cession-Fossion, A. Adam, and J. M. Hooft. Effects of muscular exercise on calcemia, the clearance of calcium and the secretion of parathyroid hormone. *Comptes Rendus Des Seances De La Societe De Biologie* (French), 1978, **172**:1245–1248.
[12] Costill, D. L., R. Cote, E. Miller, T. Miller, and S. Wynder. Water and electrolyte replacement during repeated days of work in the heat. *Aviation, Space, and Environmental Medicine,* 1975, **46**:795–800.
[13] Demers, L. M., T. S. Harrison, D. R. Halbert, and R. J. Santen. Effect of prolonged exercise on plasma prostaglandin levels. *Prostaglandins and Medicine,* 1981, **6**:413–418.
[14] Dessypris, A., G. Wagar, F. Fyhrquist, T. Makinen, M. G. Welin, and B.-A. Lamberg. Marathon run: effects on blood cortisol—ACTH, iodothyronines—TSH and vasopressin. *Acta Endocrinologica,* 1980, **95**:151–157.
[15] von Euler, U. S. Sympatho-adrenal activity in physical exercise. *Medicine and Science in Sports,* 1973, **6**:165–173.
[16] Fahey, T. D., R. Rolph, P. Moungmee, J. Nagel, and S. Mortara. Serum testosterone, body composition, and strength of young adults. *Medicine and Science in Sports,* 1976, **8**:31–34.

[17] Galbo, H. Endocrinology and metabolism in exercise. *International Journal of Sports Medicine,* 1981, **2:**203–211.

[18] Galbo, H., J. J. Holst, and N. J. Christensen. Glucagon and plasma catecholamine responses to graded and prolonged exercise in man. *Journal of Applied Physiology,* 1975, **38:**70–76.

[19] Galbo, H., L. Hummer, I. B. Petersen, N. J. Christensen, and N. Bie. Thyroid and testicular hormone responses to graded and prolonged exercise in man. *European Journal of Applied Physiology,* 1977, **36:**101–106.

[20] Gawel, M. J., J. Alaghband-Zadeh, D. M. Park, and F. C. Rose. Exercise and hormonal secretion. *Postgraduate Medical Journal,* 1979, **55:**373–376.

[21] Geyssant, A., G. Geelen, C. Denis, A. M. Allevard, M. Vincent, E. Jarsaillon, C. A. Bizollon, J. R. Lacour, and C. Gharib. Plasma vasopressin, renin activity, and aldosterone: effect of exercise and training. *European Journal of Applied Physiology,* 1981, **46:**21–30.

[22] Gyntelberg, F., M. J. Rennie, R. C. Hickson, and J. O. Holloszy. Effect of training on the response of plasma glucagon to exercise. *Journal of Applied Physiology,* 1977, **43:**302–305.

[23] Hartley, L. H. Growth hormone and catecholamine response to exercise in relation to physical training. *Medicine and Science in Sports,* 1975, **7:**34–36.

[24] Hartley, L. H., J. W. Mason, R. P. Hogan, L. G. Jones, T. A. Kotchen, E. H. Mougey, F. E. Wherry, L. L. Pennington, and P. T. Ricketts. Multiple hormonal responses to graded exercise in relation to physical training. *Journal of Applied Physiology,* 1972, **33:**602–606.

[25] Hetrick, G. A., and J. H. Wilmore. Androgen levels and muscle hypertrophy during an eight week weight training program for men/women (abstract). *Medicine and Science in Sports,* 1979, **11:**102.

[26] Jarhult, J., and J. Holst. The role of the adrenergic innervation to the pancreatic islets in the control of insulin release during exercise in man. *Pflügers Archiv,* 1979, **383:**41–45.

[27] Jurkowski, J. E. H., N. L. Jones, C. J. Toews, and J. R. Sutton. Effects of menstrual cycle on blood lactate, oxygen delivery, and performance during exercise. *Journal of Applied Physiology,* 1981, **51:**1493–1499.

[28] Jurkowski, J. E., N. L. Jones, W. C. Walker, E. V. Younglai, and J. R. Sutton. Ovarian hormonal responses to exercise. *Journal of Applied Physiology,* 1978, **44:**109–114.

[29] Keizer, H. A., J. Poortman, and G. S. J. Bunnik. Influence of physical exercise on sex-hormone metabolism. *Journal of Applied Physiology,* 1980, **48:**765–769.

[30] Kochan, R. G., and D. R. Lamb. Prostaglandin B equivalents in plasma of exercised men. In B. Samuelsson and R. Paoletti, eds., *Advances in Prostaglandin and Thromboxane Research.* New York: Raven Press, 1976, pp. 878–879.

[31] Koivisto, V. A., and R. S. Sherwin. Exercise in diabetes: therapeutic implications. *Postgraduate Medicine,* 1979, **66:**87–96.

[32] Koivisto, V. A., V. Soman, P. Conrad, R. Hendler, E. Nadel, and P. Felig. Insulin binding to monocytes in trained athletes: changes in the resting state and after exercise. *Journal of Clinical Investigation,* 1979, **64:**1011–1015.

[33] Kuoppasalmi, K., H. Naveri, M. Harkonen, and H. Adlercreutz. Plasma cortisol, androstenedione, testosterone and luteinizing hormone in running exercise of different intensities. *Scandinavian Journal of Clinical Laboratory Investigation,* 1980, **40:**403–409.

[34] Lamb, D. R. Androgens and exercise. *Medicine and Science in Sports,* 1975, **7:**1–5.

[35] Lassarre, C., F. Girard, J. Durand, and J. Raynaud. Kinetics of human growth hormone during submaximal exercise. *Journal of Applied Physiology,* 1974, **37:**826–830.

[36] Leon, A. S., W. A. Pettinger, and M. A. Saviano. Enhancement of serum renin activity by exercise in the rat. *Medicine and Science in Sports,* 1973, **5:**40–43.

[37] Maher, J. T., L. G. Jones, L. H. Hartley, G. H. Williams, and L. I. Rose. Aldosterone dynamics during graded exercise at sea level and high altitude. *Journal of Applied Physiology,* 1975, **39:**18–22.

[38] Melin, B., J. P. Eclache, G. Geelen, G. Annat, A. M. Allevard, E. Jarsaillon, A. Zebidi, J. J. Legros, and C. Gharib. Plasma AVP, neurophysin, renin activity, and aldosterone during

submaximal exercise performed until exhaustion in trained and untrained men. *European Journal of Applied Physiology,* 1980, **44:**141–151.

[39] Newmark, S. R., T. Himathongkam, R. P. Martin, K. H. Cooper, and L. I. Rose. Adrenocortical response to marathon running. *Journal of Clinical Endocrinology and Metabolism,* 1976, **42:**393–394.

[40] Nilsson, K. O., L. G. Heding, and B. Hokfelt. The influence of short-term submaximal work on the plasma concentrations of catecholamines, pancreatic glucagon and growth hormone in man. *Acta Endocrinologica,* 1975, **79:**286–294.

[41] Peronnet, F., J. Cleroux, H. Perrault, D. Cousineau, J. de Champlain, and R. Nadeau. Plasma norepinephrine response to exercise before and after training in humans. *Journal of Applied Physiology,* 1981, **51:**812–815.

[42] Pruett, E. D. R. Plasma insulin concentrations during prolonged work at near-maximal oxygen intake. *Journal of Applied Physiology,* 1970, **29:**155–158.

[43] Richter, E. A., B. Sonne, N. J. Christensen, and H. Galbo. Role of epinephrine for muscular glycogenolysis and pancreatic hormonal secretion in running rats. *American Journal of Physiology,* 1981, **240:**E526–E532.

[44] Schwartz, B., D. C. Cumming, E. Riordan, M. Selye, S. S. C. Yen, and R. W. Rebar. Exercise-associated amenorrhea: a distinct entity? *American Journal of Obstetrics and Gynecology,* 1981, **141:**662–670.

[45] Shephard, R. J., and K. H. Sidney. Effects of physical exercise on plasma growth hormone and cortisol levels in human subjects. *Exercise and Sport Sciences Reviews,* 1975, **3:**1–30.

[46] Skierska, E., J. Ustupska, B. Biczowa, and J. Lukaszewska. Effect of physical exercise on plasma cortisol, testosterone, and growth hormone levels in weight lifters. *Endokrynologia Polska,* 1976, **27:**159–165.

[47] Stromme, S. B., H. D. Meen, and A. Aakvaag. Effects of an androgenic-anabolic steroid on strength development and plasma testosterone levels in normal males. *Medicine and Science in Sports,* 1974, **6:**203–208.

[48] Sturek, M., D. R. Lamb, and A. C. Snyder. Somatomedin-like activity and muscle hypertrophy. *IRCS Medical Science: Physiology,* 1981, **9:**760.

[49] Sutton, J. R., M. J. Coleman, J. Casey, and L. Lazarus. Androgen responses during physical exercise. *British Medical Journal,* 1973, **163:**520–522.

[50] Terjung, R. Endocrine response to exercise. *Exercise and Sport Sciences Reviews,* 1979, **7:**153–180.

[51] Terjung, R. L., and C. M. Tipton. Plasma thyroxine and thyroid-stimulating hormone levels during submaximal exercise in humans. *American Journal of Physiology,* 1971, **220:**1840–1845.

[52] Tharp, G. D. The role of glucocorticoids in exercise. *Medicine and Science in Sports,* 1975, **7:**6–11.

[53] Tharp, G. D., and R. J. Buuck. Adrenal adaptation to chronic exercise. *Journal of Applied Physiology,* 1974, **37:**720–722.

[54] Wade, C. E., and J. R. Claybaugh. Plasma renin activity, vasopressin concentration, and urinary excretory responses to exercise in men. *Journal of Applied Physiology,* 1980, **49:**930–936.

[55] Wilkerson, J. E., S. M. Horvath, and B. Gutin. Plasma testosterone during treadmill exercise. *Journal of Applied Physiology,* 1980, **49:**249–253.

[56] Winder, W. W., R. C. Hickson, J. M. Hagberg, A. A. Ehsani, and J. A. McLane. Training-induced changes in hormonal and metabolic responses to submaximal exercise. *Journal of Applied Physiology,* 1979, **46:**766–771.

[57] Wirth, A., C. Diehm, H. Mayer, H. Morl, I. Vogel, P. Bjorntorp, and G. Schlierf. Plasma C-peptide and insulin in trained and untrained subjects. *Journal of Applied Physiology,* 1981, **50:**71–77.

C H A P T E R
18

Exercise and Health

IT is widely assumed by the general public that the person who exercises regularly is healthier and less subject to disease than one who does not. This assumption is especially dear to those who enjoy regular exercise. *Disease* is defined as a condition of the body in which there is incorrect or abnormal function of one or more of its parts. *Health,* on the other hand, is the condition of the body characterized by vigor, vitality, and freedom from disease. Although there is much scientific evidence that can be cited to support the view that those who exercise are healthier than those who do not, it is also true that much of the evidence regarding characteristics such as life span and susceptibility to coronary heart disease is inconclusive. Most of the data show that healthful characteristics are *associated* with populations of persons who exercise regularly, but such relationships are not necessarily cause-and-effect relationships. One might suspect, for example, that persons who exercise are less likely to suffer early heart attacks, not because they exercise, but because some other factor common to exercisers (for example, low body fat and superior hereditary qualities) has a protective effect on the heart.

Experimental and Nonexperimental Evidence

The scientist who wishes to determine whether or not regular exercise has a beneficial effect on health has essentially two avenues of investigation—experimental and non-experimental. In an experiment, the investigator can assign subjects at random to either an exercise or a sedentary group. If the study is well controlled, and if the subjects

366

who exercise regularly are healthier at the end of the study, the scientist can have a relatively high degree of confidence that the difference in health between the two groups results from the exercise and not from some other factors.

With the nonexperimental approach, the investigator typically compares the health of a population of "exercisers" to that of a population of "nonexercisers." However, the investigator does not assign the subjects to the exercise and nonexercise conditions; the populations are taken as they present themselves—as, for example, sedentary cashiers versus active foundry workers, mail carriers versus postal clerks, executives versus laborers. Accordingly, if the active population is healthier, the scientist cannot be certain that the difference in health status is due to exercise, because it is impossible to control all the other possible factors (examples include diet, heredity, and emotionality) that could account for the apparently beneficial effect of exercise on health.

It is unfortunate that all problems cannot be solved by experimentation. It is foolish, for example, to design an experiment to determine whether or not regular exercise enhances life span in humans; it is not reasonable to think that infants could be randomly assigned to active or sedentary living for their entire lives. Long-term experiments on humans are notoriously difficult to complete in a satisfactory manner because of uncontrollable changes in human life styles. Therefore, nonexperimental studies are vital to give us some evidence, albeit imperfect, on important questions that cannot be answered experimentally.

Criteria for Confidence in the Cause and Effect Nature of Nonexperimental Results

It is true that the results of a single nonexperimental study showing exercise to be associated with improved health should not be interpreted as proving that exercise *caused* the improved health. On the other hand, one can have a great deal of confidence in the cause-and-effect nature of results from nonexperimental studies if the following criteria are satisfied:

1. *The association between exercise and health must be reliable.* This means that all or nearly all studies of the same association between exercise and health must show similar results. As more studies show the same association between exercise and certain health characteristics, our confidence in the cause-and-effect nature of the association increases.

2. *The association between exercise and health must be strong.* We can place much more confidence in the cause-and-effect nature of an association, for example, if it shows that 90 per cent of the exercisers are healthier than if only 51 per cent of the exercisers are healthier than the nonexercisers.

3. *The association between exercise and health must be logical.* It would be difficult to believe that regular exercise causes a reduction in the size of warts, no matter how many studies showed a strong association of this nature. There is no logical reason to think that exercise should decrease the growth of warts.

4. *The association between exercise and health must follow an appropriate chronological sequence.* For example, before one can be certain that regular aerobic endurance exercise causes a low resting heart rate, it must be shown that the low resting heart rate does not precede the exercise training. Whenever two factors A and B are related causally, it is not only possible that A causes B but also that B could conceivably cause A.

5. *The effect on health must be shown not to be caused by some obvious factor other than exercise.* One must seek out and find wanting alternative causes for the association between exercise and health. Is it exercise *per se* that causes active populations to have less body fat, or is the reduced fat simply the result of the fact that people who exercise also happen to eat less than sedentary populations? Could the same reduction in fat be caused by dietary restriction?

Of course, it is impossible to test *all* alternative causes that might explain an association between exercise and health; many of the alternative causes are unknown. But until the obvious alternatives have been tested, one can have only limited confidence in the cause-and-effect nature of an association between exercise and health.

If the previous criteria are satisfied, one can have just as much confidence in the cause-and-effect nature of nonexperimentally discovered associations between exercise and health as one has in experimentally derived evidence. Keep these criteria in mind as you weigh the evidence presented in this chapter. Also, remember that a failure to prove absolutely that exercise has a positive effect on some health characteristics does not mean that one should abandon all physical activity performed for health purposes. *Only rarely is a properly designed exercise program harmful to health, but there is much evidence that it may be beneficial. Thus, there is a much greater risk to health from inactivity than from appropriate regular exercise.*

The remainder of this chapter is devoted to a presentation of the evidence 1) that regular exercise may influence the length and quality of human life; 2) that exercise may be useful in the prevention of disease; 3) that exercise can be useful in the treatment of disease; and 4) that *improperly designed* exercise programs may actually be harmful to one's health.

Exercise, Longevity, and Quality of Life

As mentioned earlier, in a practical sense there can be no adequately designed experiments to test the hypothesis that regular exercise throughout life can increase human longevity. Therefore, one can only compare the life spans of groups of presumably active persons with those of similar groups of presumably inactive persons. One can imagine many factors that influence life span that could easily mask any beneficial effect of lifetime exercise. Automobile accidents, wars, and infectious disease epidemics can kill many people at an early age who might otherwise have lived long, healthy lives. Accordingly, one should not expect to see a tremendous difference in the average life span of those from "active" and "sedentary" populations.

Nonexperimental Comparisons of Longevity for "Active" and "Sedentary" Human Populations

Many of the studies of exercise and longevity have included comparisons of the life spans of college athletes with those of their nonathletic classmates or of the population in general [41, 61]. Those studies in which the general population was used as a control group all showed that former college athletes lived about two years longer than the general population [61]. Unfortunately, because the life span of all university graduates (who have better nutrition, better medical care, and better jobs) tends to be longer than that of the general population, these early studies are not very useful in determining the effect of exercise on longevity.

Comparisons of the longevity of former college athletes to that of their nonathletic counterparts are more valid, but most of these studies have shown only insignificant differences between groups [44, 61]. One interesting comparison of life spans of 1,655 Japanese university athletes, 3,069 Tokyo University Medical School graduates, and the general Japanese population showed that 70 per cent of the athletes, 42 per cent of the general population, and only 35 per cent of the medical doctors reached the age range of 68–72 years [41].

It can be contended, of course, that college athletes do not necessarily remain active after college, and that no difference should be expected between life spans of former athletes and nonathletes. A study of 396 Finnish champion skiers (not necessarily university graduates), who tend to continue skiing for many years, showed that their average life span was 2.8 years longer than the median life expectation of the general male population [44]. Perhaps future investigators will be able to amass adequate data from those who jog regularly into their later years to better judge the effect of regular endurance exercise on longevity.

Experimental Studies of Exercise Effects on Longevity of Laboratory Animals

Laboratory rats typically live to about two years of age. Therefore, it is possible to conduct a longitudinal experiment on the effects of exercise on life span and to complete the study in 2–3 years. Control of diets, lighting, temperature, housing, and other factors is possible with laboratory animals, but not with humans. A number of studies has been reported where rats were randomly assigned to exercised or sedentary groups at early ages and longevity was recorded. In essentially all of these studies, the average life span of the exercised animals, both male and female, was substantially increased [18, 30, 70, 86]. The usual mode of exercise was voluntary running in a cage wheel, and the increases in life span averaged about 15–20 per cent. Therefore, we can conclude that regular exercise can markedly increase longevity in normal rats. We can only speculate about whether similar results would occur if humans could be randomly assigned to exercised and sedentary groups, but presumably the direction of the results would be the same. It should be noted that exercise caused a 15 per cent reduction in life span in rats that were genetically obese, hypertensive, blind, and affected by a number of other pathological lesions [8]. The lesson here, of course, is that exercise is not always a beneficial stressor and is not recommended for acutely ill persons or animals.

Quality of Life

Regular exercise undoubtedly plays a more important role in enhancing the quality of one's life than its length. Valid experiments on this point of enhanced quality of life are difficult to come by; men and women who participate in regular exercise do so voluntarily, usually because they are convinced that physical activity does improve the quality of their lives. Again, it is impossible to assign human beings to long-term exercise or nonexercise conditions. However, it is patently obvious that one who is physically able to do more things without assistance and with less physical and emotional strain has a better quality of life than one who is not. There are millions of persons who find it impossible to climb a flight of stairs, carry a heavy bag of groceries, shovel snow, run to catch a bus, play tennis, swim, or ride a bicycle. One need only ask a person who is bedridden if he would prefer to be active to know that regular, appropriate, physical activity enhances the quality of life.

A more serious question, but one that is impossible to answer for everyone, is: *How much* exercise is required to achieve the *optimal* quality of life? It is clear that not everyone must run 30 miles per day to experience an optimal quality of life. Each of us has different requirements for regular physical activity, depending on our hereditary endowment for withstanding disease, the physical demands of our occupations, our proclivities for recreational manual labor and sport activities, and the probabilities of unforeseen events placing unforeseen physical demands upon our bodies. Thus, it is impossible to define blanket exercise requirements for all; exercise prescription must be individualized to be most effective in the development and maintenance of overall health and well-being.

Regular Exercise and the Prevention of Disease

If disease is defined as the incorrect or abnormal function of (a) part(s) of the body, it can be vigorously asserted that regular physical activity can prevent disease. Evidence in support of this assertion has been accumulating for more than a century.

Hypokinetic Degeneration

Hypokinesis is a relative lack of movement. An extreme case of hypokinesis would be that present in a patient placed in a total body cast for recovery from multiple bone fractures. Less extreme hypokinesis is present in office workers who sit at their desks eight hours a day and then drive to their homes where they watch 5 or 6 hours of television before retiring. Hypokinetic degeneration is a disease characterized by decreased functional capacity of many organs and systems. In those who rest in bed for several weeks or months, some or all of the following may occur [6]:

1. *Osteoporosis (bone atrophy)*—Loss of bone minerals and protein makes the bones of the bed-ridden extremely susceptible to fractures.
2. *Muscle atrophy*—Gradual wasting away of skeletal muscle tissue causes progressively increasing muscular weakness. Muscle fibers assume more of the characteristics of fast twitch fibers [20]; mitochondria from atrophied muscles have a reduced capacity for aerobic metabolism.
3. *Loss of flexibility*—If joints are kept in improper positions for even a few days, connective tissue in tendons, ligaments, muscles and joint capsules becomes dense and shortened; eventually this connective tissue strongly resists any attempt at stretching to regain the lost range of motion of the joint. It is this connective tissue, especially that in the fascial sheaths of the muscles, that accounts for much of the limitation in range of motion of most joints in the body [36].
4. *Cardiovascular degeneration*—Resting heart rate increases and stroke volume is diminished; maximal oxygen uptake is markedly lowered; the circulatory system is unable to maintain normal blood pressure responses when the patient is tilted upright; blood clots in the veins sometimes develop and may lodge in the lungs to cause death; and blood volume decreases.
5. *Respiratory problems*—Lung congestion, bronchial obstruction, and even pneumonia are more common in bedridden patients.
6. *Bladder and bowel dysfunction*—Immobilization often decreases sensitivity of the bladder and bowel so that inadequate voiding of urine and feces is common.
7. *Bed sores*—Painful ulcerations of the skin occur in those who remain motionless in bed.

There is no question that some minimal exercise program can prevent hypokinetic degenerative disease: by definition, those who are reasonably active do not contract hypokinetic degenerative disease.

Earlier chapters presented ample discussion of the efficacy of training in causing improvements in the muscular and cardiovascular system. Let us now describe briefly some of the evidence that regular exercise positively affects the characteristics of bones, ligaments, connective tissue within muscles, and nerves.

Exercise and Bone Growth. Bone tissue is constantly undergoing a process of remodeling, with minerals being removed from some parts of bones and added to others. During physical activity, stress that is placed on the bone causes an increased deposition of calcium salts along the lines of stress and removal of minerals from minimally stressed areas. In rats, regular training sessions of 5 or 6 hours of light running cause few changes in either bone length or density, but more intensive exercise for shorter durations may slightly decrease bone length and increase bone density [7]. Dogs who exercised on a treadmill while carrying lead-weighted packs had significantly greater bone mineral content and tibia widths than nonexercised controls [56]. Also, bones from trained animals may have greater resistance to breaking and may heal faster after fracture [7]. In human beings, most studies show that regular moderate exercise in older persons retards the bone loss that usually accompanies advanced age [1, 84, 85]. Presumably, this effect is caused by bioelectrical currents that are generated by forces on bone. These currents alter the activity of the bone cells to reduce the net demineralization of the bone.

There is no consistent evidence that training of youngsters causes them to have shorter or taller stature.

Exercise, Ligaments, Tendons, and Intramuscular Connective Tissue. Many studies of laboratory animals show that physical training strengthens the attachments of ligaments and tendons to bones [7, 90, 95]. Trained ligaments are thicker and heavier, but the increased weight of the ligaments is not reflected in greater concentrations of collagen, the principal component of connective tissue fibers [7, 90]. The mechanism underlying the enhanced strength of ligaments and tendons with training is unclear.

When soleus and plantaris muscles of a rat are made to work harder by surgical removal of the synergistic gastrocnemius muscle, there occurs not only a hypertrophy of the soleus and plantaris muscle fibers, but also an increase in the collagen content of the connective tissues that surround the muscle fibers [7]. Perhaps the stronger connective tissue investments of the muscle allow the muscle to contract more forcefully before tears of connective tissue and capillaries result in delayed muscle soreness. The activity of an enzyme involved in collagen synthesis is increased by physical training, and this enzyme may play a part in increasing the production of collagen fibers [7]. It has been speculated that lactic acid production during exercise stimulates the enzyme activity [7].

In contrast to the growth of intramuscular connective tissue after surgical overload, moderate endurance training of rats on a treadmill produces neither muscle hypertrophy nor increased growth of intramuscular connective tissue [47]. To accelerate connective tissue growth, it appears that greater tension must be placed on the muscle fibers than is generated by treadmill training.

Maintaining Joint Range of Motion (Flexibility). The range of motion of a joint refers to the maximum ability to move the bones about the joint through an arc of a circle. For example, if one can extend the knee joint from 30 degrees at full flexion to 170 degrees at full extension, the range of motion or degree of flexibility at the knee is $170 - 30 = 140$ degrees. Joint motion is limited primarily by ligamentous joint capsules, tendons, and muscles. These tissues can be stretched to increase flexibility, and great flexibility is of obvious importance in activities such as gymnastics, diving, dance, and acrobatics and is also important in most other athletic endeavors. With advancing age, maintaining flexibility of the trunk becomes increasingly important to minimize the chance of chronic low back pain.

Fortunately, ligaments, tendons, and muscles can be stretched to improve joint range of motion. These tissues can undergo "plastic" elongation, which is a more or less permanent type of lengthening, or "elastic" elongation, which is a temporary lengthening. To improve range of motion it is desirable to increase plastic elongation. Research suggests that plastic stretch is enhanced with fewer injuries: a) when stretch is prolonged, b) when the tissue to be stretched is warmed during prolonged stretch and cooled just before release of the stretch, and c) when low tension is used to create the stretch [73]. Thus, stretching exercises should be done very slowly and with minimum involvement of forceful, jerky types of contractions by antagonist muscles. Stretches should be held for 20–60 minutes, if possible, to get the maximum plastic elongation of the connective tissues. To maintain stretch for such long periods it is obvious that only small increments in range of motion should be attempted each session. Jerky types of movements, such as violent toe touches with locked knees, invoke stretch reflexes of the stretched muscles. These reflexes facilitate contraction, not elongation in these muscles. Such jerky movements also subject the tissues to tremendous strains which can cause injury.

Contrary to the usual practice, it also appears logical to perform stretching exercises *after* a preliminary warmup of jogging, swimming, or other activity which can raise the muscle temperature. Such preliminary activities can raise the temperature of the connective tissue to increase the plastic elongation effects of the stretching activity and can decrease the risk of injury to the tissue [73]. If one is injured, muscle temperature can be increased through the use of hot packs or baths (for superficial muscles) or ultrasound (for large or deep muscles). Cooling of the tissues for the final 10–15 minutes of stretching seems to stabilize the connective tissue structure at their new length [73]. Application of bags of crushed ice around the stretched tissues seems to be an effective method of cooling the tissues during the final phase of the stretching activity.

Techniques of stretching have sometimes included active contraction of the antagonistic muscles during stretch. The idea behind this approach is that such contractions might create reciprocal inhibition nerve reflexes to minimize contractile activity in the muscle to be stretched. However, this technique does not produce any better effects than passive stretch created by body weight or by other types of weights.

Exercise and the Nervous System. It is difficult to study neural tissue with normal biochemical and histological techniques: there are very small amounts of nerve tissue to work with, and the tissue is very easily torn or otherwise disrupted because of its delicate structure. Accordingly, it is not surprising that we know little of the adaptability of the nervous system to regular exercise. Studies of laboratory animals suggest that 1) terminal axons to muscles may be lengthened with training, 2) the area of neuromuscular junctions on trained muscles may be increased, 3) increased activity of cholinesterase enzyme may occur at neuromuscular junctions of trained muscles, especially in fast-twitch fibers, 4) the size of the cell bodies, nuclei, and nucleoli of spinal motor neurons may increase with exhaustive exercise, and 5) increased activity of several enzymes of the motor neurons is present in trained animals [20]. Although the changes in neural tissue described are of unknown significance from a functional standpoint, it is clear that the nervous system can adapt to chronic exercise, and it seems highly probable that many of these neural adaptations are of major importance to the organism.

Coronary Artery Disease

Each year about one of every 100 American men 40 years of age or more will develop some symptom of coronary artery disease, the obstruction of one or more of the arteries that supply oxygen to the heart muscle. In about 60 per cent of these cases the obstruction of blood flow is so great that parts of the heart muscle are unable to function, cardiac output becomes inadequate, and the victims die immediately or within a few days. Therefore, it is clear that any significant reduction in death rate from heart disease will have to be accomplished by a greater effort to *prevent* the disease rather than by attempts to treat the disease once it has manifested itself. Many cardiologists are of the opinion that coronary artery disease begins to develop in children and that preventive efforts, including the establishment of regular aerobic exercise habits, should be emphasized at very early ages [10]. The principal question to be addressed in this section is: What role does regular exercise play in the prevention of premature heart disease?

Lack of Exercise as a Risk Factor in Coronary Artery Disease. Risk factors in coronary disease are those characteristics of persons that are associated with a large increase in susceptibility to the onset, particularly the premature onset (before age 65), of heart disease. There are many characteristics related to heart disease, but the three most powerful risk factors for the occurrence of coronary heart disease (other than age and sex) are: 1) high blood pressure, 2) high levels of blood cholesterol, and 3) cigarette smoking [9]. Physical inactivity ranks fourth on the list of significant risk factors, but it is clearly a less reliable predictor of coronary artery disease occurrence than the "big three" of high blood pressure, high blood cholesterol, and smoking [9]. Other identified risk factors include obesity, family history of coronary artery disease, diabetes mellitus, and personality patterns characterized by an exaggerated sense of time urgency and competitiveness.

Since about 1975, there has been an increasing interest in the types of fats present in the blood as risk factors for heart disease. In particular, it appears that low levels of cholesterol bound to "high density lipoproteins" (HDL) are associated with an increased risk of heart disease, and high levels of HDL cholesterol decrease the risk of heart disease [31]. High density lipoproteins seem to transport cholesterol out of the bloodstream and to the liver for metabolism. Thus, HDL seems to help clear cholesterol out of the blood more quickly so that it is less likely to become deposited in the walls of the arteries to cause atherosclerosis. Thus, one could have high levels of total cholesterol and still have a low risk of heart disease if a large fraction of that cholesterol were HDL cholesterol.

It is sobering to note that the majority of children 7–12 years of age may already exhibit at least one risk factor for heart disease [28]. Other than family history of heart disease, the most prevalent risk factors in this age group seem to be obesity and high levels of blood fat [28].

Comparisons of Heart Disease Incidence in "Active" and "Less Active" Populations. Most, but not all, comparisons of populations of presumably active workers with populations of inactive workers show that occupational physical activity predisposes one to have a lesser incidence of symptoms and early deaths from coronary artery disease. Active conductors on the double-decker busses of London tended to have less coronary heart disease than the inactive bus drivers; London and Washington, D.C., postmen had less heart disease than inactive postal clerks; active workers in Israeli kibbutzim had less heart disease than their inactive counterparts; active railroad men had less heart disease than sedentary clerks; and active utility workers and longshoremen tended to have less heart disease than less active workers [23, 24].

However, some comparisons of active and inactive populations have failed to demonstrate any protective effect of occupational physical activity. For example, Finnish workers who had physically demanding occupations had no decreased risk of heart disease, and active Los Angeles civil servants had the same risk of coronary artery disease as their less active counterparts [23].

Another finding which supports the hypothesis of a protective effect of physical activity against the early onset of heart disease is that men who engage in vigorous leisure sports and fitness activities have less early coronary artery disease than those who are not vigorously active [62]. This seems to be true not only among normal subjects but also among obese persons, smokers, those with a family history of heart disease, and those with hypertension [62]. Therefore, it appears that both occupational and leisure time exercise are beneficial in preventing early coronary disease.

As stated earlier in this chapter, positive results of large scale population comparisons do not prove a cause-and-effect relationship between more physical activity and less coronary disease. But the fact that most of these surveys implicate exercise as an independent risk factor certainly points to a high probability that regular exercise helps prevent the early onset of heart disease. Unfortunately, we need more studies of the relationship between leisure-time exercise patterns and heart disease to give us better direction for prescribing preventive exercise.

Physiological Mechanism Underlying the Probable Protective Effect of Exercise. It is reasonable to ask *how* any protective effect of regular exercise against the early onset of heart disease may be brought about. Many hypotheses that some single mechanism is responsible for this protective effect have been advanced, but none as yet has been proven. Most of the proposed mechanisms involve a presumed beneficial effect of regular exercise on 1) (blood supply to the heart muscle, 2) competency of the contractile process of the heart, 3) blood fat levels, 4) atherosclerotic lesion development, 5) blood clotting mechanisms, 6) obesity, 7) hypertension, and 8) psychological well-being. Obesity and hypertension will be considered as separate diseases in subsequent discussions in this chapter.

Regular Exercise and Blood Supply to the Heart—Coronary Blood Flow. Because heart attacks are associated with decreased circulation of blood through the coronary arteries, one of the most obvious hypotheses to explain the beneficial effects of exercise on the risk of heart disease is that exercise may enhance coronary circulation, perhaps by enlarging the main branches of the coronary arteries, by improving the distribution of capillaries in the heart muscle, or by increasing the ability of the heart to develop new branches of healthy arteries to take over the circulation to blood-starved areas of the heart.

The influence of training on blood flow in the coronary arteries is not clearly understood. For example, one study of rats trained by swimming showed an increased coronary flow in enlarged hearts but no change in flow per gram of heart weight [74]. Rats trained by treadmill running, on the other hand, showed no increase in heart weight and no increase in coronary blood flow [25]. Similarly, one dog study [87] showed no effect of treadmill training on coronary blood flow at rest or during exercise, whereas another [4] showed a reduction in coronary flow at rest and during submaximal treadmill exercise but no change with maximal exercise. No effect of training on coronary blood flow was found in pigs trained by running [72]. Most investigators use different training programs and different techniques for estimating coronary blood flow. Therefore, it is difficult to interpret the conflicting information. When changes in coronary flow are found, however, they tend to be rather small. Whether or not such changes are physiologically important is uncertain.

Regular Exercise and Blood Supply to the Heart —Coronary Tree Size. It has been repeatedly demonstrated that rats physically trained from youth by swimming or treadmill running have larger coronary arteries and a greater size of the "coronary tree" than untrained control animals [3]. Typically, in these studies, the coronary arteries of the animals are injected with a liquid plastic that rapidly hardens. The tissue around the plastic mold of the arteries is then digested away with chemicals, leaving a plastic model of the coronary tree which can be weighed or measured for arterial diameters. Some of the new coronary branches developed in the trained rat may serve areas of the heart already supplied from another artery and could be classified as coronary collaterals. It should be pointed out that the size of the coronary arteries of pigs is not increased by 10 minutes of treadmill running at 16 km/hr (10 mph), 5 days per week, for 22 months [52].

In dogs, treadmill training in one experiment did cause a small increase in the cross-sectional area of coronary arteries [94]. Also, a stable coronary flow with increased heart size after training in any animal suggests that there was coronary artery growth which accompanied the heart muscle growth [3, 74].

Regular Exercise and Blood Supply to the Heart —Cardiac Capillarization. It has often been shown by comparing the number of capillaries filled with injected India ink or other chemicals that trained animals have more coronary capillaries, a greater number of capillaries per heart muscle fiber, and a smaller diffusion distance (half the distance between two capillaries) for oxygen than untrained animals [3]. There is direct evidence that new capillaries are formed in the hearts of rats trained by swimming [53]. Thus, the increase in capillaries in trained rats is not simply the effect of opening up capillaries which were present before training began.

Dogs may not adapt to training with greater cardiac capillarization as rats do. A study which showed greater coronary artery size did not detect any change in capillarization [94].

If the increases in coronary tree size and capillarization that occur as a result of training in rats also occur in man, these changes should reduce the resistance and, therefore, increase the coronary blood flow at any given arterial pressure [3]. Also, the increased capillary development should result in the delivery of blood closer to the muscle fibers, so that oxygen can more effectively diffuse to the muscle cells. At the present time, however, we have no direct evidence that such changes do occur in man.

Regular Exercise and Blood Supply to the Heart —Coronary Collateral Circulation. Coronary collaterals are small vessels which connect two or more coronary arteries or branches of the same coronary artery. The value of these collateral channels is important to understand. If an artery is obstructed by fatty deposits or a blood clot at one point in its length, the heart tissue beyond that point will be starved of blood unless collaterals from neighboring arteries can supply the circulation beyond the point of obstruction. Therefore, the greater the development of collateral circulation, the less the risk of heart tissue damage if an arterial branch is closed off by atherosclerosis or by a clot.

It has long been known that an obstruction in a coronary artery can stimulate the growth of collaterals, probably because of the hypoxic condition that develops after blockage of the artery. This collateralization often helps people recover from a heart attack and continue to live relatively normal lives. It was thought that exercise, by placing greater oxygen demands on the heart, might be useful in stimulating the growth of coronary collaterals. In fact, more collaterals may develop in dogs that are trained after having a coronary artery tied off ("artificial" heart attack) than in nonexercised dogs [3, 75]. However, in dogs or pigs who have *normal* coronary arteries, training does not increase the development of coronary collaterals [15, 72, 75]. In rats subjected to artificial heart attacks, no effect of training was found on collateral flow to the blood-starved area of the rat hearts; however, a small increase in collateral flow was noted in adjacent areas of the hearts. [46]. It was unclear if this minor effect was of any physiological significance.

There are no studies of coronary collateral development in *normal* human subjects, but experiments have been performed with patients who have suffered heart attacks. In these studies, the coronary circulation is viewed under x-ray after a dense material has been infused into the arteries so that the vessels will stand out under the x-ray. This process is called coronary arteriography. Most of the experiments with cardiac patients have not been able to detect a significant difference in the development of coronary collaterals between trained and untrained patients [3, 22, 80]. However, the experimental method of coronary arteriography may not be sensitive enough to detect meaningful changes in collateralization [3]. Accordingly, it is too early to conclude with certainty whether exercise does or does not affect the development of coronary collateral arteries, but at this point, the bulk of the evidence is in the negative direction.

Regular Exercise and Competency of the Cardiac Contractile Process.
The oxygen uptake required by the heart to produce a given cardiac output increases with heart rate; that is, the more often the heart must contract against arterial pressure, the more oxygen must be consumed by the cardiac muscle fibers [81]. Therefore, even if regular exercise has no beneficial effect on the coronary arteries, the heart of a trained person should be able to produce a given cardiac output with somewhat less coronary blood flow than the heart of an untrained person, simply because it pumps at a lower rate with a larger stroke volume [3]. This contention is supported by the fact that a high resting heart rate is one of the risk factors associated with early death from coronary artery disease.

Greater stroke volume has been reported in trained men both with and without evidence of accompanying cardiac hypertrophy [3]. If a hypertrophied heart has a greater ventricular volume at the end of diastolic filling, it makes sense that the stroke volume of larger hearts should be increased. In trained hearts where no increase in heart volume is apparent, the increased stroke volume is most likely caused by a training-induced enhancement of cardiac contractility (strength of contraction) [3]. However, research results on the effects of training on myocardial contractility are contradictory [3, 4, 12, 24, 25, 65, 74, 89]. A majority of the evidence favors the idea that exercise has a positive effect on cardiac contractility. Any increase in contractility associated with training may be related to increases in myosin ATPase activity or to a better delivery of calcium from the sarcoplasmic reticulum to troponin during the initiation of contraction [3, 12, 89]. There seem to be no major training-induced changes in aerobic energy production mechanisms or mitochondrial structures in the heart [3].

Regardless of the mechanism involved, it is commonly observed that trained persons have greater stroke volumes and lower heart rates at rest or during a given physical load, and this training bradycardia (lower heart rate) may play an important role in the protective value of regular exercise against early death from coronary artery disease. Training bradycardia is apparently caused by an increased activity of the vagus nerves with perhaps some decrease in sympathetic stimulation to the heart [3].

Regular Exercise and Blood Fat Levels. A victim of coronary artery disease typically has fatty deposits in the walls of the coronary arteries. These deposits narrow the arterial opening and obstruct the flow of blood. They contain a large amount of cholesterol and also some triglycerides. High levels of these fats in the blood are associated with a greater risk of early heart disease.

Several investigators have studied the possibility that exercise might alter blood fat levels and, thereby, reduce the availability of cholesterol and triglycerides for deposit in the walls of the arteries. Unfortunately, in many of these studies, dietary fat intake and weight loss by the subjects were not adequately assessed. Because blood fat levels are affected both by diet and by weight loss, the interpretation of results of experiments in which these factors are not controlled becomes very difficult. Another problem of interpretation arises from the wide range of exercise programs used to study the relationship between exercise and blood fat levels. It may be that only very rigorous, long-term exercise programs of an aerobic endurance nature can lower blood fats with great reproducibility. From the studies that have been reported, we can draw several conclusions [34, 38, 83, 88, 93]. 1) Any effect of training on total blood cholesterol levels is small and not highly reproducible. 2) Endurance training is usually associated with a small increase in high-density lipoprotein cholesterol, which may be of benefit in helping degrade cholesterol in the liver. 3) Low-density lipoprotein cholesterol (LDLC) is often decreased with physical training. High levels of LDLC are positively associated with early coronary artery disease. 4) Training usually does lower triglyceride in the blood. Since triglycerides make up most of the very low density lipoproteins (VLDL), this class of blood fats is often reduced after training. 5) The alterations in blood fats that are associated with training probably last for only a few days [83]. Consequently, an exercise program designed to help lower blood fats should include an exercise frequency of at least every other day.

Regular Exercise and Development of Atherosclerosis. Heart attacks are associated with the buildup of fatty deposits in the walls of the arteries, especially the coronary arteries. Atherosclerosis is the name given to this disease whereby the openings of the arteries are narrowed by the accumulation of fat in the arterial walls. The effect of regular exercise on the development of atherosclerosis has been studied in monkeys, pigeons, geese, ducks, chickens, rabbits, dogs, rats, and pigs [48, 52].

With a few exceptions, exercise training in these studies resulted in a reduced incidence of fatty deposits in arterial walls.

A very positive effect of running exercise for one hour, three times per week, was shown in a 3–4 year experiment on monkeys [48]. In this study, the trained monkeys had higher levels of HDL cholesterol, reduced levels of LDL cholesterol and VLDL triglyceride, larger hearts, wider coronary arteries, less atherosclerosis, no signs of coronary artery narrowing or adverse ECG changes, and no incidence of sudden death. To the extent that the results of this experiment on monkeys are applicable to humans, the effect of regular moderate exercise on atherosclerosis appears highly beneficial.

In pigs (presumably good animals in which to study atherosclerosis) two different experiments produced somewhat conflicting results. In a study in which the pigs trained on a treadmill at 16 kilometers per hour, no changes were shown in blood fat levels or coronary artery size, but there was a substantial reduction in fatty deposits of the coronary arteries of the exercised pigs compared to sedentary controls [52]. In the second study, in which the pigs ran at 5.6 kilometers per hour, no changes were shown in coronary or aortic atherosclerosis or in blood fat levels [26]. However, since the exercise load in the second study was so mild that it did not even lower body weights, it seems that the results of this study should not be considered to reflect accurately the potential of exercise to reduce atherosclerosis.

Regular Exercise, Blood Clotting, and Fibrinolysis.

The final insult to the coronary circulation that leads to a heart attack is presumably the formation of a thrombus or clot in the coronary artery that has become narrowed and roughened by the buildup of fatty deposits in its walls. If physical training could somehow reduce the probability of a clot forming in the blood vessels, or if training could increase the rate at which small clots are broken down (fibrinolysis), this could perhaps explain the protective effect of regular exercise with respect to early death or illness from coronary heart disease. However, it is unclear if either of these mechanisms is of particular importance in relationship to heart disease, because a single bout of vigorous exercise is associated with a faster clotting time that seems to be offset by a faster breakdown of the fibrin threads of the clots [16, 21, 39, 51].

The increased coagulability of blood after heavy exercise is probably caused by the 200 per cent increase in the antihemophilic factor (Factor VIII) observed in the plasma of exercised persons [51]. This factor is one of the many necessary components of the blood clotting system. The increase in the antihemophilic factor does not occur in the absence of stimulation by adrenaline, so this increase is probably caused by the activation of the sympathetic nervous system that accompanies heavy exercise [51].

As tiny clots form on the walls of arteries and veins, the fibrin threads that make up the framework of the clot can be dissolved by an enzyme called *plasmin,* which is the active form of *plasminogen. Maximal* exercise results in a marked increase in fibrinolytic activity, apparently by increasing the amount of a substance that converts plasminogen to plasmin [51]. There is either no increase or only a small increase in fibrinolytic activity with *submaximal* exercise of short duration, but prolongation of the exercise for many minutes or hours causes a large rise in fibrinolytic activity. The increased fibrinolytic activity during exercise is not caused by adrenaline or by temperature elevation [51].

It is not yet possible to say with certainty whether more rapid coagulation or more rapid fibrin dissolution is physiologically more important or, indeed, if either one plays any major role in the exercising person. However, it may be significant that the increased fibrinolytic response to exercise is much more reproducible than the increased coagulability. The fact that the changes in blood clotting and clot dissolution with exercise are no longer apparent 30–60 minutes after exercise, that is, that there is no adaptation at rest with regular exercise [51], speaks against any important role for these changes in the prevention of early death or illness from coronary heart disease.

Regular Exercise and Psychological Well-Being.   There is some evidence, albeit controversial, that certain types of psychosocial tensions, personality patterns, and life styles may be significant risk factors in coronary disease [9]. It is difficult to gather conclusive evidence in this area, and it is premature to make any final judgment concerning the impact of physical training on the risk of coronary artery disease through exercise-induced changes in psychological well-being. It is clear, however, that many, but not all, of those who participate in regular exercise programs experience improvement in their outlook on life.

Hypertension

Hypertension is a chronically elevated arterial blood pressure, sometimes arbitrarily defined as any resting pressure greater than 140/90 millimeters of mercury. Hypertension is responsible for 10–15 per cent of all deaths in people over 50 years of age and is a significant risk factor not only in coronary disease but also in congestive heart disease, stroke, and kidney disease. Hypertension can now be effectively controlled by drug therapy, but many investigators have considered the possibility that hypertension might be prevented by regular physical exercise. Most comparisons of normal physically trained or occupationally active populations with untrained or inactive groups show no differences in resting blood pressures. Exercise programs in those with normal blood pressure can usually be expected to cause blood pressure reductions of only a few millimeters of mercury [69, 83]. Thus, there is no conclusive evidence that regular exercise can prevent hypertension.

Obesity

Obesity is a recognized risk factor not only in coronary artery disease, but also in diabetes, hypertension, and other ailments. As described in detail in Chapter 7, regular physical activity can prevent obesity if diet is controlled.

Stomach Ulcers

Many people who enjoy exercise have suggested that regular exercise provides an outlet for emotional tension and, therefore, can minimize the development of stomach ulcers. This hypothesis has received some support from the results of studies of laboratory rats. In these studies ulcers were artificially induced by restraining the animals or injecting them with ulcer-inducing drugs [43]. Rats that were trained usually developed less serious ulceration of the stomach, but in one study, only treadmill running, and not swimming, was *effective* [43]. It is thought that the protective effect, when it occurs, results from decreased acid secretion and increased mucous secretion in the stomach.

Whether the results of these studies on rats have any bearing on ulcer development in man is unknown.

Infectious Disease

Although laymen commonly assume that physically fit persons are less susceptible to viral and bacterial disease, there is neither any logic nor evidence that such is the case. The body's mechanisms for producing specific antibodies against disease agents is essentially unaffected by physical training.

Therapeutic Benefits of Regular Exercise

The advent of exercise programs for the rehabilitation of patients who have had heart attacks demonstrates a wide recognition that exercise therapy can play an important role in medical care. However, there are several types of disease in addition to heart disease for which exercise can be a useful tool to the clinician.

Exercise Therapy for Hypokinetic Degeneration

Essentially all of the adverse symptoms associated with prolonged bed rest or other inactivity can be reversed with a well-designed exercise program. Normal cardiovascular function can be regained with suitable aerobic endurance exercise [69]. Flexibility can be increased with little danger of injury by a gradual program of slow, static stretching rather than ballistic, jerky movements [36]. The loss of bone minerals through osteoporosis can be reduced, if not stopped, by very moderate exercise programs [1, 84]. Muscle atrophy can be reversed, bed sores eliminated, bladder and bowel dysfunction minimized, and pulmonary function improved with minimal exercise programs [6]. Physical activity can also speed recovery from surgery of torn ligaments and muscles and from repair of fractured bones [7, 11, 90, 91].

Exercise Programs in Cardiac Rehabilitation

For many years patients who had suffered heart attacks were subjected to nearly total bed rest. As a result, many of the complications of prolonged bed rest (hypokinetic degeneration) occurred in these patients; their capacity to perform work was diminished; and many were unable to return to their former jobs. More and more cardiologists are now advising minimal bed rest for patients who have suffered heart attacks and are prescribing progressive exercise programs to help their patients return to normal life [32]. Some rehabilitated cardiac patients have even been able to complete a marathon [45].

Good experimental evidence that exercised cardiac patients suffer fewer repeat heart attacks and die less frequently from heart attacks is lacking [24]. However, clinical comparisons of patients on exercise programs with those who do not exercise suggest that rates of reinfarction and mortality may be lower in exercised patients [32, 79].

In addition to the possibility that exercise programs may reduce the incidence of repeat heart attacks, benefits of the exercise training include the following: 1) increased physical working capacity, 2) increased threshold for exercise-induced angina (chest pain), 3) decreased myocardial oxygen demand at rest and during submaximal exercise with resultant decreased anginal (chest) pain, 4) decreased heart rate at rest and during submaximal work, 5) decreased symptoms of hypokinetic degeneration, 6) decreased systolic blood pressure at rest and during submaximal work, 7) decreased norepinephrine in the blood during exercise and decreased epinephrine at rest, 8) greater rate of return to gainful employment, and 9) improved psychological outlook with increased self-confidence and reduced depression [3, 24, 32, 35, 68, 80].

It should be pointed out that patients with severe damage to the left ventricle may show little or no physiologic improvement with exercise [3]. Cardiac output increases, decreases, or remains the same during submaximal work after training [3]. The bulk of the evidence available suggests that physical training does not reproducibly increase the coronary collateral circulation to the hearts of cardiac patients [3, 22, 32]. A decreased cardiac oxygen uptake at rest and during exercise may be the most important physiological benefit of exercise therapy in cardiac rehabilitation [3, 32, 80].

Exercise Therapy for Hypertension

Regular exercise training is useful for reducing blood pressure in patients with hypertension, but the blood pressure does not become normal with exercise alone [35, 69, 83]. Medication for hypertension is usually quite effective in normalizing blood pressure, but the drugs are expensive and sometimes cause undesirable side effects. Therefore, exercise training can be important as a means of minimizing the dose of drugs required to control the hypertension [29].

Exercise Therapy for Vasoregulatory Asthenia

Vasoregulatory asthenia is a circulatory disease characterized by greater than normal sympathetic stimulation of the heart and blood vessels. Physical training has been reported to increase working capacity and markedly reduce the circulatory symptoms of vasoregulatory asthenia [37].

Regular Exercise and Occlusive Arterial Disease

Arteries of the legs that are occluded by atherosclerosis often cause severe leg pain when the affected patient walks any distance. Some studies have shown that progressive walking exercises can dramatically increase the time a patient can walk before he must stop because of severe pain [14, 83]. It seems likely that this improvement is caused by enhanced blood flow in the diseased legs, but an increased tolerance to the pain should not be discounted.

Exercise Therapy for Pulmonary Disease

Patients with chronic obstructive lung disease are naturally reluctant to exercise because the increased breathing demands of exercise cause severe shortness of breath; the patient feels as though he is suffocating. This sensation results from the fact that many of the small airways in the lungs are blocked, making it extremely difficult to move an adequate volume of air through the remaining open channels. Unfortunately, physical inactivity often increases the development of airway obstruction. Therefore, patients with lung disease are usually advised to keep as active as possible to avoid hypokinetic degeneration, loss of working capacity, and loss of confidence. Exercise therapy can increase exercise tolerance and working capacity and, thereby, increase confidence and decrease the risk of hypokinetic degeneration [5, 42, 78, 82]. The mechanism for improved exercise tolerance does not necessarily involve improved cardiovascular function or obvious improvements in muscular strength or aerobic enzyme enhancement [5, 78, 82]. Thus, it is unclear exactly how training brings about its beneficial effect on exercise tolerance.

Exercise Treatment of Obesity

As described fully in Chapter 7, exercise is extremely useful in the treatment of obesity. However, it is important to understand that diet control must accompany increased energy expenditure and that few persons are able to maintain a weight control plan for a prolonged period.

Other Diseases

Exercise is sometimes used as an adjunct to insulin therapy in the treatment of *diabetes mellitus*. It has long been recognized by physicians that diabetic patients could reduce their medication when they were physically active [83]. The reason for this phenomenon seems to be that the working skeletal muscles take up more glucose during exercise with only a minimal requirement for insulin. There is no evidence that exercise affects the disease process itself; it only ameliorates the symptoms of the disease.

Chronic low back pain afflicts 70–80 per cent of the world's population at one time or another, usually between the ages of 20 and 55 [64]. The cause of this aggravating pain is usually unknown, but exercise therapy is sometimes useful in relieving it. Studies of the stresses placed on the lower back by various types of exercise suggest that isometric contraction of the abdominal muscles is the preferred exercise [64]. Strong abdominal muscles can counteract loads on the spine by increasing pressure in the abdominal cavity, but typical sit-ups with knees either bent or extended cause greater intradiscal pressures in the spinal column than do isometric contractions of the abdominal muscles [64].

Prolonged bed rest was often prescribed for *arthritic patients* as recently as 1954, but modern therapy includes mild exercise routines and passive movement of the affected joints to keep them from becoming ankylosed (frozen) [6]. Inactivity makes the joints stiffer and decreases mobility in most arthritics.

Finally, exercise therapy has proved useful in the treatment of patients with kidney failure who are undergoing hemodialysis (cleansing of the blood). In addition to improvements noted in some of the metabolic abnormalities associated with kidney failure, regular exercise improved the psychological state of some patients [29].

Potentially Harmful Effects of Exercise

As described throughout this chapter there are many potential health benefits from regular exercise, both from a preventive and from a therapeutic standpoint. But the chapter would be incomplete without some mention of the potentially harmful effects of *poorly designed* exercise programs or the potential for injury in even well-designed programs.

Fatalities in Exercise and Sport

Participation in certain sports carries with it a significant risk of death. Fatality rates for some of the most dangerous sports are listed in Table 18.1. Among the more common interscholastic and intercollegiate sports, those who play American style football suffer the greatest incidence of fatalities—about 0.005 deaths per 1,000 high school players annually and 0.01 deaths per 1,000 collegiate football players annually [63]. Thus, among about 1,400,000 football players, there are 5–10 deaths each year that are directly related to football competition.

Each year there are a few well-conditioned persons who die while exercising. These incidents attract a great deal of publicity and cause some people to question the benefit of exercise to overall health and longevity. A number of autopsy studies have been reported on presumably healthy persons who died during exercise. Typically, the results show that the deceased had severe heart disease or structural defects of the cardiovascular system [27, 54, 92]. Thus, the risk of death from ordinary exercise is quite small, and it is likely that an already defective cardiovascular system is responsible for most of the few deaths which do occur.

TABLE 18.1

Approximate Fatality Rates for Some Dangerous Sports in the United States[1]

Sport	Deaths Per 1,000 Participants Per Year
Sport Parachuting	1.64
Thoroughbred Horse Racing	1.42
Power Boat Racing	0.80
Hang Gliding	0.62
Mountaineering	0.57
Scuba Diving (Amateur)	0.42
Boxing (Professional)	0.41
Glider Flying	0.39

[1] Modified from reference 59.

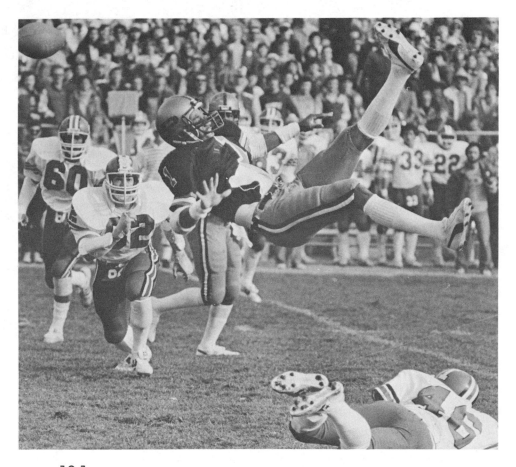

FIGURE 18.1. Each year five to ten football players die from football-related injuries. (Courtesy of Office of Public Information, Purdue University, West Lafayette, Indiana.)

Injuries to Bone, Cartilage, Ligaments, Tendons, and Muscles

The best of exercise programs can occasionally result in broken bones, torn cartilages and ligaments, and ruptured tendons and muscles, to say nothing of superficial cuts, abrasions, and bruises. Certain contact sports such as football and ice hockey are associated with a much greater incidence of severe injury than are other activities. Most football players who are active in the sport throughout junior and senior high school and college suffer a concussion, torn cartilage, pulled muscle, broken tooth, or fractured bone sometime in their careers. Most of these injuries do not cause any lasting harm, but there are thousands of former football players who now curse the sport they once loved, because it has left them with immobile knee joints resulting from torn cartilages or ligaments, and because these injuries have prevented them from enjoying sports such as tennis and racquetball later in life. Each year approximately 30 participants in American style football suffer nonfatal head and neck injuries that lead to paralysis [63]. By some estimates, 19 per cent of high school varsity football players re-

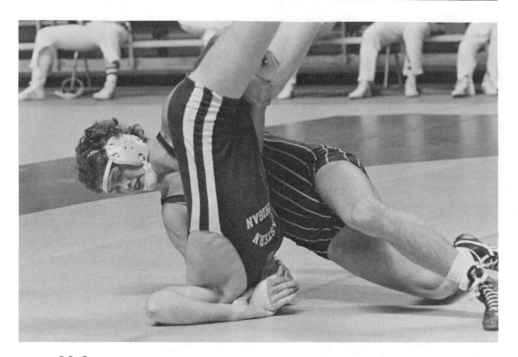

FIGURE 18.2.   Participation in wrestling can lead to shoulder and neck injuries. (Courtesy of Office of Public Information, University of Toledo, Toledo, Ohio.)

port symptoms which indicate some degree of cerebral concussion [71]. Overall injury rates in high school football have been reported to range from 40–80 per cent [60].

Stress fractures of the legs and bones of the feet are relatively common in dancers and distance runners whose bones are subjected to repeated forceful impacts. In gymnasts, weight lifters, and divers, stress fractures of spinal vertebrae and spinal arthritis are sometimes seen [60].

Competitive Sports for Children.   It has often been stated that active sports cause too much stress on bones of growing youngsters and that this stress can result in later bone deformities and osteoarthritis. Comparisons of femoral head tilt, a criterion of degenerative hip disease, between competitive male adolescent sportsmen and less active army recruits did not support this contention [66]. It is true, however, that one out of ten bone fractures at the epiphyseal plate, the zone of growth in young bones, does result in some bone deformity because of the crushing of immature bone cells and their blood supply [50]. Although relatively few children suffer such deformities, this risk should be made clear to parents of children who participate in competitive sports, and especially to parents of those who play tackle football at early ages. Compared to the risk of injury in high school football, that in Pop Warner youth football is quite small, at least partly because of the lesser impact during collision of smaller bodies [60]. The American Academy of Pediatrics believes that competitive sports for children can be beneficial if the programs are well supervised and competently conducted with the appropriate safeguards [2]. Heavy-resistance, low-repetition weight training should not be permitted in children below 16–18 years of age. A number of cases of growth plate injuries and tendon ruptures have reportedly been caused by lifting free weights, especially in the military press [60]. Well-supervised, lightweight, high-repetition lifting can be done safely by youngsters.

Minimizing Injuries in Contact Sports. There are four important principles that a coach or physical educator should stress if he wishes to minimize injuries in contact sports. First, participation should not be allowed if the appropriate protective equipment is not worn. Second, competition should be based on body weight classifications, so that small children compete against other small children. Third, safety rules should be rigidly enforced to rule out unnecessary roughness. Fourth, training should be progressive so that weak muscles and ligaments have a chance to become stronger before being subjected to severe strain. These principles are important not only to avoid injury to young bodies but also to minimize the risk of legal action being taken against the sports supervisor for failure to meet his safety responsibilities in the event of a severe injury.

Eye Injuries in Squash, Racquetball, and Handball

Participants in squash, racquetball, handball, and similar court games risk injury to the eyes by the rapidly moving ball or by the racquets used in the games. In many circumstances injuries could be prevented if players would wear impact resistant polycarbonate eye guards [17]. Regular plastic lenses or tempered glass lenses do not provide significant protection to the eyes and may easily shatter into the eye upon impact with the ball [17].

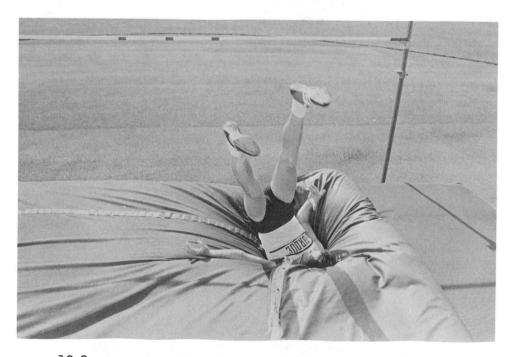

FIGURE 18.3. Protective equipment is critical to the reduction of injuries in athletics. (Courtesy of Office of Public Information, Purdue University, West Lafayette, Indiana.)

Heart Attack During Exercise

Heart attack episodes during exercise stress-testing of normal subjects and cardiac patients are extremely rare [35]. However, it is widely recognized by those who conduct such tests that persons who have recent or increasing chest pain, congestive heart failure, uncontrolled disturbances in heart rhythm or undue fatigue should not be subjected to strenuous exercise and that those who are tested should be carefully supervised to detect signs of impending heart problems [35]. Thus, it is obvious that vigorous exercise does present some risk of heart attacks, especially for those with heart disease and for those who undertake activity that is too severe for their present physical condition. The fact that some cardiac patients can eventually build up their capacities for exercise to the point where they can complete a marathon race suggests that appropriately prescribed training programs are not associated with any excessive risk of exercise-induced heart attacks. The danger arises when inappropriate exercise is undertaken by those who are not suitably prepared for the activity. For normal persons who begin a progressive exercise program, there should be little concern about suffering a heart attack during exertion; the majority of all heart attacks occur during sleep or rest [35].

Heat Illness During Exercise

As described in the chapter on temperature regulation, strenuous exercise during conditions of high environmental temperature and humidity can result in failure of the body's temperature regulating mechanisms, collapse, and even death. This risk can be minimized by consuming cool water at regular intervals during prolonged exercise or by restricting the duration of exercise under adverse environmental conditions.

Exercise-Induced Asthma

A large proportion of asthmatic persons and some sensitive normal subjects experience a narrowing of the bronchioles during exercise and a full-blown asthmatic attack 3–12 minutes following strenuous exercise [13, 40, 78]. Lung function usually returns to normal without therapy within an hour, but occasionally normal function may not resume for several hours [78]. The factors which cause these attacks are unknown, but breathing cool, dry air through the mouth is sometimes associated with the asthma attacks [13, 40]. Attacks are more common after running exercise than after bicycle exercise and are quite uncommon after swimming activity [78]. The condition can be treated with drugs, and it is widely appreciated by medical personnel that asthmatics are perfectly capable of exercising as well as normals if the appropriate medication is used.

Anaphylactic Reactions to Exercise

Anaphylactic reactions are severe allergic attacks that may result in death if not treated. Symptoms include skin rashes, fainting, bronchial constriction, nausea, diarrhea, and severe headaches [57, 58]. In one report, a person suffered anaphylactic reactions only after exercise several hours following a meal containing shellfish; the shellfish did not cause an allergic reaction when the subject did not exercise [57]. The cause of exercise-induced anaphylactic reactions is unknown.

REVIEW QUESTIONS

1. List the criteria that should be satisfied before one should conclude with a high level of confidence that Factor A caused Factor B in a nonexperimental research study.
2. Summarize the evidence bearing on the question of the influence of exercise on life span and the quality of life.
3. Describe the degenerative effects of prolonged physical inactivity and the evidence that regular exercise can both prevent and reverse these effects.
4. Defend the position that exercise is useful in preventing and treating heart disease. Include in your discussion a description of the possible mechanisms underlying the beneficial effects of exercise.
5. Defend the position that exercise is of no significant value in preventing or treating coronary disease.
6. List some of the health hazards of regular physical activity.

REFERENCES

[1] Aloia, J. F., S. H. Cohn, J. A. Ostuni, R. Cane, and K. Ellis. Prevention of involutional bone loss by exercise. *Annals of Internal Medicine,* 1978, **89:**356–358.
[2] American Academy of Pediatrics. Competitive sports for children of elementary school age. *Physician and Sportsmedicine,* 1981, **9:**140–142.
[3] Barnard, R. J. Long-term effects of exercise on cardiac function. *Exercise and Sport Sciences Reviews,* 1975, **3:**113–133.
[4] Barnard, R. J., H. W. Duncan, K. M. Baldwin, G. Grimditch, and G. D. Buckberg. Effects of intensive exercise training on myocardial performance and coronary blood flow. *Journal of Applied Physiology,* 1980, **49:**444–449.
[5] Belman, M. J., and B. A. Kendregan. Exercise training fails to increase skeletal muscle enzymes in patients with chronic obstructive pulmonary disease. *American Review of Respiratory Disease,* 1981, **123:**256–261.
[6] Bonner, C. D. Rehabilitation instead of bed rest? *Geriatrics,* 1969, **24:**109–118.
[7] Booth, F. W., and E. W. Gould. Effects of training and disuse on connective tissue. *Exercise and Sport Sciences Reviews,* 1975, **3:**84–112.
[8] Booth, F. W., W. F. MacKenzie, M. J. Seider, and E. W. Gould. Longevity of exercising obese hypertensive rats. *Journal of Applied Physiology,* 1980, **49:**634–637.
[9] Borhani, N. O. Epidemiology of coronary heart disease. In E. A. Amsterdam, J. H. Wilmore, and A. N. Demaria, eds., *Exercise In Cardiovascular Health and Disease.* New York: Yorke Medical Books, 1977, pp. 1–12.
[10] Boyer, J. L. Coronary heart disease as a pediatric problem. *American Journal of Cardiology,* 1974, **33:**784–786.
[11] Burry, H. C. Soft tissue injury in sport. *Exercise and Sport Sciences Reviews,* 1975, **3:** 275–301.
[12] Carey, R. A., C. M. Tipton, and D. R. Lund. Influence of training on myocardial responses of rats subjected to conditions of ischemia and hypoxia. *Cardiovascular Research,* 1976, **10:**359–367.
[13] Chen, W. Y., P. C. Weiser, and H. Chai. Airway cooling: stimulus for exercise-induced asthma. *Scandinavian Journal of Respiratory Disease,* 1979, **60:**144–150.
[14] Clarke, H. H. Diet and exercise relation to peripheral vascular disease. *Physical Fitness Research Digest,* Series 6, No. 2. Washington, D.C.: President's Council on Physical Fitness and Sports, 1976.

[15] Cohen, M. V., T. Yipintsoi, A. Malhotra, S. Penpargkul, and J. Scheuer. Effect of exercise on collateral development in dogs with normal cononary arteries. *Journal of Applied Physiology*, 1978, **45**:797–805.

[16] Davis, G. L., C. F. Abildgaard, E. M. Bernauer, and M. Britton. Fibrinolytic and hemostatic changes during and after maximal exercise in males. *Journal of Applied Physiology*, 1976, **40**:287–292.

[17] Easterbrook, M. Eye injuries in squash and racquetball players: an update. *Physician and Sportsmedicine*, 1982, **10**:47–56.

[18] Edington, D., A. Cosmas, and W. McCafferty. Exercise and longevity. Evidence for a threshold age. *Journal of Gerontology*, 1972, **27**:341–343.

[19] Edgerton, V. R. Exercise and the growth and development of muscle tissue. In G. L. Rarick, ed., *Physical Activity: Human Growth and Development*. New York: Academic Press, Inc., 1973, pp. 1–31.

[20] Edgerton, V. R. Neuromuscular adaptation to power and endurance work. *Canadian Journal of Applied Sport Sciences*, 1976, **1**:49–58.

[21] Ferguson, W. W., C. F. Barr, and L. L. Bernier. Fibrinogenolysis and fibrinolysis with strenuous exercise. *Journal of Applied Physiology*, 1979, **47**:1157–1161.

[22] Ferguson, R. J., G. Choquette, L. Chaniotis, R. Petitclerc, R. Huot, P. Gauthier, and L. Campeau. Coronary arteriography and treadmill exercise capacity before and after 13 months physical training. *Medicine and Science in Sports*, 1973, **5**:67–68.

[23] Fox, S. M., and W. L. Haskell. Population studies. *Canadian Medical Association Journal*, 1967, **96**:806–811.

[24] Froelicher, V., A. Battler, and M. D. McKirnan. Physical activity and coronary heart disease. *Cardiology*, 1980, **65**:153–190.

[25] Fuller, E. O., and D. O. Nutter. Endurance training in the rat II. Performance of isolated and intact heart. *Journal of Applied Physiology*, 1981, **51**:941–947.

[26] Gass, G. C., F. E. Romack, and T. G. Lohman. The effect of exercise on atherosclerosis in the coronary artery and abdominal aorta of mature female swine. *European Journal of Applied Physiology*, 1979, **42**:235–246.

[27] Gibbons, L. W., J. H. Cooper, B. M. Meyer, and R. C. Ellison. The acute cardiac risk of strenuous exercise. *Journal of the American Medical Association*, 1980, **244**:1799–1801.

[28] Gilliam, T. B., V. L. Katch, W. Thorland, and A. Weltman. Prevalence of coronary heart disease risk factors in active children, 7 to 12 years of age. *Medicine and Science in Sports*, 1977, **9**:21–25.

[29] Goldberg, A. P., J. Hagberg, J. A. Delmez, R. M. Carney, P. M. McKegitt, A. A. Ehsani, and H. R. Harter. The metabolic and psychological effects of exercise training in hemodialysis patients. *American Journal of Clinical Nutrition*, 1980, **33**:1620–1628.

[30] Goodrick, C. L. Effects of long-term voluntary wheel exercise on male and female Wistar rats. Gerontology, **26**:22–33, 1980.

[31] Gordon, T., W. P. Castelli, M. C. Hjortland, W. B. Kannel, and T. R. Dawber. High density lipoprotein as a protective factor against coronary heart disease. The Framingham Study. *American Journal of Medicine*, 1977, **62**:707–714.

[32] Haskell, W. L. Physical activity after myocardial infarction. *American Journal of Cardiology*, 1974, **33**:776–783.

[33] Haskell, W. L., and S. N. Blair. The physical activity component of health promotion in occupational settings. *Public Health Reports*, 1980, **95**:109–118.

[34] Haskell, W. L., H. L. Taylor, P. D. Wood, H. Schrott, and G. Heiss. Strenuous physical activity, treadmill exercise test performance and plasma high-density lipoprotein cholesterol. The lipid research clinics program prevalence study. *Circulation*, 1980, **62** (suppl. IV):53–59.

[35] Hellerstein, H. K. Relation of exercise to acute myocardial infarction. *Circulation*, 1969, **39–40** (suppl. 4):124–129.

[36] Holland, G. The physiology of flexibility: a review of the literature. *Kinesiology Review*, 1968, **1**:49–62.

[37] Holmgren, A. Vasoregulatory asthenia. *Canadian Medical Association Journal,* 1967, **96:**904–905.

[38] Huttunen, J. K., E. Lansimies, E. Voutilainen, C. Ehnholm, E. Hietanen, I. Penttila, O. Siitonen, and R. Rauramaa. Effect of moderate physical exercise on serum lipoproteins. A controlled clinical trial with special reference to serum high-density lipoproteins. *Circulation,* 1979, **60:**1220:1229.

[39] Hyers, T. M., B. J. Martin, D. S. Pratt, R. B. Dreisin, and J. J. Franks. Enhanced thrombin and plasmin activity with exercise in man. *Journal of Applied Physiology,* 1980, **48:**821–825.

[40] Inbar, O., R. Dotan, R. A. Dlin, I. Neuman, and O. Bar-Or. Breathing dry or humid air and exercise-induced asthma during swimming. *European Journal of Applied Physiology,* 1980, **44:**43–50.

[41] Ishiko, T. Commentary. *Canadian Medical Association Journal,* 1967, **96:**821.

[42] Jankowski, L. W., L. Roy, R. Soucy, and J. Vallee. Aquatic exercise therapy for rehabilitation of chronic obstructive pulmonary disease. *Medicine and Science in Sports,* 1974, **6:**82.

[43] Johnson, T. H., and G. D. Tharp. The effect of chronic exercise on reserpine-induced gastric ulceration in rats. *Medicine and Science in Sports,* 1974, **6:**188–190.

[44] Karvonen, M. J., H. Klemola, J. Virkajarvi, and A. Kekkonen. Longevity of endurance skiers. *Medicine and Science in Sports,* 1974, **6:**49–51.

[45] Kavanagh, T., R. H. Shephard, and V. Pandit. Marathon running after myocardial infarction. *Journal of the American Medical Association,* 1974, **229:**1,602–1,605.

[46] Koerner, J. E., and R. L. Terjung. Effect of physical training on coronary colateral circulation of the rat. *Journal of Applied Physiology,* 1982, **52:**376–387.

[47] Kovanen, V., H. Suominen, and E. Heikkinen. Connective tissue of "fast" and "slow" skeletal muscle in rats—effects of endurance training. *Acta Physiologica Scandinavica,* 1980, **108:**173–180.

[48] Kramsch, D. M., A. J. Aspen, B. M. Abramowitz, T. Kreimendahl, and W. B. Hood. Reduction of coronary atherosclerosis by moderate conditioning exercise in monkeys on an atherogenic diet. *New England Journal of Medicine,* 1981, **305:**1483–1489.

[49] Kramsch, D. M., A. J. Aspen, and L. J. Rozler. Atherosclerosis: prevention by agents not affecting abnormal levels of blood lipids. *Science,* 1981, **213:**1511–1512.

[50] Larson, R. L. Physical activity and the growth and development of bone and joint structures. In G. L. Rarick, ed., *Physical Activity: Human Growth and Development.* New York: Academic Press, Inc., 1973, pp. 32–59.

[51] Lee, G., E. A. Amsterdam, A. N. DeMaria, G. Davis, T. LaFave, and D. T. Mason. Effect of exercise on hemostatic mechanisms. In E. A. Amsterdam, J. H. Wilmore, and A. N. DeMaria, eds., *Exercise in Cardiovascular Health and Disease.* New York: Yorke Medical Books, 1977, pp. 122–136.

[52] Link, R. P., W. M. Pedersoli, and A. H. Safanie. Effect of exercise on development of atherosclerosis in swine. *Atherosclerosis,* 1972, **15:**107–122.

[53] Ljungqvist, A., and G. Unge. Capillary proliferative activity in myocardium and skeletal muscle of exercised rats. *Journal of Applied Physiology,* 1977, **43:**306–307.

[54] Maron, B. J., W. C. Roberts, H. A. McAllister, D. R. Rosing, and S. E. Epstein. Sudden death in young athletes. *Circulation,* 1980, **62:**218–229.

[55] Martin, B. J. Effect of sleep deprivation on tolerance of prolonged exercise. *European Journal of Applied Physiology,* 1981, **47:**345–354.

[56] Martin, R. K., J. P. Albright, W. R. Clarke, and J. A. Niffenegger. Load-carrying effects on the adult beagle tibia. *Medicine and Science in Sports and Exercise,* 1981, **13:**343–349.

[57] Maulitz, R. M., D. S. Pratt, and A. L. Schocket. Exercise-induced anaphylactic reaction to shellfish. *Journal of Allergy and Clinical Immunology,* 1979, **63:**433–434.

[58] McCann, C. Exercise-induced anaphylaxis reported. *Physician and Sportsmedicine,* 1979, **7:**14.

[59] Metropolitan Life Insurance Company. Sports hazards. *Statistical Bulletin,* 1979, **60:**2–5.

[60] Micheli, L. J. Sports injuries in children and adolescents. In R. H. Strauss, ed., *Sports Medicine And Physiology*. Philadelphia: W. B. Saunders Company, 1979, pp. 288–303.

[61] Montoye, H. J. Participation in athletics. *Canadian Medical Association Journal*, 1967, **96**:813–820.

[62] Morris, J. N., M. G. Everitt, R. Pollard, S. P. W. Chave, and A. M. Semmence. Vigorous exercise in leisure-time: protection against coronary heart disease. *Lancet*, 1980, Dec. 6: 1207–1210.

[63] Mueller, F. O., and C. S. Blyth. Football injury update—1979 season. *Physician and Sportsmedicine*, 1980, **8**:53–55.

[64] Nachemson, A. L. Low back pain—its etiology and treatment. *Clinical Medicine*, 1971, **78**:18–24.

[65] Nutter, D. O., R. E. Priest, and E. O. Fuller. Endurance training in the rat I. Myocardial mechanics and biochemistry. *Journal of Applied Physiology*, 1981, **51**:934–940.

[66] Oka, M., and S. Hatanpaa. Degenerative hip disease in adolescent athletes. *Medicine and Science in Sports*, 1976, **8**:77–80.

[67] Oscai, L. B. The role of exercise in weight control. *Exercise and Sport Sciences Reviews*, 1973, **1**:103–123.

[68] Paterson, D. H., R. J. Shephard, D. Cunningham, N. L. Jones, and G. Andrew. Effects of physical training on cardiovascular function following myocardial infarction. *Journal of Applied Physiology*, 1979, **47**:482–489.

[69] Pollock, M. L. The quantification of endurance training programs. *Exercise and Sport Sciences Reviews*, 1973, **1**:155–188.

[70] Retzlaff, E. J., J. Fontaine, and W. Furuta. Effect of daily exercise on life span of albino rats. *Geriatrics*, 1966, **21**:171–177.

[71] Ryan, A. J. 19% report head injury in high school football. *Physician and Sportsmedicine*, 1981, **9**:21.

[72] Sanders, M., F. C. White, T. M. Peterson, and C. M. Bloor. Effects of endurance exercise on coronary collateral blood flow in miniature swine. *American Journal of Physiology*, 1978, **234**:H614–H619.

[73] Sapega, A. A., T. C. Quedenfeld, R. A. Moyer, and R. A. Butler. Biophysical factors in range-of-motion exercise. *Physician and Sportsmedicine*, 1981, **9**:57–65.

[74] Schaible, T. F., and J. Scheuer. Cardiac function in hypertrophied hearts from chronically exercised female rats. *Journal of Applied Physiology*, 1981, **50**:1140–1145.

[75] Scheel, K. W., L. A. Ingram, and J. L. Wilson. Effects of exercise on the coronary and collateral vasculature of beagles with and without coronary occlusion. *Circulation Research*, 1981, **48**:523–530.

[76] Shapiro, C. M., R. Bortz, D. Mitchell, P. Bartel, and P. Jooste. Slow-wave sleep: a recovery period after exercise. *Science*, 1981, **214**:1253–1254.

[77] Shephard, R. J. Exercise-induced bronchospasm—a review. *Medicine and Science in Sports*, 1977, **9**:1–10.

[78] Shephard, R. J. Exercise and chronic obstructive lung disease. *Exercise and Sport Sciences Reviews*, 1976, **4**:263–296.

[79] Shephard, R. J., P. Corey, and T. Kavanagh. Exercise compliance and the prevention of a recurrence of myocardial infarction. *Medicine and Science in Sports and Exercise*, 1981, **13**:1–5.

[80] Sim, D. N., and W. A. Neill. Investigation of the physiological basis for increased exercise threshold for angina pectoris after physical conditioning. *Journal of Clinical Investigation*, 1974, **54**:763–770.

[81] Simonson, E. Evaluation of cardiac performance in exercise. *American Journal of Cardiology*, 1972, **30**:722–726.

[82] Sinclair, D. J. M., and C. G. Ingram. Controlled trial of supervised exercise training in chronic bronchitis. *British Medical Journal*, 1980, **280**:519–521.

[83] Skinner, J. S. Longevity, general health, and exercise. In H. B. Falls, ed., *Exercise Physiology*. New York: Academic Press, Inc., 1968, pp. 219–238.

[84] Smith, E. L., and S. W. Babcock. Effects of physical activity on bone loss in the aged. *Medicine and Science in Sports,* 1973, **5:**68.

[85] Smith, Jr., E. L., W. Reddan, and P. E. Smith. Physical activity and calcium modalities for bone mineral increase in aged women. *Medicine and Science in Sports and Exercise,* 1981, **13:**60–64.

[86] Sperling, G. A., J. K. Loosli, P. Lupien, and C. M. McCay. Effect of sulfamerazine and exercise on life span of rats and hamsters. *Gerontology,* 1978, **24:**220–224.

[87] Stone, H. L. Coronary flow, myocardial oxygen consumption, and exercise training in dogs. *Journal of Applied Physiology,* 1980, **49:**759–768.

[88] Thorland, W. G., and T. B. Gilliam. Comparison of serum lipids between habitually high and low active preadolescent males. *Medicine and Science in Sports and Exercise,* 1981, **13:**316–321.

[89] Tibbits, G., B. J. Koziol, N. K. Roberts, K. M. Baldwin, and R. J. Barnard. Adaptation of the rat myocardium to endurance training. *Journal of Applied Physiology,* 1978, **44:**85–89.

[90] Tipton, C. M., R. D. Matthes, J. A. Maynard, and R. A. Carey. The influence of physical activity on ligaments and tendons. *Medicine and Science in Sports,* 1975, **7:**165–175.

[91] Tipton, C. M., R. D. Matthes, A. C. Vailas, and P. M. Gross. Effect of immobilization, surgical repair and training on the strength of isolated knee ligaments of rats. *Medicine and Science in Sports,* 1976, **8:**61.

[92] Waller, B. F., and W. C. Roberts. Sudden death while running in conditioned runners aged 40 years or over. *American Journal of Cardiology,* 1980, **45:**1292–1300.

[93] Wood, P. D., and W. L. Haskell. The effect of exercise on plasma high density lipoproteins. *Lipids,* 1979, **14:**417–427.

[94] Wyatt, H. L., and J. Mitchell. Influences of physical conditioning and deconditioning on coronary vasculature of dogs. *Journal of Applied Physiology,* 1978, **45:**619–625.

[95] Zuckerman, J., and G. A. Stull. Ligamentous separation force in rats as influenced by training, detraining, and cage restriction. *Medicine and Science in Sports,* 1973, **5:**44–49.

CHAPTER 19

Aids and Impediments to Physical Performance: Fact and Fiction

FOR hundreds and probably thousands of years athletes have ingested, injected, inhaled, or applied to the skin substances that were thought to have a beneficial effect on physical performance. In earlier times it was taught that blood sucking by leeches and water deprivation would improve performance. Now, some would promote the injection of blood into the veins of endurance athletes, and it is widely recognized that water *supplementation* rather than deprivation should be encouraged. Thus, the use of various presumed performance aids tends to wax and wane with the positive and negative testimonials of currently successful and popular athletes and coaches. If an Olympic champion in the marathon promoted a prerace potion of bat blood and buffalo saliva, one could safely predict that bats and buffaloes would soon become endangered species as thousands of distance runners attempted to get an edge on their opponents. The truth of the matter is that nothing is absolutely certain to aid athletic performance in *every* person; very few things are beneficial to many; most have no effect on anyone; and some things are harmful and potentially deadly to all. It is the purpose of this chapter to describe the reasons why some substances or regimens have been presumed to be beneficial to performance and to summarize the evidence that supports or discounts such claims.

Diet

In an earlier chapter on performance and diet, it was emphasized that the important fuels for muscular exercise are carbohydrates and fats. Protein contributes insignificantly to the exercise effort from an energy standpoint. Accordingly, any promotion of protein supplementation must stand on the merit of the possible effect of extra protein on increasing the muscle mass of the athlete. This effect is unlikely unless the athlete has been deprived of adequate protein intake in his normal diet, but such deprivation could occur in athletes living in underdeveloped countries or in poverty areas of developed nations. In a normal, well-fed person, however, dietary protein supplements are not ordinarily effective in promoting extra muscular development.

High Carbohydrate Diet

There does seem to be a beneficial effect of a high carbohydrate diet on performance time in endurance events lasting longer than 30–40 minutes. With vigorous, long-duration activity, there is a severe depletion of glycogen in the working muscles that seems to limit performance. With a high carbohydrate diet, the muscle glycogen stores can be filled to capacity so that exercise can be prolonged for as long as possible. The suggested regimen for application of the high carbohydrate diet in a training program is described in an earlier chapter.

As described in Chapter 5, the consumption of sugar 30 minutes to an hour before endurance competition is ineffective in improving endurance and could lead to lowered blood glucose levels after insulin is secreted in response to the sugar feeding. Sugar feedings *immediately before or during* prolonged exercise can maintain blood glucose levels which might otherwise decline after 90–120 minutes of exercise. The extent to which this maintenance of blood glucose is of benefit to the muscles or the nervous system is controversial.

Vitamins and Minerals

There is no proven value of vitamin or mineral supplementation for the purpose of enhancing athletic performance. Those persons living in poverty or consuming fad diets could possibly benefit from vitamin and mineral supplementation, but this does not seem likely for those on normal diets in well-developed countries. A more detailed discussion of performance related to vitamins and minerals is presented in Chapter 5.

Gelatin (Glycine)

Gelatin contains high concentrations of the amino acid glycine, which is structurally related to creatine. Believing that feeding gelatin supplements would increase the body's stores of creatine phosphate, an important energy source for intense exercise, some have recommended gelatin as an aid to athletic performance. However, well-designed studies have disclosed no beneficial effect of gelatin or glycine supplementation on performance [23].

Aspartic Acid

Aspartic acid is an amino acid that is thought to be useful in reducing ammonia levels in the body. Since high levels of ammonia have been implicated in fatigue [24], it is not surprising that there have been several investigations of the influence of potassium or magnesium salts of aspartic acid on physical performance. The results of such studies on both men and laboratory animals have been contradictory [6, 24]. If aspartic acid is beneficial, it apparently does not work at the level of the exercising muscles, since it has been shown that levels of muscle ammonia are not reduced by the administration of aspartic acid [24]. In one study the aspartic acid seemed to lower blood ammonia by increasing the liver production of urea from circulating ammonia [24]. Overall, however, we must reserve judgment on whether or not aspartic acid salts can improve performance.

Dehydration

Whenever athletes are classified by weight for competition, as in such sports as wrestling, boxing, and junior football, there will always be those who will attempt to gain the advantages of maturity, leverage, strength, and reach by rapidly reducing their normal body weights before weighing in so they might qualify for lower-weight classes. Much of this weight reduction is brought about by a few days of water deprivation and by water loss through sweating during exercise and exposure to heat in steam rooms, saunas, and so on. Thus, dehydration is indirectly viewed as a means by which athletic performance can be improved.

If less than about 5 per cent of the body weight is rapidly lost prior to athletic performance of short duration, it is unlikely that much of an effect on performance will be observed [6]. For example, if Cedric Slumpsnuffer, whose normal weight is 140 pounds, loses 5 per cent (7 pounds) of his body weight just prior to his wrestling match with Phelonius Assult, he will not be faced with a reduction in strength or anaerobic muscular endurance and probably will experience only a small drop in aerobic endurance. Greater percentages of weight loss through dehydration, however, are associated with performance decrements, especially in aerobic endurance [6]. With prolonged work in the heat, severe dehydration can lead to marked impairment in performance and a failure of normal temperature regulation mechanisms. As described in an earlier chapter on temperature regulation during exercise, the temperature rise in the body during prolonged heavy exercise in the heat requires that some of the blood normally distributed to working muscles must be diverted to the skin for cooling purposes. This, along with poor psychological tolerance to heat, probably accounts for the decline in performance. The precise mechanism for this increased body temperature during dehydration is unknown [6].

Because dehydration never improves and may actually diminish physical performance or even cause illness or death in certain cases, it is incorrect to consider dehydration an aid to performance. If dehydration allows an athlete to compete in a lower weight class, inappropriate to his body build, it is true that the athlete may win more contests. But this effect of dehydration should be looked upon as taking advantage of a smaller opponent, not as a means of improving athletic performance.

Water Intake Before and During Exercise

In short-term exercise during which the body is able to maintain its temperature within acceptable limits quite easily, it makes little sense to fill up with water prior to or during exercise. But with prolonged exercise of 30 minutes or more, especially in a hot environment, it has been quite conclusively shown that water intake prior to exercise allows the participant to exercise more comfortably for longer durations with lower heart rates and body temperatures [6]. There is no evidence that drinking a quart or more of water a few minutes prior to athletic performance has any deleterious effect because of a full feeling in the stomach [6]. Accordingly, water intake prior to prolonged exercise in the heat can often facilitate performance. It requires about 24–36 hours to voluntarily rehydrate oneself following dehydration of 4.0–7.5 per cent of body weight [6].

In a similar fashion, replenishment of body water by drinking water at intervals during prolonged exercise also has been shown to be of value for improving performance [6, 7]. This beneficial effect on endurance time seems to be mostly the result of maintaining the body temperature at a lower level than is possible in a dehydrated condition. Because voluntary thirst does not drive one to refill his water stores during prolonged exercise in the heat, it may be necessary for coaches to insist that athletes drink about 200 milliliters of cool liquid approximately every 15 minutes to insure peak performance and, more importantly, to minimize the risk of heat illness.

Supplementary Salt Intake

While it is true that salt (sodium chloride) is lost in the sweat during exercise, relatively small amounts are lost compared to the loss of water. Consequently, the blood fluids during prolonged exercise usually have greater than normal *concentrations* of salt. Thus, salt supplementation without adequate water supplementation can actually be harmful to salt and fluid balance. Except under the most severe, prolonged types of work in the heat, such as occurs in foundries and in hot, humid mines, it is doubtful that any extra salt is required during the work itself. Extra salt sprinkled on table food seems to be just as effective as salt supplementation in maintaining body fluid salt levels with repeated days of work in the heat [7]. The effect of supplementary salt intake on most types of athletic performance is negligible and is probably more apt to be harmful than beneficial.

Commercial salt solutions containing minerals and glucose are unlikely to be detrimental to performance when taken in moderation, but athletes should not expect greater benefits from such solutions than from ordinary drinking water [6, 7]. Solutions which have too much sugar and/or minerals per volume of water are only slowly emptied from the stomach during exercise, so if glucose or salts are dissolved in water to be drunk during exercise, they should be used sparingly [6].

Oxygen

Because it has long been known that oxygen deprivation quickly brings exercise to a halt, it is not surprising that many studies have been undertaken to discover whether or not the inhalation of greater than normal concentrations of oxygen might enhance athletic performance. Such studies have investigated the breathing of oxygen-enriched gas mixtures before, during, and after exercise.

Oxygen Inhalation Before Exercise

There is evidence that breathing extra oxygen just before exercise in which the breath is held allows one to perform more exercise before he must take a breath [42]. The normal stores of oxygen in the blood and body fluids, the oxygen bound to myoglobin, and the muscle stores of creatine phosphate and glycogen should be adequate to supply energy for these short periods (usually less than a minute); thus, it seems likely that this beneficial effect of oxygen inhalation prior to brief exercise is the result of a decreased desire to breathe. There would be a decreased stimulation to the respiratory control centers of the brain if oxygen levels in the extracellular fluids were raised and carbon dioxide levels were lowered during the period of oxygen inhalation. It is also likely to have a strong positive psychological effect on performance when exercisers know they have inhaled oxygen [42]. There is little practical value in oxygen inhalation prior to performance, however, because the oxygen breathing must take place within about one minute of the start of exercise, and in nearly all athletic competitions that much time and more is taken up by preliminary starting instructions. After a few breaths during competition, any effect of the oxygen inhalation is quickly lost.

Oxygen Inhalation During Exercise

With exercise periods shorter than 2 minutes there is no beneficial effect of breathing high concentrations of oxygen during the work [42]. This is so, presumably, because anaerobic fuel reserves adequately meet the energy needs of brief exercise, because blood flow to the working muscles is not maximal until after a short period of exercise, and because it takes some time for adequate concentrations of ADP to build up in the mitochondria and stimulate oxygen consumption. During longer periods of exercise, oxygen inhalation usually is accompanied by better endurance, subjective feelings that the work is easier, reduced blood lactic acid levels, lower ventilation rates, and lower exercise heart rates for submaximal work [31, 42, 43]. During maximal work, maximal oxygen uptake is usually increased by about 10 per cent when one breathes higher concentrations of oxygen [31]. However, in recent studies no increase in oxygen uptake or in carbon dioxide production was observed in subjects who breathed oxygen-enriched gas mixtures [1, 4, 43], even though endurance was enhanced [1, 43]. It is suspected that improved performance in this case is caused by a decreased work of breathing and/or a reduced production of lactic acid [1, 4, 43]. Since no increase in oxygen uptake (aerobic metabolism) or glycogen breakdown was observed, it was suggested that less lactic acid was produced because pyruvic acid was more readily changed to alanine in the glucose-alanine cycle [4]. The decreased ventilation and decreased heart rates typically seen when persons breathe high concentrations of oxygen can be explained by the depressing effect of high oxygen levels on the arterial chemoreceptors and on the respiratory centers of the brain [42].

In normal athletic competition the positive effect of oxygen inhalation during exercise has no use because it is impractical to wear an oxygen supply unit during competition. In noncompetitive situations, however, oxygen breathing during physical activity has great value. This is especially true for high altitude mountaineers, for fire fighters, and for those with lung disease who would remain bedridden if it were not for their portable oxygen canisters.

Oxygen Inhalation During Recovery

Oxygen inhalation during recovery would be of benefit to a performer only if he were a participant in a subsequent competition that demanded quick recovery from the previous activity. Although it is commonly asserted that oxygen breathing hastens recovery from exercise, the conclusions from the scientific literature are contradictory [42]. It seems likely that any positive effects of oxygen inhalation on recovery stem from psychological, rather than physiological, factors.

High Altitude Training

It is known that persons who live at high altitudes generally have increased concentrations of circulating red blood cells and that such persons have much better exercise endurance at high altitudes than those who live at sea level. Some people also suspect that tissue hypoxia is an important stimulus to the adaptations in aerobic metabolism that occur after aerobic endurance training. Accordingly, it is not surprising that many have investigated the possibility that endurance athletes might have better endurance performances at sea level if they first train at high altitudes to increase the presumed hypoxia in their tissues and to bring about an increased production of red blood cells that might enhance oxygen delivery to their muscles during exercise.

Although a few early studies indicated that endurance performance at sea level was somewhat enhanced by altitude training, more recent work points out that an exercise training effect independent of any altitude effect might have been responsible for the early results [2]. Experiments in which the exercise training effect was well controlled found no beneficial effect of altitude training at 2,300 meters for 3 weeks over a similar period of training at sea level [2]. It appears that any effect of high altitude training that may exist is quite small, is difficult to reproduce, and is more likely to occur at altitudes greater than 2,300 meters.

Blood Doping

Some endurance athletes have attempted to increase the oxygen transport capacity of their blood by completing the following regimen. First, a pint or more of blood is withdrawn from the veins, and the red blood cells are stored. Second, the athlete resumes training, during which time the body replenishes the blood volume, including the red blood cells. Third, a short time prior to competition the stored red blood cells are injected back into the circulation to increase the number of circulating red cells. It is assumed that the increased amount of red blood cells will transfer more oxygen from the blood to the working muscles so that more ATP can be produced aerobically to give the athlete improved endurance performance.

If only a pint (about 500 ml) of blood is withdrawn for blood doping purposes, there is usually no significant effect on performance [40]. On the other hand, if 800–1200 ml (about 2 pints) are withdrawn and stored for 6 weeks or more, a significant improvement in hemoglobin level and aerobic endurance performance usually results [11, 41]. For example, in one well-designed study 5-mile run times decreased from 30:17 to 29:26 in the blood doping condition [41]. It is illegal in Olympic competition to dope oneself with physiological solutions in abnormal amounts for the purpose of improving competitive performance. Also, there is always danger of infection in blood transfusions, especially when performed by untrained personnel.

Heat and Cold Applications

The idea that applications of heat or cold to the skin might have some positive effect on muscular performance is usually based on the belief that 1) heat will increase enzyme activities in the working muscles so that ATP can be more rapidly replenished and muscle contraction can occur more quickly, 2) heat will increase blood flow to the working muscles to enhance aerobic ATP replenishment, 3) heat will decrease the viscosity or resistance of the muscles to changes in length so that less energy will have to be spent to overcome this factor, or 4) cold will decrease blood flow to the skin so that more blood can be diverted to the working muscles. At normal physiological temperatures, it seems that the latter factor is much more important than the former ones, especially with prolonged work. Over the years researchers have experimented with hot and cold baths and showers, cold sprays and cold packs on the abdominal area, cold towels over the head, and water- or air-cooled suits as possible aids to work and athletic performance.

In general, pre-exercise heat application that is sufficient to warm the muscles seems to have a slight (1–2 per cent) beneficial effect on the performance of athletic events such as short sprints, which have a significant anaerobic component. On the other hand, longer, aerobic events are often benefitted by the application of cold [14]. However, there are contradictory reports in the literature that show no demonstrated improvement in performance with heat or cold applications, so one should expect to see many individual differences in response to these maneuvers. It is true that in certain industrial situations (work in foundries, for example) it is possible for a worker to be clothed in a water- or air-cooled suit or to have cold air directed to his head, but in ordinary athletic competitions these procedures are impractical. One exception is the use of cold towels and water sprays to cool competitors in distance events in running, cycling, and rowing. Even though it may be difficult to demonstrate a significant effect of such coolants on performance time, the brief psychological lift they provide to most distance athletes makes their use commendable.

Although there are not many practical ways to apply cold during athletic competition, it is very feasible to do so in recovery periods between exercise bouts. Abdominal cold packs, cold sprays, cold towels, and even cold showers and baths can hasten recovery time and make subsequent work periods easier [14]. Consequently, some of these techniques could be used in football, basketball, soccer, track, boxing, tennis, and in any other athletic event characterized by rest periods and/or substitution practices. The optimal temperature for cold water baths is 18–24°C [14]. Cooling the skin to temperatures above or below this range is not likely to be effective.

Active Warmup

A common behavior observed in students and athletes prior to physical education classes, athletic practices, and sports competitions is the participants' actively "warming up" by stretching, performing calisthenics, jogging, and/or practicing the skills in which they are about to participate. The traditional reasons given for this "warmup" include the factors related to heat application described in the previous section, plus a desire to "loosen up" the muscles, tendons, and ligaments so that there will be less chance of injury to these tissues. Another reason more recently added to this list is that without warmup, there is a greater possibility that blood flow to the heart muscle might be inadequate during the first seconds of all-out physical activity.

It is unlikely that warmup activities that increase body temperature substantially are beneficial to performance lasting more than a few minutes because the increased body temperature causes a shift of blood flow away from working muscles to the skin. There are, however, some reports of a beneficial effect of warmup in strength and sprint events, which can be performed with little blood flow to the working muscles because of the emphasis on anaerobic ATP production for such activities [15]. Such a positive effect of warmup on athletic performance is quite difficult to demonstrate; about 50 per cent of the available studies have reported that warmup was either ineffective or, in a few cases, was actually harmful to performance [15]. Any beneficial effect of warmup is small and can be easily obscured by differences in motivation, pain tolerance, techniques of performance, and strategy.

The facts that 1) there is no overwhelming evidence that warmup is advantageous to athletic performance, and 2) there is no scientific evidence that athletes are less apt to suffer injury after warmup do not mean that warmup practices should be discouraged. There is minimal evidence that warmup is harmful to performance, and the personal empirical experience of thousands of athletes and coaches suggests that warmup does help prevent injuries. Accordingly, warmup practices should be promoted with greatest use being made of practice of the actual physical activity in which the exerciser is about to participate. Supposedly, these preliminary trials will help to establish the appropriate neural patterns for the final performance of the activity. Warmup is particularly to be encouraged in those who are about to participate in very heavy exercise that places sudden demands on the heart and circulation. The warmup should minimize the risk of inadequate coronary blood flow during the first few seconds of heavy exercise.

Music

Music is often part of the scene at athletic competitions. Whether the pounding bass drum or the blaring trumpets have any stimulating effect on athletic performance or whether music arouses only the spectators may never be proven. In any attempt to study the effects of music, one should minimize the possibility that the subjects realize that the addition or deletion of music from the performance setting is being evaluated; subjects may unconsciously respond positively to music because they assume they

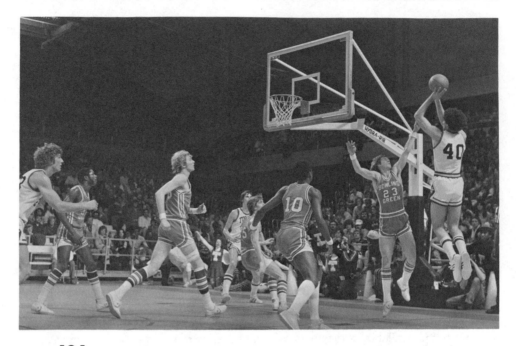

FIGURE 19.1. It is doubtful that these athletes would be conscious of any background music. (Courtesy of Office of Public Information, University of Toledo, Toledo, Ohio.

should. It is very difficult to accomplish this degree of experimental control when music is the variable of interest. Therefore, when a study without such control shows a beneficial effect of music on performance, the results are open to question.

Intuitively, it seems likely that rousing musical selections might be helpful to many athletes during the first minute or so of a contest because such music is associated with heightened emotions. But most athletes express the belief that once a contest is underway, they are generally oblivious to background music. This belief seems to be supported by the meager experimental evidence available: neither athletic performance nor industrial production seems to benefit from background music [29]. Nevertheless, most factory workers and athletes prefer the presence of music to its absence, and performance is rarely adversely affected by music.

Hypnosis and Suggestion

Stories of fantastic achievements in muscular performance under conditions of emotional stress and countless examples of suddenly superior athletic performances by previously "run-of-the-mill" competitors have led to many investigations of the role of hypnosis and suggestion on physical performance. As with most of the literature on other so-called aids to performance, the evidence regarding any beneficial effect of hypnosis and suggestion is contradictory, and much of the research suffers from inadequate controls.

The vast majority of studies dealing with the possibility that performance can be improved by suggesting to the performer that he has a great capacity or by having the performer exercise while in a hypnotic state have tested strength or short duration anaerobic endurance of a few muscle groups. No strong conclusions can be stated about the effectiveness of hypnosis or suggestion on performance in tests of grip strength, dynamic elbow-flexion endurance, and isometric endurance because the evidence is about equally divided between positive and negative results [18, 33]. It seems that only certain types of persons are responsive to either waking or hypnotic suggestion; the effects of such procedures are very unpredictable.

There is clinical evidence that some athletes can be helped by hypnosis if their performances are adversely affected by chronic pain or various psychological problems [33]. Hypnotherapy is not always effective, however.

Drugs

The use of most drugs as aids to performance is forbidden by athletic regulary agencies; the drugs can sometimes become physiologically and/or psychologically addictive; and they may lead to severe injury, disease, or even death. Therefore, no athlete should consider the use of any agent described in this section as a potential aid to performance. The purpose of the following discussion is to provide some insight into why these drugs are ineffective or potentially harmful.

Amphetamines

Activation of the sympathetic nervous system causes increased cardiac output, vaso-constriction of blood vessels, a rise in blood pressure, and stimulation of the psychological arousal mechanisms in the brain stem. Each of these actions should be a useful response during many types of exercise and athletic competition. Therefore, it is not surprising that drugs which mimic the effects of sympathetic stimulation are often used by athletes who wish to improve their performances [30, 32]. The most popular of these drugs are amphetamines, methamphetamines, and hydroxyamphetamines (trade names include: Benzedrine, Dexedrine and, Isophan). It is widely recognized that the amphetamines can help one stay awake by delaying the sense of fatigue and can help persons concentrate on accomplishing long, tedious tasks. However, it is also known that these drugs are commonly abused and that this abuse often leads to psychological dependence on the drugs. In addition, excessive doses of the drug can lead to circulatory collapse and death.

Although there are many exceptions, the majority of studies testing the effect of amphetamines on work performances such as prolonged marching, hiking, and cycling show that the drugs allow the exerciser to work longer with less sense of fatigue [28]. It should be pointed out, however, that there is no firm evidence that the work can be performed faster than in the nondrugged condition [16]. One study showed that amphetamine treatment improved knee extension strength, running acceleration, and time to exhaustion in a treadmill test which lasted about seven minutes [5]. In this same study, however, elbow flexion strength, leg power, sprinting speed, and maximal oxygen uptake were not significantly affected by the drug. Thus, the effects of amphetamines on short duration performance are somewhat inconclusive.

The most likely types of events to be positively influenced by amphetamines are long-distance cycling and running. But it is precisely these events that amphetamines are most dangerous. The drug can mask the sensation of oncoming circulatory collapse resulting from heat stress so that severe heat illness and even death may ensue [16].

In summary, amphetamines cause emotional arousal in many persons, but this arousal and other physiological effects are not enough to result in reproducible benefits to most types of athletic performance. When weighed against the possibility of 1) developing psychological dependence on the drug, 2) masking symptoms of potentially lethal circulatory collapse, and 3) being discovered by sports governing bodies, it seems foolish to even consider the use of amphetamines as a potential aid to athletic performance.

Cocaine

Cocaine is a highly addictive drug that acts on the brain to markedly inhibit the sensation of fatigue during prolonged work, thereby allowing substantially greater quantities of work to be performed [23]. Any use of this drug is illegal and highly dangerous.

Caffeine

Coffee, tea, and cola drinks contain caffeine, with a cup of coffee containing about 150 milligrams, a cup of tea about 120 milligrams, and a glass of cola about 50 milligrams. Caffeine is noted especially for its stimulation of the brain so that the sense of fatigue is diminished, but in large doses it can also increase cardiac output and stimulate the metabolism of skeletal muscles. About 300–500 milligrams of caffeine consumed an hour or two before endurance exercise may [8] or may not [35] improve performance. In those subjects for whom caffeine treatment is beneficial, the effect has been attributed to increased fatty acid mobilization, a psychostimulatory effect, and a sparing of glycogen in the muscle [8, 12]. Caffeine ordinarily has no noticeable effect on anaerobic types of performance [23].

Fencamfamine

This drug is a psychostimulant. In mice it causes restlessness, aggressive behavior, and better motor coordination, but a 40 per cent reduction in swimming endurance [13].

Epinephrine (Adrenaline)

Injections of epinephrine increase heart rate, cardiac output, and blood pressure and may raise the level of blood glucose by increasing the breakdown of glycogen to glucose in the liver. There is little evidence that epinephrine injections are beneficial to endurance performance in humans [23].

Anabolic Steroids

In young boys and girls there is little difference in muscle mass and strength. But at puberty, in concert with a marked acceleration in the secretion of testosterone, males rapidly outdistance most females in muscle growth and in strength. This association between male sex hormone and strength has led to the belief that supplemental administration of drugs that have the muscle building characteristics of testosterone might lead to improved athletic performance, especially in those events where strength and body mass are of great importance. Testosterone, besides promoting muscular development, also enhances the male secondary sex characteristics; this latter property is called the *androgenic* effect of a drug, whereas the growth promoting property is called the *anabolic* effect. Since testosterone has a structure typical of the group of chemicals called steroids, it is thus referred to as an *androgenic-anabolic steroid.* Drug manufacturers have synthesized steroid-like drugs that have strong anabolic properties but weak androgenic properties. These synthetic drugs, the anabolic steroids, include those with the following trade names: Dianabol, Androyd, Nilevor, Maxibolen, and Winstrol. Some of these drugs have greater androgenic effects than others.

Testimonial evidence by athletes indicates that anabolic steroids are very widely used, especially by shot putters, discus throwers, hammer throwers, weight lifters, and others who must rely heavily on strength for success [16]. Most of these athletes are convinced that the drug has a beneficial effect on their athletic performances. It appears that many users of anabolic steroids take the drug at ten to twenty times the recommended therapeutic dose [16, 44].

The scientific evidence regarding the effectiveness of anabolic steroids in stimulating weight gain and strength improvements is contradictory [16, 21, 26, 39, 44]. Apparently well-designed studies have shown both a lack of effect and a positive effect of anabolic steroid treatment.

A majority of the reasonably well-designed studies show a gain in body weight of about 2 kilograms (5 pounds), but it is not clear that this increased weight can be entirely attributed to greater muscle mass; there have been too few body composition analyses performed with acceptable procedures [26]. About half the studies show substantial strength gains, usually amounting to 8–10 kilograms (17–22 pounds) in bench press and squat lifts [26]. There does not seem to be any consistent effect of type of drug used, dosage of drug administered, diet consumed, or training program employed that can account for the different results. It seems likely that there are great individual differences in sensitivity to anabolic steroids that account for much of the great variability in drug effects.

There is abundant clinical evidence that long-term use of anabolic steroids is associated with liver dysfunction, liver cancer, infertility, menstrual dysfunction, male-pattern baldness, deepening of the voice in women, and other health problems [20, 44]. It is clear that the use of anabolic steroids in an attempt to obtain rather unpredictable improvements in athletic performance is not warranted when one considers the potential health risks involved.

Alcohol

Alcohol is the most widely abused drug in modern societies. Alcohol is sometimes thought to be a nervous system stimulant because it tends to remove social inhibitions by depressing the brain centers responsible for those inhibitions. In actuality, of course, alcohol is a central nervous system depressant and in large doses can produce total stupor. In small doses there is no consistent effect of alcohol on work performance, but in larger doses, such as six ounces of whiskey, athletic performance is impaired [23].

Tobacco

Most people believe that tobacco smoking has a detrimental effect on athletic performance. The facts that the carbon monoxide in tobacco smoke can displace oxygen from the red blood cells and that smoking is associated with airway constriction in the small bronchioles lend some support to this possible adverse effect of smoking on athletic performance. However, there seem to be no consistent effects, positive or negative, of smoking on athletic performance [23]. The common experience of young students returning to athletic training after a relatively sedentary summer is that ". . . the summer's smoking definitely cuts the wind." This experience is mostly caused by the absence of regular physical training and not by the practice of smoking.

Smoking should be actively discouraged because of its terrible long-range effects on increasing the risk of contracting lung cancer and heart disease, not because it will cause a dramatic decrement in athletic performance.

Marijuana

Marijuana smoking tends to increase heart rate and cause a feeling of relaxation and/or exhilaration. When smoked just before exercise, marijuana seems to have no effect on grip strength or on lung function, but it does require the heart to beat faster at a given submaximal workload, so that working capacity at a standard heart rate is reduced [38]. Marijuana smoking does not improve athletic performance and poses a long-term risk to the lungs and heart similar to that of tobacco.

Dichloroacetic Acid

Dichloroacetic acid is a drug which activates pyruvic acid dehydrogenase, the enzyme responsible for beginning the aerobic breakdown of pyruvic acid to carbon dioxide and water in the mitochondria. Theoretically, the drug might enhance endurance by speeding up the aerobic breakdown of pyruvic acid, thereby decreasing the production of lactic acid. Rats treated with dichloroacetic acid swam 40 per cent longer than control rats when the animals were forced to swim with loads equivalent to 10 per cent of their body weights fastened to their trunks [36]. Accumulation of lactic acid in muscle and blood was slower in the drug-treated rats. Unfortunately, rats weighted so heavily can only swim 4–7 minutes before exhaustion, and it is doubtful that swim time to exhaustion in such circumstances is a reliable measure of endurance. It would be interesting to know if dichloroacetic acid has beneficial effects on endurance in man.

Alkalinizing Buffers

There is substantial evidence that accumulation of acid contributes to fatigue in many types of exercise. Thus, it is logical to assume that pre-exercise ingestion of a solution which would buffer the acid and raise the pH of the body fluids should extend endurance. In two studies in which subjects consumed 18–20 grams of sodium bicarbonate over a 2–3 hour period before exercise, different results were obtained, perhaps because of the different tests used. In one experiment subjects cycled at 95 per cent of their maximal power output for 270 seconds in the control condition and 438 seconds in the buffered condition [22]. In the other experiment, no effect of the buffer was shown on time (about 62 seconds) to sprint 400 meters [25]. Since the shorter test presumably is more limited by lactic acid accumulation than the longer one, it might be questioned whether the effect observed in the longer test is a reproducible one. Further experiments should be performed. It should be noted that vomiting and diarrhea are potential side effects of ingestion of sodium bicarbonate in large doses.

Ginseng

Ancient Chinese medicines include the extract of ginseng root, which is purported to have many properties, including the reduction of fatigue during exercise. One study of rats showed that animals treated with the drug had less muscle glycogen depletion during prolonged swimming than control animals, but no differences were shown in endurance to swimming [3].

Air Pollution

Air pollution, both in closed rooms [37] and out of doors [9], can cause irritation of the eyes and nose and disturbances in respiration. However, under conditions of moderate pollution, maximal oxygen uptake is unaffected, and treadmill walking endurance in the heat is only slightly reduced [9]. The chronic effects of exercise in polluted environments have not been adequately studied, but there are clearly long-term implications for the development of lung cancer and other diseases.

REVIEW QUESTIONS

1. Explain why the following items have been thought to be potential aids to athletic performance, describe any possible harmful effects associated with their use, and state your views concerning their use in athletics: high protein diets, high carbohydrate diets, vitamin and mineral supplementation, gelatin, aspartic acid, dehydration, water, salt, oxygen, high-altitude training, blood doping, heat and cold applications, active warmup, music, hypnosis and suggestion, amphetamines, cocaine, caffeine, adrenaline, alcohol, tobacco, marijuana, anabolic steroids.

2. Discuss the difference between testimonial evidence and scientific evidence pertaining to presumed aids to muscular performance. Ask your instructor or someone familiar with research design and statistics why it is so difficult to "prove" that some so-called "ergogenic aid" does not improve athletic performance. Would you always prefer scientific evidence when it conflicts with testimonial evidence? What if you are the one giving testimony?

REFERENCES

[1] Adams, R. P., and H. G. Welch. Oxygen uptake, acid-base status, and performance with varied inspired oxygen fractions. *Journal of Applied Physiology,* 1980, **49:**863–868.

[2] Adams, W. C., E. M. Bernauer, D. B. Dill, and J. B. Bomar, Jr. Effects of equivalent sea-level and altitude training on VO_2 max and running performance. *Journal of Applied Physiology,* 1975, **39:**262–266.

[3] Avakian, E. V., Jr., and E. Evonuk. Effect of Panax ginseng extract on tissue glycogen and adrenal cholesterol depletion during prolonged exercise. *Planta Medica,* 1979, **36:**43–48.

[4] Byrnes, W. C., and J. P. Mullin. Metabolic effects of breathing hyperoxic gas mixtures during heavy exercise. *International Journal of Sports Medicine,* 1981, **4:**236–239.

[5] Chandler, J. V., and S. N. Blair. The effect of amphetamines on selected physiological components related to athletic success. *Medicine and Science in Sports and Exercise,* 1980, **12:**65–69.

[6] Costill, D. L. Water and electrolytes. In W. P. Morgan, ed., *Ergogenic Aids and Muscular Performance.* New York: Academic Press, Inc., 1972, pp. 293–320.

[7] Costill, D. L., R. Cote, E. Miller, T. Miller, and S. Wynder. Water and electrolyte replacement during repeated days of work in the heat. *Aviation, Space, and Environmental Medicine,* 1975, **46:**795–800.

[8] Costill, D. L., G. P. Dalsky, and W. J. Fink. Effects of caffeine ingestion on metabolism and exercise performance. *Medicine and Science in Sports,* 1978, **10:**155–158.

[9] Drinkwater, B. L., P. B. Raven, S. M. Horvath, J. A. Gliner, R. O. Ruhling, N. W. Bolduan, and S. Taguchi. Air pollution, exercise, and heat stress. *Archives of Environmental Health,* 1974, **28:**177–182.

[10] Ehn, L., B. Carlmark, and S. Hoglund. Iron status in athletes involved in intense physical activity. *Medicine and Science in Sports and Exercise,* 1980, **12:**61–64.

[11] Ekblom, B., A. N. Goldbarg, and B. Gullbring. Response to exercise after blood loss and reinfusion. *Journal of Applied Physiology,* 1972, **33:**175–180.

[12] Essig, D., D. L. Costill, and P. J. Van Handel. Effects of caffeine ingestion on utilization of muscle glycogen and lipid during leg ergometer cycling. *International Journal of Sports Medicine,* 1980, **1:**86–90.

[13] Estler, C.-J., and M. K. Gabrys. Swimming capacity of mice after prolonged treatment with psychostimulants. *Psychopharmacology,* 1979, **63:**281–284.

[14] Falls, H. B. Heat and cold applications. In W. P. Morgan, ed., *Ergogenic Aids and Muscular Performance.* New York: Academic Press, Inc., 1972, pp. 119–158.

[15] Franks, B. D. Physical warm-up. In W. P. Morgan, ed., *Ergogenic Aids and Muscular Performance.* New York: Academic Press, Inc., 1972, pp. 160–191.

[16] Golding, L. A. Drugs and hormones. In W. P. Morgan, ed., *Ergogenic Aids and Muscular Performance.* New York: Academic Press, Inc., 1972, pp. 367–397.

[17] Gustafsson, L., L. Appelgren, and H. E. Myrvold. The effect of polycythemia on blood flow in working and non-working skeletal muscle. *Acta Physiologica Scandinavica,* 1980, **109:**143–148.

[18] Hyvarinen, J., P. V. Komi, and P. Puhakka. Endurance of muscle contraction under hypnosis. *Acta Physiologica Scandinavica,* 1977, **100:**485–487.

[19] Ingjer, F., and S. B. Stromme. Effects of active, passive or no warm-up on the physiological response to heavy exercise. *European Journal of Applied Physiology,* 1979, **40:**273–282.

[20] Johnson, F. L. The association of oral androgenic-anabolic steroids and life-threatening disease. *Medicine and Science in Sports,* 1975, **7:**284–286.

[21] Johnson, L. C., E. S. Roundy, P. E. Allsen, A. G. Fisher, and L. J. Silvester. Effect of anabolic steroid treatment on endurance. *Medicine and Science in Sports*, 1975, **7**:287–289.

[22] Jones, N. L., J. R. Sutton, R. Taylor, and C. J. Toews. Effect of pH on cardiorespiratory and metabolic responses to exercise. *Journal of Applied Physiology*, 1977, **43**:959–964.

[23] Karpovich, P. V., and W. E. Sinning. *Physiology of Muscular Activity.* Philadelphia: W. B. Saunders Company, 1971, pp. 321–338.

[24] Kendrick, Z. V., S. Tangsakul, A. Goldfarb, and P. A. Molé. Potassium aspartate treatment: effects on blood ammonia, urea, and exercise to exhaustion. *Medicine and Science in Sports*, 1976, **8**:70.

[25] Kindermann, W., J. Keul, and G. Huber. Physical exercise after induced alkalosis (bicarbonate or Tris-buffer). *European Journal of Applied Physiology*, 1977, **37**:197–204.

[26] Lamb, D. R. Anabolic steroids. In M. Williams, ed., *Ergogenics in Sport.* Champaign, Ill.: Human Kinetics Publishers, (In press).

[27] Lamb, D. R. Androgens and exercise. *Medicine and Science in Sports*, 1975, **7**:1–5.

[28] Laties, V. G., and B. Weiss. The amphetamine margin in sports. *Federation Proceedings*, 1981, **40**:2689–2692.

[29] Lucaccini, L. F., and L. H. Kreit. Music. In W. P. Morgan, ed., *Ergogenic Aids and Muscular Performance.* New York: Academic Press, Inc., 1972, pp. 235–262.

[30] Mandell, A. J., K. D. Stewart, and P. V. Russo. The Sunday syndrome: from kinetics to altered consciousness. *Federation Proceedings*, 1981, **40**:2693–2698.

[31] Margaria, R., E. Camporesi, P. Aghemo, and G. Sassi. The effect of O_2 breathing on maximal aerobic power. *Pflügers Archiv*, 1972, **336**:225–235.

[32] Marshall, E. Drugging of football players curbed by central monitoring plan, NFL claims. *Science*, 1979, **203**:626–628.

[33] Morgan, W. P. Hypnosis and muscular performance. In W. P. Morgan, ed., *Ergogenic Aids and Muscular Performance.* New York: Academic Press, Inc., 1972, pp. 193–233.

[34] Pate, R. R., M. Maguire, and J. Van Wyk. Dietary iron supplementation in women athletes. *Physician and Sportsmedicine*, 1979, **7**:81–86.

[35] Schade, D., C. Simonelli, J. C. Standerer, and R. P. Eaton. Caffeine-induced hormonal changes during running (abstract). *Federation Proceedings*, 1979, **38**:944.

[36] Schneider, S. H., P. M. Komanicky, M. N. Goodman, and N. B. Ruderman. Dichloroacetate: effects on exercise endurance in untrained rats. *Metabolism*, 1981, **30**:590–595.

[37] Shephard, R. J., R. Collins, and F. Silverman. Responses of exercising subjects to acute "passive" cigarette smoke exposure. *Environmental Research*, 1979, **19**:279–291.

[38] Steadward, R. D., and M. Singh. The effects of smoking marihuana on physical performance. *Medicine and Science in Sports*, 1975, **7**:309–311.

[39] Stromme, S. B., H. D. Meen, and A. Aakvaag. Effects of an androgenic-anabolic steroid on strength development and plasma testosterone levels in normal males. *Medicine and Science in Sports*, 1974, **6**:203–208.

[40] Williams, M. H., A. R. Goodwin, R. Perkins, and J. Bocrie. Effect of blood reinjection upon endurance capacity and heart rate. *Medicine and Science in Sports*, 1973, **5**:181–186.

[41] Williams, M. H., S. Wesseldine, T. Somma, and R. Schuster. The effect of induced erythrocythemia upon 5-mile run time. *Medicine and Science in Sports and Exercise*, 1981, **13**:169–175.

[42] Wilmore, J. H. Oxygen. In W. P. Morgan, ed., *Ergogenic Aids and Muscular Performance.* New York: Academic Press, Inc., 1972, pp. 321–342.

[43] Wilson, G. D., and H. G. Welch. Effects of varying concentrations of N_2/O_2 and He/O_2 on exercise tolerance in man. *Medicine and Science in Sports and Exercise*, 1980, **12**:380–384.

[44] Wright, J. E. Anabolic steroids and athletics. *Exercise and Sport Sciences Reviews*, 1980, **8**:149–202.

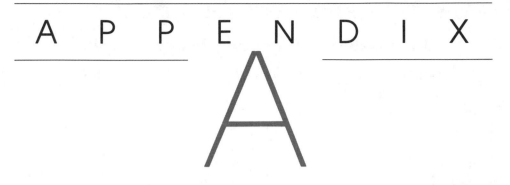

A P P E N D I X

Units of Measurement and Conversion Factors

The International System of Units (SI)

The internationally preferred system of measurement units uses the metric system and has been increasingly adopted by scientific publishing houses since the *International System of Units (Système International d'Unités)* was developed in 1960. For exercise physiology, the most important SI units are as follows:

For length .... meter (m)
For area .... square meter (m²)
For volume .... cubic meter (m³)
For mass .... kilogram (kg)
For density .... kg per cubic meter (kg m⁻³)
For time .... second (s)
For plane angle .... radian (rad)
For linear velocity .... meter per second (m s⁻¹)
For angular velocity .... radian per sec (rad s⁻¹)
For acceleration .... meter/sec squared (m s⁻²)
For angular acceleration .... rad/sec squared (rad s⁻²)
For force .... newton (N)
For energy, work, heat .... joule (J)
For power .... watt (W)
For pressure .... Pascal (P)
For temperature .... kelvin (K)
For frequency .... hertz (Hz)
For amount of chemical .... mole (mol)

Multiples and Submultiples of SI Units

The following prefixes should be used with the SI units where appropriate:

exa (E)	for 10^{18}	deci (d)	for 10^{-1}
peta (P)	for 10^{15}	centi (c)	for 10^{-2}
tera (T)	for 10^{12}	milli (m)	for 10^{-3}
giga (G)	for 10^9	micro (μ)	for 10^{-6}
mega (M)	for 10^6	nano (n)	for 10^{-9}
kilo (k)	for 10^3	pico (p)	for 10^{-12}
hecto (h)	for 10^2	femto (f)	for 10^{-15}
deca (da)	for 10^1	atto (a)	for 10^{-18}

As examples, a millimeter is a thousandth of a meter, and a megajoule is a million joules.

Length Units

1 millimeter (mm) = 0.1 centimeter = 0.001 meter = 0.039 inch

1 centimeter (cm) = 10 millimeters = 0.01 meter = 0.394 inch

1 meter (m) = 1,000 millimeters = 100 centimeters = 39.37 inches = 3.281 feet = 1.09 yards

1 kilometer (km) = 1,000 meters = 0.621 miles

1 inch (in) = 25.4 millimeters = 2.54 centimeters

1 foot (ft) = 304.8 millimeters = 30.48 centimeters = 0.3048 meter = 12 inches = 0.333 yard

1 yard (yd) = 914.4 millimeters = 91.44 centimeters = 0.9144 meter = 36 inches = 3 feet

1 mile (mi) = 1,609 meters = 1.609 kilometers = 5,280 feet = 1,760 yards

Area Units

1 square centimeter (cm²) = 100 square millimeters = 0.0001 square meter = 0.1550 square inch

1 square meter (m²) = 1 million square millimeters = 10 thousand square centimeters = 1,550 square inches = 10.76 square feet = 1.196 square yards

1 square inch (in²) = 645.2 square millimeters = 6.452 square centimeters

1 square foot (ft²) = 92,900 square millimeters = 929 square centimeters = 0.0929 square meter = 144 square inches = 0.1111 square yards

1 square yard (yd²) = 0.8361 square meters = 9.0 square feet

1 acre (A) = 4,047 square meters = 0.4047 hectare = 43,560 square feet = 4,840 square yards

1 square mile (mi²) = 2.590 square kilometers = 640 acres

Volume Units

1 cubic millimeter (mm³) = 0.001 cubic centimeter = 1 microliter = 0.001 milliliter = 10^{-6} liter

1 cubic centimeter (cm³,cc) = 1 milliliter = 0.001 liter = 1,000 microliters = 1,000 cubic millimeters = 0.061 cubic inch

1 cubic meter (m³) = 1 million cubic centimeters = 1,000 liters = 35.314 cubic feet = 1.308 cubic yards = 264.2 gallons (U.S. liquid)

1 microliter (μL) = 1 cubic millimeter = 0.001 milliliter = 10^{-6} liter

1 milliliter (mL) = 1,000 microliters = 1 cubic centimeter = 0.001 liter = 0.03381 ounces (U.S. fluid)

1 deciliter (dL) = 100 milliliters = 0.1 liter

1 liter (L) = 1 million cubic milliliters = 1,000 cubic centimeters = 0.001 cubic meters = 61.02 cubic inches = 0.03531 cubic feet = 2.113 pints (U.S. liquid) = 1.057 quarts (U.S. liquid) = 0.2642 gallons (U.S. liquid)

1 cubic inch (in³) = 16.39 cubic centimeters

1 cubic foot (ft³) = 28,320 cubic centimeters = 0.02832 cubic meter = 28.32 liters = 59.84 pints (U.S. liquid) = 29.92 quarts (U.S. liquid) = 7.481 gallons (U.S. liquid)

1 U.S. fluid ounce (fl oz) = 29.5735 milliliters = 0.0296 liter = 0.0625 pint = 0.03125 quart

1 U.S. liquid pint (liq pt) = 473.2 milliliters = 0.4732 liter = 0.5 quart (U.S. liquid) = 0.125 gallon (U.S. liquid)

1 U.S. liquid quart (liq qt) = 946.4 milliliters = 0.9464 liter = 2 pints (U.S. liquid) = 0.25 gallons (U.S. liquid)

1 U.S. liquid gallon (gal) = 3,785 milliliters = 3.785 liters = 8 pints (U.S. liquid) = 4 quarts (U.S. liquid)

Mass Units

1 attogram (ag) = 10^{-3} femtogram = 10^{-6} picogram = 10^{-9} nanogram = 10^{-12} microgram = 10^{-15} milligram = 10^{-18} gram = 10^{-21} kilogram

1 femtogram (fg) = 1,000 attograms = 10^{-3} picogram = 10^{-6} nanogram = 10^{-9} microgram = 10^{-12} milligram = 10^{-15} gram = 10^{-18} kilogram

1 picogram (pg) = 10^{6} attograms = 1,000 femtograms = 10^{-3} nanogram = 10^{-6} microgram = 10^{-9} milligram = 10^{-12} gram = 10^{-15} kilogram

1 nanogram (ng) = 10^{9} attograms = 10^{6} femtograms = 1,000 picograms = 10^{-3} microgram = 10^{-6} milligram = 10^{-9} gram = 10^{-12} kilogram

1 microgram (μg) = 10^{12} attograms = 10^{9} femtograms = 10^{6} picograms = 1,000 nanograms = 10^{-3} milligram = 10^{-6} gram = 10^{-9} kilogram

1 milligram (mg) = 10^{15} attograms = 10^{12} femtograms = 10^{9} picograms = 10^{6} nanograms = 1,000 micrograms = 10^{-3} gram = 10^{-6} kilogram

1 gram (g) = 10^{18} attograms = 10^{15} femtograms = 10^{12} picograms = 10^{9} nanograms = 10^{6} micrograms = 1,000 milligrams = 10^{-3} kilograms = 0.03527 ounces

1 kilogram (kg) = 10^{21} attograms = 10^{18} femtograms = 10^{15} picograms = 10^{12} nanograms $= 10^9$ micrograms $= 10^6$ milligrams $= 1,000$ grams $= 35.28$ ounces $= 2.205$ pounds

1 ounce (oz) $= 28.3495$ grams $= 0.0625$ pounds

1 pound (lb) $= 453.59$ grams $= 16$ ounces $= 0.4536$ kilograms

Density Units

1 gram per cubic centimeter (g $\times$ cm^{-3}) $= 1$ gram per milliliter $= 1$ kilogram per liter $= 1,000$ kilograms per cubic meter $= 62.43$ pounds per cubic foot

1 kilogram per cubic meter (kg $\times$ m^{-3}) $= 10^{-3}$ grams per cubic centimeter $= 10^{-3}$ grams per milliliter $= 1$ gram per liter $= 10^{-3}$ kilogram per liter $= 0.06243$ pounds per cubic foot

Time Units

1 second (s) $= 1.6 \times 10^{-2}$ minute $= 2.7 \times 10^{-4}$ hour $= 1.5740 \times 10^{-5}$ day

1 minute (min) $= 60$ seconds $= 1.6 \times 10^{-2}$ hour $= 6.94 \times 10^{-4}$ day

1 hour (h) $= 3,600$ seconds $= 60$ minutes $= 4.16 \times 10^{-2}$ day

1 day (d) $= 8.64 \times 10^4$ seconds $= 1.44 \times 10^3$ minutes $= 24$ hours

Plane Angle Units

The *radian* is defined as the plane angle that, as the central angle of a circle of radius $= 1$ meter, cuts an arc of 1 meter out of the circumference.

The *degree* is defined as the plane angle that, as the central angle of a circle, cuts out one 360th part of the circumference. Each degree can be divided into 60 minutes which can be further divided into 60 seconds.

1 radian (rad) $= 2.063 \times 10^5$ seconds $= 3,438$ minutes $= 57.30$ degrees

1 degree (°) $= 0.01745329$ radian $= 3,600$ seconds $= 60$ minutes

Linear Velocity Units

1 centimeter per second (cm $\times$ s^{-1}) $= 0.01$ meters per second $= 0.6$ meters per minute $= 0.036 \times$ kilometers per hour $= 0.033$ feet per second $= 1.1969$ feet per minute

1 meter per second (m $\times$ s^{-1}) $= 100$ centimeters per second $= 60$ meters per minute $= 3.6$ kilometers per hour $= 3.281$ feet per second $= 196.8$ feet per minute $= 2.237$ miles per hour

1 meter per minute (m × min⁻¹) = 1.667 centimeters per second = 0.0167 meters per second = 0.06 kilometers per hour = 0.0547 feet per second = 3.281 feet per minute = 0.0373 miles per hour

1 kilometer per hour (km × h⁻¹) = 0.2778 meter per second = 16 meters per minute = 54.68 feet per minute = 0.6214 miles per hour

1 foot per second (ft × s⁻¹) = 30.48 centimeters per second = 0.3048 meters per second = 18.29 meters per minute = 1.097 kilometers per hour = 60 feet per minute = 0.6818 miles per hour

1 foot per minute (ft × min⁻¹) = 0.508 centimeter per second = 0.0051 meter per second = 0.3048 meter per minute = 0.0183 kilometer per hour = 0.0114 mile per hour

1 mile per hour (mi × h⁻¹) = 26.82 meters per minute = 1.609 kilometers per hour

10-minute mile = 6 miles per hour = 9.65 kilometers per hour = 160.92 meters per minute = 2.68 meters per second

9-minute mile = 6.67 miles per hour = 10.73 kilometers per hour = 178.78 meters per minute = 2.98 meters per second

8-minute mile = 7.5 miles per hour = 12.07 kilometers per hour = 201.12 meters per minute = 3.35 meters per second

7-minute mile = 8.57 miles per hour = 13.79 kilometers per hour = 229.86 meters per minute = 3.83 meters per second

6-minute mile = 10 miles per hour = 16.09 kilometers per hour = 268.17 meters per minute = 4.47 meters per second

5-minute mile = 12 miles per hour = 19.31 kilometers per hour = 321.80 meters per minute = 5.36 meters per second

4-minute mile = 15 miles per hour = 24.14 kilometers per hour = 402.25 meters per minute = 6.70 meters per second

Angular Velocity Units

1 radian per sec (rad × s⁻¹) = 57.2958 degrees per second = 9.549 revolutions per minute

1 degree per sec (° × s⁻¹) = 0.017453 radian per second = 0.1667 revolution per minute

Acceleration Units

1 meter per second squared (m × s⁻²) = 3.2841 feet per second squared

1 foot per second squared (ft × s⁻²) = 0.3048 meter per second squared

Acceleration due to gravity (g_n) = 9.80665 meters per second squared = 32.174 feet per second squared

Angular Acceleration Units

1 radian per second squared (rad $\times$ s^{-2}) = 5.7296 degrees per second squared
1 degree per second squared ($^\circ \times$ s^{-2}) = 1.7453 radians per second squared

Force

The *newton* (*N*), the preferred international unit of force, is defined as the force that imparts an acceleration of one meter per second per second on a mass of one kilogram (1 N = 1 kg m $\times$ s^{-2}). Multiples (kilo-, mega-, etc.) and submultiples (milli-, micro-, etc.) of newtons are used where appropriate.

The English system's *poundal* (*pdl*) is defined as the force that imparts an acceleration of one foot per second per second on a mass of one pound (1 pdl = 1 ft lb $\times$ s^{-2}).

The *pond* (*p*) is an older unit defined as the force that imparts the standard acceleration of gravity (9.807 m $\times$ s^{-2}) to a mass of one gram, and the *kilopond* (*kp*) is the force that imparts the acceleration of gravity to a mass of one kilogram (1 kp = $g_n \times$ 1 kg).

1 newton (N) = 7.233 poundals = 101.97 ponds = 0.102 kilopond
1 poundal (pdl) = 0.1383 newtons = 14.1 ponds = 0.014 kilopond
1 pond (p) = 0.001 kilopond = 0.0098 newtons = 0.0709 poundals
1 kilopond (kp) = 1,000 ponds = 9.8067 newtons = 70.9316 poundals

Energy, Work, and Heat Units

The *joule* (*J*) is defined as the work performed when the point of application of a force of one newton is moved one meter in the direction of the force (1 J = 1 N m = 1 kg m$^2 \times$ s^{-2}). Multiples (kilo-, mega-, etc.) and submultiples (milli-, micro-, etc.) of joules are used where appropriate.

The *foot poundal* (*ft pdl*) is defined as the work performed when the point of application of a force of one poundal is moved one foot in the direction of the force (1 ft pdl = 1 ft^2 lb s^{-2}).

1 joule (J) = 0.000239 kilocalorie = 1 newton meter = 0.102 kilopond meter = 1 kilogram meter squared per second squared = 2.373 foot poundals
1 kilojoule (kJ) = 0.239 kilocalorie = 1,000 newton meters = 102 kilopond meters = 1,000 kilogram meters squared per second squared = 2,373 foot poundals
1 megajoule (MJ) = 238.92 kilocalories
1 kilocalorie (kcal) = 4,185.5 joules = 4.1855 kilojoules = 0.0042 megajoules = 426.85 kilopond meters
1 kilopond meter (kpm) = 9.8066 joules = 0.0098 kilojoules = 0.0023 kilocalories

Power Units

Power is the rate of performing work (force × distance/time) or the rate of expending energy. The preferred unit of power is the *watt,* which is defined as the power required to transform one joule of energy in one second.

1 watt (W) = 1 joule per second = 1 newton meter per second = 6.12 kilopond meters per minute = 0.1433 kilocalories per minute = 8.6 kilocalories per hour

1 kilopond meter per minute (kpm × min^{-1}) = 0.1634 watt = 0.1634 joule per second = 0.1634 newton meter per second = 0.0234 kilocalorie per minute = 1.4049 kilocalories per hour

1 kilocalorie per minute (kcal × min^{-1}) = 6.978 watts = 6.978 joules per second = 6.978 newton meters per second = 42.735 kilopond meters per minute

1 kilocalorie per hour (kcal × h^{-1}) = 0.1163 watts = 0.1163 joules per second = 0.1163 newton meters per second = 0.7122 kilopond meters per minute

Pressure Units

The *pascal* is defined as the pressure that exerts a force of one newton vertically on one square meter of area.

An *atmosphere* (*atm*) is defined as 101,325 pascals.

The *torr* is defined as 1/760th of 1 atmosphere or 133.322 pascals. Atmospheric pressure at sea level is 760 millimeters of mercury under specified conditions, and one torr is, therefore, essentially equivalent to a pressure of one millimeter of mercury under those conditions. However, since the torr is independent of temperature and other material constants, its use is preferred over that of millimeters of mercury.

1 pascal (Pa) = 0.0075 torr = 0.102 millimeters of water = 0.01 millibar = 9.8 × 10^{-6} atmosphere

1 torr (torr) = 133.3224 pascals = 1 millimeter of mercury = 13.6 millimeters of water = 1.33 millibars = 0.0013 atmosphere

1 millibar (mbar) = 100 pascals

1 atmosphere (atm) = 101,325 pascals = 760 torr = 1013.25 millibars

Temperature Conversions

Kelvin temp. (°K) = Celsius temp. + 273.15
= 5/9 (Fahrenheit temp. + 459.67)

Celsius temp. (°C) = Kelvin temp. −273.15
= 5/9 (Fahrenheit temp. −32)

Fahrenheit temp. (°F) = (9/5 Kelvin temp.) − 459.67
(9/5 Celsius temp.) + 32

Frequency Units

The *hertz* is defined as the frequency of a periodic process with the period equal to one second. The older terminology is *cycle per second*.

1 hertz (Hz) = 1 cycle per second   **1 megahertz (MHz)** = 10^6 hertz
1 kilohertz (kHz) = 1,000 hertz   **1 cycle per second (cps)** = 1 hertz

Units for Amount of Chemical Substance in Solution

A *mole* (*mol*) of a substance is defined as the molecular weight of the substance in grams. For example, one mole of glucose (molecular weight = 180) weighs 180 grams, whereas one mole of lactic acid (molecular weight = 90) weighs 90 grams. A *millimole* is one thousandth the weight of a mole (or the molecular weight of the substance in milligrams), a *micromole* is one millionth the weight of a mole (or the molecular weight of the substance in micrograms), and so on.

A *molar* (*M*) *solution* of a substance contains one mole of the substance dissolved in each liter of solution. Thus, to make up two liters of a 1 M solution of glucose, enough water would have to be added to $2 \times 180 = 360$ grams of glucose to produce two liters of solution. Similarly, a *millimolar* (*mM*) *solution* of a substance contains one millimole of the substance dissolved in each liter of solution. In the case of glucose, 180 milligrams would be dissolved to obtain one liter of a 1 mM solution.

Many times, concentrations of substances are expressed in grams per liter, per deciliter (100 milliliters), or per milliliter. For example, blood glucose and lactic acid levels are commonly expressed as a per cent, e.g., glucose = 90 mg % and lactate = 10 mg%. In this case, the % symbol means "per 100 milliliters." Thus, a 90 mg% concentration of blood glucose contains 90 milligrams of glucose per 100 milliliters of blood. If one knows the molecular weight of the substance in question, it is simple to convert from these older expressions to molar concentrations or from molar to the older expressions of concentration. Some examples follow:

Given: Lactic acid has a molecular weight of 90.
Problems:

1. What is the molar concentration of a 100 mg% solution of lactic acid? **Answer:** If there are 100 mg of lactic acid in 100 ml, there are 1,000 mg (1 g) in a liter. A mole of lactic acid weighs 90 grams, so there is $1/90 = 0.0111$ mole per liter of solution. This concentration could be expressed as 1.11×10^{-2} M or as 11.1 mM.

2. What is the molar concentration of an 18% solution of lactic acid? **Answer:** A 20% solution of lactic acid contains 18 g of lactic acid per 100 ml of solution or 180 g per liter of solution. Because lactic acid has a molecular weight of 90, the molarity of an 18% solution is $180/90 = 2$ M.

3. What is the concentration in mg % of a 10 mM solution of lactic acid? **Answer:** A 10 mM solution of lactic acid contains 10 millimoles (0.010 moles) of lactic acid in each liter. Because the molecular weight of lactic acid is 90 grams, there are $90 \times 0.010 = 0.9$ grams of lactate per liter or 0.09 g per 100 ml. Since 0.09 g = 90 mg, the concentration of the solution is 90 mg%.

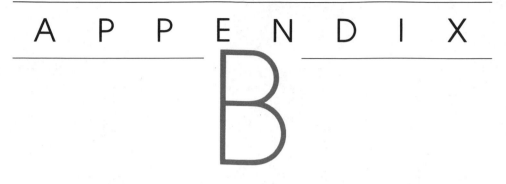

A P P E N D I X
B

Nutritive Values of the Edible Part of Foods[*]

* From "Nutritive Value of Foods." Home and Garden Bulletin No. 72, U.S. Department of Agriculture, April, 1981.

(Dashes (—) denote lack of reliable data for a constituent believed to be present in measurable amount)

DAIRY PRODUCTS (CHEESE, CREAM, IMITATION CREAM, MILK, RELATED PRODUCTS)

Butter. See Fats, oils; related products, items 103-108.

Item No. (A)	Foods, approximate measures, units, and weight (edible part unless footnotes indicate otherwise) (B)	Grams	Water (C) Percent	Food energy (D) Calories	Protein (E) Grams	Fat (F) Grams	Saturated (total) (G) Grams	Oleic (H) Grams	Linoleic (I) Grams	Carbohydrate (J) Grams	Calcium (K) Milligrams	Phosphorus (L) Milligrams	Iron (M) Milligrams	Potassium (N) Milligrams	Vitamin A value (O) International units	Thiamin (P) Milligrams	Riboflavin (Q) Milligrams	Niacin (R) Milligrams	Ascorbic acid (S) Milligrams
	Cheese:																		
	Natural:																		
1	Blue------ 1 oz	28	42	100	6	8	5.3	1.9	0.2	1	150	110	0.1	73	200	0.01	0.11	0.3	0
2	Camembert (3 wedges per 4-oz container). 1 wedge	38	52	115	8	9	5.8	2.2	.2	Trace	147	132	.1	71	350	.01	.19	.2	0
	Cheddar:																		
3	Cut pieces------ 1 oz	28	37	115	7	9	6.1	2.1	.2	Trace	204	145	.2	28	300	.01	.11	Trace	0
4	1 cu in	17.2	37	70	4	6	3.7	1.3	.1	Trace	124	88	.1	17	180	Trace	.06	Trace	0
5	Shredded------ 1 cup	113	37	455	28	37	24.2	8.5	.7	1	815	579	.8	111	1,200	.03	.42	.1	0
	Cottage (curd not pressed down):																		
	Creamed (cottage cheese, 4% fat):																		
6	Large curd------ 1 cup	225	79	235	28	10	6.4	2.4	.2	6	135	297	.3	190	370	.05	.37	.3	Trace
7	Small curd------ 1 cup	210	79	220	26	9	6.0	2.2	.2	6	126	277	.3	177	340	.04	.34	.3	Trace
8	Low fat (2%)------ 1 cup	226	79	205	31	4	2.8	1.0	.1	8	155	340	.4	217	160	.05	.42	.3	Trace
9	Low fat (1%)------ 1 cup	226	82	165	28	2	1.5	.5	.1	6	138	302	.3	193	80	.05	.37	.3	Trace
10	Uncreamed (cottage cheese dry curd, less than 1/2% fat). 1 cup	145	80	125	25	1	.4	.1	Trace	3	46	151	.3	47	40	.04	.21	.2	0
11	Cream------ 1 oz	28	54	100	2	10	6.2	2.4	.2	1	23	30	.3	34	400	Trace	.06	Trace	0
	Mozzarella, made with—																		
12	Whole milk------ 1 oz	28	48	90	6	7	4.4	1.7	.2	1	163	117	.1	21	260	Trace	.08	Trace	0
13	Part skim milk------ 1 oz	28	49	80	8	5	3.1	1.2	.1	1	207	149	.1	27	180	.01	.10	Trace	0
	Parmesan, grated:																		
14	Cup, not pressed down------ 1 cup	100	18	455	42	30	19.1	7.7	.3	4	1,376	807	1.0	107	700	.05	.39	.3	0
15	Tablespoon------ 1 tbsp	5	18	25	2	2	1.0	.4	Trace	Trace	69	40	Trace	5	40	Trace	.02	Trace	0
16	Ounce------ 1 oz	28	18	130	12	9	5.4	2.2	.1	1	390	229	.3	30	200	.01	.11	.1	0
17	Provolone------ 1 oz	28	41	100	7	8	4.8	1.7	.1	1	214	141	.1	39	230	.01	.09	Trace	0
	Ricotta, made with—																		
18	Whole milk------ 1 cup	246	72	430	28	32	20.4	7.1	.7	7	509	389	.9	257	1,210	.03	.48	.3	0
19	Part skim milk------ 1 cup	246	74	340	28	19	12.1	4.7	.5	13	669	449	1.1	308	1,060	.05	.46	.2	0
20	Romano------ 1 oz	28	31	110	9	8				1	302	215	.1		160		.11	.1	0
21	Swiss------ 1 oz	28	37	105	8	8	5.0	1.7	.2	1	272	171	Trace	31	240	.01	.10	Trace	0
	Pasteurized process cheese:																		
22	American------ 1 oz	28	39	105	6	9	5.6	2.1	.2	Trace	174	211	.1	46	340	.01	.10	Trace	0
23	Swiss------ 1 oz	28	42	95	7	7	4.5	1.7	.1	1	219	216	.2	61	230	Trace	.08	Trace	0
24	Pasteurized process cheese food, American. 1 oz	28	43	95	6	7	4.4	1.7	.2	2	163	130	.2	79	260	.01	.13	Trace	0
25	Pasteurized process cheese spread, American. 1 oz	28	48	80	5	6	3.8	1.5	.1	2	159	202	.1	69	220	.01	.12	Trace	0
	Cream, sweet:																		
26	Half-and-half (cream and milk)- 1 cup	242	81	315	7	28	17.3	7.0	.6	10	254	230	.2	314	260	.08	.36	.2	2
27	1 tbsp	15	81	20	Trace	2	1.1	.4	Trace	Trace	16	14	Trace	19	20	.01	.02	Trace	Trace
28	Light, coffee, or table------ 1 cup	240	74	470	6	46	28.8	11.7	1.0	9	231	192	.1	292	1,730	.08	.36	.1	2
29	1 tbsp	15	74	30	Trace	3	1.8	.7	.1	1	14	12	Trace	18	110	Trace	.02	Trace	Trace

(A)	(B)		(C)	(D)	(E)	(F)	(G)	(H)	(I)	(J)	(K)	(L)	(M)	(N)	(O)	(P)	(Q)	(R)	(S)
	Whipping, unwhipped (volume about double when whipped):																		
30	Light	1 cup	239	64	700	5	74	46.2	18.3	1.5	7	166	146	0.1	231	2,690	0.06	0.30	0.1	1
31		1 tbsp	15	64	45	Trace	5	2.9	1.1	.1	Trace	10	10	Trace	15	170	Trace	.02	Trace	Trace
32	Heavy	1 cup	238	58	820	5	88	54.8	22.2	2.0	7	154	149	.1	179	3,500	.05	.26	.1	1
33		1 tbsp	15	58	80	Trace	6	3.5	1.4	.1	Trace	10	10	Trace	11	220	Trace	.02	.1	Trace
34	Whipped topping, (pressurized)	1 cup	60	61	155	2	13	8.3	3.4	.3	7	61	54	Trace	88	550	.02	.04	Trace	0
35		1 tbsp	3	61	10	Trace	1	.4	.2	Trace	Trace	3	3	Trace	4	30	Trace	Trace	Trace	0
36	Cream, sour	1 cup	230	71	495	7	48	30.0	12.1	1.1	10	268	195	.1	331	1,820	.08	.34	.2	2
37		1 tbsp	12	71	25	Trace	3	1.6	.6	.1	1	14	10	Trace	17	90	Trace	.02	Trace	Trace
	Cream products, imitation (made with vegetable fat): Sweet: Creamers:																		
38	Liquid (frozen)	1 cup	245	77	335	2	24	22.8	.3	Trace	28	23	157	.1	467	[1]220	0	0	0	0
39		1 tbsp	15	77	20	Trace	1	1.4	Trace	0	2	2	9	Trace	29	[1]10	0	0	0	0
40	Powdered	1 cup	94	2	515	5	33	30.6	.9	Trace	52	21	397	.1	763	[1]190	0	[1].16	0	0
41		1 tsp	2	2	10	Trace	1	.7	Trace	0	1	Trace	8	Trace	16	[1]Trace	0	[1]Trace	0	0
	Whipped topping:																		
42	Frozen	1 cup	75	50	240	1	19	16.3	1.0	.2	17	5	6	.1	14	[1]650	Trace	Trace	0	0
43		1 tbsp	4	50	15	Trace	1	.9	.1	Trace	1	Trace	Trace	Trace	1	[1]30	0	0	0	0
44	Powdered, made with whole milk.	1 cup	80	67	150	3	10	8.5	.6	.1	13	72	69	Trace	121	[1]290	.02	.09	Trace	1
45		1 tbsp	4	67	10	Trace	Trace	.4	Trace	Trace	1	4	3	Trace	6	[1]10	Trace	Trace	Trace	Trace
46	Pressurized	1 cup	70	60	185	1	16	13.2	1.4	.2	11	4	13	Trace	13	[1]330	0	0	0	0
47		1 tbsp	4	60	10	Trace	1	.8	.1	Trace	1	Trace	1	Trace	1	[1]20	0	0	0	0
48	Sour dressing (imitation sour cream) made with nonfat dry milk.	1 cup	235	75	415	8	39	31.2	4.4	1.1	11	266	205	.1	380	[1]20	.09	.38	.2	2
49		1 tbsp	12	75	20	Trace	2	1.6	.2	.1	1	14	10	Trace	19	[1]Trace	.01	.02	Trace	Trace
	Ice cream. See Milk desserts, frozen (items 75-80).																		
	Ice milk. See Milk desserts, frozen (items 81-83).																		
	Milk: Fluid:																		
50	Whole (3.3% fat)	1 cup	244	88	150	8	8	5.1	2.1	.2	11	291	228	.1	370	[2]310	.09	.40	.2	2
51	Lowfat (2%): No milk solids added	1 cup	244	89	120	8	5	2.9	1.2	.1	12	297	232	.1	377	500	.10	.40	.2	2
52	Milk solids added: Label claim less than 10 g of protein per cup.	1 cup	245	89	125	9	5	2.9	1.2	.1	12	313	245	.1	397	500	.10	.42	.2	2
53	Label claim 10 or more grams of protein per cup (protein fortified).	1 cup	246	88	135	10	5	3.0	1.2	.1	14	352	276	.1	447	500	.11	.48	.2	3
54	Lowfat (1%): No milk solids added	1 cup	244	90	100	8	3	1.6	.7	.1	12	300	235	.1	381	500	.10	.41	.2	2
55	Milk solids added: Label claim less than 10 g of protein per cup.	1 cup	245	90	105	9	2	1.5	.6	.1	12	313	245	.1	397	500	.10	.42	.2	2
56	Label claim 10 or more grams of protein per cup (protein fortified).	1 cup	246	89	120	10	3	1.8	.7	.1	14	349	273	.1	444	500	.11	.47	.2	3
57	Nonfat (skim): No milk solids added	1 cup	245	91	85	8	Trace	.3	.1	Trace	12	302	247	.1	406	500	.09	.34	.2	2

[1]Vitamin A value is largely from beta-carotene used for coloring. Riboflavin value for items 40-41 apply to products with added riboflavin.

[2]Applies to product without added vitamin A. With added vitamin A, value is 500 International Units (I.U.).

							Fatty Acids												
								Unsaturated								NUTRIENTS IN INDICATED QUANTITY			
Item No.	Foods, approximate measures, units, and weight (edible part unless footnotes indicate otherwise)		Water	Food energy	Pro-tein	Fat	Satu-rated (total)	Oleic	Lino-leic	Carbo-hydrate	Calcium	Phos-phorus	Iron	Potas-sium	Vitamin A value	Thiamin	Ribo-flavin	Niacin	Ascorbic acid
(A)	(B)	Grams	(C) Per-cent	(D) Cal-ories	(E) Grams	(F) Grams	(G) Grams	(H) Grams	(I) Grams	(J) Grams	(K) Milli-grams	(L) Milli-grams	(M) Milli-grams	(N) Milli-grams	(O) Inter-national units	(P) Milli-grams	(Q) Milli-grams	(R) Milli-grams	(S) Milli-grams

DAIRY PRODUCTS (CHEESE, CREAM, IMITATION CREAM, MILK; RELATED PRODUCTS)—Con.

Milk—Continued
Fluid—Continued
Nonfat (skim)—Continued
Milk solids added:

(A)	(B)	Grams	(C)	(D)	(E)	(F)	(G)	(H)	(I)	(J)	(K)	(L)	(M)	(N)	(O)	(P)	(Q)	(R)	(S)
58	Label claim less than 10 g of protein per cup. 1 cup	245	90	90	9	1	0.4	0.1	Trace	12	316	255	0.1	418	500	0.10	0.43	0.2	2
59	Label claim 10 or more grams of protein per cup (protein fortified). 1 cup	246	89	100	10	1	.4	.1	Trace	14	352	275	.1	446	500	.11	.48	.2	3
60	Buttermilk. 1 cup	245	90	100	8	2	1.3	.5	Trace	12	285	219	.1	371	[3]80	.08	.38	.1	2
	Canned: Evaporated, unsweetened:																		
61	Whole milk. 1 cup	252	74	340	17	19	11.6	5.3	0.4	25	657	510	.5	764	[3]610	.12	.80	.5	5
62	Skim milk. 1 cup	255	79	200	19	1	.3	.1	Trace	29	738	497	.7	845	[4]1,000	.11	.79	.4	3
63	Sweetened, condensed. 1 cup	306	27	980	24	27	16.8	6.7	.7	166	868	775	.6	1,136	[3]1,000	.28	1.27	.6	8
	Dried:																		
64	Buttermilk. 1 cup	120	3	465	41	7	4.3	1.7	.2	59	1,421	1,119	.4	1,910	[3]260	.47	1.90	1.1	7
	Nonfat instant:																		
65	Envelope, net wt., 3.2 oz[5]. 1 envelope	91	4	325	32	1	.4	.1	Trace	47	1,120	896	.3	1,552	[6]2,160	.38	1.59	.8	5
66	Cup[7]. 1 cup	68	4	245	24	Trace	.3	.1	Trace	35	837	670	.2	1,160	[6]1,610	.28	1.19	.6	4
	Milk beverages: Chocolate milk (commercial):																		
67	Regular. 1 cup	250	82	210	8	8	5.3	2.2	.2	26	280	251	.6	417	[3]300	.09	.41	.3	2
68	Lowfat (2%). 1 cup	250	84	180	8	5	3.1	1.3	.1	26	284	254	.6	422	500	.10	.42	.3	2
69	Lowfat (1%). 1 cup	250	85	160	8	3	1.5	.7	.1	26	287	257	.6	426	500	.10	.40	.2	2
70	Eggnog (commercial). 1 cup	254	74	340	10	19	11.3	5.0	.6	34	330	278	.5	420	890	.09	.48	.3	4
	Malted milk, home-prepared with 1 cup of whole milk and 2 to 3 heaping tsp of malted milk powder (about 3/4 oz):																		
71	Chocolate. 1 cup of milk plus 3/4 oz of powder	265	81	235	9	9	5.5	—	—	29	304	265	.5	500	330	.14	.43	.7	2
72	Natural. 1 cup of milk plus 3/4 oz of powder	265	81	235	11	10	6.0	—	—	27	347	307	.3	529	380	.20	.54	1.3	2
	Shakes, thick:[8]																		
73	Chocolate, container, net wt., 10.6 oz. 1 container	300	72	355	9	8	5.0	2.0	.2	63	396	378	.9	672	260	.14	.67	.4	0
74	Vanilla, container, net wt., 11 oz. 1 container	313	74	350	12	9	5.9	2.4	.2	56	457	361	.3	572	360	.09	.61	.5	0
	Milk desserts, frozen: Ice cream: Regular (about 11% fat):																		
75	Hardened. 1/2 gal	1,064	61	2,155	38	115	71.3	28.8	2.6	254	1,406	1,075	1.0	2,052	4,340	.42	2.63	1.1	6
76	1 cup	133	61	270	5	14	8.9	3.6	.3	32	176	134	.1	257	540	.05	.33	.1	1
77	3-fl oz container	50	61	100	2	5	3.4	1.4	.1	12	66	51	Trace	96	200	.02	.12	.1	Trace
78	Soft serve (frozen custard). 1 cup	173	60	375	7	23	13.5	5.9	.6	38	236	199	.4	338	790	.08	.45	.2	1
	Rich (about 16% fat):																		
79	1/2 gal	1,188	59	2,805	33	190	118.3	47.8	4.3	256	1,213	927	.8	1,771	7,200	.36	2.27	.9	5
80	1 cup	148	59	350	4	24	14.7	6.0	.5	32	151	115	.1	221	900	.04	.28	.1	1
	Ice milk: Hardened (about 4.3% fat):																		
81	1/2 gal	1,048	69	1,470	41	45	28.1	11.3	1.0	232	1,409	1,035	1.5	2,117	1,710	.61	2.78	.9	6
82	1 cup	131	69	185	5	6	3.5	1.4	.1	29	176	129	.1	265	210	.08	.35	.1	1

(A)	(B)	(C)	(D)	(E)	(F)	(G)	(H)	(I)	(J)	(K)	(L)	(M)	(N)	(O)	(P)	(Q)	(R)	(S)
83	Soft serve (about 2.6% fat)------ 1 cup	175	70	225	8	5	2.9	1.2	0.1	38	274	202	0.3	412	180	0.12	0.54	0.2	1
84	Sherbet (about 2% fat)----------- 1/2 gal	1,542	66	2,160	17	31	19.0	7.7	.7	469	827	594	2.5	1,585	1,480	.26	.71	1.0	31
85	1 cup	193	66	270	2	4	2.4	1.0	.1	59	103	74	.3	198	190	.03	.09	.1	4
	Milk desserts, other:																		
	Custard, baked:																		
86	1 cup	265	77	305	14	15	6.8	5.4	.7	29	297	310	1.1	387	930	.11	.50	.3	1
	Puddings:																		
	From home recipe:																		
	Starch base:																		
87	Chocolate------ 1 cup	260	66	385	8	12	7.6	3.3	.3	67	250	255	1.3	445	390	.05	.36	.3	1
88	Vanilla (blancmange)--- 1 cup	255	76	285	9	10	6.2	2.5	.2	41	298	232	Trace	352	410	.08	.41	.3	2
89	Tapioca cream------ 1 cup	165	72	220	8	8	4.1	2.5	.5	28	173	180	.7	223	480	.07	.30	.2	2
	From mix (chocolate) and milk:																		
90	Regular (cooked)---- 1 cup	260	70	320	9	8	4.3	2.6	.2	59	265	247	.8	354	340	.05	.39	.3	2
91	Instant---- 1 cup	260	69	325	8	7	3.6	2.2	.3	63	374	237	1.3	335	340	.08	.39	.3	2
	Yogurt:																		
	With added milk solids:																		
	Made with lowfat milk:																		
92	Fruit-flavored - 1 container, net wt., 8 oz	227	75	230	10	3	1.8	.6	.1	42	343	269	.2	439	[10]120	.08	.40	.2	1
93	Plain - 1 container, net wt., 8 oz	227	85	145	12	4	2.3	.8	.1	16	415	326	.2	531	[10]150	.10	.49	.3	2
94	Made with nonfat milk - 1 container, net wt., 8 oz	227	85	125	13	Trace	.3	.1	Trace	17	452	355	.2	579	[1]120	.11	.53	.3	2
	Without added milk solids:																		
95	Made with whole milk - 1 container, net wt., 8 oz	227	88	140	8	7	4.8	1.7	.1	11	274	215	.1	351	280	.07	.32	.2	1

EGGS

(A)	(B)	(C)	(D)	(E)	(F)	(G)	(H)	(I)	(J)	(K)	(L)	(M)	(N)	(O)	(P)	(Q)	(R)	(S)
	Eggs, large (24 oz per dozen):																		
	Raw:																		
96	Whole, without shell----- 1 egg	50	75	80	6	6	1.7	2.0	.6	1	28	90	1.0	65	260	.04	.15	Trace	0
97	White---- 1 white	33	88	15	3	Trace	0	0	0	Trace	4	4	Trace	45	0	Trace	.09	Trace	0
98	Yolk---- 1 yolk	17	49	65	3	6	1.7	2.1	.6	Trace	26	86	.9	15	310	.04	.07	Trace	0
	Cooked:																		
99	Fried in butter---- 1 egg	46	72	85	5	6	2.4	2.2	.6	1	26	80	.9	58	290	.03	.13	Trace	0
100	Hard-cooked, shell removed- 1 egg	50	75	80	6	6	1.7	2.0	.6	1	28	90	.9	65	260	.04	.14	Trace	0
101	Poached---- 1 egg	50	74	80	6	6	1.7	2.0	.6	1	28	90	1.0	65	260	.04	.13	Trace	0
102	Scrambled (milk added) in butter. Also omelet. 1 egg	64	76	95	6	7	2.8	2.3	.6	1	47	97	.9	85	310	.04	.16	Trace	0

FATS, OILS; RELATED PRODUCTS

(A)	(B)	(C)	(D)	(E)	(F)	(G)	(H)	(I)	(J)	(K)	(L)	(M)	(N)	(O)	(P)	(Q)	(R)	(S)
	Butter:																		
	Regular (1 brick or 4 sticks per lb):																		
103	Stick (1/2 cup)------ 1 stick	113	16	815	1	92	57.3	23.1	2.1	Trace	27	26	.2	29	[11]3,470	.01	.04	Trace	0
104	Tablespoon (about 1/8 stick)- 1 tbsp	14	16	100	Trace	12	7.2	2.9	.3	Trace	3	3	Trace	4	[11]430	Trace	Trace	Trace	0
105	Pat (1 in square, 1/3 in high; 90 per lb)- 1 pat	5	16	35	Trace	4	2.5	1.0	.1	Trace	1	1	Trace	1	[11]150	Trace	Trace	Trace	0
	Whipped (6 sticks or two 8-oz containers per lb):																		
106	Stick (1/2 cup)------ 1 stick	76	16	540	1	61	38.2	15.4	1.4	Trace	18	17	.1	20	[11]2,310	Trace	.03	Trace	0
107	Tablespoon (about 1/8 stick)- 1 tbsp	9	16	65	Trace	8	4.7	1.9	.2	Trace	2	2	Trace	2	[11]290	Trace	Trace	Trace	0
108	Pat (1 1/4 in square, 1/3 in high; 120 per lb)- 1 pat	4	16	25	Trace	3	1.9	.8	.1	Trace	1	1	Trace	1	[11]120	0	Trace	Trace	0

[3] Applies to product without vitamin A added.
[4] Applies to product with added vitamin A. Without added vitamin A, value is 20 International Units (I.U.).
[5] Yields 1 qt of fluid milk when reconstituted according to package directions.
[6] Applies to product with added vitamin A.
[7] Weight applies to product with label claim of 1 1/3 cups equal 3.2 oz.
[8] Applies to products made from thick shake mixes and that do not contain added ice cream. Products made from milk shake mixes are higher in fat and usually contain added ice cream.
[9] Content of fat, vitamin A, and carbohydrate varies. Consult the label when precise values are needed for special diets
[10] Applies to products made from thick shake mixes and that do not contain added ice cream.
[10] Applies to product made with milk containing no added vitamin A.
[11] Based on year-round average.

(Dashes (—) denote lack of reliable data for a constituent believed to be present in measurable amount)

							Fatty Acids			NUTRIENTS IN INDICATED QUANTITY									
								Unsaturated											
Item No.	Foods, approximate measures, units, and weight (edible part unless footnotes indicate otherwise)		Water	Food energy	Pro-tein	Fat	Satu-rated (total)	Oleic	Lino-leic	Carbo-hydrate	Calcium	Phos-phorus	Iron	Potas-sium	Vitamin A value	Thiamin	Ribo-flavin	Niacin	Ascorbic acid
(A)	(B)		(C)	(D)	(E)	(F)	(G)	(H)	(I)	(J)	(K)	(L)	(M)	(N)	(O)	(P)	(Q)	(R)	(S)
		Grams	Per cent	Cal-ories	Grams	Grams	Grams	Grams	Grams	Grams	Milli-grams	Milli-grams	Milli-grams	Milli-grams	Inter-national units	Milli-grams	Milli-grams	Milli-grams	Milli-grams

FATS, OILS; RELATED PRODUCTS—Con.

(A)	(B)		(C)	(D)	(E)	(F)	(G)	(H)	(I)	(J)	(K)	(L)	(M)	(N)	(O)	(P)	(Q)	(R)	(S)
109	Fats, cooking (vegetable shortenings). 1 cup----	200	0	1,770	0	200	48.8	88.2	48.4	0	0	0	0	0	—	0	0	0	0
110	1 tbsp---	13	0	110	0	13	3.2	5.7	3.1	0	0	0	0	0	0	0	0	0	0
111	Lard---- 1 cup---	205	0	1,850	0	205	81.0	83.8	20.5	0	0	0	0	0	0	0	0	0	0
112	1 tbsp---	13	0	115	0	13	5.1	5.3	1.3	0	0	0	0	0	0	0	0	0	0
	Margarine (1 brick or 4 sticks per lb):																		
113	Stick (1/2 cup)----	113	16	815	1	92	16.7	42.9	24.9	Trace	27	26	.2	29	[12]3,750	.01	.04	Trace	0
114	Tablespoon (about 1/8 stick)-	14	16	100	Trace	12	3.2	5.3	3.1	Trace	3	3	Trace	4	[12]470	Trace	Trace	Trace	0
115	Pat (1 in square, 1/3 in high; 90 per lb). 1 pat---	5	16	35	Trace	4	.7	1.9	1.1	Trace	1	1	Trace	1	[12]170	Trace	Trace	Trace	0
116	Soft, two 8-oz containers per lb. 1 container---	227	16	1,635	1	184	32.5	71.5	65.4	Trace	53	52	.4	59	[12]7,500	.01	.08	.1	0
117	1 tbsp---	14	16	100	Trace	12	2.0	4.5	4.1	Trace	3	3	Trace	4	[12]470	Trace	Trace	Trace	0
	Whipped (6 sticks per lb):																		
118	Stick (1/2 cup)----	76	16	545	Trace	61	11.2	28.7	16.7	Trace	18	17	.1	20	[12]2,500	Trace	.03	Trace	0
119	Tablespoon (about 1/8 stick)-	9	16	70	Trace	8	1.4	3.6	2.1	Trace	2	2	Trace	2	[12]310	Trace	Trace	Trace	0
	Oils, salad or cooking:																		
120	Corn--- 1 cup---	218	0	1,925	0	218	27.7	53.6	125.1	0	0	0	0	0	—	0	0	0	0
121	1 tbsp---	14	0	120	0	14	1.7	3.3	7.8	0	0	0	0	0	—	0	0	0	0
122	Olive--- 1 cup---	216	0	1,910	0	216	30.7	154.4	17.7	0	0	0	0	0	—	0	0	0	0
123	1 tbsp---	14	0	120	0	14	1.9	9.7	1.1	0	0	0	0	0	—	0	0	0	0
124	Peanut--- 1 cup---	216	0	1,910	0	216	37.4	98.5	67.0	0	0	0	0	0	—	0	0	0	0
125	1 tbsp---	14	0	120	0	14	2.3	6.2	4.2	0	0	0	0	0	—	0	0	0	0
126	Safflower--- 1 cup---	218	0	1,925	0	218	20.5	25.9	159.8	0	0	0	0	0	—	0	0	0	0
127	1 tbsp---	14	0	120	0	14	1.3	1.6	10.0	0	0	0	0	0	—	0	0	0	0
128	Soybean oil, hydrogenated (partially hardened). 1 cup---	218	0	1,925	0	218	31.8	93.1	75.6	0	0	0	0	0	—	0	0	0	0
129	1 tbsp---	14	0	120	0	14	2.0	5.8	4.7	0	0	0	0	0	—	0	0	0	0
130	Soybean-cottonseed oil blend, hydrogenated. 1 cup---	218	0	1,925	0	218	38.2	63.0	99.6	0	0	0	0	0	—	0	0	0	0
131	1 tbsp---	14	0	120	0	14	2.4	3.9	6.2	0	0	0	0	0	—	0	0	0	0
	Salad dressings:																		
	Commercial:																		
	Blue cheese:																		
132	Regular--- 1 tbsp---	15	32	75	1	8	1.6	1.7	3.8	1	12	11	Trace	6	30	Trace	.02	Trace	Trace
133	Low calorie (5 Cal per tsp) 1 tbsp---	16	84	10	Trace	1	.5	.3	Trace	1	10	8	Trace	5	30	Trace	.01	Trace	Trace
	French:																		
134	Regular--- 1 tbsp---	16	39	65	Trace	6	1.1	1.3	3.2	3	2	2	.1	13	—	—	—	—	—
135	Low calorie (5 Cal per tsp) 1 tbsp---	16	77	15	Trace	1	.1	.1	.4	2	2	2	.1	13	—	—	—	—	—
	Italian:																		
136	Regular--- 1 tbsp---	15	28	85	Trace	9	1.6	1.9	4.7	1	2	1	Trace	2	Trace	Trace	Trace	Trace	—
137	Low calorie (2 Cal per tsp) 1 tbsp---	15	90	10	Trace	1	.1	.1	.4	1	2	1	Trace	2	Trace	Trace	Trace	Trace	—
138	Mayonnaise--- 1 tbsp---	14	15	100	Trace	11	2.0	2.4	5.6	Trace	3	4	.1	5	40	Trace	.01	Trace	—
	Mayonnaise type:																		
139	Regular--- 1 tbsp---	15	41	65	Trace	6	1.1	1.4	3.2	2	2	4	Trace	1	30	Trace	Trace	Trace	—
140	Low calorie (8 Cal per tsp) 1 tbsp---	16	81	20	Trace	2	.4	.4	1.0	2	3	4	Trace	1	40	Trace	Trace	Trace	—
141	Tartar sauce, regular--- 1 tbsp---	14	34	75	Trace	8	1.5	1.8	4.1	1	3	4	Trace	11	30	Trace	Trace	Trace	Trace
	Thousand Island:																		
142	Regular--- 1 tbsp---	16	32	80	Trace	8	1.4	1.7	4.0	2	2	3	.1	18	50	Trace	Trace	Trace	Trace
143	Low calorie (10 Cal per tsp) 1 tbsp---	15	68	25	Trace	2	.4	.4	1.0	2	2	3	.1	17	50	Trace	Trace	Trace	Trace
	From home recipe:																		
144	Cooked type[13]--- 1 tbsp---	16	68	25	1	2	.5	.6	.3	2	14	15	.1	19	80	.01	.03	Trace	Trace

FISH, SHELLFISH, MEAT, POULTRY; RELATED PRODUCTS

(A)	(B)	(C)	(D)	(E)	(F)	(G)	(H)	(I)	(J)	(K)	(L)	(M)	(N)	(O)	(P)	(Q)	(R)	(S)
	Fish and shellfish:																	
145	Bluefish, baked with butter or margarine. 3 oz (85 g)	68	135	22	4	—	—	—	0	25	244	.6	—	40	0.09	0.08	1.6	—
	Clams:																	
146	Raw, meat only. 3 oz (85 g)	82	65	11	1	—	—	—	2	59	138	5.2	154	90	.08	.15	1.1	8
147	Canned, solids and liquid. 3 oz (85 g)	86	45	7	1	—	—	—	2	47	116	3.5	119	—	.01	.09	.9	—
148	Crabmeat (white or king), canned, not pressed down. 1 cup (135 g)	77	135	24	3	—	—	—	1	61	246	1.1	149	—	.11	.11	2.6	—
149	Fish sticks, breaded, cooked, frozen (stick, 4 by 1 by 1/2 in). 1 fish stick or 1 oz (28 g)	66	50	5	3	—	—	—	2	3	47	.1	—	0	.01	.02	.5	—
150	Haddock, breaded, fried[14]. 3 oz (85 g)	66	140	17	5	1.4	2.2	1.2	5	34	210	1.0	296	—	.03	.06	2.7	2
151	Ocean perch, breaded, fried[14]. 1 fillet (85 g)	59	195	16	11	2.7	4.4	2.3	6	28	192	1.1	242	—	.10	.10	1.6	—
152	Oysters, raw, meat only (13-19 medium Selects). 1 cup (240 g)	85	160	20	4	1.3	.2	.1	8	226	343	13.2	290	740	.34	.43	6.0	—
153	Salmon, pink, canned, solids and liquid. 3 oz (85 g)	71	120	17	5	.9	.8	.1	0	[15]167	243	.7	307	60	.03	.16	6.8	—
154	Sardines, Atlantic, canned in oil, drained solids. 3 oz (85 g)	62	175	20	9	3.0	2.5	.5	0	372	424	2.5	502	190	.02	.17	4.6	—
155	Scallops, frozen, breaded, fried, reheated. 6 scallops (90 g)	60	175	16	8	—	—	—	9	—	—	—	—	—	—	—	—	—
156	Shad, baked with butter or margarine, bacon. 3 oz (85 g)	64	170	20	10	—	—	—	0	20	266	.5	320	30	.11	.22	7.3	—
	Shrimp:																	
157	Canned meat. 3 oz (85 g)	70	100	21	1	—	—	—	1	98	224	2.6	104	50	.01	.03	1.5	—
158	French fried[16]. 3 oz (85 g)	57	190	17	9	2.3	3.7	2.0	9	61	162	1.7	195	—	.03	.07	2.3	—
159	Tuna, canned in oil, drained solids. 3 oz (85 g)	61	170	24	7	1.7	1.7	.7	0	7	199	1.6	—	70	.04	.10	10.1	—
160	Tuna salad[17]. 1 cup (205 g)	70	350	30	22	4.3	6.3	5.7	7	41	291	2.7	—	590	.08	.23	10.3	2
	Meat and meat products:																	
161	Bacon, (20 slices per lb, raw), broiled or fried, crisp. 2 slices (15 g)	8	85	4	8	2.5	3.7	.7	Trace	2	34	.5	35	0	.08	.05	.8	—
	Beef,[18] cooked: Cuts braised, simmered or pot roasted:																	
162	Lean and fat (piece, 2 1/2 by 2 1/2 by 3/4 in). 3 oz (85 g)	53	245	23	16	6.8	6.5	.4	0	10	114	2.9	184	30	.04	.18	3.6	—
163	Lean only from item 162. 2.5 oz (72 g)	62	140	22	5	2.1	1.8	.2	0	10	108	2.7	176	10	.04	.17	3.3	—
	Ground beef, broiled:																	
164	Lean with 10% fat. 3 oz or patty 3 by 5/8 in (85 g)	60	185	23	10	4.0	3.9	.3	0	10	196	3.0	261	20	.08	.20	5.1	—
165	Lean with 21% fat. 2.9 oz or patty 3 by 5/8 in (82 g)	54	235	20	17	7.0	6.7	.4	0	9	159	2.6	221	30	.07	.17	4.4	—
	Roast, oven cooked, no liquid added: Relatively fat, such as rib:																	
166	Lean and fat (2 pieces, 4 1/8 by 2 1/4 by 1/4 in). 3 oz (85 g)	40	375	17	33	14.0	13.6	.8	0	8	158	2.2	189	70	.05	.13	3.1	—
167	Lean only from item 166. 1.8 oz (51 g)	57	125	14	7	3.0	2.5	.3	0	6	131	1.8	161	10	.04	.11	2.6	—
	Relatively lean, such as heel of round:																	
168	Lean and fat (2 pieces, 4 1/8 by 2 1/4 by 1/4 in). 3 oz (85 g)	62	165	25	7	2.8	2.7	.2	0	11	208	3.2	279	10	.06	.19	4.5	—

[12] Based on average vitamin A content of fortified margarine. Federal specifications for fortified margarine require a minimum of 15,000 International Units (I.U.) of vitamin A per pound.

[13] Fatty acid values apply to product made with regular-type margarine.

[14] Dipped in egg, milk or water, and breadcrumbs; fried in vegetable shortening.

[15] If bones are discarded, value for calcium will be greatly reduced.

[16] Dipped in egg, breadcrumbs, and flour or batter.

[17] Prepared with tuna, celery, salad dressing (mayonnaise type), pickle, onion, and egg.

[18] Outer layer of fat on the cut was removed to within approximately 1/2 in of the lean. Deposits of fat within the cut were not removed.

FISH, SHELLFISH, MEAT, POULTRY; RELATED PRODUCTS-Con.

NUTRIENTS IN INDICATED QUANTITY

Item No.	Foods, approximate measures, units, and weight (edible part unless footnotes indicate otherwise)		Water	Food energy	Protein	Fat	Fatty Acids Saturated (total)	Unsaturated Oleic	Unsaturated Linoleic	Carbohydrate	Calcium	Phosphorus	Iron	Potassium	Vitamin A value	Thiamin	Riboflavin	Niacin	Ascorbic acid
(A)	(B)	Grams	(C) Percent	(D) Calories	(E) Grams	(F) Grams	(G) Grams	(H) Grams	Grams	(I) Grams	(K) Milligrams	(L) Milligrams	(M) Milligrams	(N) Milligrams	(O) International units	(P) Milligrams	(Q) Milligrams	(R) Milligrams	(S) Milligrams
	Meat and meat products-Continued																		
	Beef,[8] cooked-Continued																		
	Roast, oven cooked, no liquid added-Continued																		
	Relatively lean such as heel of round-Continued																		
169	Lean only from item 168--- 2.8 oz	78	65	125	24	3	1.2	1.0	0.1	0	10	199	3.0	268	Trace	0.06	0.18	4.3	---
	Steak:																		
	Relatively fat-sirloin, broiled:																		
170	Lean and fat (piece, 2 1/2 by 2 1/2 by 3/4 in). 3 oz	85	44	330	20	27	11.3	11.1	.6	0	9	162	2.5	220	50	.05	.15	4.0	---
171	Lean only from item 170--- 2.0 oz	56	59	115	18	4	1.8	1.6	.2	0	7	146	2.2	202	10	.05	.14	3.6	---
	Relatively lean-round, braised:																		
172	Lean and fat (piece, 4 1/8 by 2 1/4 by 1/2 in). 3 oz	85	55	220	24	13	5.5	5.2	.4	0	10	213	3.0	272	20	.07	.19	4.8	---
173	Lean only from item 172--- 2.4 oz	68	61	130	21	4	1.7	1.5	.2	0	9	182	2.5	238	10	.05	.16	4.1	---
	Beef, canned:																		
174	Corned beef--- 3 oz	85	59	185	22	10	4.9	4.5	.2	0	17	90	3.7	440	---	.01	.20	2.9	---
175	Corned beef hash--- 1 cup	220	67	400	19	25	11.9	10.9	.5	24	29	147	4.4	142	---	.02	.20	4.6	---
176	Beef, dried, chipped--- 2 1/2-oz jar	71	48	145	24	4	2.1	2.0	.1	0	14	287	3.6	142	---	.05	.23	2.7	---
177	Beef and vegetable stew--- 1 cup	245	82	220	16	11	4.9	4.5	.2	15	29	184	2.9	613	2,400	.15	.17	4.7	17
178	Beef potpie (home recipe), baked[9] (piece, 1/3 of 9-in diam. pie). 1 piece	210	55	515	21	30	7.9	12.8	6.7	39	29	149	3.8	334	1,720	.30	.30	5.5	6
179	Chili con carne with beans, canned. 1 cup	255	72	340	19	16	7.5	6.8	.3	31	82	321	4.3	594	150	.08	.18	3.3	---
180	Chop suey with beef and pork (home recipe). 1 cup	250	75	300	26	17	8.5	6.2	.7	13	60	248	4.8	425	600	.28	.38	5.0	33
181	Heart, beef, lean, braised--- 3 oz	85	61	160	27	5	1.5	1.1	.6	1	5	154	5.0	197	20	.21	1.04	6.5	1
	Lamb, cooked:																		
	Chop, rib (cut 3 per lb with bone), broiled:																		
182	Lean and fat--- 3.1 oz	89	43	360	18	32	14.8	12.1	1.2	0	8	139	1.0	200	---	.11	.19	4.1	---
183	Lean only from item 182--- 2 oz	57	60	120	16	6	2.5	2.1	.2	0	6	121	1.1	174	---	.09	.15	3.4	---
	Leg, roasted:																		
184	Lean and fat (2 pieces, 4 1/8 by 2 1/4 by 1/4 in). 3 oz	85	54	235	22	16	7.3	6.0	.6	0	9	177	1.4	241	---	.13	.23	4.7	---
185	Lean only from item 184--- 2.5 oz	71	62	130	20	5	2.1	1.8	.2	0	9	169	1.4	227	---	.12	.21	4.4	---
	Shoulder, roasted:																		
186	Lean and fat (3 pieces, 2 1/2 by 2 1/2 by 1/4 in). 3 oz	85	50	285	18	23	10.8	8.8	.9	0	9	146	1.0	206	---	.11	.20	4.0	---
187	Lean only from item 186--- 2.3 oz	64	61	130	17	6	3.6	2.3	.2	0	8	140	1.0	193	---	.10	.18	3.7	---
188	Liver, beef, fried[20] (slice, 6 1/2 by 2 3/8 by 3/8 in). 3 oz	85	56	195	22	9	2.5	3.5	.9	5	9	405	7.5	323	[2]45,390	.22	3.56	14.0	23
	Pork, cured, cooked:																		
	Ham, light cure, lean and fat, roasted (2 pieces, 4 1/8 by 2 1/4 by 1/4 in).[22]																		
189	3 oz	85	54	245	18	19	6.8	7.9	1.7	0	8	146	2.2	199	0	.40	.15	3.1	---
	Luncheon meat:																		
190	Boiled ham, slice (8 per 8-oz pkg.). 1 oz	28	59	65	5	5	1.7	2.0	.4	0	3	47	.8	---	0	.12	.04	.7	---
191	Canned, spiced or unspiced: Slice, approx. 3 by 2 by 1/2 in. 1 slice	60	55	175	9	15	5.4	6.7	1.0	1	5	65	1.3	133	0	.19	.13	1.8	---

(A)	(B)		(C)	(D)	(E)	(F)	(G)	(H)	(I)	(J)	(K)	(L)	(M)	(N)	(O)	(P)	(Q)	(R)	(S)
	Pork, fresh,[18] cooked:																		
	Chop, loin (cut 3 per lb with bone), broiled:																		
192	Lean and fat ---- 2.7 oz	78	42	305	19	25	8.9	10.4	2.2	0	9	209	2.7	216	0	0.75	0.22	4.5	—
193	Lean only from item 192 --- 2 oz	56	53	150	17	9	3.1	3.6	.8	0	7	181	2.2	192	0	.63	.18	3.8	—
194	Roast, oven cooked, no liquid added: Lean and fat (piece, 2 1/2 by 2 1/2 by 3/4 in). 3 oz	85	46	310	21	24	8.7	10.2	2.2	0	9	218	2.7	233	0	.78	.22	4.8	—
195	Lean only from item 194 ---- 2.4 oz	68	55	175	20	10	3.5	4.1	.8	0	3	211	2.6	224	0	.73	.21	4.4	—
196	Shoulder cut, simmered: Lean and fat (3 pieces, 2 1/2 by 2 1/2 by 1/4 in). 3 oz	85	46	320	20	26	9.3	10.9	2.3	0	9	118	2.6	158	0	.46	.21	4.1	—
197	Lean only from item 196 ---- 2.2 oz	63	60	135	18	6	2.2	2.6	.6	0	8	111	2.3	146	0	.42	.19	3.7	—
	Sausages (see also Luncheon meat (items 190-191)):																		
198	Bologna, slice (8 per 8-oz pkg.). 1 slice	28	56	85	3	8	3.0	3.4	.5	Trace	2	36	.5	65	—	.05	.06	.7	—
199	Braunschweiger, slice (6 per 6-oz pkg.). 1 slice	28	53	90	4	8	2.6	3.4	.8	1	3	69	1.7	—	1,850	.05	.41	2.3	—
200	Brown and serve (10-11 per 8-oz pkg.), browned. 1 link	17	40	70	3	6	2.3	2.8	.7	Trace	—	—	—	—	—	—	—	—	—
201	Deviled ham, canned---- 1 tbsp	13	51	45	2	4	1.5	1.8	.4	0	1	12	.3	—	0	.02	.01	.2	—
202	Frankfurter (8 per 1-lb pkg.), cooked (reheated). 1 frankfurter	56	57	170	7	15	5.6	6.5	1.2	1	3	57	.8	—	—	.08	.11	1.4	—
203	Meat, potted (beef, chicken, turkey), canned. 1 tbsp	13	61	30	2	2				0				35		Trace	.03	.2	—
204	Pork link (16 per 1-lb pkg.), cooked. 1 link	13	35	60	2	6	2.1	2.4	.5	Trace	1	21	.3	—	0	.10	.04	.5	—
	Salami:																		
205	Dry type, slice (12 per 4-oz pkg.). 1 slice	10	30	45	2	4	1.6	1.6	.1	Trace	1	28	.4	—	—	.04	.03	.5	—
206	Cooked type, slice (8 per 8-oz pkg.). 1 slice	28	51	90	5	7	3.1	3.0	.2	Trace	3	57	.7	—	—	.07	.07	1.2	—
207	Vienna sausage (7 per 4-oz can). 1 sausage	16	63	40	2	3	1.2	1.4	.2	Trace	1	24	.3	—	—	.01	.02	.4	—
	Veal, medium fat, cooked, bone removed:																		
208	Cutlet (4 1/8 by 2 1/4 by 1/2 in), braised or broiled. 3 oz	85	60	185	23	9	4.0	3.4	.4	0	9	196	2.7	258	—	.06	.21	4.6	—
209	Rib (2 pieces, 4 1/8 by 2 1/4 by 1/4 in), roasted. 3 oz	85	55	230	23	14	6.1	5.1	.6	0	10	211	2.9	259	—	.11	.26	6.6	—
	Poultry and poultry products: Chicken, cooked:																		
210	Breast, fried,[21] bones removed, 1/2 breast (3.3 oz with bones). 2.8 oz	79	58	160	26	5	1.4	1.8	1.1	1	9	218	1.3	—	70	.04	.17	11.6	—
211	Drumstick, fried,[21] bones removed (2 oz with bones). 1.3 oz	38	55	90	12	4	1.1	1.3	.9	Trace	6	89	.9	—	50	.03	.15	2.7	—
212	Half broiler, broiled, bones removed (10.4 oz with bones). 6.2 oz	176	71	240	42	7	2.2	2.5	1.3	0	16	355	3.0	483	160	.09	.34	15.5	—
213	Chicken, canned, boneless---- 3 oz	85	65	170	18	10	3.2	3.8	2.0	0	18	210	1.3	117	200	.03	.11	3.7	3
214	Chicken a la king, cooked (home recipe). 1 cup	245	68	470	27	34	12.7	14.3	3.3	12	127	358	2.5	404	1,130	.10	.42	5.4	12
215	Chicken and noodles, cooked (home recipe). 1 cup	240	71	365	22	18	5.9	7.1	3.5	26	26	247	2.2	149	430	.05	.17	4.3	Trace

[18] Outer layer of fat on the cut was removed to within approximately 1/2 in of the lean. Deposits of fat within the cut were not removed.
[19] Crust made with vegetable shortening and enriched flour.
[20] Regular-type margarine used.
[21] Value varies widely.
[22] About one-fourth of the outer layer of fat on the cut was removed. Deposits of fat within the cut were not removed.
[23] Vegetable shortening used.

427

(Dashes (—) denote lack of reliable data for a constituent believed to be present in measurable amount)

Item No. (A)	Foods, approximate measures, units, and weight (edible part unless footnotes indicate otherwise) (B)	Grams	Water (C) Percent	Food energy (D) Calories	Protein (E) Grams	Fat (F) Grams	Fatty Acids Saturated (total) (G) Grams	Unsaturated Oleic (H) Grams	Unsaturated Linoleic (I) Grams	Carbohydrate (J) Grams	Calcium (K) Milligrams	Phosphorus (L) Milligrams	Iron (M) Milligrams	Potassium (N) Milligrams	Vitamin A value (O) International units	Thiamin (P) Milligrams	Riboflavin (Q) Milligrams	Niacin (R) Milligrams	Ascorbic acid (S) Milligrams
	FISH, SHELLFISH, MEAT, POULTRY, RELATED PRODUCTS—Con.																		
	Poultry and poultry products—Continued																		
	Chicken chow mein:																		
216	Canned --- 1 cup	250	89	95	7	Trace	—	—	—	18	45	35	1.3	418	150	0.05	0.10	1.0	13
217	From home recipe --- 1 cup	250	78	255	31	10	2.4	3.4	3.1	10	58	293	2.5	473	280	.08	.23	4.3	10
218	Chicken potpie (home recipe), baked, piece (1/3 or 9-in diam. pie). --- 1 piece	232	57	545	23	31	11.3	10.9	5.6	42	70	232	3.0	343	3,090	.34	.31	5.5	5
	Turkey, roasted, flesh without skin:																		
219	Dark meat, piece, 2 1/2 by 1 5/8 by 1/4 in. --- 4 pieces	85	61	175	26	7	2.1	1.5	1.5	0	—	—	2.0	338	—	.03	.20	3.6	—
220	Light meat, piece, 4 by 2 by 1/4 in. --- 2 pieces	85	62	150	28	3	.9	.6	.7	0	—	—	1.0	349	—	.04	.12	9.4	—
	Light and dark meat:																		
221	Chopped or diced --- 1 cup	140	61	265	44	9	2.5	1.7	1.8	0	11	351	2.5	514	—	.07	.25	10.8	—
222	Pieces (1 slice white meat, 4 by 2 by 1/4 in with 2 slices dark meat, 2 1/2 by 1 5/8 by 1/4 in). --- 3 pieces	85	61	160	27	5	1.5	1.0	1.1	0	7	213	1.5	312	—	.04	.15	6.5	—
	FRUITS AND FRUIT PRODUCTS																		
	Apples, raw, unpeeled, without cores:																		
223	2 3/4-in diam. (about 3 per lb with cores). --- 1 apple	138	84	80	Trace	1	—	—	—	20	10	14	.4	152	120	.04	.03	.1	6
224	3 1/4-in diam. (about 2 per lb with cores). --- 1 apple	212	84	125	Trace	1	—	—	—	31	15	21	.6	233	190	.06	.04	.2	8
225	Applejuice, bottled or canned[24] --- 1 cup	248	88	120	Trace	Trace	—	—	—	30	15	22	1.5	250	—	.02	.05	.2	2[52]
	Applesauce, canned:																		
226	Sweetened --- 1 cup	255	76	230	1	Trace	—	—	—	61	10	13	1.3	166	100	.05	.03	.1	2[53]
227	Unsweetened --- 1 cup	244	89	100	Trace	Trace	—	—	—	26	10	12	1.2	190	100	.05	.02	.1	2[52]
	Apricots:																		
228	Raw, without pits (about 12 per lb with pits). --- 3 apricots	107	85	55	1	Trace	—	—	—	14	18	25	.5	301	2,890	.03	.04	.6	11
229	Canned in heavy sirup (halves and sirup). --- 1 cup	258	77	220	2	Trace	—	—	—	57	28	39	.8	604	4,490	.05	.05	1.0	10
	Dried:																		
230	Uncooked (28 large or 37 medium halves per cup). --- 1 cup	130	25	340	7	1	—	—	—	86	87	140	7.2	1,273	14,170	.01	.21	4.3	16
231	Cooked, unsweetened, fruit and liquid. --- 1 cup	250	76	215	4	1	—	—	—	54	55	88	4.5	795	7,500	.01	.13	2.5	8
232	Apricot nectar, canned --- 1 cup	251	85	145	1	Trace	—	—	—	37	23	30	.5	379	2,380	.03	.03	.5	2[6]36
	Avocados, raw, whole, without skins and seeds:																		
233	California, mid- and late-winter (with skin and seed, 3 1/8-in diam.; wt., 10 oz). --- 1 avocado	216	74	370	5	37	5.5	22.0	3.7	13	22	91	1.3	1,303	630	.24	.43	3.5	30
234	Florida, late summer and fall (with skin and seed, 3 5/8-in diam.; wt., 1 lb). --- 1 avocado	304	78	390	4	33	6.7	15.7	5.3	27	30	128	1.8	1,836	880	.33	.61	4.9	43
235	Banana without peel (about 2.6 per lb with peel). --- 1 banana	119	76	100	1	Trace	—	—	—	26	10	31	.8	440	230	.06	.07	.8	12
236	Banana flakes --- 1 tbsp	6	3	20	Trace	Trace	—	—	—	5	2	6	.2	92	50	.01	.01	.2	Trace

(A)	(B)		(C)	(D)	(E)	(F)	(G)	(H)	(I)	(J)	(K)	(L)	(M)	(N)	(O)	(P)	(Q)	(R)	(S)
237	Blackberries, raw	1 cup	144	85	85	2	1	—	—	—	19	46	27	1.3	245	290	0.04	0.06	0.6	30
238	Blueberries, raw	1 cup	145	83	90	1	1	—	—	—	22	22	19	1.5	117	150	.04	.09	.7	20
	Cantaloup. See Muskmelons (item 271).																			
	Cherries:																			
239	Sour (tart), red, pitted, canned, water pack.	1 cup	244	88	105	2	Trace	—	—	—	26	37	32	.7	317	1,660	.07	.05	.5	12
240	Sweet, raw, without pits and stems.	10 cherries	68	80	45	1	Trace	—	—	—	12	15	13	.3	129	70	.03	.04	.3	7
241	Cranberry juice cocktail, bottled, sweetened.	1 cup	253	83	165	Trace	Trace	—	—	—	42	13	8	.8	25	Trace	.03	.03	.1	[27]81
242	Cranberry sauce, sweetened, canned, strained.	1 cup	277	62	405	Trace	1	—	—	—	104	17	11	.6	83	60	.03	.03	.1	6
	Dates:																			
243	Whole, without pits	10 dates	80	23	220	2	Trace	—	—	—	58	47	50	2.4	518	40	.07	.08	1.8	0
244	Chopped	1 cup	178	23	490	4	1	—	—	—	130	105	112	5.3	1,153	90	.16	.18	3.9	0
245	Fruit cocktail, canned, in heavy sirup.	1 cup	255	80	195	1	Trace	—	—	—	50	23	31	1.0	411	360	.05	.03	1.0	5
	Grapefruit: Raw, medium, 3 3/4-in diam. (about 1 lb 1 oz):																			
246	Pink or red	1/2 grapefruit with peel[28]	241	89	50	1	Trace	—	—	—	13	20	20	.5	166	540	.05	.02	.2	44
247	White	1/2 grapefruit with peel[28]	241	89	45	1	Trace	—	—	—	12	19	19	.5	159	10	.05	.02	.2	44
248	Canned, sections with sirup	1 cup	254	81	180	2	Trace	—	—	—	45	33	36	.8	343	30	.08	.05	.5	76
	Grapefruit juice:																			
249	Raw, pink, red, or white	1 cup	246	90	95	1	Trace	—	—	—	23	22	37	.5	399	(30)	.10	.05	.5	93
	Canned, white:																			
250	Unsweetened	1 cup	247	89	100	1	Trace	—	—	—	24	20	35	1.0	400	20	.07	.05	.5	84
251	Sweetened	1 cup	250	86	135	1	Trace	—	—	—	32	20	35	1.0	405	30	.08	.05	.5	78
	Frozen concentrate, unsweetened:																			
252	Undiluted, 6-fl oz can	1 can	207	62	300	4	1	—	—	—	72	70	124	.8	1,250	60	.29	.12	1.4	286
253	Diluted with 3 parts water by volume.	1 cup	247	89	100	1	Trace	—	—	—	24	25	42	.2	420	20	.10	.04	.5	96
254	Dehydrated crystals, prepared with water (1 lb yields about 1 gal).	1 cup	247	90	100	1	Trace	—	—	—	24	22	40	.2	412	20	.10	.05	.5	91
	Grapes, European type (adherent skin), raw:																			
255	Thompson Seedless	10 grapes	50	81	35	Trace	Trace	—	—	—	9	6	10	.2	87	50	.03	.02	.2	2
256	Tokay and Emperor, seeded types	10 grapes[29]	60	81	40	Trace	Trace	—	—	—	10	7	11	.2	99	60	.03	.02	.2	2
	Grapejuice:																			
257	Canned or bottled	1 cup	253	83	165	1	Trace	—	—	—	42	28	30	.8	293	—	.10	.05	.5	[25]Trace
	Frozen concentrate, sweetened:																			
258	Undiluted, 6-fl oz can	1 can	216	53	395	1	Trace	—	—	—	100	22	32	.9	255	40	.13	.22	1.5	[31]32
259	Diluted with 3 parts water by volume.	1 cup	250	86	135	1	Trace	—	—	—	33	8	10	.3	85	10	.05	.08	.5	[31]10
260	Grape drink, canned	1 cup	250	86	135	Trace	Trace	—	—	—	35	8	10	.3	88	—	[32].03	[32].03	.3	(32)
261	Lemon, raw, size 165, without peel and seeds (about 4 per lb with peels and seeds).	1 lemon	74	90	20	1	Trace	—	—	—	6	19	12	.4	102	10	.03	.01	.1	39
	Lemon juice:																			
262	Raw	1 cup	244	91	60	1	Trace	—	—	—	20	17	24	.5	344	50	.07	.02	.2	112
263	Canned, or bottled, unsweetened	1 cup	244	92	55	1	Trace	—	—	—	19	17	24	.5	344	50	.07	.02	.2	102
264	Frozen, single strength, unsweetened, 6-fl oz can.	1 can	183	92	40	1	Trace	—	—	—	13	13	16	.5	258	40	.05	.02	.2	81
	Lemonade concentrate, frozen:																			
265	Undiluted, 6-fl oz can	1 can	219	49	425	Trace	Trace	—	—	—	112	9	13	.4	153	40	.05	.06	.7	66
266	Diluted with 4 1/3 parts water by volume.	1 cup	248	89	105	Trace	Trace	—	—	—	28	2	3	.1	40	10	.01	.02	.2	17

[19] Crust made with vegetable shortening and enriched flour.
[24] Also applies to pasteurized apple cider.
[25] Applies to product without added ascorbic acid. For value of product with added ascorbic acid, refer to label.
[26] Based on product with label claim of 45% of U.S. RDA in 6 fl oz.
[27] Based on product with label claim of 100% of U.S. RDA in 6 fl oz.
[28] Weight includes peel and membranes between sections. Without these parts, the weight of the edible portion is 123 g for item 246 and 118 g for item 247.
[29] Weight includes seeds. Without seeds, weight of the edible portion is 57 g.
[30] For white-fleshed varieties, value is about 20 International Units (I.U.) per cup; for red-fleshed varieties, 1,080 I.U.
[31] Applies to product without added ascorbic acid. With added ascorbic acid, based on claim that 6 fl oz of reconstituted juice contain 45% or 50% of the U.S. RDA, value in milligrams is 108 or 120 for a 6-fl oz can (item 258), 36 or 40 for 1 cup of diluted juice (item 259).
[32] For products with added thiamin and riboflavin but without added ascorbic acid, values in milligrams would be 0.60 for thiamin, 0.80 for riboflavin, and trace for ascorbic acid. For products with only ascorbic acid added, value varies with the brand. Consult the label.

(Dashes (—) denote lack of reliable data for a constituent believed to be present in measurable amount)

						Fatty Acids												
							Unsaturated											
Item No.	Foods, approximate measures, units, and weight (edible part unless footnotes indicate otherwise)		Water	Food energy	Pro-tein	Fat	Satu-rated (total)	Oleic	Lino-leic	Carbo-hydrate	Calcium	Phos-phorus	Iron	Potas-sium	Vitamin A value	Thiamin	Ribo-flavin	Niacin	Ascorbic acid
(A)	(B)		(C)	(D)	(E)	(F)	(G)	(H)	(I)	(J)	(K)	(L)	(M)	(N)	(O)	(P)	(Q)	(R)	(S)
		Grams	Per-cent	Cal-ories	Grams	Grams	Grams	Grams	Grams	Grams	Milli-grams	Milli-grams	Milli-grams	Milli-grams	Inter-national units	Milli-grams	Milli-grams	Milli-grams	Milli-grams

FRUITS AND FRUIT PRODUCTS—Con.

Item No.	Foods	Grams	Water	Food energy	Pro-tein	Fat	Sat.	Oleic	Lino.	Carbo.	Calcium	Phos.	Iron	Potas-sium	Vit. A	Thiamin	Ribo-flavin	Niacin	Ascorbic acid
	Limeade concentrate, frozen:																		
267	Undiluted, 6-fl oz can — 1 can	218	50	410	Trace	Trace	—	—	—	108	11	13	0.2	129	Trace	0.02	0.02	0.2	26
268	Diluted with 4 1/3 parts water by volume — 1 cup	247	89	100	Trace	Trace	—	—	—	27	3	3	Trace	32	Trace	Trace	Trace	Trace	6
	Lime juice:																		
269	Raw — 1 cup	246	90	65	1	Trace	—	—	—	22	22	27	.5	256	20	.05	.02	.2	79
270	Canned, unsweetened — 1 cup	246	90	65	1	Trace	—	—	—	22	22	27	.5	256	20	.05	.02	.2	52
	Muskmelons, raw, with rind, without seed cavity:																		
271	Cantaloup, orange-fleshed (with rind and seed cavity, 5-in diam., 2 1/3 lb) — 1/2 melon with rind[33]	477	91	80	2	Trace	—	—	—	20	38	44	1.1	682	9,240	.11	.08	1.6	90
272	Honeydew (with rind and seed cavity, 6 1/2-in diam., 5 1/4 lb) — 1/10 melon with rind[33]	226	91	50	1	Trace	—	—	—	11	21	24	.6	374	60	.06	.04	.9	34
	Oranges, all commercial varieties, raw:																		
273	Whole, 2 5/8-in diam., without peel and seeds (about 2 1/2 per lb with peel and seeds) — 1 orange	131	86	65	1	Trace	—	—	—	16	54	26	.5	263	260	.13	.05	.5	66
274	Sections without membranes — 1 cup	180	86	90	2	Trace	—	—	—	22	74	36	.7	360	360	.18	.07	.7	90
	Orange juice:																		
275	Raw, all varieties — 1 cup	248	88	110	2	Trace	—	—	—	26	27	42	.5	496	500	.22	.07	1.0	124
276	Canned, unsweetened — 1 cup	249	87	120	2	Trace	—	—	—	28	25	45	1.0	496	500	.17	.05	.7	100
	Frozen concentrate:																		
277	Undiluted, 6-fl oz can — 1 can	213	55	360	5	Trace	—	—	—	87	75	126	.9	1,500	1,620	.68	.11	2.8	360
278	Diluted with 3 parts water by volume — 1 cup	249	87	120	2	Trace	—	—	—	29	25	42	.2	503	540	.23	.03	.9	120
279	Dehydrated crystals, prepared with water (1 lb yields about 1 gal) — 1 cup	248	88	115	1	Trace	—	—	—	27	25	40	.5	518	500	.20	.07	1.0	109
	Orange and grapefruit juice: Frozen concentrate:																		
280	Undiluted, 6-fl oz can — 1 can	210	59	330	4	1	—	—	—	78	61	99	.8	1,308	800	.48	.06	2.3	302
281	Diluted with 3 parts water by volume — 1 cup	248	88	110	1	Trace	—	—	—	26	20	32	.2	439	270	.15	.02	.7	102
282	Papayas, raw, 1/2-in cubes — 1 cup	140	89	55	1	Trace	—	—	—	14	28	22	.4	328	2,450	.06	.06	.4	78
	Peaches: Raw:																		
283	Whole, 2 1/2-in diam., peeled, pitted (about 4 per lb with peels and pits) — 1 peach	100	89	40	1	Trace	—	—	—	10	9	19	.5	202	[34]1,330	.02	.05	1.0	7
284	Sliced — 1 cup	170	89	65	1	Trace	—	—	—	16	15	32	.9	343	[34]2,260	.03	.09	1.7	12
	Canned, yellow-fleshed, solids and liquid (halves or slices):																		
285	Sirup pack — 1 cup	256	79	200	1	Trace	—	—	—	51	10	31	.8	333	1,100	.03	.05	1.5	8
286	Water pack — 1 cup	244	91	75	1	Trace	—	—	—	20	10	32	.7	334	1,100	.02	.07	1.5	7
	Dried:																		
287	Uncooked — 1 cup	160	25	420	5	1	—	—	—	109	77	187	9.6	1,520	6,240	.02	.30	8.5	29
288	Cooked, unsweetened, halves and juice — 1 cup	250	77	205	3	1	—	—	—	54	38	93	4.8	743	3,050	.01	.15	3.8	5

(A)	(B)		(C)	(D)	(E)	(F)	(G)	(H)	(I)	(J)	(K)	(L)	(M)	(N)	(O)	(P)	(Q)	(R)	(S)
	Frozen, sliced, sweetened:																		
289	10-oz container	1 container	284	250	1	Trace	—	—	—	64	11	37	1.4	352	1,850	0.03	0.11	2.0	35116
290	Cup	1 cup	250	220	1	Trace	—	—	—	57	10	33	1.3	310	1,630	.03	.10	1.8	35103
	Pears:																		
	Raw, with skin, cored:																		
291	Bartlett, 2 1/2-in diam. (about 2 1/2 per lb with cores and stems).	1 pear	164	100	1	1	—	—	—	25	13	18	.5	213	30	.03	.07	.2	7
292	Bosc, 2 1/2-in diam. (about 3 per lb with cores and stems).	1 pear	141	85	1	1	—	—	—	22	11	16	.4	83	30	.03	.06	.1	6
293	D'Anjou, 3-in diam. (about 2 per lb with cores and stems).	1 pear	200	120	1	1	—	—	—	31	16	22	.6	260	40	.04	.08	.2	8
294	Canned, solids and liquid, sirup pack, heavy (halves or slices).	1 cup	255	195	1	1	—	—	—	50	13	18	.5	214	10	.03	.05	.3	3
	Pineapple:																		
295	Raw, diced.	1 cup	155	80	1	Trace	—	—	—	21	26	12	.8	226	110	.14	.05	.3	26
	Canned, heavy sirup pack, solids and liquid:																		
296	Crushed, chunks, tidbits	1 cup	255	190	1	Trace	—	—	—	49	28	13	.8	245	130	.20	.05	.5	18
	Slices and liquid:																		
297	Large	1 slice; 2 1/4 tbsp liquid.	105	80	Trace	Trace	—	—	—	20	12	5	.3	101	50	.08	.02	.2	7
298	Medium	1 slice; 1 1/4 tbsp liquid.	58	45	Trace	Trace	—	—	—	11	6	3	.2	56	30	.05	.01	.1	4
299	Pineapple juice, unsweetened, canned.	1 cup	250	140	1	Trace	—	—	—	34	38	23	.8	373	130	.13	.05	.5	2780
	Plums:																		
	Raw, without pits:																		
300	Japanese and hybrid (2 1/8-in diam., about 6 1/2 per lb with pits).	1 plum	66	30	Trace	Trace	—	—	—	8	8	12	.3	112	160	.02	.02	.3	4
301	Prune-type (1 1/2-in diam., about 15 per lb with pits).	1 plum	28	20	Trace	Trace	—	—	—	6	3	5	.1	48	80	.01	.01	.1	1
	Canned, heavy sirup pack (Italian prunes), with pits and liquid:																		
302	Cup	1 cup[36]	272	215	1	Trace	—	—	—	56	23	26	2.3	367	3,130	.05	.05	1.0	5
303	Portion	3 plums; 2 3/4 tbsp liquid.[36]	140	110	1	Trace	—	—	—	23	12	13	1.2	189	1,610	.03	.03	.5	3
	Prunes, dried, "softenized," with pits:																		
304	Uncooked	4 extra large or 5 large prunes.[36]	49	110	1	Trace	—	—	—	29	22	34	1.7	298	690	.04	.07	.7	1
305	Cooked, unsweetened, all sizes, fruit and liquid.	1 cup[36]	250	255	2	1	—	—	—	57	51	79	3.8	695	1,590	.07	.15	1.5	2
306	Prune juice, canned or bottled	1 cup	256	195	1	Trace	—	—	—	49	36	51	1.8	602	—	.03	.03	1.0	5
	Raisins, seedless:																		
307	Cup, not pressed down	1 cup	145	420	4	Trace	—	—	—	112	90	146	5.1	1,106	30	.16	.12	.7	1
308	Packet, 1/2 oz (1 1/2 tbsp)	1 packet	14	40	Trace	Trace	—	—	—	11	9	14	.5	107	Trace	.02	.01	.1	Trace
	Raspberries, red:																		
309	Raw, capped, whole	1 cup	123	70	1	1	—	—	—	17	27	27	1.1	207	160	.04	.11	1.1	31
310	Frozen, sweetened, 10-oz container	1 container	284	280	2	1	—	—	—	70	37	48	1.7	284	200	.06	.17	1.7	60
	Rhubarb, cooked, added sugar:																		
311	From raw	1 cup	270	380	1	Trace	—	—	—	97	211	41	1.6	548	220	.05	.14	.8	16
312	From frozen, sweetened	1 cup	270	385	1	Trace	—	—	—	98	211	32	1.9	475	190	.05	.11	.5	16

27 Based on product with label claim of 100% of U.S. RDA in 6 fl oz.

33 Weight includes rind. Without rind, the weight of the edible portion is 272 g for item 271 and 149 g for item 272.

34 Represents yellow-fleshed varieties. For white-fleshed varieties, value is 50 International Units (I.U.) for 1 peach, 90 I.U. for 1 cup of slices.

35 Value represents products with added ascorbic acid. For products without added ascorbic acid, value in milligrams is 116 for a 10-oz container, 103 for 1 cup.

36 Weight includes pits. After removal of the pits, the weight of the edible portion is 258 g for item 302, 133 g for item 304, and 213 g for item 305.

431

(Dashes (—) denote lack of reliable data for a constituent believed to be present in measurable amount)

Item No.	Foods, approximate measures, units, and weight (edible part unless footnotes indicate otherwise)		(Grams)	Water (Per cent)	Food energy (Cal-ories)	Pro-tein (Grams)	Fat (Grams)	Fatty Acids: Satu-rated (total) (Grams)	Unsaturated: Oleic (Grams)	Lino-leic (Grams)	Carbo-hydrate (Grams)	Calcium (Milli-grams)	Phos-phorus (Milli-grams)	Iron (Milli-grams)	Potas-sium (Milli-grams)	Vitamin A value (International units)	Thiamin (Milli-grams)	Ribo-flavin (Milli-grams)	Niacin (Milli-grams)	Ascorbic acid (Milli-grams)
(A)	(B)			(C)	(D)	(E)	(F)	(G)	(H)	(I)	(J)	(K)	(L)	(M)	(N)	(O)	(P)	(Q)	(R)	(S)
	FRUITS AND FRUIT PRODUCTS—Con.																			
	Strawberries:																			
313	Raw, whole berries, capped	1 cup	149	90	55	1	1	—	—	—	13	31	31	1.5	244	90	0.04	0.10	0.9	88
	Frozen, sweetened:																			
314	Sliced, 10-oz container	1 container	284	71	310	1	1	—	—	—	79	40	48	2.0	318	90	.06	.17	1.4	151
315	Whole, 1-lb container (about 1 3/4 cups)	1 container	454	76	415	2	1	—	—	—	107	59	73	2.7	472	140	.09	.27	2.3	249
316	Tangerine, raw, 2 3/8-in diam., size 176, without peel (about 4 per lb with peels and seeds)	1 tangerine	86	87	40	1	Trace	—	—	—	10	34	15	.3	108	360	.05	.02	.1	27
317	Tangerine juice, canned, sweetened	1 cup	249	87	125	1	Trace	—	—	—	30	44	35	.5	440	1,040	.15	.05	.2	54
318	Watermelon, raw, 4 by 8 in wedge with rind and seeds (1/16 of 32 2/3-lb melon, 10 by 16 in).	1 wedge with rind and seeds[37]	926	93	110	2	1	—	—	—	27	30	43	2.1	426	2,510	.13	.13	.9	30
	GRAIN PRODUCTS																			
	Bagel, 3-in diam.:																			
319	Egg	1 bagel	55	32	165	6	2	0.5	0.9	0.8	28	9	43	1.2	41	30	.14	.10	1.2	0
320	Water	1 bagel	55	29	165	6	2	.2	.4	.6	30	8	41	1.2	42	0	.15	.11	1.4	0
321	Barley, pearled, light, uncooked	1 cup	200	11	700	16	2	.3	.2	.8	158	32	378	4.0	320	0	.24	.10	6.2	0
	Biscuits, baking powder, 2-in diam. (enriched flour, vegetable shortening):																			
322	From home recipe	1 biscuit	28	27	105	2	5	1.2	2.0	1.2	13	34	49	.4	33	Trace	.08	.08	.7	Trace
323	From mix	1 biscuit	28	29	90	2	3	.6	1.1	.7	15	19	65	.6	32	Trace	.09	.08	.8	Trace
324	Breadcrumbs (enriched):[38] Dry, grated	1 cup	100	7	390	13	5	1.0	1.6	1.4	73	122	141	3.6	152	Trace	.35	.35	4.8	Trace
	Breads: Soft. See White bread (items 349–350).																			
325	Boston brown bread, canned, slice, 3 1/4 by 1/2 in.[38]	1 slice	45	45	95	2	1	.1	.2	.2	21	41	72	.9	131	[39]0	.06	.04	.7	0
	Cracked-wheat bread (3/4 enriched wheat flour, 1/4 cracked wheat):[38]																			
326	Loaf, 1 lb	1 loaf	454	35	1,195	39	10	2.2	3.0	3.9	236	399	581	9.5	608	Trace	1.52	1.13	14.4	Trace
327	Slice (18 per loaf)	1 slice	25	35	65	2	1	.1	.2	.2	13	22	32	.5	34	Trace	.08	.06	.8	Trace
	French or vienna bread, enriched:[38]																			
328	Loaf, 1 lb	1 loaf	454	31	1,315	41	14	3.2	4.7	4.6	251	195	386	10.0	408	Trace	1.80	1.10	15.0	Trace
	Slice:																			
329	French (5 by 2 1/2 by 1 in)	1 slice	35	31	100	3	1	.2	.4	.4	19	15	30	.8	32	Trace	.14	.08	1.2	Trace
330	Vienna (4 3/4 by 4 by 1/2 in)	1 slice	25	31	75	2	1	.2	.3	.3	14	11	21	.6	23	Trace	.10	.06	.8	Trace
	Italian bread, enriched:																			
331	Loaf, 1 lb	1 loaf	454	32	1,250	41	4	.6	.3	1.5	256	77	349	10.0	336	0	1.80	1.10	15.0	0
332	Slice, 4 1/2 by 3 1/4 by 3/4 in.	1 slice	30	32	85	3	Trace	Trace	Trace	.1	17	5	23	.7	22	0	.12	.07	1.0	0
	Raisin bread, enriched:[38]																			
333	Loaf, 1 lb	1 loaf	454	35	1,190	30	13	3.0	4.7	3.9	243	322	395	10.0	1,057	Trace	1.70	1.07	10.7	Trace
334	Slice (18 per loaf)	1 slice	25	35	65	2	1	.2	.3	.2	13	18	22	.6	58	Trace	.09	.06	.6	Trace

NUTRIENTS IN INDICATED QUANTITY

Rye Bread:

(A)	(B)	g	(C)	(D)	(E)	(F)	(G)	(H)	(I)	(J)	(K)	(L)	(M)	(N)	(O)	(P)	(Q)	(R)	(S)
	Rye Bread:																		
	American, light (2/3 enriched wheat flour, 1/3 rye flour):																		
335	Loaf, 1 lb — 1 loaf	454	36	1,100	41	5	0.7	0.5	2.2	236	340	667	9.1	658	0	1.35	0.98	12.9	0
336	Slice (4 3/4 by 3 3/4 by 7/16 in) — 1 slice	25	36	60	2	Trace	Trace	Trace	.1	13	19	37	.5	36	0	.07	.05	.7	0
	Pumpernickel (2/3 rye flour, 1/3 enriched wheat flour):																		
337	Loaf, 1 lb — 1 loaf	454	34	1,115	41	5	.7	.5	2.4	241	381	1,039	11.8	2,059	0	1.30	.93	8.5	0
338	Slice (5 by 4 by 3/8 in) — 1 slice	32	34	80	3	Trace	Trace	Trace	.2	17	27	73	.8	145	0	.09	.07	.6	0
	White bread, enriched:[38]																		
	Soft-crumb type:																		
339	Loaf, 1 lb — 1 loaf	454	36	1,225	39	15	3.4	5.3	4.6	229	381	440	11.3	476	Trace	1.80	1.10	15.0	Trace
340	Slice (18 per loaf) — 1 slice	25	36	70	2	1	.2	.3	.3	13	21	24	.6	26	Trace	.10	.06	.8	Trace
341	Slice, toasted — 1 slice	22	25	70	2	1	.2	.3	.3	13	21	24	.6	26	Trace	.08	.06	.8	Trace
342	Slice (22 per loaf) — 1 slice	20	36	55	2	1	.2	.2	.2	10	17	19	.5	21	Trace	.08	.05	.7	Trace
343	Slice, toasted — 1 slice	17	25	55	2	1	.2	.2	.2	10	17	19	.5	21	Trace	.06	.05	.7	Trace
344	Loaf, 1 1/2 lb — 1 loaf	680	36	1,835	59	22	5.2	7.9	6.9	343	571	660	17.0	714	Trace	2.70	1.65	22.5	Trace
345	Slice (24 per loaf) — 1 slice	28	36	75	2	1	.2	.3	.3	14	24	27	.7	29	Trace	.11	.07	.9	Trace
346	Slice, toasted — 1 slice	24	24	75	2	1	.2	.3	.3	14	24	27	.7	29	Trace	.09	.07	.9	Trace
347	Slice (28 per loaf) — 1 slice	24	36	65	2	1	.2	.2	.2	12	20	23	.6	25	Trace	.10	.06	.8	Trace
348	Slice, toasted — 1 slice	21	25	65	2	1	.2	.2	.2	12	20	23	.6	25	Trace	.08	.06	.8	Trace
349	Cubes — 1 cup	30	36	80	3	1	.3	.3	.3	15	25	29	.8	32	Trace	.12	.07	1.0	Trace
350	Crumbs — 1 cup	45	36	120	4	4	.3	.5	.5	23	38	44	1.1	47	Trace	.18	.11	1.5	Trace
	Firm-crumb type:																		
351	Loaf, 1 lb — 1 loaf	454	35	1,245	41	17	3.9	5.9	5.2	228	435	463	11.3	549	Trace	1.80	1.10	15.0	Trace
352	Slice (20 per loaf) — 1 slice	23	35	65	2	2	.2	.3	.3	12	22	23	.6	28	Trace	.09	.06	.8	Trace
353	Slice, toasted — 1 slice	20	24	65	2	2	.2	.3	.3	12	22	23	.6	28	Trace	.07	.06	.8	Trace
354	Loaf, 2 lb — 1 loaf	907	35	2,495	82	34	7.2	11.8	10.4	455	371	925	22.7	1,097	Trace	3.60	2.20	30.0	Trace
355	Slice (34 per loaf) — 1 slice	27	35	75	2	1	.2	.3	.3	14	26	28	.7	33	Trace	.11	.06	.9	Trace
356	Slice, toasted — 1 slice	23	24	75	2	1	.2	.3	.3	14	26	28	.7	33	Trace	.09	.06	.9	Trace
	Whole-wheat bread:[38]																		
	Soft-crumb type:[38]																		
357	Loaf, 1 lb — 1 loaf	454	36	1,095	41	12	2.2	2.9	4.2	224	381	1,152	13.6	1,161	Trace	1.37	.45	12.7	Trace
358	Slice (16 per loaf) — 1 slice	28	36	65	3	1	.1	.2	.2	14	24	71	.8	72	Trace	.09	.03	.8	Trace
359	Slice, toasted — 1 slice	24	24	65	3	1	.1	.2	.2	14	24	71	.8	72	Trace	.07	.03	.8	Trace
	Firm-crumb type:[38]																		
360	Loaf, 1 lb — 1 loaf	454	36	1,100	48	14	2.5	3.3	4.9	216	449	1,034	13.6	1,238	Trace	1.17	.54	12.7	Trace
361	Slice (18 per loaf) — 1 slice	25	36	60	3	1	.1	.2	.3	12	25	57	.8	68	Trace	.06	.03	.7	Trace
362	Slice, toasted — 1 slice	21	24	60	3	1	.1	.2	.3	12	25	57	.8	68	Trace	.05	.03	.7	Trace
	Breakfast cereals:																		
	Hot type, cooked:																		
	Corn (hominy) grits, degermed:																		
363	Enriched — 1 cup	245	87	125	3	Trace	Trace	.1	.1	27	2	25	.7	27	[40]Trace	.10	.07	1.0	0
364	Unenriched — 1 cup	245	87	125	3	Trace	Trace	.1	.1	27	2	25	.2	27	[40]Trace	.05	.02	.5	0
365	Farina, quick-cooking, enriched — 1 cup	245	89	105	3	Trace	Trace	.1	.1	22	147	[41]113	([42])	25	0	.12	.07	1.0	0
366	Oatmeal or rolled oats — 1 cup	240	87	130	5	2	.4	.8	.9	23	22	137	1.4	146	0	.19	.05	.2	0
367	Wheat, rolled — 1 cup	240	80	180	5	1	—	—	—	41	19	182	1.7	202	0	.17	.07	2.2	0
368	Wheat, whole-meal — 1 cup	245	88	110	4	1	—	—	—	25	25	127	1.2	118	0	.15	.05	1.5	0
	Ready-to-eat:																		
369	Bran flakes (40% bran), added sugar, salt, iron, vitamins. — 1 cup	35	3	105	4	1	—	—	—	28	19	125	5.6	137	1,540	.46	.52	6.2	0
370	Bran flakes with raisins, added sugar, salt, iron, vitamins. — 1 cup	50	7	145	4	1	—	—	—	40	28	146	7.9	154	[43]2,200	([44])	([44])	6.2	0

[37]Weight includes rind and seeds. Without rind and seeds, weight of the edible portion is 426 g.
[38]Made with vegetable shortening.
[39]Applies to product made with white cornmeal. With yellow cornmeal, value is 30 International Units (I.U.).
[40]Applies to white varieties. For yellow varieties, value is 150 International Units (I.U.).
[41]Applies to products that do not contain di-sodium phosphate. If di-sodium phosphate is an ingredient, value is 162 mg.
[42]Value may range from less than 1 mg to about 8 mg depending on the brand. Consult the label.
[43]Applies to product with added nutrient. Without added nutrient, value is trace.
[44]Value varies with the brand. Consult the label.

(Dashes (—) denote lack of reliable data for a constituent believed to be present in measurable amount)

							Fatty Acids												
(A)	(B)	(C)	(D)	(E)	(F)	Saturated (total) (G)	Unsaturated Oleic (H)	Linoleic (I)	(J)	(K)	(L)	(M)	(N)	(O)	(P)	(Q)	(R)	(S)
Item No.	Foods, approximate measures, units, and weight (edible part unless footnotes indicate otherwise)	Water	Food energy	Protein	Fat				Carbo-hydrate	Calcium	Phos-phorus	Iron	Potas-sium	Vitamin A value	Thiamin	Ribo-flavin	Niacin	Ascorbic acid
		Per-cent	Cal-ories	Grams	Grams	Grams	Grams	Grams	Grams	Milli-grams	Milli-grams	Milli-grams	Milli-grams	Inter-national units	Milli-grams	Milli-grams	Milli-grams	Milli-grams
	Grams																	

GRAIN PRODUCTS—Con.

Breakfast cereals—Continued
Ready-to-eat—Continued
Corn flakes:

(A)	(B)	Grams	(C)	(D)	(E)	(F)	(G)	(H)	(I)	(J)	(K)	(L)	(M)	(N)	(O)	(P)	(Q)	(R)	(S)
371	Plain, added sugar, salt, iron, vitamins. 1 cup	25	4	95	2	Trace	—	—	—	21	([44])	9	([44])	30	([44])	([44])	([44])	([44])	[4,5]13
372	Sugar-coated, added salt, iron, vitamins. 1 cup	40	2	155	2	Trace	—	—	—	37	1	10	([44])	27	1,760	.53	.50	7.1	[4]21
373	Corn, oat flour, puffed, added sugar, salt, iron, vitamins. 1 cup	20	4	80	2	1	—	—	—	16	4	18	5.7	—	880	.26	.30	3.5	11
374	Corn, shredded, added sugar, salt, iron, thiamin, niacin. 1 cup	25	3	95	2	Trace	—	—	—	22	1	10	.6	—	0	.33	.05	4.4	13
375	Oats, puffed, added sugar, salt, minerals, vitamins. 1 cup	25	3	100	3	1	—	—	—	19	44	102	4.0	—	1,100	.33	.38	4.4	13
	Rice, puffed:																		
376	Plain, added iron, thiamin, niacin. 1 cup	15	4	60	1	Trace	—	—	—	13	3	14	.3	15	0	.07	.01	.7	0
377	Presweetened, added salt, iron, vitamins. 1 cup	28	3	115	1	0	—	—	—	26	3	14	([44])	43	[4,5]1,240	([44])	([44])	([44])	[4,5]15
378	Wheat flakes, added sugar, salt, iron, vitamins. 1 cup	30	4	105	3	Trace	—	—	—	24	12	83	4.8	81	1,320	.40	.45	5.3	16
	Wheat, puffed:																		
379	Plain, added iron, thiamin, niacin. 1 cup	15	3	55	2	Trace	—	—	—	12	4	48	.6	51	0	.08	.03	1.2	0
380	Presweetened, added salt, iron, vitamins. 1 cup	38	3	140	3	Trace	—	—	—	33	7	52	([44])	63	1,680	.50	.57	6.7	[4,5]20
381	Wheat, shredded, plain. 1 oblong biscuit or 1/2 cup spoon-size biscuits.	25	7	90	2	1	—	—	—	20	11	97	.9	87	0	.06	.03	1.1	0
382	Wheat germ, without salt and sugar, toasted. 1 tbsp	6	4	25	2	1	—	—	—	3	3	70	.5	57	10	.11	.05	.3	1
383	Buckwheat flour, light, sifted. 1 cup	98	12	340	6	1	—	—	—	78	11	86	1.0	314	0	.08	.04	.4	0
384	Bulgur, canned, seasoned. 1 cup	135	56	245	8	4		0.4	0.4	44	27	263	1.9	151	0	.08	.05	4.1	0
	Cake icings. See Sugars and Sweets (items 532-536). Cakes made from cake mixes with enriched flour:[46]																		
	Angelfood:																		
385	Whole cake (9 3/4-in diam. tube cake). 1 cake	635	34	1,645	36	1	—	—	—	377	603	756	2.5	381	0	.37	.95	3.6	0
386	Piece, 1/12 of cake. 1 piece	53	34	135	3	Trace	—	—	—	32	50	63	.2	32	0	.03	.08	.3	0
	Coffeecake:																		
387	Whole cake (7 3/4 by 5 5/8 by 1 1/4 in). 1 cake	430	30	1,385	27	41	11.7	16.3	8.8	225	262	748	6.9	469	690	.82	.91	7.7	1
388	Piece, 1/6 of cake. 1 piece	72	30	230	5	7	2.0	2.7	1.5	38	44	125	1.2	78	120	.14	.15	1.3	Trace
	Cupcakes, made with egg, milk, 2 1/2-in diam.:																		
389	Without icing. 1 cupcake	25	26	90	1	3	.8	1.2	.7	14	40	59	.3	21	40	.05	.05	.4	Trace
390	With chocolate icing. 1 cupcake	36	22	130	2	5	2.0	1.6	.6	21	47	71	.4	42	60	.05	.06	.4	Trace
	Devil's food with chocolate icing:																		
391	Whole, 2 layer cake (8- or 9-in diam.). 1 cake	1,107	24	3,755	49	136	50.0	44.9	17.0	645	653	1,162	16.6	1,439	1,660	1.06	1.65	10.1	1
392	Piece, 1/16 of cake. 1 piece	69	24	235	3	8	3.1	2.8	1.1	40	41	72	1.0	90	100	.07	.10	.6	Trace
393	Cupcake, 2 1/2-in diam. 1 cupcake	35	24	120	2	4	1.6	1.4	.5	20	21	37	.5	46	50	.03	.05	.3	Trace

(A)	(B)			(C)	(D)	(E)	(F)	(G)	(H)	(I)	(J)	(K)	(L)	(M)	(N)	(O)	(P)	(Q)	(R)	(S)
	Gingerbread:																			
394	Whole cake (8-in square)-------	1 cake-------------------	570	37	1,575	18	39	9.7	16.6	10.0	291	513	570	8.6	1,562	Trace	0.84	1.00	7.4	Trace
395	Piece, 1/9 of cake-------------	1 piece------------------	63	37	175	2	4	1.1	1.8	1.1	32	57	63	.9	173	Trace	.09	.11	.8	Trace
	White, 2 layer with chocolate icing:																			
396	Whole cake (8- or 9-in diam.)--	1 cake-------------------	1,140	21	4,000	44	122	48.2	46.4	20.0	716	1,129	2,041	11.4	1,322	680	1.50	1.77	12.5	2
397	Piece, 1/16 of cake------------	1 piece------------------	71	21	250	3	8	3.0	2.9	1.2	45	70	127	.7	82	40	.09	.11	.8	Trace
	Yellow, 2 layer with chocolate icing:																			
398	Whole cake (8- or 9-in diam.)--	1 cake-------------------	1,108	26	3,735	45	125	47.8	47.8	20.3	638	1,008	2,017	12.2	1,208	1,550	1.24	1.67	10.6	2
399	Piece, 1/16 of cake------------	1 piece------------------	69	26	235	3	8	3.0	3.0	1.3	40	63	126	.8	75	100	.08	.10	.7	Trace
	Cakes made from home recipes using enriched flour:[47]																			
	Boston cream pie with custard filling:																			
400	Whole cake (8-in diam.)--------	1 cake-------------------	825	35	2,490	41	78	23.0	30.1	15.2	412	553	833	8.2	[48]734	1,730	1.04	1.27	9.6	2
401	Piece, 1/12 of cake------------	1 piece------------------	69	35	210	3	6	1.9	2.5	1.3	34	46	70	.7	[48]61	140	.09	.11	.8	Trace
	Fruitcake, dark:																			
402	Loaf, 1-lb (7 1/2 by 2 by 1 1/2 in).	1 loaf-------------------	454	18	1,720	22	69	14.4	33.5	14.8	271	327	513	11.8	2,250	540	.72	.73	4.9	2
403	Slice, 1/30 of loaf------------	1 slice------------------	15	18	55	1	2	.5	1.1	.5	9	11	17	.4	74	20	.02	.02	.2	Trace
	Plain, sheet cake:																			
	Without icing:																			
404	Whole cake (9-in square)-----	1 cake-------------------	777	25	2,830	35	108	29.5	44.4	23.9	434	497	793	8.5	[48]614	1,320	1.21	1.40	10.2	2
405	Piece, 1/9 of cake-----------	1 piece------------------	86	25	315	4	12	3.3	4.9	2.6	48	55	88	.9	[48]68	150	.13	.15	1.1	Trace
	With uncooked white icing:																			
406	Whole cake (9-in square)-----	1 cake-------------------	1,096	21	4,020	37	129	42.2	49.5	24.4	694	543	822	8.2	[48]669	2,190	1.22	1.47	10.2	2
407	Piece, 1/9 of cake-----------	1 piece------------------	121	21	445	4	14	4.7	5.5	2.7	77	61	91	.8	[48]74	240	.14	.16	1.1	Trace
	Pound:[49]																			
408	Loaf, 8 1/2 by 3 1/2 by 3 1/4 in.	1 loaf-------------------	565	16	2,725	31	170	42.9	73.1	39.6	273	107	418	7.9	345	1,410	.90	.99	7.3	0
409	Slice, 1/17 of loaf------------	1 slice------------------	33	16	160	2	10	2.5	4.3	2.3	16	6	24	.5	20	80	.05	.06	.4	0
	Spongecake:																			
410	Whole cake (9 3/4-in diam. tube cake).	1 cake-------------------	790	32	2,345	60	45	13.1	15.8	5.7	427	237	885	13.4	687	3,560	1.10	1.64	7.4	Trace
411	Piece, 1/12 of cake------------	1 piece------------------	66	32	195	5	4	1.1	1.3	.5	36	20	74	1.1	57	300	.09	.14	.6	Trace
	Cookies made with enriched flour:[50] [51]																			
	Brownies with nuts:																			
	Home-prepared, 1 3/4 by 1 3/4 by 7/8 in:																			
412	From home recipe-------------	1 brownie----------------	20	10	95	1	6	1.5	3.0	1.2	10	8	30	.4	38	40	.04	.03	.2	Trace
413	From commercial recipe-------	1 brownie----------------	20	11	85	1	4	.9	1.4	1.3	13	9	27	.4	34	20	.03	.02	.2	Trace
414	Frozen, with chocolate icing,[52] 1 1/2 by 1 3/4 by 7/8 in.	1 brownie----------------	25	13	105	1	5	2.0	2.2	.7	15	10	31	.4	44	50	.03	.03	.2	Trace
	Chocolate chip:																			
415	Commercial, 2 1/4-in diam., 3/8 in thick.	4 cookies----------------	42	3	200	2	9	2.8	2.9	2.2	29	16	48	1.0	56	50	.10	.17	.9	Trace
416	From home recipe, 2 1/3-in diam.	4 cookies----------------	40	3	205	2	12	3.5	4.5	2.9	24	14	40	.8	47	40	.06	.06	.5	Trace
417	Fig bars, square (1 5/8 by 1 5/8 by 3/8 in) or rectangular (1 1/2 by 1 3/4 by 1/2 in).	4 cookies----------------	56	14	200	2	3	.8	1.2	.7	42	44	34	1.0	111	60	.04	.14	.9	Trace
418	Gingersnaps, 2-in diam., 1/4 in thick.	4 cookies----------------	28	3	90	2	2	.7	1.0	.6	22	20	13	.7	129	20	.08	.06	.7	0
419	Macaroons, 2 3/4-in diam., 1/4 in thick.	2 cookies----------------	38	4	180	2	9	—	—	—	25	10	32	.3	176	0	.02	.06	.2	0
420	Oatmeal with raisins, 2 5/8-in diam., 1/4 in thick.	4 cookies----------------	52	3	235	3	8	2.0	3.3	2.0	38	11	53	1.4	192	30	.15	.10	1.0	Trace

[44]Value varies with the brand. Consult the label.
[45]Applies to product with added nutrient. Without added nutrient, value is trace.
[46]Excepting angelfood cake, cakes were made from mixes containing vegetable shortening; icings, with butter.
[47]Excepting spongecake, vegetable shortening used for cake portion; butter, for icing. If butter or margarine used for cake portion, vitamin A values would be higher.
[48]Applies to product made with a sodium aluminum-sulfate type baking powder. With a low-sodium type baking powder containing potassium, value would be about twice the amount shown.
[49]Equal weights of flour, sugar, eggs, and vegetable shortening.
[50]Products are commercial unless otherwise specified.
[51]Made with enriched flour and vegetable shortening except for macaroons which do not contain flour or shortening.
[52]Icing made with butter.

(Dashes (—) denote lack of reliable data for a constituent believed to be present in measurable amount)

Item No. (A)	Foods, approximate measures, units, and weight (edible part unless footnotes indicate otherwise) (B)	Grams	Water (C) Percent	Food energy (D) Calories	Protein (E) Grams	Fat (F) Grams	Fatty Acids Saturated (total) (G) Grams	Unsaturated Oleic (H) Grams	Linoleic (I) Grams	Carbohydrate (J) Grams	Calcium (K) Milligrams	Phosphorus (L) Milligrams	Iron (M) Milligrams	Potassium (N) Milligrams	Vitamin A value (O) International units	Thiamin (P) Milligrams	Riboflavin (Q) Milligrams	Niacin (R) Milligrams	Ascorbic acid (S) Milligrams
	GRAIN PRODUCTS—Con.																		
	Cookies made with enriched flour[50][51]—Continued																		
421	Plain, prepared from commercial chilled dough, 2 1/2-in diam., 1/4 in thick. 4 cookies	48	5	240	2	12	3.0	5.2	2.9	31	17	35	0.6	23	30	0.10	0.08	0.9	0
422	Sandwich type (chocolate or vanilla), 1 3/4-in diam., 3/8 in thick. 4 cookies	40	2	200	2	9	2.2	3.9	2.2	28	10	96	.7	15	0	.06	.10	.7	0
423	Vanilla wafers, 1 3/4-in diam., 1/4 in thick. 10 cookies	40	3	185	2	6	—	—	—	30	16	25	.6	29	50	.10	.09	.8	0
	Cornmeal:																		
424	Whole-ground, unbolted, dry form. 1 cup	122	12	435	11	5	.5	1.0	2.5	90	24	312	2.9	346	5 620	.46	.13	2.4	0
425	Bolted (nearly whole-grain), dry form. 1 cup	122	12	440	11	4	.5	.9	2.1	91	21	272	2.2	303	5 590	.37	.10	2.3	0
	Degermed, enriched:																		
426	Dry form 1 cup	138	12	500	11	2	.2	.4	.9	108	8	137	4.0	166	5 610	.61	.36	4.8	0
427	Cooked 1 cup	240	88	120	3	Trace	Trace	.1	.2	26	2	34	1.0	38	5 140	.14	.10	1.2	0
	Degermed, unenriched:																		
428	Dry form 1 cup	138	12	500	11	2	.2	.4	.9	108	8	137	1.5	166	5 610	.19	.07	1.4	0
429	Cooked 1 cup	240	88	120	3	Trace	Trace	.1	.2	26	2	34	.5	38	5 140	.05	.02	.2	0
	Crackers:[38]																		
430	Graham, plain, 2 1/2-in square 2 crackers	14	6	55	1	1	.3	.5	.3	10	6	21	.5	55	0	.02	.08	.5	0
431	Rye wafers, whole-grain, 1 7/8 by 3 1/2 in. 2 wafers	13	6	45	2	Trace	—	—	—	10	7	50	.5	78	0	.04	.03	.5	0
432	Saltines, made with enriched flour. 4 crackers or 1 packet	11	4	50	1	1	.3	.5	.4	8	2	10	.5	13	0	.05	.05	.4	0
	Danish pastry (enriched flour), plain without fruit or nuts:[54]																		
433	Packaged ring, 12 oz 1 ring	340	22	1,435	25	80	24.3	31.7	16.5	155	170	371	6.1	381	1,050	.97	1.01	8.6	Trace
434	Round piece, about 4 1/4-in diam. by 1 in. 1 pastry	65	22	275	5	15	4.7	6.1	3.2	30	33	71	1.2	73	200	.18	.19	1.7	Trace
435	Ounce 1 oz	28	22	120	2	7	2.0	2.7	1.4	13	14	31	.5	32	90	.08	.08	.7	Trace
	Doughnuts, made with enriched flour:[38]																		
436	Cake type, plain, 2 1/2-in diam., 1 in high. 1 doughnut	25	24	100	1	5	1.2	2.0	1.1	13	10	48	.4	23	20	.05	.05	.4	Trace
437	Yeast-leavened, glazed, 3 3/4-in diam., 1 1/4 in high. 1 doughnut	50	26	205	3	11	3.3	5.8	3.3	22	16	33	.6	34	25	.10	.10	.8	0
	Macaroni, enriched, cooked (cut lengths, elbows, shells):																		
	Firm stage (hot):																		
438	1 cup	130	64	190	7	1	—	—	—	39	14	85	1.4	103	0	.23	.13	1.8	0
	Tender stage:																		
439	Cold macaroni 1 cup	105	73	115	4	Trace	—	—	—	24	8	53	.9	64	0	.15	.08	1.2	0
440	Hot macaroni 1 cup	140	73	155	5	1	—	—	—	32	11	70	1.3	85	0	.20	.11	1.5	0
	Macaroni (enriched) and cheese:																		
441	Canned[55] 1 cup	240	80	230	9	10	4.2	3.1	1.4	26	199	182	1.0	139	260	.12	.24	1.0	Trace
442	From home recipe (served hot)[56] 1 cup	200	58	430	17	22	8.9	8.8	2.9	40	362	322	1.8	240	860	.20	.40	1.8	Trace
	Muffins made with enriched flour:[38]																		
	From home recipe:																		
443	Blueberry, 2 3/8-in diam., 1 1/2 in high. 1 muffin	40	39	110	3	4	1.1	1.4	.7	17	34	53	.6	46	90	.09	.10	.7	Trace
444	Bran 1 muffin	40	35	105	3	4	1.2	1.4	.8	17	57	162	1.5	172	90	.07	.10	1.7	Trace
445	Corn (enriched degermed cornmeal and flour), 2 3/8-in diam., 1 1/2 in high. 1 muffin	40	33	125	3	4	1.2	1.6	.9	19	42	68	.7	54	[57]120	.10	.10	.7	Trace

436

(A)	(B)	(C)	(D)	(E)	(F)	(G)	(H)	(I)	(J)	(K)	(L)	(M)	(N)	(O)	(P)	(Q)	(R)	(S)
446	Plain, 3-in diam., 1 1/2 in high. 1 muffin	40	38	120	3	4	1.0	1.7	1.0	17	42	60	0.6	50	40	0.09	0.12	0.9	Trace
	From mix, egg, milk:																		
447	Corn, 2 3/8-in diam., 1 1/2 in high.[58] 1 muffin	40	30	130	3	4	1.2	1.7	.9	20	96	152	.6	44	[57]100	.08	.09	.7	Trace
448	Noodles (egg noodles), enriched, cooked. 1 cup	160	71	200	7	2	—	—	—	37	16	94	1.4	70	110	.22	.13	1.9	0
449	Noodles, chow mein, canned. 1 cup	45	1	220	6	11	—	—	—	26	—	—	—	—	—	—	—	—	—
450	Pancakes, (4-in diam.),[38] Buckwheat, made from mix (with buckwheat and enriched flours), egg and milk added. 1 cake	27	58	55	2	2	.8	.9	.4	6	59	91	.4	66	60	.04	.05	.2	Trace
	Plain:																		
-51	Made from home recipe using enriched flour. 1 cake	27	50	60	2	2	.5	.8	.5	9	27	38	.4	33	30	.06	.07	.5	Trace
452	Made from mix with enriched flour, egg and milk added. 1 cake	27	51	60	2	2	.7	.7	.3	9	58	70	.3	42	70	.04	.06	.2	Trace
	Pies, piecrust made with enriched flour, vegetable shortening (9-in diam.):																		
	Apple:																		
453	Whole. 1 pie	945	48	2,420	21	105	27.0	44.5	25.2	360	73	208	6.6	756	280	1.06	.79	9.3	9
454	Sector, 1/7 of pie. 1 sector	135	48	345	3	15	3.9	6.4	3.6	51	11	30	.9	108	40	.15	.11	1.3	2
	Banana cream:																		
455	Whole. 1 pie	910	54	2,010	41	85	26.7	33.2	16.2	279	601	746	7.3	1,847	2,280	.77	1.51	7.0	9
456	Sector, 1/7 of pie. 1 sector	130	54	285	6	12	3.8	4.7	2.3	40	86	107	1.0	264	330	.11	.22	1.0	1
	Blueberry:																		
457	Whole. 1 pie	945	51	2,285	23	102	24.8	43.7	25.1	330	134	217	9.5	614	280	1.03	.80	10.0	28
458	Sector, 1/7 of pie. 1 sector	135	51	325	4	15	3.5	6.2	3.6	47	15	31	1.4	88	40	.15	.11	1.4	4
	Cherry:																		
459	Whole. 1 pie	945	47	2,465	25	107	28.2	45.0	25.3	363	132	236	6.6	992	4,160	1.09	.84	9.8	Trace
460	Sector, 1/7 of pie. 1 sector	135	47	350	4	15	4.0	6.4	3.6	52	19	34	.9	142	590	.16	.12	1.4	Trace
	Custard:																		
461	Whole. 1 pie	910	58	1,985	56	101	33.9	38.5	17.5	213	374	1,028	8.2	1,247	2,090	.79	1.92	5.6	0
462	Sector, 1/7 of pie. 1 sector	130	58	285	8	14	4.8	5.5	2.5	30	125	147	1.2	178	300	.11	.27	.8	0
	Lemon meringue:																		
463	Whole. 1 pie	840	47	2,140	31	86	26.1	33.8	16.4	317	118	412	6.7	420	1,430	.61	.84	5.2	25
464	Sector, 1/7 of pie. 1 sector	120	47	305	4	12	3.7	4.8	2.3	45	17	59	1.0	60	200	.09	.12	.7	4
	Mince:																		
465	Whole. 1 pie	945	43	2,560	24	109	28.0	45.9	25.2	389	265	359	13.3	1,682	20	.96	.86	9.8	9
466	Sector, 1/7 of pie. 1 sector	135	43	365	3	16	4.0	6.6	3.6	56	38	51	1.9	240	Trace	.14	.12	1.4	1
	Peach:																		
467	Whole. 1 pie	945	48	2,410	24	101	24.8	43.7	25.1	361	95	274	8.5	1,408	6,900	1.04	.97	14.0	28
468	Sector, 1/7 of pie. 1 sector	135	48	345	3	14	3.5	6.2	3.6	52	14	39	1.2	201	990	.15	.14	2.0	4
	Pecan:																		
469	Whole. 1 pie	825	20	3,450	42	189	27.8	101.0	44.2	423	388	850	25.6	1,015	1,320	1.80	.95	6.9	Trace
470	Sector, 1/7 of pie. 1 sector	118	20	495	6	27	4.0	14.4	6.3	61	55	122	3.7	145	190	.26	.14	1.0	Trace
	Pumpkin:																		
471	Whole. 1 pie	910	59	1,920	36	102	37.4	37.5	16.6	223	464	628	7.3	1,456	22,480	.78	1.27	7.0	Trace
472	Sector, 1/7 of pie. 1 sector	130	59	275	5	15	5.4	5.4	2.4	32	66	90	1.0	208	3,210	.11	.18	1.0	Trace
473	Piecrust (home recipe) made with enriched flour and vegetable shortening, baked. 1 pie shell, 9-in diam.	180	15	900	11	60	14.8	26.1	14.9	79	25	90	3.1	89	0	.47	.40	5.0	0
474	Piecrust mix with enriched flour and vegetable shortening, 10-oz pkg. prepared and baked. Piecrust for 2-crust pie, 9-in diam.	320	19	1,485	20	93	22.7	39.7	23.4	141	131	272	6.1	179	0	1.07	.79	9.9	0

[38] Made with vegetable shortening.
[50] Products are commercial unless otherwise specified.
[51] Made with enriched flour and vegetable shortening except for macaroons which do not contain flour or shortening.
[52] Applies to yellow varieties; white varieties contain only a trace.
[53] Made with corn oil.
[54] Contains vegetable shortening and butter.
[55] Made with regular margarine.
[56] Made with yellow cornmeal.
[57] Applies to product made with yellow cornmeal.
[58] Made with enriched degermed cornmeal and enriched flour.

NUTRIENTS IN INDICATED QUANTITY

Item No. (A)	Foods, approximate measures, units, and weight (edible part unless footnotes indicate otherwise) (B)	Grams	Water (C) Per-cent	Food energy (D) Cal-ories	Pro-tein (E) Grams	Fat (F) Grams	Fatty Acids Satu-rated (total) (G) Grams	Unsaturated Oleic (H) Grams	Lino-leic (I) Grams	Carbo-hydrate (J) Grams	Calcium (K) Milli-grams	Phos-phorus (L) Milli-grams	Iron (M) Milli-grams	Potas-sium (N) Milli-grams	Vitamin A value (O) Inter-national units	Thiamin (P) Milli-grams	Ribo-flavin (Q) Milli-grams	Niacin (R) Milli-grams	Ascorbic acid (S) Milli-grams
	GRAIN PRODUCTS—Con.																		
475	Pizza (cheese) baked, 4 3/4-in sector; 1/8 of 12-in diam. pie.[13] — 1 sector	60	45	145	6	4	1.7	1.5	0.6	22	86	89	1.1	67	230	0.16	0.18	1.6	4
	Popcorn, popped:																		
476	Plain, large kernel — 1 cup	6	4	25	1	Trace	Trace	.1	.2	5	1	17	.2	—	—	—	.01	.1	0
477	With oil (coconut) and salt added, large kernel. — 1 cup	9	3	40	1	2	1.5	.2	.2	5	1	19	.2	—	—	—	.01	.2	0
478	Sugar coated — 1 cup	35	4	135	2	1	.5	.2	.4	30	2	47	.5	—	—	—	.02	.4	0
	Pretzels, made with enriched flour:																		
479	Dutch, twisted, 2 3/4 by 2 5/8 in. — 1 pretzel	16	5	60	2	1				12	4	21	.2	21	0	.05	.04	.7	0
480	Thin, twisted, 3 1/4 by 2 1/4 by 1/4 in. — 10 pretzels	60	5	235	6	3				46	13	79	.9	78	0	.20	.15	2.5	0
481	Stick, 2 1/4 in long — 10 pretzels	3	5	10	Trace	Trace				2	1	4	Trace	4	0	.01	.01	.1	0
	Rice, white, enriched:																		
482	Instant, ready-to-serve, hot — 1 cup	165	73	180	4	Trace	Trace	Trace	Trace	40	5	31	1.3	—	0	.21	(59)	1.7	0
	Long grain:																		
483	Raw — 1 cup	185	12	670	12	1	.2	.2	.2	149	44	174	5.4	170	0	.81	.06	6.5	0
484	Cooked, served hot — 1 cup	205	73	225	4	Trace	.1	.1	.1	50	21	57	1.8	57	0	.23	.02	2.1	0
	Parboiled:																		
485	Raw — 1 cup	185	10	685	14	1	.2	.1	.2	150	111	370	5.4	278	0	.81	.07	6.5	0
486	Cooked, served hot — 1 cup	175	73	185	4	Trace	.1	.1	.1	41	33	100	1.4	75	0	.19	.02	2.1	0
	Rolls, enriched:[38] Commercial:																		
487	Brown-and-serve (12 per 12-oz pkg.), browned. — 1 roll	26	27	85	2	2	.4	.7	.5	14	20	23	.5	25	Trace	.10	.06	.9	Trace
488	Cloverleaf or pan, 2 1/2-in diam., 2 in high. — 1 roll	28	31	85	2	2	.4	.6	.4	15	21	24	.5	27	Trace	.11	.07	.9	Trace
489	Frankfurter and hamburger (8 per 11 1/2-oz pkg.). — 1 roll	40	31	120	3	2	.5	.8	.6	21	30	34	.8	38	Trace	.16	.10	1.3	Trace
490	Hard, 3 3/4-in diam., 2 in high. — 1 roll	50	25	155	5	2	.4	.6	.5	30	24	46	1.2	49	Trace	.20	.12	1.7	Trace
491	Hoagie or submarine, 11 1/2 by 3 by 2 1/2 in. — 1 roll	135	31	390	12	4	.9	1.4	1.4	75	58	115	3.0	122	Trace	.54	.32	4.5	Trace
	From home recipe:																		
492	Cloverleaf, 2 1/2-in diam., 2 in high. — 1 roll	35	26	120	3	3	.8	1.1	.7	20	16	36	.7	41	30	.12	.12	1.2	Trace
	Spaghetti, enriched, cooked:																		
493	Firm stage, "al dente," served hot. — 1 cup	130	64	190	7	1				39	14	85	1.4	103	0	.23	.13	1.8	0
494	Tender stage, served hot — 1 cup	140	73	155	5	1				32	11	70	1.3	85	0	.20	.11	1.5	0
	Spaghetti (enriched) in tomato sauce with cheese:																		
495	From home recipe — 1 cup	250	77	260	9	9	2.0	5.4	.7	37	80	135	2.3	408	1,080	.25	.18	2.3	13
496	Canned — 1 cup	250	80	190	6	2	.5	.3	.4	39	40	88	2.8	303	930	.35	.28	4.5	10
	Spaghetti (enriched) with meat balls and tomato sauce:																		
497	From home recipe — 1 cup	248	70	330	19	12	3.3	6.3	.9	39	124	236	3.7	665	1,590	.25	.30	4.0	22
498	Canned — 1 cup	250	78	260	12	10	2.2	3.3	3.9	29	53	113	3.3	245	1,000	.15	.18	2.3	5
499	Toaster pastries — 1 pastry	50	12	200	3	6				36	[65]54	[66]67	1.9	[66]74	500	.16	.17	2.1	(60)
	Waffles, made with enriched flour, 7-in diam.:[38]																		
500	From home recipe — 1 waffle	75	41	210	7	7	2.3	2.8	1.4	28	85	130	1.3	109	250	.17	.23	1.4	Trace
501	From mix, egg and milk added — 1 waffle	75	42	205	7	8	2.8	2.9	1.2	27	179	257	1.0	146	170	.14	.22	.9	Trace

(A)	(B)		(C)	(D)	(E)	(F)	(G)	(H)	(I)	(J)	(K)	(L)	(M)	(N)	(O)	(P)	(Q)	(R)	(S)
	Wheat flours:																		
	All-purpose or family flour, enriched:																		
502	Sifted, spooned	1 cup	115	420	12	1	0.2	0.1	0.5	88	1E	100	3.3	109	0	0.74	0.46	6.1	0
503	Unsifted, spooned	1 cup	125	455	13	1	.2	.1	.5	95	2C	109	3.6	119	0	.80	.50	6.6	0
504	Cake or pastry flour, enriched, sifted, spooned.	1 cup	96	350	7	1	.1	.1	.3	76	1€	70	2.8	91	0	.61	.38	5.1	0
505	Self-rising, enriched, unsifted, spooned.	1 cup	125	440	12	1	.2	.1	.5	93	334	583	3.6	—	0	.80	.50	6.6	0
506	Whole-wheat, from hard wheats, stirred.	1 cup	120	400	16	2	.4	.2	1.0	85	49	446	4.0	444	0	.66	.14	5.2	0
	LEGUMES (DRY), NUTS, SEEDS; RELATED PRODUCTS																		
	Almonds, shelled:																		
507	Chopped (about 130 almonds)	1 cup	130	775	24	70	5.6	47.7	12.8	25	304	655	6.1	1,005	0	.31	1.20	4.6	Trace
508	Slivered, not pressed down (about 115 almonds).	1 cup	115	690	21	62	5.0	42.2	11.3	22	269	580	5.4	889	0	.28	1.06	4.0	Trace
	Beans, dry:																		
	Common varieties as Great Northern, navy, and others:																		
	Cooked, drained:																		
509	Great Northern	1 cup	180	210	14	1	—	—	—	38	90	266	4.9	749	0	.25	.13	1.3	0
510	Pea (navy)	1 cup	190	225	15	1	—	—	—	40	95	281	5.1	790	0	.27	.13	1.3	0
	Canned, solids and liquid:																		
	White with—																		
511	Frankfurters (sliced)	1 cup	255	365	19	18	2.4	2.8	.6	32	94	303	4.8	668	330	.13	.15	3.3	Trace
512	Pork and tomato sauce	1 cup	255	310	16	7	4.3	5.0	1.1	48	138	235	4.6	536	330	.20	.08	1.5	5
513	Pork and sweet sauce	1 cup	255	385	16	12	—	—	—	54	161	291	5.9	—	10	.15	.10	1.3	—
514	Red kidney	1 cup	255	230	15	1	—	—	—	42	74	278	4.6	673	10	.13	.10	1.5	—
515	Lima, cooked, drained	1 cup	190	260	16	1	—	—	—	49	55	293	5.9	1,163	—	.25	.10	1.5	—
516	Blackeye peas, dry, cooked (with residual cooking liquid).	1 cup	250	190	13	1	—	—	—	35	43	238	3.3	573	30	.40	.10	1.0	—
517	Brazil nuts, shelled (6-8 large kernels).	1 oz	28	185	4	19	4.8	6.2	7.1	3	53	196	1.0	203	Trace	.27	.03	.5	—
518	Cashew nuts, roasted in oil	1 cup	140	785	24	64	12.9	36.8	10.2	41	53	522	5.3	650	140	.60	.35	2.5	—
	Coconut meat, fresh:																		
519	Piece, about 2 by 2 by 1/2 in	1 piece	45	155	2	16	14.0	.9	.3	4	6	43	.8	115	0	.02	.01	.2	1
520	Shredded or grated, not pressed down.	1 cup	80	275	3	28	24.8	1.6	.5	8	10	76	1.4	205	0	.04	.02	.4	2
521	Filberts (hazelnuts), chopped (about 60 kernels).	1 cup	115	730	14	72	5.1	55.2	7.3	19	240	388	3.9	810	—	.53	—	1.0	Trace
522	Lentils, whole, cooked	1 cup	200	210	16	Trace	13.7	33.0	20.7	3%	50	238	4.2	498	40	.14	.12	1.2	0
523	Peanuts, roasted in oil, salted (whole, halves, chopped).	1 cup	144	840	37	72	13.7	33.0	20.7	27	107	577	3.0	971	—	.46	.19	24.8	0
524	Peanut butter	1 tbsp	16	95	4	8	1.5	3.7	2.3	3	9	61	.3	100	—	.02	.02	2.4	0
525	Peas, split, dry, cooked	1 cup	200	230	16	1	—	—	—	42	22	178	3.4	592	80	.30	.18	1.8	0
526	Pecans, chopped or pieces (about 120 large halves).	1 cup	118	810	11	84	7.2	50.5	20.0	77	86	341	2.8	712	150	1.01	.15	1.1	2
527	Pumpkin and squash kernels, dry, hulled.	1 cup	140	775	41	65	11.8	23.5	27.5	51	71	1,602	15.7	1,386	100	.34	.27	3.4	—
528	Sunflower seeds, dry, hulled	1 cup	145	810	35	69	8.2	13.7	43.2	29	174	1,214	10.3	1,334	70	2.84	.33	7.8	—
	Walnuts:																		
	Black:																		
529	Chopped or broken kernels	1 cup	125	785	26	74	6.3	13.3	45.7	19	Trace	713	7.5	575	380	.28	.14	.9	—
530	Ground (finely)	1 cup	80	500	16	47	4.0	8.5	29.2	12	Trace	456	4.8	368	240	.18	.09	.6	—
531	Persian or English, chopped (about 60 halves).	1 cup	120	780	18	77	8.4	11.8	42.2	19	119	456	3.7	540	40	.40	.16	1.1	2

[19] Crust made with vegetable shortening and enriched flour.
[38] Made with vegetable shortening.
[59] Product may or may not be enriched with riboflavin. Consult the label.
[60] Value varies with the brand. Consult the label.

(Dashes (—) denote lack of reliable data for a constituent believed to be present in measurable amount)

NUTRIENTS IN INDICATED QUANTITY

Item No. (A)	Foods, approximate measures, units, and weight (edible part unless footnotes indicate otherwise) (B)	Grams	Water (C) Per-cent	Food energy (D) Cal-units	Pro-tein (E) Grams	Fat (F) Grams	Fatty Acids Satu-rated (total) (G) Grams	Unsaturated Oleic (H) Grams	Unsaturated Lino-leic (I) Grams	Carbo-hydrate (J) Grams	Calcium (K) Milli-grams	Phos-phorus (L) Milli-grams	Iron (M) Milli-grams	Potas-sium (N) Milli-grams	Vitamin A value (O) Inter-national units	Thiamin (P) Milli-grams	Ribo-flavin (Q) Milli-grams	Niacin (R) Milli-grams	Ascorbic acid (S) Milli-grams
	SUGARS AND SWEETS																		
	Cake icings:																		
	Boiled, white:																		
532	Plain--- 1 cup---	94	18	295	1	0	0			75	2	2	Trace	17	0	Trace	0.03	Trace	0
533	With coconut--- 1 cup---	166	15	605	3	13	11.0	.9	Trace	124	10	50	0.8	277	0	0.02	.07	0.3	0
	Uncooked:																		
534	Chocolate made with milk and butter. 1 cup---	275	14	1,035	9	38	23.4	11.7	1.0	185	165	305	3.3	536	580	.06	.28	.6	1
535	Creamy fudge from mix and water. 1 cup---	245	15	830	7	16	5.1	6.7	3.1	183	96	218	2.7	238	Trace	.05	.20	.7	Trace
536	White--- 1 cup---	319	11	1,200	2	21	12.7	5.1	.5	260	48	38	Trace	57	860	Trace	.06	Trace	Trace
	Candy:																		
537	Caramels, plain or chocolate--- 1 oz---	28	8	115	1	3	1.6	1.1	.1	22	42	35	.4	54	Trace	.01	.05	.1	Trace
	Chocolate:																		
538	Milk, plain--- 1 oz---	28	1	145	2	9	5.5	3.0	.3	16	65	65	.3	109	80	.02	.10	.1	Trace
539	Semisweet, small pieces (60 per oz). 1 cup or 6-oz pkg---	170	1	860	7	61	36.2	19.8	1.7	97	51	255	4.4	553	30	.02	.14	.9	0
540	Chocolate-coated peanuts--- 1 oz---	28	1	160	5	12	4.0	4.7	2.1	11	33	84	.4	143	Trace	.10	.05	2.1	Trace
541	Fondant, uncoated (mints, candy corn, other). 1 oz---	28	8	105	Trace	1	.1	.3	.1	25	4	2	.3	1	0	Trace	Trace	Trace	0
542	Fudge, chocolate, plain--- 1 oz---	28	8	115	Trace	3	1.3	1.4	.6	21	22	24	.3	42	Trace	.01	.03	.1	Trace
543	Gum drops--- 1 oz---	28	12	100	Trace	Trace	---	---	---	25	2	Trace	.1	1	0	0	Trace	Trace	0
544	Hard--- 1 oz---	28	1	110	0	Trace	---	---	---	28	6	2	.5	1	0	0	0	0	0
545	Marshmallows--- 1 oz---	28	17	90	1	Trace	---	---	---	23	5	2	.5	2	0	0	Trace	Trace	0
	Chocolate-flavored beverage powders (about 4 heaping tsp per oz):																		
546	With nonfat dry milk--- 1 oz---	28	2	100	5	1	.5	.3	Trace	20	167	155	.5	227	10	.04	.21	.2	1
547	Without milk--- 1 oz---	28	1	100	1	1	.4	.2	Trace	25	9	48	.6	142	---	.01	.03	.1	0
548	Honey, strained or extracted--- 1 tbsp---	21	17	65	Trace	0	0	0	0	17	1	1	.1	11	0	Trace	.01	.1	Trace
549	Jams and preserves--- 1 tbsp---	20	29	55	Trace	Trace	---	---	---	14	4	2	.2	18	Trace	Trace	.01	Trace	Trace
550	1 packet---	14	29	40	Trace	Trace	---	---	---	10	3	1	.1	12	Trace	Trace	Trace	Trace	Trace
551	Jellies--- 1 tbsp---	18	29	50	Trace	Trace	---	---	---	13	4	1	.3	14	Trace	Trace	.01	Trace	1
552	1 packet---	14	29	40	Trace	Trace	---	---	---	10	3	1	.2	11	Trace	Trace	Trace	Trace	Trace
	Sirups:																		
	Chocolate-flavored sirup or topping:																		
553	Thin type--- 1 fl oz or 2 tbsp---	38	32	90	1	1	.5	.3	Trace	24	6	35	.6	106	Trace	.01	.03	.2	0
554	Fudge type--- 1 fl oz or 2 tbsp---	38	25	125	2	5	3.1	1.6	.1	20	48	60	.5	107	60	.02	.08	.2	Trace
	Molasses, cane:																		
555	Light (first extraction)--- 1 tbsp---	20	24	50	---	---	---	---	---	13	33	9	.9	183	---	.01	.01	Trace	---
556	Blackstrap (third extraction)--- 1 tbsp---	20	24	45	---	---	---	---	---	11	137	17	3.2	585	---	.02	.04	.4	---
557	Sorghum--- 1 tbsp---	21	23	55	---	---	---	---	---	14	35	5	2.6	1	---	---	.02	Trace	---
558	Table blends, chiefly corn, light and dark. 1 tbsp---	21	24	60	0	0	0	0	0	15	9	3	.8	1	0	0	0	0	0
	Sugars:																		
559	Brown, pressed down--- 1 cup---	220	2	820	0	0	0	0	0	212	187	42	7.5	757	0	.02	.07	.4	0
	White:																		
560	Granulated--- 1 cup---	200	1	770	0	0	0	0	0	199	0	0	.2	6	0	0	0	0	0
561	1 tbsp---	12	1	45	0	0	0	0	0	12	0	0	Trace	Trace	0	0	0	0	0
562	1 packet---	6	1	23	0	0	0	0	0	6	0	0	Trace	Trace	0	0	0	0	0
563	Powdered, sifted, spooned into cup. 1 cup---	100	1	385	0	0	0	0	0	100	0	0	.1	3	0	0	0	0	0

VEGETABLE AND VEGETABLE PRODUCTS

(A)	(B)	grams (C)→	(C)	(D)	(E)	(F)	(G)	(H)	(I)	(J)	(K)	(L)	(M)	(N)	(O)	(P)	(Q)	(R)	(S)
	Asparagus, green:																		
	Cooked, drained:																		
	Cuts and tips, 1 1/2- to 2-in lengths:																		
564	From raw---------------- 1 cup----	145	94	30	3	Trace	—	—	—	5	30	73	0.9	265	1,310	0.23	0.26	2.0	38
565	From frozen------------- 1 cup----	180	93	40	6	Trace	—	—	—	6	40	115	2.2	396	1,530	.25	.23	1.8	41
	Spears, 1/2-in diam. at base:																		
566	From raw---------------- 4 spears--	60	94	10	1	Trace	—	—	—	2	13	30	.4	110	540	.10	.11	.8	16
567	From frozen------------- 4 spears--	60	92	15	2	Trace	—	—	—	2	13	40	.7	143	470	.10	.08	.7	16
568	Canned, spears, 1/2-in diam, at base. 4 spears--	80	93	15	2	Trace	—	—	—	3	15	42	1.5	133	640	.05	.08	.6	12
	Beans:																		
	Lima, immature seeds, frozen, cooked, drained:																		
569	Thick-seeded types (Fordhooks) 1 cup----	170	74	170	10	Trace	—	—	—	32	34	153	2.9	724	390	.12	.09	1.7	29
570	Thin-seeded types (baby limas) 1 cup----	180	69	210	13	Trace	—	—	—	40	63	227	4.7	709	400	.16	.09	2.2	22
	Snap:																		
	Green:																		
	Cooked, drained:																		
571	From raw (cuts and French style). 1 cup----	125	92	30	2	Trace	—	—	—	7	63	46	.8	189	680	.09	.11	.6	15
	From frozen:																		
572	Cuts------------------- 1 cup----	135	92	35	2	Trace	—	—	—	8	54	43	.9	205	780	.09	.12	.5	7
573	French style----------- 1 cup----	130	92	35	2	Trace	—	—	—	8	49	39	1.2	177	690	.08	.10	.4	9
574	Canned, drained solids (cuts). 1 cup----	135	92	30	2	Trace	—	—	—	7	61	34	2.0	128	630	.04	.07	.4	5
	Yellow or wax:																		
	Cooked, drained:																		
575	From raw (cuts and French style). 1 cup----	125	93	30	2	Trace	—	—	—	6	63	46	.8	189	290	.09	.11	.6	16
576	From frozen (cuts)------ 1 cup----	135	92	35	2	Trace	—	—	—	3	47	42	.9	221	140	.09	.11	.5	8
577	Canned, drained solids (cuts). 1 cup----	135	92	30	2	Trace	—	—	—	7	61	34	2.0	128	140	.04	.07	.4	7
	Beans, mature. See Beans, dry (items 509-515) and Blackeye peas, dry (item 516).																		
	Bean sprouts (mung):																		
578	Raw---------------------- 1 cup----	105	89	35	4	Trace	—	—	—	7	20	67	1.4	234	20	.14	.14	.8	20
579	Cooked, drained---------- 1 cup----	125	91	35	4	Trace	—	—	—	7	21	60	1.1	195	30	.11	.13	.9	8
	Beets:																		
	Cooked, drained, peeled:																		
580	Whole beets, 2-in diam--- 2 beets---	100	91	30	1	Trace	—	—	—	7	14	23	.5	208	20	.03	.04	.3	6
581	Diced or sliced---------- 1 cup----	170	91	55	2	Trace	—	—	—	12	24	39	.9	354	30	.05	.07	.5	10
	Canned, drained solids:																		
582	Whole beets, small------- 1 cup----	160	89	60	2	Trace	—	—	—	14	30	29	1.1	267	20	.02	.05	.2	5
583	Diced or sliced---------- 1 cup----	170	89	65	2	Trace	—	—	—	15	32	31	1.2	284	30	.02	.05	.2	5
584	Beet greens, leaves and stems, cooked, drained. 1 cup----	145	94	25	2	Trace	—	—	—	5	144	36	2.8	481	7,400	.10	.22	.4	22
	Blackeye peas, immature seeds, cooked and drained:																		
585	From raw----------------- 1 cup----	165	72	180	13	1	—	—	—	30	40	241	3.5	625	580	.50	.18	2.3	28
586	From frozen-------------- 1 cup----	170	66	220	15	1	—	—	—	40	43	286	4.8	573	290	.68	.19	2.4	15
	Broccoli, cooked, drained:																		
	From raw:																		
587	Stalk, medium size------- 1 stalk---	180	91	45	6	1	—	—	—	8	158	112	1.4	481	4,500	.16	.36	1.4	162
588	Stalks cut into 1/2-in pieces- 1 cup----	155	91	40	5	Trace	—	—	—	7	136	96	1.2	414	3,880	.14	.31	1.2	140
	From frozen:																		
589	Stalk, 4 1/2 to 5 in long- 1 stalk---	30	91	10	1	Trace	—	—	—	1	12	17	.2	66	570	.02	.03	.2	22
590	Chopped------------------ 1 cup----	185	92	50	5	1	—	—	—	9	100	104	1.3	392	4,810	.11	.22	.9	105
	Brussels sprouts, cooked, drained:																		
591	From raw, 7-8 sprouts (1 1/4- to 1 1/2-in diam.). 1 cup----	155	88	55	7	1	—	—	—	10	50	112	1.7	423	810	.12	.22	1.2	135
592	From frozen-------------- 1 cup----	155	89	50	5	Trace	—	—	—	10	33	95	1.2	457	880	.12	.16	.9	126

(Dashes (—) denote lack of reliable data for a constituent believed to be present in measurable amount)

							Fatty Acids												
							Saturated (total)	Unsaturated											
Item No.	Foods, approximate measures, units, and weight (edible part unless footnotes indicate otherwise)		Water	Food energy	Protein	Fat		Oleic	Lino-leic	Carbo-hydrate	Calcium	Phos-phorus	Iron	Potas-sium	Vitamin A value	Thiamin	Ribo-flavin	Niacin	Ascorbic acid
(A)	(B)		(C)	(D)	(E)	(F)	(G)	(H)	(I)	(J)	(K)	(L)	(M)	(N)	(O)	(P)	(Q)	(R)	(S)
		Grams	Per-cent	Cal-ories	Grams	Grams	Grams	Grams	Grams	Grams	Milli-grams	Milli-grams	Milli-grams	Milli-grams	Inter-national units	Milli-grams	Milli-grams	Milli-grams	Milli-grams

VEGETABLE AND VEGETABLE PRODUCTS—Con.

	Cabbage:																		
	Common varieties:																		
	Raw:																		
593	Coarsely shredded or sliced— 1 cup	70	92	15	1	Trace	—	—	—	4	34	20	0.3	163	90	0.04	0.04	0.2	33
594	Finely shredded or chopped— 1 cup	90	92	20	1	Trace	—	—	—	5	44	26	.4	210	120	.05	.05	.3	42
595	Cooked, drained— 1 cup	145	94	30	2	Trace	—	—	—	6	64	29	.4	236	190	.06	.06	.4	48
596	Red, raw, coarsely shredded or sliced. 1 cup	70	90	20	1	Trace	—	—	—	5	29	25	.6	188	30	.06	.04	.3	43
597	Savoy, raw, coarsely shredded or sliced. 1 cup	70	92	15	2	Trace	—	—	—	3	47	38	.6	188	140	.04	.06	.2	39
598	Cabbage, celery (also called pe-tsai or wongbok), raw, 1-in pieces. 1 cup	75	95	10	1	Trace	—	—	—	2	32	30	.5	190	110	.04	.03	.5	19
599	Cabbage, white mustard (also called bokchoy or pakchoy), cooked, drained. 1 cup	170	95	25	2	Trace	—	—	—	4	252	56	1.0	364	5,270	.07	.14	1.2	26
	Carrots:																		
	Raw, without crowns and tips, scraped:																		
600	Whole, 7 1/2 by 1 1/8 in, or strips, 2 1/2 to 3 in long. 1 carrot or 18 strips	72	88	30	1	Trace	—	—	—	7	27	26	.5	246	7,930	.04	.04	.4	6
601	Grated— 1 cup	110	88	45	1	Trace	—	—	—	11	41	40	.8	375	12,100	.07	.06	.7	9
602	Cooked (crosswise cuts), drained. 1 cup	155	91	50	1	Trace	—	—	—	11	51	48	.9	344	16,280	.08	.08	.8	9
	Canned:																		
603	Sliced, drained solids— 1 cup	155	91	45	1	Trace	—	—	—	10	47	34	1.1	186	23,250	.03	.05	.6	3
604	Strained or junior (baby food)— 1 oz (1 3/4 to 2 tbsp)—	28	92	10	Trace	Trace	—	—	—	2	7	6	.1	51	3,690	.01	.01	.1	1
	Cauliflower:																		
605	Raw, chopped— 1 cup	115	91	31	3	Trace	—	—	—	6	29	64	1.3	339	70	.13	.12	.8	90
	Cooked, drained:																		
606	From raw (flower buds)— 1 cup	125	93	30	3	Trace	—	—	—	5	26	53	.9	258	80	.11	.10	.8	69
607	From frozen (flowerets)— 1 cup	180	94	30	3	Trace	—	—	—	6	31	68	.9	373	50	.07	.09	.7	74
	Celery, Pascal type, raw:																		
608	Stalk, large outer, 8 by 1 1/2 in, at root end. 1 stalk	40	94	5	Trace	Trace	—	—	—	2	16	11	.1	136	110	.01	.01	.1	4
609	Pieces, diced— 1 cup	120	94	20	1	Trace	—	—	—	5	47	34	.4	409	320	.04	.04	.4	11
	Collards, cooked, drained:																		
610	From raw (leaves without stems)— 1 cup	190	90	65	7	1	—	—	—	10	357	99	1.5	498	14,820	.21	.38	2.3	144
611	From frozen (chopped)— 1 cup	170	90	50	5	1	—	—	—	10	299	87	1.7	401	11,560	.10	.24	1.0	56
	Corn, sweet:																		
	Cooked, drained:																		
612	From raw, ear 5 by 1 3/4 in— 1 ear[61]	140	74	70	2	1	—	—	—	16	2	69	.5	151	[62]310	.09	.08	1.1	7
	From frozen:																		
613	Ear, 5 in long— 1 ear[61]	229	73	120	4	1	—	—	—	27	4	121	1.0	291	[62]440	.18	.10	2.1	9
614	Kernels— 1 cup	165	77	130	5	1	—	—	—	31	5	120	1.3	304	[62]580	.15	.10	2.5	8
	Canned:																		
615	Cream style— 1 cup	256	76	210	5	2	—	—	—	51	8	143	1.5	248	[62]840	.08	.13	2.6	13
	Whole kernel:																		
616	Vacuum pack— 1 cup	210	76	175	5	1	—	—	—	43	6	153	1.1	204	[62]740	.06	.13	2.3	11
617	Wet pack, drained solids— 1 cup	165	76	140	4	1	—	—	—	33	8	81	.8	160	[62]580	.05	.08	1.5	7
	Cowpeas. See Blackeye peas. (Items 585-586).																		
	Cucumber slices, 1/8 in thick (large, 2 1/8-in diam.; small, 1 3/4-in diam.):																		
618	With peel— 6 large or 8 small slices	28	95	5	Trace	Trace	—	—	—	1	7	8	.3	45	70	.01	.01	.1	3

442

(A)	(B)	(C)	(D)	(E)	(F)	(G)	(H)	(I)	(I)	(K)	(L)	(M)	(N)	(O)	(P)	(Q)	(R)	(S)
619	Without peel---- 6 1/2 large or 9 small pieces.	96	5	Trace	Trace	—	—	—	1	5	5	0.1	45	Trace	0.01	0.01	0.1	3
620	Dandelion greens, cooked, drained-- 1 cup	90	35	2	1	—	—	—	7	147	44	1.9	244	12,290	.14	.17	1.9	19
621	Endive, curly (including escarole), 1 cup raw, small pieces.	93	10	1	Trace	—	—	—	2	41	27	.9	147	1,650	.04	.07	.3	5
	Kale, cooked, drained.																	
622	From raw (leaves without stems and midribs)-- 1 cup	88	45	5	1	—	—	—	7	206	64	1.8	243	9,130	.11	.20	1.8	102
623	From frozen (leaf style)-- 1 cup	91	40	4	1	—	—	—	7	157	62	1.3	251	10,660	.08	.20	.9	49
	Lettuce, raw: Butterhead, as Boston types:																	
624	Head, 5-in diam---- 1 head	95	25	2	Trace	—	—	—	4	57	42	3.3	430	1,580	.10	.10	.5	13
625	Leaves---- outer or 2 inner or 3 heart leaves.	95	Trace	Trace	Trace	—	—	—	Trace	5	4	.3	40	150	.01	.01	Trace	1
	Crisphead, as Iceberg:																	
626	Head, 6-in diam---- 1 head	96	70	5	1	—	—	—	16	108	118	2.7	943	1,780	.32	.32	1.6	32
627	Wedge, 1/4 of head-- 1 wedge	96	20	1	Trace	—	—	—	4	27	30	.7	236	450	.08	.08	.4	8
628	Pieces, chopped or shredded-- 1 cup	96	5	Trace	Trace	—	—	—	2	12	12	.3	96	180	.03	.03	.2	3
629	Looseleaf (bunching varieties including romaine or cos), chopped or shredded pieces. 1 cup	94	10	1	Trace	—	—	—	2	37	14	.8	145	1,050	.03	.04	.2	10
630	Mushrooms, raw, sliced or chopped-- 1 cup	90	20	2	Trace	—	—	—	3	4	81	.6	290	Trace	.07	.32	2.9	2
631	Mustard greens, without stems and midribs, cooked, drained-- 1 cup	93	30	3	1	—	—	—	6	193	45	2.5	308	8,120	.11	.20	.8	67
632	Okra pods, 3 by 5/8 in, cooked-- 10 pods	91	30	2	Trace	—	—	—	6	98	43	.5	184	520	.14	.19	1.0	21
	Onions: Mature: Raw:																	
633	Chopped---- 1 cup	89	65	3	Trace	—	—	—	15	46	61	.9	267	65Trace	.05	.07	.3	17
634	Sliced---- 1 cup	89	45	2	Trace	—	—	—	10	31	41	.6	181	65Trace	.03	.05	.2	12
635	Cooked (whole or sliced), 1 cup drained.	92	60	3	Trace	—	—	—	14	50	61	.8	231	65Trace	.06	.06	.4	15
636	Young green, bulb (3/8 in diam.) 6 onions and white portion of top.	88	15	Trace	Trace	—	—	—	3	12	12	.2	69	Trace	.02	.01	.1	8
637	Parsley, raw, chopped-- 1 tbsp	85	Trace	Trace	Trace	—	—	—	Trace	7	2	.2	25	300	Trace	.01	Trace	6
638	Parsnips, cooked (diced or 2-in 1 cup lengths).	82	100	2	1	—	—	—	23	70	96	.9	587	50	.11	.12	.2	16
	Peas, green: Canned:																	
639	Whole, drained solids-- 1 cup	77	150	8	1	—	—	—	29	44	129	3.2	163	1,170	.15	.10	1.4	14
640	Strained (baby food)-- 1 oz (1 3/4 to 2 tbsp)-	86	15	1	Trace	—	—	—	3	3	18	.3	28	140	.02	.03	.3	3
641	Frozen, cooked, drained-- 1 cup	82	110	8	Trace	—	—	—	19	30	138	3.0	216	960	.43	.14	2.7	21
642	Peppers, hot, red, without seeds, 1 tsp dried (ground chili powder, added seasonings).	9	5	Trace	Trace	—	—	—	1	5	4	.3	20	1,300	Trace	.02	.2	Trace
	Peppers, sweet (about 5 per lb, whole), stem and seeds removed:																	
643	Raw---- 1 pod	93	15	1	Trace	—	—	—	4	7	16	.5	157	310	.06	.06	.4	94
644	Cooked, boiled, drained-- 1 pod	95	15	1	Trace	—	—	—	3	7	12	.4	109	310	.05	.05	.4	70
	Potatoes, cooked:																	
645	Baked, peeled after baking (about 1 potato 2 per lb, raw).	75	145	4	Trace	—	—	—	33	14	101	1.1	782	Trace	.15	.07	2.7	31
	Boiled (about 3 per lb, raw):																	
646	Peeled after boiling-- 1 potato	80	105	3	Trace	—	—	—	23	10	72	.8	556	Trace	.12	.05	2.0	22
647	Peeled before boiling-- 1 potato	83	90	3	Trace	—	—	—	20	8	57	.7	385	Trace	.12	.05	1.6	22
	French-fried, strip, 2 to 3 1/2 in long:																	
648	Prepared from raw-- 10 strips	45	135	2	7	1.7	1.2	3.3	18	8	56	.7	427	Trace	.07	.04	1.6	11
649	Frozen, oven heated-- 10 strips	53	110	2	4	1.1	.8	2.1	17	5	43	.9	326	Trace	.07	.01	1.3	11
650	Hashed brown, prepared from 1 cup frozen.	56	345	3	18	4.6	3.2	9.0	45	28	78	1.9	439	Trace	.11	.03	1.6	12
	Mashed, prepared from— Raw:																	
651	Milk added---- 1 cup	83	135	4	2	.7	.4	Trace	27	50	103	8	548	40	.17	.11	2.1	21

[61] Weight includes cob. Without cob, weight is 77 g for item 612, 126 g for item 613.
[62] Based on yellow varieties. For white varieties, value is trace.
[63] Weight includes refuse of outer leaves and core. Without these parts, weight is 163 g.
[64] Weight includes core. Without core, weight is 539 g.
[65] Value based on white-fleshed varieties. For yellow-fleshed varieties, value in International Units (I.U.) is 70 for item 633, 50 for item 634, and 80 for item 635.

(Dashes (—) denote lack of reliable data for a constituent believed to be present in measurable amount)

| | | | | | | | Fatty Acids | | | NUTRIENTS IN INDICATED QUANTITY | | | | | | | | | |
Item No. (A)	Foods, approximate measures, units, and weight (edible part unless footnotes indicate otherwise) (B)	Grams	Water (C) Per cent	Food energy (D) Cal-ories	Pro-tein (E) Grams	Fat (F) Grams	Satu-rated (total) (G) Grams	Unsaturated Oleic (H) Grams	Unsaturated Lino-leic (I) Grams	Carbo-hydrate (J) Grams	Calcium (K) Milli-grams	Phos-phorus (L) Milli-grams	Iron (M) Milli-grams	Potas-sium (N) Milli-grams	Vitamin A value (O) Inter-national units	Thiamin (P) Milli-grams	Ribo-flavin (Q) Milli-grams	Niacin (R) Milli-grams	Ascorbic acid (S) Milli-grams
	VEGETABLE AND VEGETABLE PRODUCTS—Con.																		
	Potatoes, cooked—Continued																		
	Mashed, prepared from—Continued																		
	Raw—Continued																		
652	Milk and butter added — 1 cup	210	80	195	4	9	5.6	2.3	0.2	26	50	101	0.8	525	360	0.17	0.11	2.1	19
653	Dehydrated flakes (without milk), water, milk, butter, and salt added. — 1 cup	210	79	195	4	7	3.6	2.1	.2	30	65	99	.6	601	270	.08	.08	1.9	11
654	Potato chips, 1 3/4 by 2 1/2 in oval cross section. — 10 chips	20	2	115	1	8	2.1	1.4	4.0	10	8	28	.4	226	Trace	.04	.01	1.0	3
655	Potato salad, made with cooked salad dressing. — 1 cup	250	76	250	7	7	2.0	2.7	1.3	41	80	160	1.5	798	350	.20	.18	2.8	28
656	Pumpkin, canned — 1 cup	245	90	80	2	1	—	—	—	19	61	64	1.0	588	15,680	.07	.12	1.5	12
657	Radishes, raw (prepackaged) stem ends, rootlets cut off. — 4 radishes	18	95	5	Trace	Trace	—	—	—	1	5	6	.2	58	Trace	.01	.01	.1	5
658	Sauerkraut, canned, solids and liquid. — 1 cup	235	93	40	2	Trace	—	—	—	9	85	42	1.2	329	120	.07	.09	.5	33
	Southern peas. See Blackeye peas (items 585-586).																		
	Spinach:																		
659	Raw, chopped — 1 cup	55	91	15	2	Trace	—	—	—	2	51	28	1.7	259	4,460	.06	.11	.3	28
660	Cooked, drained: From raw — 1 cup	180	92	40	5	1	—	—	—	6	167	68	4.0	583	14,580	.13	.25	.9	50
	From frozen:																		
661	Chopped — 1 cup	205	92	45	6	1	—	—	—	8	232	90	4.3	683	16,200	.14	.31	.8	39
662	Leaf — 1 cup	190	92	45	6	1	—	—	—	7	200	84	4.8	688	15,390	.15	.27	1.0	53
663	Canned, drained solids — 1 cup	205	91	50	6	1	—	—	—	7	242	53	5.3	513	16,400	.04	.25	.6	29
	Squash, cooked:																		
664	Summer (all varieties), diced, drained. — 1 cup	210	96	30	2	Trace	—	—	—	7	53	53	.8	296	820	.11	.17	1.7	21
665	Winter (all varieties), baked, mashed. — 1 cup	205	81	130	4	1	—	—	—	32	57	98	1.6	945	8,610	.10	.27	1.4	27
	Sweetpotatoes:																		
	Cooked (raw, 5 by 2 in; about 2 1/2 per lb):																		
666	Baked in skin, peeled — 1 potato	114	64	160	2	1	—	—	—	37	46	66	1.0	342	9,230	.10	.08	.8	25
667	Boiled in skin, peeled — 1 potato	151	71	170	3	1	—	.8	—	40	48	71	1.1	367	11,940	.14	.09	.9	26
668	Candied, 2 1/2 by 2-in piece — 1 piece	105	60	175	1	3	2.0	.8	.1	36	39	45	.9	200	6,620	.06	.04	.4	11
	Canned:																		
669	Solid pack (mashed) — 1 cup	255	72	275	5	1	—	—	—	63	64	105	2.0	510	19,890	.13	.10	1.5	36
670	Vacuum pack, piece 2 3/4 by 1 in. — 1 piece[66]	40	72	45	1	Trace	—	—	—	10	10	16	.3	80	3,120	.02	.02	.2	6
	Tomatoes:																		
671	Raw, 2 3/5-in diam. (3 per 12 oz pkg.). — 1 tomato[66]	135	94	25	1	Trace	—	—	—	6	16	33	.6	300	1,110	.07	.05	.9	[6][7]28
672	Canned, solids and liquid — 1 cup	241	94	50	2	Trace	—	—	—	10	[6][8]14	46	1.2	523	2,170	.12	.07	1.7	41
673	Tomato catsup — 1 cup	273	69	290	5	1	—	—	—	69	60	137	2.2	991	3,820	.25	.19	4.4	41
674	— 1 tbsp	15	69	15	Trace	Trace	—	—	—	4	3	8	.1	54	210	.01	.01	.2	2
	Tomato juice, canned:																		
675	Cup — 1 cup	243	94	45	2	Trace	—	—	—	10	17	44	2.2	552	1,940	.12	.07	1.9	39
676	Glass (6 fl oz) — 1 glass	182	94	35	2	Trace	—	—	—	8	13	33	1.6	413	1,460	.09	.05	1.5	29
677	Turnips, cooked, diced — 1 cup	155	94	35	1	Trace	—	—	—	8	54	37	.6	291	Trace	.06	.08	.5	34
	Turnip greens, cooked, drained:																		
678	From raw (leaves and stems) — 1 cup	145	94	30	3	Trace	—	—	—	5	252	49	1.5	—	8,270	.15	.33	.7	68
679	From frozen (chopped) — 1 cup	165	93	40	4	Trace	—	—	—	6	195	64	1.6	246	11,390	.08	.15	.7	31
680	Vegetables, mixed, frozen, cooked— — 1 cup	182	83	115	6	1	—	—	—	24	46	115	2.4	348	9,010	.22	.13	2.0	15

MISCELLANEOUS ITEMS

(A)	(B)	(C)	(D)	(E)	(F)	(G)	(H)	(I)	(J)	(K)	(L)	(M)	(N)	(O)	(P)	(Q)	(R)	(S)
	Baking powders for home use:																	
681	Sodium aluminum sulfate:																	
	With monocalcium phosphate monohydrate.	1 tsp	3.0	2	5	Trace	Trace	0	0	0	1	58	87	—	5	0	0	0	0	0
682	With monocalcium phosphate monohydrate, calcium sulfate.	1 tsp	2.9	1	5	Trace	Trace	0	0	0	1	183	45	—	—	0	0	0	0	0
683	Straight phosphate	1 tsp	3.8	2	5	Trace	Trace	0	0	0	1	239	359	—	6	0	0	0	0	0
684	Low sodium	1 tsp	4.3	2	5	Trace	Trace	0	0	0	2	207	314	—	471	0	0	0	0	0
685	Barbecue sauce	1 cup	250	81	230	4	17	2.2	4.3	10.0	20	53	50	2.0	435	900	.03	.03	.8	13
686	Beverages, alcoholic:																		
	Beer	12 fl oz	360	92	150	1	0	0	0	0	14	18	108	Trace	90	—	.01	.11	2.2	—
	Gin, rum, vodka, whisky:																		
687	80-proof	1 1/2-fl oz jigger	42	67	95	—	—	—	—	—	Trace	—	—	—	1	—	—	—	—	—
688	86-proof	1 1/2-fl oz jigger	42	64	105	—	—	—	—	—	Trace	—	—	—	1	—	—	—	—	—
689	90-proof	1 1/2-fl oz jigger	42	62	110	—	—	—	—	—	Trace	—	—	—	1	—	—	—	—	—
	Wines:																		
690	Dessert	3 1/2-fl oz glass	103	77	140	Trace	0	0	0	0	8	8	—	—	77	—	.01	.02	.2	—
691	Table	3 1/2-fl oz glass	102	86	85	Trace	0	0	0	0	4	9	10	.4	94	—	Trace	.01	.1	—
	Beverages, carbonated, sweetened, nonalcoholic:																		
692	Carbonated water	12 fl oz	366	92	115	0	0	0	0	0	29	—	—	—	—	0	0	0	0	0
693	Cola type	12 fl oz	369	90	145	0	0	0	0	0	37	—	—	—	—	0	0	0	0	0
694	Fruit-flavored sodas and Tom Collins mixer.	12 fl oz	372	88	170	0	0	0	0	0	45	—	—	—	—	0	0	0	0	0
695	Ginger ale	12 fl oz	366	92	115	0	0	0	0	0	29	—	—	—	0	0	0	0	0	0
696	Root beer	12 fl oz	370	90	150	0	0	0	0	0	39	—	—	—	0	0	0	0	0	0
	Chili powder. See Peppers, hot, red (item 642).																		
697	Chocolate: Bitter or baking	1 oz	28	2	145	3	15	8.9	4.9	.4	8	22	109	1.9	235	20	.01	.07	.4	0
	Sweet, see Candy, chocolate (item 539).																		
698	Gelatin, dry	1 7-g envelope	7	13	25	6	Trace	0	0	0	0	—	—	—	—	—	—	—	—	—
699	Gelatin dessert prepared with gelatin dessert powder and water.	1 cup	240	84	140	4	0	0	0	0	34	—	—	—	—	—	—	—	—	—
700	Mustard, prepared, yellow	1 tsp or individual serving pouch or cup.	5	80	5	Trace	Trace	—	—	—	Trace	4	4	.1	7	0	—	—	—	—
	Olives, pickled, canned:																		
701	Green	4 medium or 3 extra large or 2 giant.[69]	16	78	15	Trace	2	.2	1.2	.1	Trace	8	2	.2	7	40	—	—	—	—
702	Ripe, Mission	3 small or 2 large[69]	10	73	15	Trace	2	.2	1.2	.1	Trace	9	1	.1	2	10	Trace	Trace	—	—
	Pickles, cucumber:																		
703	Dill, medium, whole, 3 3/4 in long, 1 1/4-in diam.	1 pickle	65	93	5	Trace	Trace	—	—	—	1	17	14	.7	130	70	Trace	.01	Trace	4
704	Fresh-pack, slices 1 1/2-in diam., 1/4 in thick.	2 slices	15	79	10	Trace	Trace	—	—	—	3	5	4	.3	—	20	Trace	Trace	Trace	1
705	Sweet, gherkin, small, whole, about 2 1/2 in long, 3/4-in diam.	1 pickle	15	61	20	Trace	Trace	—	—	—	5	2	2	.2	—	10	Trace	Trace	Trace	1
706	Relish, finely chopped, sweet.	1 tbsp	15	63	20	Trace	Trace	—	—	—	5	3	2	.1	—	—	—	—	—	—
	Popcorn. See items 476-478.																		
707	Popsicle, 3-fl oz size	1 popsicle	95	80	70	0	0	0	0	0	18	0	—	Trace	—	0	0	0	0	0

[66] Weight includes cores and stem ends. Without these parts, weight is 123 g.
[67] Based on year-round average. For tomatoes marketed from November through May, value is about 12 mg; from June through October, 32 mg.
[68] Applies to product with calcium salts added. Value for products with calcium salts added may be as much as 63 mg for whole tomatoes, 241 mg for cut forms.
[69] Weight includes pits. Without pits, weight is 13 g for item 701, 9 g for item 702.

(Dashes (—) denote lack of reliable data for a constituent believed to be present in measurable amount)

Item No. (A)	Foods, approximate measures, units, and weight (edible part unless footnotes indicate otherwise) (B)		Water (C) Per-cent	Food energy (D) Cal-ories	Pro-tein (E) Grams	Fat (F) Grams	Fatty Acids Satu-rated (total) (G) Grams	Unsaturated Oleic (H) Grams	Lino-leic (I) Grams	Carbo-hydrate (J) Grams	Calcium (K) Milli-grams	Phos-phorus (L) Milli-grams	Iron (M) Milli-grams	Potas-sium (N) Milli-grams	Vitamin A value (O) Inter-national units	Thiamin (P) Milli-grams	Ribo-flavin (Q) Milli-grams	Niacin (R) Milli-grams	Ascorbic acid (S) Milli-grams
		Grams																	
	MISCELLANEOUS ITEMS—Con.																		
	Soups:																		
	Canned, condensed:																		
	Prepared with equal volume of milk:																		
708	Cream of chicken --- 1 cup ---	245	85	180	7	10	4.2	3.6	1.3	15	172	152	0.5	260	610	0.05	0.27	0.7	2
709	Cream of mushroom --- 1 cup ---	245	83	215	7	14	5.4	2.9	4.6	16	191	169	.5	279	250	.05	.34	.7	1
710	Tomato --- 1 cup ---	250	84	175	7	7	3.4	1.7	1.0	23	168	155	.8	418	1,200	.10	.25	1.3	15
	Prepared with equal volume of water:																		
711	Bean with pork --- 1 cup ---	250	84	170	8	6	1.2	1.8	2.4	22	63	128	2.3	395	650	.13	.08	1.0	3
712	Beef broth, bouillon, consomme. --- 1 cup ---	240	96	30	5	0	0	0	0	3	Trace	31	.5	130	Trace	Trace	.02	1.2	
713	Beef noodle --- 1 cup ---	240	93	65	4	3	.6	.7	.8	7	7	48	1.0	77	50	.05	.07	1.0	Trace
714	Clam chowder, Manhattan type (with tomatoes, without milk). --- 1 cup ---	245	92	80	2	3	.5	.4	1.3	12	34	47	1.0	184	880	.02	.02	1.0	
715	Cream of chicken --- 1 cup ---	240	92	95	3	6	1.6	2.3	1.1	8	24	34	.5	79	410	.02	.05	.5	Trace
716	Cream of mushroom --- 1 cup ---	240	90	135	2	10	2.6	1.7	4.5	10	41	50	.5	98	70	.02	.12	.7	Trace
717	Minestrone --- 1 cup ---	245	90	105	5	3	.7	.9	1.3	14	37	59	1.0	314	2,350	.07	.05	1.0	
718	Split pea --- 1 cup ---	245	85	145	9	3	1.1	1.2	.4	21	29	149	1.5	270	440	.25	.15	1.5	1
719	Tomato --- 1 cup ---	245	91	90	2	3	.5	.5	1.0	16	15	34	.7	230	1,000	.05	.05	1.2	12
720	Vegetable beef --- 1 cup ---	245	92	80	5	2	—	—	—	10	12	49	.7	162	2,700	.05	.05	1.0	
721	Vegetarian --- 1 cup ---	245	92	80	2	2	—	—	—	13	20	39	1.0	172	2,940	.05	.05	1.0	
	Dehydrated:																		
722	Bouillon cube, 1/2 in --- 1 cube ---	4	4	5	1	Trace	—	—	—	Trace	—	—	—	4	—	—	—	—	
	Mixes:																		
	Unprepared:																		
723	Onion --- 1 1/2-oz pkg ---	43	3	150	6	5	1.1	2.3	1.0	23	42	49	.6	238	30	.05	.03	.3	6
	Prepared with water:																		
724	Chicken noodle --- 1 cup ---	240	95	55	2	1	—	—	—	8	7	19	.2	19	50	.07	.05	.5	Trace
725	Onion --- 1 cup ---	240	96	35	1	1	—	—	—	6	10	12	.2	58	Trace	Trace	Trace	Trace	2
726	Tomato vegetable with noodles. --- 1 cup ---	240	93	65	1	1	—	—	—	12	7	19	.2	29	480	.05	.02	.5	5
727	Vinegar, cider --- 1 tbsp ---	15	94	Trace	Trace	0	0	0	0	1	1	1	.1	15	—	—	—	—	
728	White sauce, medium, with enriched flour. --- 1 cup ---	250	73	405	10	31	19.3	7.8	.8	22	288	233	.5	348	1,150	.12	.43	.7	2
	Yeast:																		
729	Baker's, dry, active --- 1 pkg ---	7	5	20	3	Trace	—	—	—	3	3	90	1.1	140	Trace	.16	.38	2.6	Trace
730	Brewer's, dry --- 1 tbsp ---	8	5	25	3	Trace	—	—	—	3	[7]17	140	1.4	152	Trace	1.25	.34	3.0	Trace

[7]Value may vary from 6 to 60 mg.

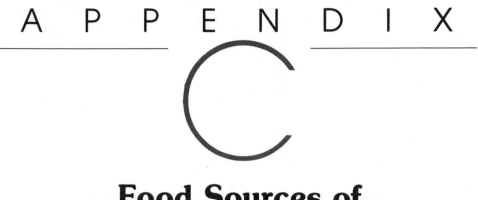

APPENDIX C

Food Sources of Additional Nutrients

Vitamins

Vitamin B₆	Vitamin B₁₂	Vitamin E
Bananas	(present in foods of animal origin only)	Vegetable oils
Whole-grain cereals		Margarine
Chicken	Kidney	Whole-grain cereals
Dry legumes	Liver	Peanuts
Most dark-green leafy vegetables	Meat	
Most fish and shellfish	Milk	
Muscle meats, liver and kidney	Most cheese	
Peanuts, walnuts, filberts, and peanut butter	Most fish	
Potatoes and sweet potatoes	Shellfish	
Prunes and raisins	Whole egg and egg yolk	
Yeast		

Vitamin D	Folacin
Vitamin D milks	Liver
Egg yolk	Dark-green vegetables
Saltwater fish	Dry beans
Liver	Peanuts
	Wheat germ

Minerals

Iodine	Magnesium	Zinc
Iodized salt	Bananas	Shellfish
Seafood	Whole-grain cereals	Meat
	Dry beans	Poultry
	Milk	Cheese
	Most dark-green vegetables	Whole-grain cereals
	Nuts	Dry beans
	Peanuts and peanut butter	Cocoa
		Nuts

APPENDIX

D

Standard Symbols in Pulmonary Gas Exchange

	Symbol	Definition	Example
Quantitative variables	P	Gas pressure	$P_{O_2} = 100$ mm Hg
	V	Gas volume	$V_{Tidal} = 500$ ml
	$\dot{V}$	Gas volume (flow) per unit time	$\dot{V}_{Expired} = 6$ L/min
	f	Frequency of respiration	$f = 10$ breaths/min
	F	Fractional concentration of gas in dry gas phase	F_{O_2} in air $= 0.2094$
	C	Concentration in blood or other aqueous phase	$C_{O_2 Arterial} = 0.3$ vol%
	$\dot{Q}$	Blood volume flow per unit time	$\dot{Q}_{Bronchial} = 100$ ml/min
	R	Respiratory exchange ratio (RQ)	$\dot{V}_{CO_2}/\dot{V}_{O_2} = 0.80$
	D	Diffusing capacity	$D_{LO_2} =$ 50 ml O_2/min/mm Hg ΔP_{O_2}
Qualifying terms Gas	A	Alveolar	$P_{O_2} = 100$ mm Hg
	D	Dead space	$V_D = 150$ ml
	T	Tidal	$V_T = 500$ ml
	I	Inspired	$F_I O_2 = 0.2094$
	E	Expired	$F_E CO_2 = 0.045$
Blood	a	Arterial	$P_{O_2} = 95$
	v	Venous	$P_{O_2} = 40$
	c	Capillary	$P_{O_2} = 60$
	b	Unspecified site	

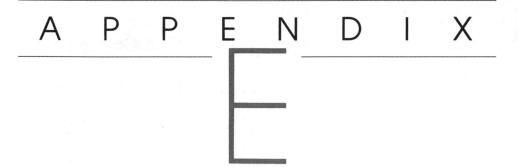

A P P E N D I X E

STPD (Standard Temperature, Pressure, Dry) Correction Factors for Expired Gas Volumes

Tabled values are multiplication factors used to correct volumes of moist exhaled gas to volumes occupied by dry gas at 0°C, 760 torr. Values in the left hand column are observed barometric pressures at the time of gas collection, whereas values across the top are observed temperatures of gas collected. Because this table assumes that the gas volume is saturated with water vapor, the table should only be used when volumes of *expired* gas are to be corrected. See Appendix F for correction of inspired gas volumes.

STPD (Standard Temperature, Pressure, Dry) Correction Factors

| | | | | | | | | | Temperature of Expired Air (°C) | | | | | | | | | |
Observed Barometric Reading, Uncorrected for Temperature (torr)	15°	16°	17°	18°	19°	20°	21°	22°	23°	24°	25°	26°	27°	28°	29°	30°	31°	32°
700	0.855	851	847	842	838	834	829	825	821	816	812	807	802	797	793	788	783	778
702	857	853	849	845	840	836	832	827	823	818	814	809	805	800	795	790	785	780
704	860	856	852	847	843	839	834	830	825	821	816	812	807	802	797	792	787	783
706	862	858	854	850	845	841	837	832	828	823	819	814	810	804	800	795	790	785
708	865	861	856	852	848	843	839	834	830	825	821	816	812	807	802	797	792	787
710	867	863	859	855	850	846	842	837	833	828	824	819	814	809	804	799	795	790
712	870	866	861	857	853	848	844	839	836	830	826	821	817	812	807	802	797	792
714	872	868	864	859	855	851	846	842	837	833	828	824	819	814	809	804	799	794
716	875	871	866	862	858	853	849	844	840	835	831	826	822	816	812	807	802	797
718	877	873	869	864	860	856	851	847	842	838	833	828	824	819	814	809	804	799
720	880	876	871	867	863	858	854	849	845	840	836	831	826	821	816	812	807	802
722	882	878	874	869	865	861	856	852	847	843	838	833	829	824	819	814	809	804
724	885	880	876	872	867	863	858	854	849	845	840	835	831	826	821	816	811	806
726	887	883	879	874	870	866	861	856	852	847	843	838	833	829	824	818	813	808
728	890	886	881	877	872	868	863	859	854	850	845	840	836	831	826	821	816	811
730	892	888	884	879	875	871	866	861	857	852	847	843	838	833	828	823	818	813
732	895	890	886	882	877	873	868	864	859	854	850	845	840	836	831	825	820	815

734	818	823	828	833	838	843	847	852	857	862	866	871	875	880	884	889	893	897
736	820	825	830	835	840	845	850	855	859	864	869	873	878	882	887	891	895	900
738	822	828	833	838	843	848	852	857	862	866	871	876	880	885	889	894	898	902
740	825	830	835	840	845	850	855	860	864	869	874	878	883	887	892	896	900	905
742	827	832	837	842	847	852	857	862	867	871	876	881	885	890	894	898	903	907
744	829	834	840	845	850	855	859	864	869	874	878	883	888	892	897	901	906	910
746	832	837	842	847	852	857	862	867	872	876	881	886	890	895	899	903	908	912
748	834	839	845	850	854	860	864	869	874	879	883	888	892	897	901	906	910	915
750	837	842	847	852	857	862	867	872	876	881	886	890	895	900	904	908	913	917
752	839	844	849	854	859	864	869	874	879	883	888	893	897	902	906	911	915	920
754	841	846	852	857	862	867	872	876	881	886	891	895	900	904	909	913	918	922
756	844	849	854	859	864	869	874	879	883	888	893	898	902	907	911	916	920	925
758	846	851	856	861	866	872	876	881	886	891	896	900	905	909	914	918	923	927
760	848	854	859	864	869	874	879	883	888	893	898	902	907	912	916	921	925	930
762	851	856	861	866	871	876	881	886	891	896	900	905	910	914	919	923	928	932
764	853	858	864	869	874	879	884	888	893	898	903	907	912	916	921	926	930	936
766	855	861	866	871	876	881	886	891	896	900	905	910	915	919	924	928	933	937
768	858	863	868	873	878	883	888	893	898	903	908	912	917	922	926	931	935	940
770	860	865	871	876	881	886	891	896	901	905	910	915	919	924	928	933	938	942
772	862	868	873	878	883	888	893	898	903	908	912	917	922	926	931	936	940	945
774	865	870	875	880	886	891	896	901	905	910	915	920	924	929	933	938	943	947
776	867	872	878	883	888	893	898	903	908	912	917	922	927	931	936	941	945	950
778	869	875	880	885	890	895	900	905	910	915	920	924	929	934	938	943	948	952
780	872	877	882	887	892	898	903	908	912	917	922	927	932	936	941	945	950	955

Peters, J. P., and Van Slyke, D. D.: Quantitative Clinical Chemistry. Vol. II (Methods) Baltimore: The Williams and Wilkins Co., 1932.

F

Calculation of STPD Correction Factors for Volumes of Inspired Air

Unlike volumes of expired air, inspired air is typically not saturated with water vapor. Therefore, various values of water vapor saturation must be considered along with barometric pressure and temperature values to derive a factor which can be used to correct inspired air volumes to STPD conditions of standard temperature (0°C), standard pressure (760 torr) and dry (free of water vapor). The following equation can be used to correct the appropriate correction factor.

$$\textbf{STPD factor} = \left[\frac{273}{273 + °C_{insp}} \right] \times \left[\frac{P_B - P_{H_2O}}{760} \right]$$

In the above equation,

$°C_{insp}$ = the observed temperature of the inspired air
P_B = the observed barometric pressure (torr), corrected for temperature
P_{H_2O} = the water vapor pressure (torr) of the inspired air

The water vapor pressure of the inspired air is found by multiplying the vapor pressure value for air saturated with water vapor at $°C_{insp}$ (Appendix G) by the relative humidity of the room air expressed as a fraction. In equation form:

$$P_{H_2O} = \text{(Saturated Vapor Pressure (torr) at } °C_{insp})}$$
$$\times \text{(Relative Humidity (\%)/100)}$$

As an illustration of the calculation of an STPD correction factor, consider the following case:

$°C_{insp}$ = 25.2°C
P_B = 770.68 torr

Relative Humidity = 50%

Saturated Vapor Pressure at 25.2℃ = 24.039 torr (from Appendix G)

$$\text{Thus, } P_{H_2O} = 24.039 \times (50/100)$$
$$= 12.0195.$$

$$\text{Therefore, } \textbf{STPD factor} = \frac{273}{273 + 25.2} \times \frac{770.68 - 12.0195}{760}$$

$$= 0.915 \times 0.998$$

$$\textbf{STPD factor} = 0.913$$

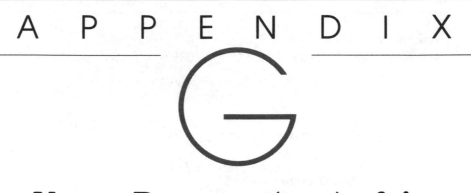

Vapor Pressure (torr) of Air Saturated with Water Vapor

°C	0.0	0.2	0.4	0.6	0.8
10	9.209	9.333	9.458	9.585	9.714
11	9.844	9.976	10.109	10.244	10.380
12	10.518	10.658	10.799	10.941	11.085
13	11.231	11.379	11.528	11.680	11.833
14	11.987	12.144	12.302	12.462	12.624
15	12.788	12.953	13.121	13.290	13.461
16	13.634	13.809	13.987	14.166	14.347
17	14.530	14.715	14.903	15.092	15.284
18	15.477	15.673	15.871	16.071	16.272
19	16.477	16.685	16.894	17.105	17.319
20	17.535	17.753	17.974	18.197	18.422
21	18.650	18.880	19.113	19.349	19.587
22	19.827	20.070	20.316	20.565	20.815
23	21.068	21.324	21.583	21.845	22.110
24	22.377	22.648	22.922	23.198	23.476
25	23.756	24.039	24.326	24.617	24.912
26	25.209	25.509	25.812	26.117	26.426
27	26.739	27.055	27.374	27.696	28.021
28	28.349	28.680	29.015	29.354	29.697
29	30.043	30.392	30.745	31.102	31.461
30	31.824	32.191	32.561	32.934	33.312
31	33.695	34.082	34.471	34.864	35.261
32	35.663	36.068	36.477	36.891	37.308

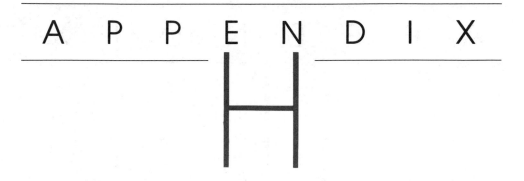

APPENDIX H

BTPS (Body Temperature, Ambient Pressure Saturated) Correction Factors

Tabled values are multiplication factors used to correct volumes of exhaled air to volumes occupied at 37°C with the air saturated with water vapor. These are called BTPS correction factors (Body Temperature, Ambient Pressure, Saturated) and should be used to report all lung volumes and capacities.

Temperature of Exhaled Air	Factors to Convert Air Volume to 37°C Saturated
20	1.102
20.5	1.099
21	1.096
21.5	1.093
22	1.091
22.5	1.089
23	1.085
23.5	1.082
24	1.079
24.5	1.077
25	1.074
25.5	1.071
26	1.069
26.5	1.065
27	1.062
27.5	1.060

Factors for Correction of Gas Volumes from STPD Conditions to BTPS Conditions at Various Barometric Pressures[1]

Sometimes it is necessary to convert volumes of gas from STPD conditions (0°C, 760 torr, dry) to BTPS conditions (37°C, ambient pressure, saturated with water vapor). The factors in the following table should be used as multipliers of STPD volumes to convert to BTPS volumes.

[1] Modified from "Clinical Spirometry," Boston, Mass.: Warren E. Collins, Inc., 1957, p. 17.

Observed Barometric Pressure (torr)	Factors for Correction of Gas Volume from STPD to BTPS Conditions
740	1.245
741	1.243
742	1.241
743	1.240
744	1.238
745	1.236
746	1.235
747	1.234
748	1.232
749	1.230
750	1.227
751	1.225
752	1.224
753	1.223
754	1.221
755	1.218
756	1.217
757	1.216
758	1.214
759	1.212
760	1.211
761	1.210
762	1.208
763	1.206
764	1.203
765	1.201
766	1.200
767	1.198
768	1.196
769	1.195
770	1.193
771	1.191
772	1.190
773	1.189
774	1.188
775	1.185
776	1.183
777	1.182
778	1.181

A P P E N D I X

J

Density of Water at Various Temperatures[1]

Water Temperature (°C)	Density of Water (grams per cubic centimeter)
20	0.9982
21	0.9980
22	0.9978
23	0.9975
24	0.9973
25	0.9970
26	0.9968
27	0.9965
28	0.9962
29	0.9959
30	0.9956
31	0.9953
32	0.9950
33	0.9947
34	0.9944
35	0.9940
36	0.9937
37	0.9933
38	0.9930

[1] Modified from R. C. Weast and S. M. Selby, eds., *Handbook of Chemistry and Physics,* 48th ed., Cleveland, Ohio: The Chemical Rubber Co., 1967, p. F-4.

A P P E N D I X

K

American College of
Sports Medicine Position
Stand on Weight Loss
in Wrestlers[1]

Despite repeated admonitions by medical, educational and athletic groups [2, 8, 17, 22, 33], most wrestlers have been inculcated by instruction or accepted tradition to lose weight in order to be certified for a class that is lower than their preseason weight [34]. Studies [34, 40] of weight losses in high school and college wrestlers indicate that from 3–20% of the preseason body weight is lost before certification or competition occurs. Of this weight loss, most of the decrease occurs in the final days or day before the official weigh-in [34, 40] with the youngest and/or lightest members of the team losing the highest percentage of their body weight [34]. Under existing rules and practices, it is not uncommon for an individual to repeat this weight losing process many times during the season because successful wrestlers compete in 15–30 matches/year [13].

Contrary to existing beliefs, most wrestlers are not "fat" before the season starts [35]. In fact, the fat content of high school and college wrestlers weighing less than 190 pounds has been shown to range from 1.6 to 15.1 per cent of their body weight with the majority possessing less than 8% [14, 28, 31]. It is well known and documented that wrestlers lose body weight by a combination of food restriction, fluid deprivation and sweating induced by thermal or exercise procedures [20, 22, 34, 40]. Of these methods, dehydration through sweating appears to be the method most frequently chosen.

Careful studies on the nature of the weight being lost show that water, fats and proteins are lost when food restriction and fluid deprivation procedures are followed [10]. Moreover, the proportionality between these constituents will change with continued restriction and deprivation. For example, if food restriction is held constant

[1] Reprinted from *Med. Sci. Sports* 8(2):1–2, 1976.

when the volume of fluid being consumed is decreased, more water will be lost from the tissues of the body than before the fluid restriction occurred. The problem becomes more acute when thermal or exercise dehydration occurs because electrolyte losses will accompany the water losses [16]. Even when 1–5 hours are allowed for purposes of rehydration after the weigh-in, this time interval is insufficient for fluid and electrolyte homeostasis to be completely reestablished [11, 37, 39, 40].

Since the "making of weight" occurs by combinations of food restriction, fluid deprivation and dehydration, responsible officials should realize that the single or combined effects of these practices are generally associated with 1) a reduction in muscular strength [4, 15, 30]; 2) a decrease in work performance times [24, 26, 27, 30]; 3) lower plasma and blood volumes [6, 7, 24, 27]; 4) a reduction in cardiac functioning during sub-maximal work conditions which are associated with higher heart rates [1, 19, 23, 24, 27], smaller stroke volumes [27], and reduced cardiac outputs [27]; 5) a lower oxygen consumption, especially with food restriction [15, 30]; 6) an impairment of thermoregulatory processes [3, 9, 24]; 7) a decrease in renal blood flow [21, 25] and in the volume of fluid being filtered by the kidney [21]; 8) a depletion of liver glycogen stores [12]; and 9) an increase in the amount of electrolytes being lost from the body [6, 7, 16].

Since it is possible for these changes to impede normal growth and development, there is little physiological or medical justification for the use of the weight reduction methods currently followed by many wrestlers. These sentiments have been expressed in part within Rule 1, Section 3, Article 1 of the **Official Wrestling Rule Book** [18] published by the National Federation of State High School Associations which states, "The Rules Committee recommends that individual state high school associations develop and utilize an effective weight control program which will discourage severe weight reduction and/or wide variations in weight, because this may be harmful to the competitor . . .". However, until the National Federation of State High School Associations defines the meaning of the terms "severe" and "wide variations," this rule will be ineffective in reducing the abuses associated with the "making of weight."

Therefore, it is the position of the American College of Sports Medicine* that the potential health hazards created by the procedures used to "make weight" by wrestlers can be eliminated if state and national organizations will:

1. Assess the body composition of each wrestler several weeks in advance of the competitive season [5, 14, 28, 31, 38]. Individuals with a fat content less than five per cent of their certified body weight should receive medical clearance before being allowed to compete.

2. Emphasize the fact that the daily caloric requirements of wrestlers should be obtained from a balanced diet and determined on the basis of age, body surface area, growth and physical activity levels [29]. The minimal caloric needs of wrestlers in high schools and colleges will range from 1200 to 2400 KCal/day [32]; therefore, it is the responsibility of coaches, school officials, physicians and

---

* The services of the American College of Sports Medicine are available to assist local and national organizations in implementing these recommendations.

parents to discourage wrestlers from securing less than their minimal needs without prior medical approval.

3. Discourage the practice of fluid deprivation and dehydration. This can be accomplished by:

   a. Educating the coaches and wrestlers on the physiological consequences and medical complications that can occur as a result of these practices.

   b. Prohibiting the single or combined use of rubber suits, steam rooms, hot boxes, saunas, laxatives, and diuretics to "make weight."

   c. Scheduling weigh-ins just prior to competition.

   d. Scheduling more official weigh-ins between team matches.

4. Permit more participants/team to compete in those weight classes (119–145 pounds) which have the highest percentages of wrestlers certified for competition [36].

5. Standardize regulations concerning the eligibility rules at championship tournaments so that individuals can only participate in those weight classes in which they had the highest frequencies of matches throughout the season.

6. Encourage local and county organizations to systematically collect data on the hydration state [39, 40] of wrestlers and its relationship to growth and development.

REFERENCES

[1] Ahlman, K. and M. J. Karvonen. Weight reduction by sweating in wrestlers and its effect on physical fitness. *J. Sports Med. Phys. Fit.* **1:**58–62, 1961.

[2] AMA Committee on the Medical Aspects of Sports, Wrestling and Weight Control. *JAMA* **201:**541–543, 1967.

[3] Bock, W. E., E. L. Fox and R. Bowers. The effect of acute dehydration upon cardiorespiratory endurance. *J. Sports Med. Phys. Fit.* **7:**62–72, 1967.

[4] Bosco, J. S., R. L. Terjung and J. E. Greenleaf. Effects of progressive hypohydration on maximal isometric muscular strength. *J. Sports Med. Phys. Fit.* **8:**81–86, 1968.

[5] Clarke, K. S. Predicting certified weight of young wrestlers: a field study of the Tcheng-Tipton method. *Med. Sci. Sports* **6:**52–57, 1974.

[6] Costill, D. L. and K. E. Sparks. Rapid fluid replacement following thermal dehydration. *J. Appl. Physiol.* **34:**299–303, 1973.

[7] Costill, D. L., R. Cote, E. Miller, T. Miller and S. Wynder. Water and electrolyte replacement during repeated days of work in the heat. *Aviat. Space Environ. Med.* **46:**795–800, 1975.

[8] Eriksen, F. G. Interscholastic wrestling and weight control: Current plans and their loopholes. *Proceedings of the Eighth National Conference on The Medical Aspects of Sports.* Chicago: AMA, 1967, pp. 34–39.

[9] Grande, F., J. E. Monagle, E. R. Buskirk and H. L. Taylor. Body temperature responses to exercise in man on restricted food and water intake. *J. Appl. Physiol.* **14:**194–198, 1959.

[10] Grande, F. Nutrition and energy balance in body composition studies. *Techniques for Measuring Body Composition,* edited by J. Brôzek and A. Henschel. Washington, D.C., National Acad. Sci. & Nat. Res. Council, pp. 168–188, 1961.

[11] Herbert, W. G. and P. M. Ribisl. Effects of dehydration upon physical work capacity of wrestlers under competitive conditions. *Res. Quart.* **43:**416–422, 1972.

[12] Hultman, E. and L. Nilsson. Liver glycogen as glucose-supplying source during exercise. *Limiting Factors of Physical Performance,* edited by J. Keul. Stuttgart: Georg Thieme, pp. 179–189, 1973.

[13] *1975 Program for the 55th State Wrestling Tournament.* Iowa High School Athletic Association., pp. 7–9.
[14] Katch, F. I. and E. D. Michael, Jr. Body composition of high school wrestlers according to age and wrestling weight category. *Med. Sci. Sports* **3:**190–194, 1971.
[15] Keys, A. L., J. Brôzek, A. Henschel, O. Mickelsen and H. L. Taylor. *The Biology of Human Starvation.* Minneapolis: U. of Minn. Press, Vol. 1, pp. 718–748, 1950.
[16] Kozlowski, S. and B. Saltin. Effect of sweat loss on body fluids. *J. Appl. Physiol.* **19:**1119–1124, 1964.
[17] Kroll, W. Guidelines for rules and practices. *Proceedings of the Eighth National Conference on the Medical Aspects of Sports.* Chicago: AMA, pp. 40–44, 1967.
[18] *The National Federation 1974–75 Wrestling Rule Book.* The National Federation Publications. Elgin, Illinois, p. 6.
[19] Palmer, W. Selected physiological responses of normal young men following dehydration and rehydration. *Res. Quart.* **39:**1054–1059, 1968.
[20] Paul, W. D. Crash diets in wrestling. *J. Iowa Med. Soc.* **56:**835–840, 1966.
[21] Radigan, L. R. and S. Robinson. Effect of environmental heat stress and exercise on renal blood flow and filtration rate. *J. Appl. Physiol.* **2:**185–191, 1949.
[22] Rasch, P. G. and W. Kroll. *What Research Tells the Coach About Wrestling.* Washington: AAHPER, pp. 41–50, 1964.
[23] Ribisl, P. M. and W. G. Herbert. Effect of rapid weight reduction and subsequent rehydration upon the physical working capacity of wrestlers. *Res. Quart.* **41:**536–541, 1970.
[24] Robinson, S. The effect of dehydration on performance. *Football Injuries.* Washington: Nat. Acad. Sci., pp. 191–197, 1970.
[25] Rowell, L. B. Human cardiovascular adjustments to exercise and thermal stress. *Physiol. Rev.* **54:**75–159, 1974.
[26] Saltin, B. Aerobic and anaerobic work capacity after dehydration. *J. Appl. Physiol.* **19:**1114–1118, 1964.
[27] Saltin, B. Circulatory response to submaximal and maximal exercise after thermal dehydration. *J. Appl. Physiol.* **19:**1125–1132, 1964.
[28] Sinning, W. E. Body composition assessment of college wrestlers. *Med. Sci. Sports* **6:**139–145, 1974.
[29] Suggested Daily Dietary Requirements, National Research Council Data, published in Oser, B. O. *Hawk's Physiological Chemistry.* 14th Edition, New York: McGraw-Hill, pp. 1370–1371, 1965.
[30] Taylor, H. L., E. R. Buskirk, J. Brôzek, J. T. Anderson and F. Grande. Performance capacity and effects of caloric restriction with hard physical work on young men. *J. Appl. Physiol.* **10:**421–429, 1957.
[31] Tcheng, T. K. and C. M. Tipton. Iowa wrestling study: Anthropometric measurements and the prediction of a "minimal" body weight for high school wrestlers. *Med. Sci. Sports* **5:**1–10, 1973.
[32] Tipton, C. M. Unpublished calculations on Iowa High School Wrestlers using a height and weight surface area nomogram. (Consalazio, C. F., R. E. Johnson and L. J. Pecora. *Physiological Measurements of Metabolic Functions in Man.* New York: McGraw-Hill, 1963, p. 27, that was constructed from the Dubois-Meech formula published in Arch. Int. Med. **17:**863–871, 1916) plus the metabolic standards for age used by the Mayo Foundation Standards that were published by Boothby, Berkson and Dunn in *Am. J. Physiol.* **116:**467–484, 1936.
[33] Tipton, C. M., T. K. Tcheng and W. D. Paul. Evaluation of the Hall Method for determining minimum wrestling weights. *J. Iowa Med. Soc.* **59:**571–574, 1969.
[34] Tipton, C. M. and T. K. Tcheng. Iowa wrestling study: Weight loss in high school students. *JAMA* **2114:**1269–1274, 1970.
[35] Tipton, C. M. Current status of the Iowa Wrestling Study. *The Predicament,* 12-30-73, p. 7.

[36] Tipton, C. M., T. K. Tcheng and E. J. Zambraski. Iowa Wrestling Study: Weight classification systems. *Med. Sci. Sports* **8**:101–104, 1976.

[37] Vaccaro, P., C. W. Zauner and J. R. Cade. Changes in body weight, hematocrit and plasma protein concentration due to dehydration and rehydration in wrestlers. *Med. Sci. Sports* **7**:76, 1975.

[38] Wilmore, J. H. and A. Behnke. An anthropometric estimation of body density and lean body weight in young men. *J. Appl. Physiol.* **27**:25–31, 1969.

[39] Zambraski, E. J., C. M. Tipton, T. K. Tcheng, H. R. Jordan, A. C. Vailas and A. K. Callahan. Changes in the urinary profiles of wrestlers prior to and after competition. *Med. Sci. Sports* **7**:217–220, 1975.

[40] Zambraski, E. J., D. T. Foster, P. M. Gross and C. M. Tipton. Iowa wrestling study: Weight loss and urinary profiles of collegiate wrestlers. *Med. Sci. Sports* **8**:105–108, 1976.

GLOSSARY

A bands—the darkly striped areas seen in longitudinal slices of skeletal muscle tissue. A bands contain overlapping thick and thin filaments.

Acetylcholine—a chemical released from certain nerve endings, especially those innervating skeletal muscles.

Acetyl group—a two carbon molecule produced by the removal of carbon dioxide from pyruvic acid; used to generate acetyl coenzyme A for use in the Krebs cycle.

Actin—one of the contractile protein filaments in muscles.

Action potential—a sudden change in electrical activity across a nerve or muscle membrane, usually due to a rapid flow of sodium ions across the membrane into the cell.

Actomyosin—the interaction of actin and myosin protein filaments in muscle.

Adaptation—a more or less persistent change in structure or function, especially as caused by repeated bouts of physical exercise.

Adenosine diphosphate (ADP)—one of the chemical products of the breakdown of adenosine triphosphate (ATP) for energy during muscle contraction.

Adenosine triphosphate (ATP)—a chemical that serves as the immediate source of chemical energy for most of the energy-consuming reactions of the body, especially for muscle contraction. ATP is split into adenosine diphosphate and phosphate to produce energy.

Adipose tissue—fat tissue.

Adrenaline—See epinephrine.

Adrenal cortex—outer portion of the adrenal gland. The cortex produces many hormones, especially cortisol and aldosterone.

Adrenal medulla—inner portion of the adrenal gland. The medulla produces epinephrine and norepinephrine in a ratio of about 3:1.

464

Adrenocorticotrophic hormone (ACTH)—See corticotropin.

Aerobic—utilizing oxygen.

Aerobic endurance—the ability to persist in physical activities that rely heavily upon oxygen for energy production.

Aerobic power—the maximal volume of oxygen consumed per unit of time. Also known as maximal oxygen uptake or maximal oxygen consumption.

Afferent fibers—sensory nerve fibers, i.e., those which conduct impulses toward the central nervous system and especially the brain.

Alactic acid oxygen debt—that part of the oxygen debt which is not accompanied by an increase of lactic acid in the blood.

Alanine—an amino acid that is converted to blood glucose in the liver (See: Glucose-alanine cycle).

Aldosterone—a hormone released from the adrenal cortex. Aldosterone causes sodium retention by the kidney.

All or none law—a phenomenon whereby a motor unit either contracts maximally or not at all under similar environmental conditions.

Alpha motor neurons—nerves that cause skeletal muscle fibers (extrafusal fibers) to contract.

Alpha-tocopherol—vitamin E.

Alveolus—tiny air sacs of the lungs. Plural: alveoli.

Amino acids—compounds that are the building blocks of proteins.

Amphetamine—a synthetic drug related to epinephrine. Amphetamines cause stimulation of the central nervous system.

Anabolic—pertaining to the synthesis of complex substances from simpler substances, especially to the synthesis of body proteins from amino acids.

Anabolic steroids—chemical substances with a steroid structure that promote protein synthesis.

Anaerobic—without oxygen.

Anaerobic capacity—the ability to persist at the maintenance or repetition of strenuous muscular contractions that rely substantially upon anaerobic mechanisms of energy supply.

Anaerobic power—the maximal rate at which energy can be produced or work can be performed without a significant contribution of aerobic energy production.

Anaerobic threshold—the level of exercise at which the anaerobic production of energy through glycolysis leads to the rapid accumulation of lactic acid in the blood.

Anaphylactic reaction—a serious allergic reaction often characterized by bronchial constriction, skin eruptions, and falling blood pressure.

Androgen—a class of hormones associated with masculine development.

Antidiuretic hormone (ADH, Vasopressin)—a hormone released by the posterior pituitary. Antidiuretic hormone causes water retention by the kidneys.

Anuria—absence of urine production.

Arteriovenous oxygen difference—the difference in oxygen content between the arterial blood and the mixed venous blood in the right atrium of the heart.

Ascorbic acid—vitamin C.

Athletic pseudonephritis—urinary changes after severe exercise that are similar to those seen in kidney pathology. Exercise-induced changes are transient and apparently not pathological.

Atrophy—reduction in size of cells and tissues.

Autoregulation—the regulation of blood flow to an organ or tissue by direct effects of localized changes of chemicals or temperature in the organ or tissue.

Basal ganglia—clusters of nerve cells located at the base of the brain that help to control movements.

Basal metabolic rate—energy expenditure at rest after a 12 hour fast and a good night's sleep.

Beta oxidation cycle—a series of metabolic reactions in which fatty acids are broken down for energy.

Biopsy—the extraction of small pieces of tissue for chemical analysis.

Blood doping—the practice of injecting previously withdrawn and stored blood cells to increase the number of circulating red blood cells.

Body composition—the proportion of fat and lean constituents of the human body.

Body density—the weight of the body per unit volume; typically expressed in grams per cubic centimeter.

Bradycardia—decreased heart rate, especially at rest.

Calcitonin—a hormone released from the thyroid. Calcitonin decreases levels of blood calcium.

Calorie—a unit of heat energy required to raise the temperature of a kilogram of water 1 degree Celsius under specified conditions. (Also known as a large calorie or kilocalorie.)

Carbohydrate—a chemical compound consisting of carbon, hydrogen and oxygen atoms in specified arrangements. Carbohydrates are major components of foods such as bread, potatoes, and rice.

Cardiac—pertaining to the heart.

Cardiac output—the volume of blood pumped from a ventricle of the heart per unit of time; cardiac output is the product of heart rate and stroke volume.

Cardiorespiratory endurance—See aerobic endurance.

Cardiovascular—pertaining to the heart and blood vessels.

Carotid sinus—a widening of the carotid artery where it divides into internal and external branches.

Catabolism—the degradation of complex substances into simpler structures, for example, the breakdown of fats and carbohydrates for energy production.

Catecholamines—a class of chemicals that includes epinephrine and norepinephrine.

Central nervous system—the brain and spinal cord.

Cerebellum—a large bulbar structure at the rear of the brain that helps control voluntary movement and maintain balance.

Cerebral cortex—the large outer portions of the cerebral hemispheres.

Chemoreceptors—sensory nerve endings sensitive to changes in their chemical environment. Such receptors are located in the aortic arch and the carotid sinuses.

Citric acid cycle—Krebs cycle.

Coenzyme—a nonprotein molecule that is required in enzyme–catalyzed reactions.

Collagen—a fibrous protein that serves as the major component of ligaments and tendons.

Concentric contraction—contraction of a muscle resulting in shortening of the muscle.

Conduction—the transfer of heat energy from a warm to a cooler object by direct physical contact.

Continuous work—work uninterrupted by rest pauses.

Convection—the transfer of heat by circulation or movement. Convective heat loss from the surface of the body to the surrounding air (or water, if one is swimming) is enhanced by increased air or water currents.

Core temperature—the temperature of the deep muscles and viscera of the body.

Cori cycle—a sequence of metabolic reactions whereby lactic acid released by muscle is transported to the liver, transformed to glycogen, and then released from the liver as glucose to be transported back to the muscle.

Corticotropin—a hormone released by the anterior pituitary. Corticotropin stimulates the growth and secretory activities of the adrenal cortex.

Cortisol—a hormone secreted by the adrenal cortex. Cortisol results in conservation of carbohydrate stores in the body at the expense of fat and protein.

Creatine phosphate (phosphocreatine)—a chemical that can donate its phosphate to adenosine diphosphate to rapidly replenish tissue stores of adenosine triphosphate.

Cross bridges—the linkages between thick and thin filaments during muscle contraction.

Cyanocobalamin—vitamin B_{12}.

Cyclic adenosine monophosphate (cyclic AMP)—a chemical implicated in the action of many hormones.

Cytochromes—proteins in the electron transport system of the mitochondria.

Dehydration—the condition that results from excessive loss of water.

Delta-aminolevulinic acid synthetase—an enzyme that is vital to the production of mitochondrial proteins.

Depolarization—reduction in the electrical charge across the resting cell membrane.

Diastole—relaxation of the heart.

Diffusion—the net movement of chemicals such as oxygen, carbon dioxide and sodium from an area of high concentration to an area of lower concentration.

Dry bulb thermometer—an ordinary temperature recording instrument.

Dynamic contraction—a muscle contraction that causes a change in joint angle; isokinetic, isotonic, eccentric, and concentric contractions are special types of dynamic contractions.

Eccentric contraction—a muscle contraction incapable of overcoming the resistance imposed; the overall muscle length increases.

Efferent nerve—a motor nerve.

Electrocardiogram (EKG, ECG)—a recording of the transmission of an action potential through the heart.

Electrolyte—any substance that dissociates into positively and negatively charged ions when dissolved in water.

Electromyography (EMG)—the recording of the electrical activity of muscles.

Electron transport system—a series of biochemical reactions in the mitochondria whereby energy present in electrons is used to generate adenosine triphosphate.

Endomysium—the connective tissue that surrounds muscle fibers and binds them together to form bundles.

Endorphins—peptides (amino acid chains) released by the pituitary gland; they may counteract pain.

Energy—the capacity to perform work.

Endurance—the ability to persist in performing some physical activity.

Enzyme—a protein molecule that serves as a catalyst for biochemical reactions.

Epinephrine—a chemical liberated from the adrenal medulla and from sympathetic nerve endings. Important effects include cardiac stimulation and constriction of blood vessels with a consequent rise in blood pressure.

Ergometer—a device which can measure work done, e.g., a bicycle ergometer.

Erythropoiesis—the production of red blood cells.

Erythropoietin—a hormone secreted by the kidneys. Erythropoietin stimulates the bone marrow cells to produce red blood cells.

Estradiol—a hormone secreted by the ovary; important in regulation of female sexual function and development of female secondary sex characteristics.

Estrogen—a class of hormones associated with feminine development.

Excitatory neurons—neurons that excite other neurons, tending to cause the other neurons to fire.

Extracellular fluid—fluid not within the cells, e.g., interstitial fluid, blood plasma.

Extrafusal muscle fibers—ordinary muscle fibers that lie outside muscle spindles.

Fasiculus (pl: fasiculi)—a bundle of muscle fibers bound together and connected to other fasiculi by connective tissue called the perimysium.

Fast twitch fibers—skeletal muscle fibers most active in short-duration, intensive exercise, e.g., in sprints and jumps.

Fatigue—the inability to maintain a given level of physical performance.

Fatty acids—long-chain organic acids associated with glycerol in fat molecules. Fatty acids are used extensively for muscular fuel, especially in prolonged exercise.

Fibrinolysis—the breakdown of fibrin strands produced during the clotting of blood.

Flavin adenine dinucleotide (FAD, FADH$_2$)—a coenzyme used to accept (FAD) or donate (FADH$_2$) electrons in biochemical oxidation-reduction reactions.

Flexibility—the range of motion of the body's joints.

Follicle-stimulating hormone (FSH)—See follitropin.

Follitropin—a hormone secreted by the anterior pituitary. Follitropin causes increased growth and hormone-secreting activity of the ovaries and testes.

Force vector—magnitude and direction of force as represented by an arrow, the direction of which indicates the direction of force and the length of which indicates the magnitude of force.

Frank-Starling effect—the increased contraction of the heart muscle caused by stretching of the muscle fibers upon increased filling of the chambers.

Free fatty acids—fatty acids that circulate in the blood and are only loosely attached to proteins. Free fatty acids are used extensively for energy in long-duration exercise.

Gamma motor nerve—a nerve that innervates the intrafusal fibers within muscle spindles.

Ginseng—a plant native to China and Korea thought by some to have various curative and restorative powers.

Glomerular filtration rate—the rate at which fluid is filtered from the glomeruli of the kidney into the nephrons.

Glomerulus—capillary bed lying in Bowman's capsule of the kidney.

Glucagon—a hormone that is secreted by the pancreas. Glucagon causes more glucose to be released from the liver into the blood.

Glucocorticoids—a class of hormones secreted from the adrenal cortex. Glucocorticoids tend to spare carbohydrate at the expense of protein and fat. Cortisol is the most important glucocorticoid in man.

Gluconeogenesis—the synthesis of glycogen or glucose from amino acids and other substances.

Glucose—blood sugar.

Glucose-alanine cycle—a series of metabolic reactions whereby pyruvic acid in the muscle is transformed into the amino acid, alanine. Alanine is delivered to the liver where it is changed to glucose. This glucose then can be delivered to the muscle for use in glycolysis.

Glycerol—a three-carbon compound associated with fatty acids in molecules of fat.

Glycogen—a polymer of glucose. Glycogen is the storage form of carbohydrate in animals.

Glycogen loading—the filling of liver and muscle glycogen stores to greater than normal levels by consumption of a high carbohydrate diet following the depletion of glycogen stores through exhaustive exercise and a low carbohydrate diet.

Glycogen phosphorylase—an enzyme involved in the breakdown of glycogen.

Glycogen supercompensation—See glycogen loading.

Glycogenolysis—the breakdown of glycogen to glucose.

Glycolysis—the breakdown of glucose to pyruvic or lactic acid. Also, sometimes used to describe the breakdown of glucose to carbon dioxide and water.

Golgi tendon organs—receptors at the junctions of muscles and tendons that report force changes to the brain and spinal cord.

Growth hormone—a hormone released from the anterior pituitary; causes growth of many body cells.

H zone—the central portion of an A band. The H zone contains only thick filaments at rest and usually disappears during contraction when thin filaments overlap the central portions of thick filaments.

Heat cramps—muscle cramps associated with heat-induced changes in electrolyte balance in muscle tissue. May be relieved after administration of salt water.

Heat exhaustion—extreme fatigue, collapse, or fainting caused by heat-induced reduction in cardiac output.

Heat stroke—serious heat illness wherein the body loses its ability to regulate body temperature.

Heat syncope—See heat exhaustion.

Hematocrit—the percentage of blood volume that is made up of red blood cells.

Hemoconcentration—an increase in the concentration of red blood cells in the total blood volume; usually caused by a loss of plasma water to the tissue spaces.

Hemoglobin—a protein found in red blood cells. Hemoglobin combines with oxygen.

Hexokinase—the enzyme that changes blood glucose to glucose-6-phosphate in muscle.

High density lipoproteins (HDL)—relatively heavy complexes of fat and protein in the blood; associated with a reduced incidence of coronary artery disease.

Homeostasis—the tendency of the body to maintain its internal environment within narrow ranges of temperature, acidity, osmolarity, etc.

Hormonal pathway—a response or adaptation that involves changes in hormonal activity.

Humoral—found in body fluids.

Hydrostatic weighing—underwater weighing used to determine body volume, which in turn is used to determine body density and body composition.

Hyperplasia—increased cell number.

Hyperpnea—significantly increased breathing.

Hypertension—chronically high arterial blood pressure.

Hypertrophy—increased cell size leading to increased tissue size.

Hyperventilation—a rate of ventilation in excess of physiological demand.

Hypokinesis—relative lack of exercise.

Hypothalamus—a group of nerve cells at the base of the brain that has many complex functions, including regulation of temperature, appetite, emotional reactions, and hormonal responses.

Hypothermia—lowering of the core temperature of the body.

Hypoxia—a relative lack of oxygen.

Inhibitory neurons—neurons that inhibit other neurons, tending to keep the other neurons quiet.

Insulin—a hormone secreted by the pancreas. Insulin lowers blood glucose by increasing the uptake of glucose by the tissues of the body.

Intermittent exercise—exercise sessions interrupted by rest sessions.

Interval training—periods of exercise interspersed with regular rest or recovery periods.

Intrafusal fibers—muscle fibers located within muscle spindles.

Interstitial fluid—the fluid that lies between cells in the tissue spaces.

Intrinsic pathway—a response or adaptation pathway located within an organ or tissue; that organ both senses and reacts to a homeostatic disturbance.

Ischemia—a lack of blood flow.

Isokinetic contraction—a muscular contraction through a range of motion at a constant velocity.

Isometric (static) contraction—a muscular contraction in which there is no change in the angle of the involved joint(s) and little or no change in the length of the contracting muscle.

Isotonic contraction—a muscular contraction in which a constant load is moved through a range of motion of the involved joint(s).

Joint receptors—nerve receptor organs located in and around joints of the limbs.

Joint receptors provide information about limb position to the brain and spinal cord.

Joule—a unit of measurement of energy (A kilojoule equals approximately 4.2 kilocalories.).

Karvonen formula—a formula for prescribing exercise heart rate.

Kilocalorie (kcal)—the heat required to raise the temperature of 1 kilogram of water 1 degree Celsius under specified conditions.

Kilogram—a unit of mass equivalent to 2.2 pounds.

Kilopond-meter (kpm)—the work done when a mass of one kilogram is lifted one meter against the force of gravity.

Kinesthetic sense—the sense of orientation of the body and its parts in space and to each other.

Krebs cycle—a series of enzyme-catalyzed reactions in the mitochondria of cells; involved in the catabolism of fats, carbohydrates, and proteins to carbon dioxide and water.

Lactic acid (lactate)—the end-product of anaerobic glycolysis.

Lactic acid oxygen debt—that portion of the oxygen debt that is associated with a rise in blood lactic acid.

Lean body mass—the body mass that does not include fat tissue.

Ligament—the tough connective tissue that binds bones together at joints.

Limbic lobe—a portion of the medial and ventral surfaces of each cerebral hemisphere that is associated with emotions and other "automatic" types of behavior.

Limbic system—the hypothalamus and the limbic lobe of the cerebral cortex. The limbic system is involved in emotions; during exercise it activates nerve fibers leading to the cardiac control centers of the brain.

Lipase—a class of enzymes that splits fatty acid molecules from fats.

Lipid—fat, especially triglycerides.

Lipoprotein lipase—an enzyme that splits fatty acids from fat-protein complexes.

Longitudinal studies—studies that involve the same subjects for several months or years.

Low density lipoproteins (LDL)—relatively light complexes of fat and protein in the blood; associated with a high incidence of coronary artery disease.

Lymph—fluid transported in the lymphatic channels from the tissues to the blood circulatory system. Lymph consists of water, electrolytes, proteins and other substances found in most body fluids.

Maximal oxygen uptake (maximal oxygen consumption, $\dot{V}_{O_2}$ max., maximal oxygen intake, maximal aerobic power)—the greatest volume of oxygen used by the cells of the body per unit of time.

Mechanism—the physical and chemical events underlying biological processes; knowledge of mechanisms is required for complete understanding of how a process occurs.

Metabolites—chemical substances generated from the degradation of larger molecules, e.g., carbon dioxide and water are metabolites generated from the breakdown of fats, carbohydrates and proteins.

METS (Metabolic equivalents)—an expression of energy cost relative to an individual's resting energy expenditure. The rate of energy expenditure in a task that requires 10 METS is 10 times that required to support the energy needs of a subject at rest. One MET is equivalent to 3.5 milliliters of oxygen per kilogram of body weight.

Mitochondria—the structures located within the cells. Mitochondria contain the enzymes responsible for the generation of adenosine triphosphate by aerobic mechanisms.

Motor neuron—a nerve cell that conducts an impulse from the central nervous system to muscles or glands.

Motor cortex—that portion of the cerebral cortex that generates the nerve impulses leading to voluntary movement.

Motor unit—a motor neuron and all the muscle fibers which it innervates.

Muscle spindle—a sensory organ imbedded in skeletal muscle. The spindle is sensitive to changes in muscle length and especially to stretch.

Myofibril—element of muscle which contains the contractile actin and myosin proteins.

Myofilaments—minute protein threads within a myofibril.

Myoglobin—oxygen-binding protein in skeletal muscle.

Myokinase reaction—a chemical reaction in which two molecules of adenosine diphosphate are combined to form one molecule of adenosine triphosphate plus one molecule of adenosine monophosphate.

Myosin—contractile protein in muscle. Myosin molecules make up the thick filaments in muscle.

Myosin ATPase—the name given to the activity of myosin in catalyzing the breakdown of adenosine triphosphate to adenosine diphosphate and phosphate during muscle contraction.

Negative feedback regulation—a system whereby the body opposes (negates) homeostatic disturbances.

Nephron—the tubular structure that is the functional unit of the kidney.

Net caloric cost of exercise—the caloric cost of both exercise and recovery less the calories that would have been expended had the subject remained at rest during the period of exercise and recovery.

Net oxygen cost of exercise—the amount of oxygen consumed during both exercise and recovery less the oxygen that would have been consumed had the subject remained at rest during the period of exercise and recovery.

Neural pathway—a response or adaptation that involves changes in nerve activity.

Neurogenic—resulting from nerve impulses.

Neuromuscular fatigue—inability to sustain or repeat the production of a given muscular force. Also, the inability to sustain the production of a given power.

Neuromuscular junction (motor endplate)—the junction between motor nerve ending and the sarcolemmal membrane of a muscle fiber.

Neuron—a nerve cell, consisting of cell body, axon, and dendrites.

Neurotrophic substance—a chemical transmitted by nerves; causes some growth or development of the structure innervated.

Newton (N)—the force that imparts an acceleration of one meter per second on a mass of one kilogram.

Niacin—vitamin B_3.

Nicotinamide adenine dinucleotide (NAD, NADH)—an electron acceptor (NAD) or donor (NADH) used in metabolic oxidation-reduction reactions.

Noradrenaline—See norepinephrine.

Norepinephrine—a chemical secreted by sympathetic nerve endings and by the adrenal medulla. Norepinephrine increases cardiac output, vasoconstriction, and blood pressure.

Obesity—excess body fat.

Osmolarity—a measure of the dissolved particles in a solution that can create osmotic force in the presence of a semipermeable membrane.

Osteoporosis—wasting of bones; especially prevalent in older women.

Oxidation—the removal of electrons from a chemical.

Oxidative phosphorylation—the production of adenosine triphosphate dependent upon oxidative processes in the electron transport system of the mitochondria.

Oxygen debt—the oxygen uptake during recovery from exercise in excess of the oxygen uptake normally observed during a rest period of similar duration.

Oxygen deficit—the difference between the theoretical oxygen requirement of a physical activity and the oxygen actually used during the activity.

Oxygen uptake—the oxygen used up by the mitochondria of all the body's cells.

Parathyroid hormone—a hormone secreted by the parathyroid glands; increases the level of calcium in the blood.

Partial pressure—in a mixture of gases, the pressure exerted by one of the gases in the mixture. The pressure is due to the heat energy of the gas molecules.

Perimysium—connective tissue that surrounds bundles of muscle fibers and binds them to other bundles within a skeletal muscle.

Peripheral nervous system—nerve tissue located outside the brain and spinal cord.

pH—a measure of the acidity of a solution. The possible values of pH range between 0–14, with 7.0 representing a balance between acid and base. Values lower than 7.0 become progressively more acidic, and values above 7.0 become progressively more basic.

Phosphofructokinase—an enzyme involved in the breakdown of glucose to pyruvic acid. The enzyme is especially important in regulation of glycolysis because small changes in its activity can slow or speed the rate of glycolysis.

Phosphorylase—an enzyme involved in the breakdown of glycogen to glucose-6-phosphate. Small changes in the activity of this enzyme help regulate the rate of glycogen breakdown.

Plasma—the fluid portion of the blood.

Polyunsaturated fat—a fat, many of whose fatty acid carbon atoms are not saturated with hydrogen atoms but are bonded together by double bonds. Polyunsaturated fats are usually liquid at room temperature and are derived from plant sources.

Power—work performed per unit time.

Precapillary sphincters—smooth muscle cells located at the entrances of many capillaries; they control blood flow into the capillaries.

Prostaglandins—a class of chemical substances derived from arachidonic acid; involved in regulation of blood flow in arteries, blood clotting, and many other functions.

Pyruvic acid—a three carbon molecule produced by the breakdown of glycogen or glucose.

Radiation—the transfer of heat energy through space from one object to another.

Renin—an enzyme secreted by the kidney; catalyzes the production of angiotensin I from a plasma protein, angiotensinogen.

Repolarization—the reestablishment of resting membrane potential following depolarization.

Residual volume of air—the volume of air in the lungs and gastrointestinal tract that must be taken into account when determining body composition.

Respiratory exchange ratio (R)—the ratio between carbon dioxide produced and oxygen consumed.

Respiratory quotient (RQ)—the ratio between the carbon dioxide produced and oxygen consumed during the metabolism of foodstuffs. Often used as synonym for respiratory exchange ratio (R) even though R may reflect processes other than foodstuff metabolism, e.g., hyperventilation due to acidosis.

Response—a sudden temporary adjustment in physiological function brought on by a single exposure to exercise, e.g., the rise in heart rate associated with an exercise bout.

Rest (recovery) intervals—in an interval training program, the periods of recovery between exercise intervals.

Sarcolemma—muscle fiber membrane.

Sarcomere—the distance between Z lines; sarcomeres shorten when muscles contract.

Sarcoplasm—the cytoplasm of muscle fibers.

Sarcoplasmic reticulum—a network of channels extending throughout muscle fibers; regulates the availability of calcium to the troponin molecules of the thin filaments.

Saturated fat—a fat whose fatty acid carbon atoms are saturated with hydrogen atoms. Typically, saturated fats are solid at room temperature and are often derived from animal sources.

Sensory fibers—nerve fibers that conduct impulses from the periphery to the central nervous system.

Serum—the fluid exuded from clotted blood.

Sinoatrial node—specialized cells in the right atrium of the heart that serve as the pacemaker of the heart beat because of their rapid rates of depolarization and repolarization.

Siri equation—a formula for converting body density to percentage of body fat.

Skin fold technique—a method of estimating body fat by measuring subcutaneous fat with skin fold calipers.

Sling psychrometer—a device used to measure relative humidity.

Slow-twitch fibers—skeletal muscle fibers characterized by relatively slow contraction times and great capacity for the aerobic production of adenosine triphosphate.

Somatomedins—amino acid chains that promote cell growth; they are usually released from liver and other tissues upon stimulation by growth hormone.

Somatotropin—See growth hormone.

Splanchnic circulation—circulation to the viscera, especially the liver.

Static contraction—a muscular contraction that does not involve changes in the angle of the joint(s) involved.

Steady state—that state of physiological stability wherein the energy demands of the body can be met relatively easily for a prolonged period of time.

Stearic acid—an 18 carbon fatty acid.

STPD—standard temperature (0°C), pressure (760 mm Hg), and dry.

Strength—the ability to exert muscular force briefly.

Stroke volume—the amount of blood pumped out of the heart ventricles with each beat.

Submaximal exercise—usually exercise at less than maximal intensity, but may also refer to exercise of less than maximal duration.

Sympathetic nervous system—that portion of the autonomic nervous system with nerves leaving the spinal cord at the thoracic and lumbar levels. In most tissues, the chemical transmitters secreted from sympathetic nerve endings are norepinephrine and epinephrine.

Systole—contraction, usually of the heart ventricles.

T-tubules—channels that conduct action potentials from the surface of a muscle fiber to the interior of the fiber.

Teleology—the study of purposes underlying events. Teleological reasoning is used to explain why an event occurs.

Testosterone—a hormone secreted by the testes; causes the secondary sex characteristics of the male and is involved in muscle growth.

Tetanic contractions—contractions of muscle fibers at such high frequencies that fibers do not have time to return to their resting lengths between contractions.

Tetanus—the state of apparently continuous contraction of a muscle fiber that is being stimulated at such high frequency that it does not have time to return to its resting length between contractions.

Thiamine—vitamin B_1.

Thyroxine—the primary hormone secreted by the thyroid gland; increases oxygen uptake by the mitochondria and works with somatotropin to cause cell growth.

Transverse tubules—See T-tubules.

Triacylglycerol—See triglyceride.

Triglyceride—a fat consisting of a molecule of glycerol and three molecules of fatty acid.

Tropomyosin—a protein in the thin filaments of skeletal muscle; blocks attachment sites on actin.

Troponin—a protein in the thin filaments of skeletal muscle; inhibits myosin ATPase activity until troponin is inactivated by calcium ions released from the sarcoplasmic reticulum.

Twitch—a single, brief muscle contraction caused by a single stimulus.

Uridine triphosphate—an energy-rich compound whose breakdown is required for the synthesis of glycogen from glucose.

Vagus nerve—the tenth cranial nerve.

Vasoconstriction—narrowing of the opening of blood vessels caused by contraction of the smooth muscle cells in the walls of the vessels.

Vasodilation—widening of the opening of blood vessels caused by a relaxation of the smooth muscle cells in the walls of the vessels.

Vasopressin—See antidiuretic hormone.

Vasoregulatory asthenia—a disease characterized by the inability to alter blood flow to and from various regions of the body.

Ventilation breaking point—the level of exercise at which the accumulation of lactic acid in the blood stimulates a marked increase in ventilation that is out of proportion to oxygen uptake.

Very low density lipoproteins (VLDL)—very light complexes of fat (primarily triglycerides) and protein in the blood; associated with a high incidence of coronary artery disease.

Vestibular nuclei—clusters of nerve cells in the brain that help to maintain balance.

Viscera—the internal organs of the body.

$\dot{V}_{O_2}$ max.—See maximal oxygen uptake.

Watt—a unit of power equivalent to one joule per second or one newton meter per second.

Wet bulb thermometer—a thermometer whose mercury bulb is encased in a wetted cloth wick.

Work (exercise) intervals—in an interval training program, the intermittent periods of exercise.

Z line or disc—the structure which bisects the I bands of skeletal muscle and anchors the thin filaments.

INDEX